Volume - 2

CURRENT PRACTICE OF PEDIATRIC CARDIOLOGY

Incorporating Fetus, Newborn, Infants, Children & Adolescents

Useful for Pediatric postgraduate students /Cardiologists/Pediatricians and General Physicians

Dr. K C VERMA

notionpress.com

INDIA • SINGAPORE • MALAYSIA

ISBN
Hardcase 979-8-89544-544-0
Paperback 979-8-89519-811-7

Current Practice of Pediatric Cardiology

Incorporating Fetus,Newborn,infants, children & Adolescents

Useful for Pediatric postgraduate students /Cardiologists/Pediatricians and General Physicians

Prof.(Dr) K.C.VERMA

MBBS, DCH, MD, DM (CARDIOLOGY) FICP (USA),
FRSTM & H (Lond), FCSI (India)
Senior Consulting Heart Specialist and Formerly
Prof. in Cardiovascular and Thoracic Unit
Govt. Medical College, Jammu (J&K)

notionpress.com

INDIA • SINGAPORE • MALAYSIA

Acknowledgement

I am very grateful to my wife Dr (Mrs) Urmil Kanta Verma, Formerly Prof. in department of Blood transfusion medicine and pathology for providing me a perfect congenial atmosphere and all material and moral support needed for writing such a speciality book on "**Current Practice of Pediatric Cardiology**"

To my lovely grand children—Adwita, Sidhant, Deven, Leena and Meera. I also appreciate the support of concerned staff of Renu Publishers, New Delhi for their timely guidance in its perfect designing, type setting, preparation of lucid figures and line diagrames, which itself was a big challenging task and is therefore, joyfully acknowledged.

Dedication

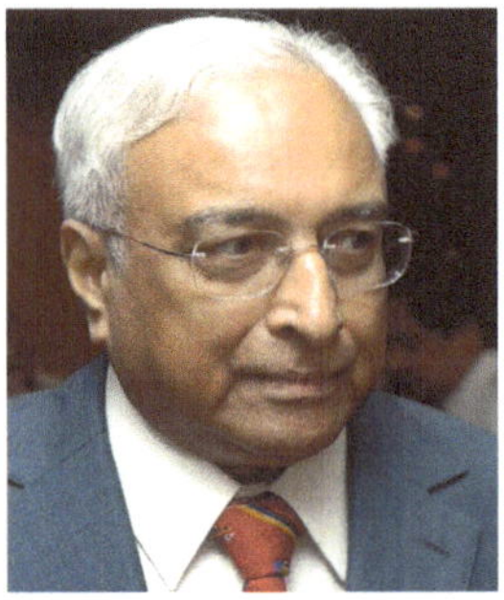

Honorable Dr. M. R. Girinath
MBBS,MS(GeneralSurgery),
MCh (CardioThoracic Surgery)

Dr. M. R. Girinath is a Cardiothoracic Surgeon at Apollo Hospitals Chennai with a prior work experience of 45 years including 3 years of working in Auckland. He is the head of Cardiac surgery unit of Apollo hospitals, Chennai since 1984. Under the guidance of Dr Girinath M R Cardio Thoracic Surgeon in Chennai, the unit has done 40,000 heart operations of which 29,000 have been coronary bypass operations including 14,000 on a beating heart. The Cardiovascular surgeon at Apollo Hospitals, Chennai has pioneered congenital heart surgery and heart valve surgery in India and trained 30 heart surgeons in India. The Cardiothoracic Surgery specialist in Chennai has performed over 25,000 open heart surgeries in the last 16 years.The Best Cardiac Surgeon of India is one of the first surgeons to receive MCh degree in India and a pioneer in cardiac surgery for infants, coronary bypass surgery, multivalve replacement and cardiac transplantation. He has presentated over 275 papers at national and international conderences and participated in the first multi-organ transplant in India (Heart, Liver, Kidneys and Cornea). Dr. Girinath has made around 20 orations and has been a member of various prestigious groups. His major surgeries include surgeries of coronary artery, valves, carotid arteries, aortic aneurysm, cardiomyoplasty, cardiac arrhythmias, total arterial myocardial revascularization, transmyocardial laser revascularisation and least invasive coronary artery surgery on a beating heart and reduction ventriculoplasty (Batista Operation) with excellent results. Some of these operations have been performed by him for the first time in India.

This book is also dedicated to those scientists and research workers whose conclusive reviews has become the platefarm of writing this manuscript. Their names alongwith their respective journals have been depicticted in the comprehensive bibliography section at the end of each chapter. This manuscript is also being dedicated to the various patients whose photographs have been utilized in making this book more authoritative and illustrative as seen different sections To those great medical teachers of India who have produced hundreds and thousands of specialists in the field of pediatric cardiology and guided them in their respective research studies. To those medical artists who have applied their best skill in the preparation of various line diagrams utilized in this book.

Author

Preface

There are a number of commonly encountered acute cardiac presentations in older infants and children that are essential to recognise early in order to institute appropriate emergency care. Many of these will be the first clinical presentation of a child; therefore the attending doctor or nurse, with no specific diagnosis, will need to know the basic physiology of the cardiovascular system and the common derangements that may occur. For children with a known diagnosis, such as the above-mentioned one, attending practitioners must be able to manage life-threatening complications, as these patients will often be seen in a non-tertiary setting. This book ,therefore,begins with brief over view of history taking, physical examination, and investigative techniques just as in any other book in discipline of Medicine/cardiology

Cardiac arrhythmias in children are not only difficult to diagnose but also to manage these rhythm disturbances with emergent treatment, this book therefore, describes in detail their respective management. The heart failure which is often the terminal event of many congenital and acquired heart disorders is yet an other cardiac emergency which attracts physician/cardiologist/cardiac surgeon's attention in emergency department. This subject has been written with utmost care giving details of its recognition , medical and surgical interventions in its management. A brief description of cardiac complications such as myocarditis, endocarditis, pericarditis, cardiac tamponade, DCM, valvular and vascular emergencies, hypothermia and sudden cardiac death syndrome, have been included in this manuscript.Percutaneous catheter interventions remains the cornerstone in the management of both valvular and congenital cardiovascular anomalies, hence a brief description of these procedures has been recorded in this book.

Cardiac resuscitation is the most essential part of management of cardiac emergencies both on road side and inside ICU, hence the author has been able to describe in details of the techniques including "ECMO therapy" in acute cardio-pulmonary failure. In emergency department attending physician/duty medical officer may find young children and adolescents admitted with either heart failure, cardiac arrhythmias, intoxicated with frequently prescribed drugs such as Digitalis, Calcium channel blockers, beta-blockers and other antiarrhythmics for their respective treatment or others with addictions of alcohol and cocaine. The brief account of the role of toxicological substances affecting heart in pediatric age group has been highlighted.

Over the past a few years ,there had been many advances in the field of cardiovascular medicine and therefore,a few reviewed chapters such as Artificial intelligence in Pediatric Cardiology., Transformative technology Of 3D Printing in congenital heart disease ,Nano-technology innovations in Pediatric Cardiology. Advances in the prenatal management of fetal cardiac disease, Tropical diseases affecting cardiovascular system and comprehensive review on Heart Transplantation in Pediatric Cardiology have been added for readers

In view of the above mentioned chapters included in this book of current practice of pediatric cardiology , the author is very confident that readers would find it a most valuable and perfect guide and would act as ready rechnor in obtaining knowledge for the day to day management of cardiac problems at any level of postings in their service. Besides, it would be very useful book for medical officers,undergraduate and postgraduate pediatric medicine and cardiology , cardiac fellows, and physicians.

(K C Verma)

Contents

Volume - 1

Volume - 2

Chapter No.	Name of the chapter	Page No.

29 ECMO (Extra Corporeal Membrane Oxygenation) Support in Critically Ill Children

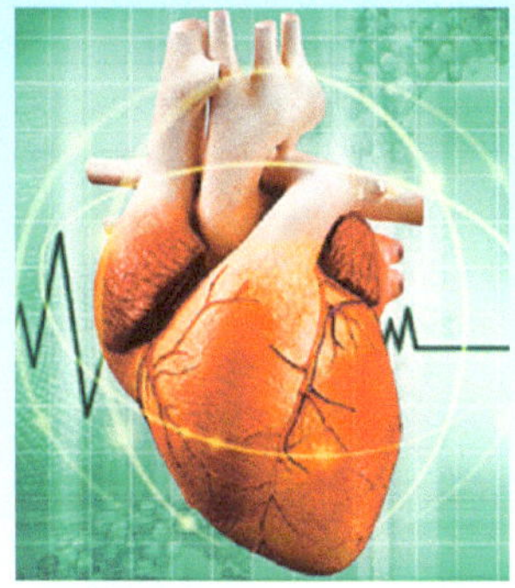

The term extracorporeal membrane oxygenation (ECMO) was initially used to describe long-term extracorporeal support that focused on the function of oxygenation. Subsequently, in some patients, the emphasis shifted to carbon dioxide removal, and the term extracorporeal carbon dioxide removal was coined. Extracorporeal support was later used for postoperative support in patients following cardiac surgery. Other variations of its capabilities have been tested and used over the last few years, making it an important tool in the armamentarium of life and organ support measures for clinicians. With all of these uses for extracorporeal circuitry, a new term, extracorporeal life support (ECLS), has come into vogue to describe this technology.

In emergency medicine, extracorporeal membrane oxygenation (ECMO) is an extracorporeal technique of providing both cardiac and respiratory support oxygen to patients whose heart and lungs are so severely diseased or damaged that they can no longer serve their function. Initial cannulation of a patient receiving ECMO is performed by a surgeon and maintenance of the patient is the responsibility of the ECMO Specialist and gives 24/7 monitoring care for the duration of the ECMO treatment (Fig. 26.1).

The differences between ECMO and cardiopulmonary bypass are as follows:

- ECMO is frequently instituted using only cervical cannulation, which can be performed under local anesthesia; standard cardiopulmonary bypass is usually instituted by transthoracic cannulation under general anesthesia
- Unlike standard cardiopulmonary bypass, which is used for short-term support measured in hours, ECMO is used for longer-term support ranging from 3–10 days
- The purpose of ECMO is to allow time for intrinsic recovery of the lungs and heart; a standard cardiopulmonary bypass provides support during various types of cardiac surgical procedures.

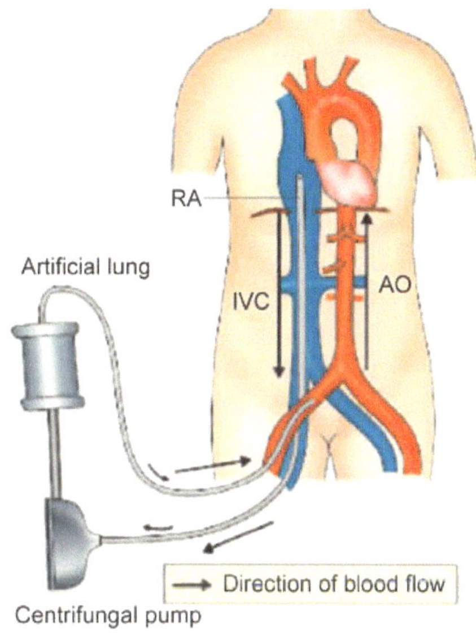

Fig. 29.1: Diagram of ECMO system. RA=right atrium; IVC=inferior venacava; Ao=aorta.

TYPES OF ECMO

1. Single site Veno-venous (VV) ECMO for respiratory failure
2. Two-site venovenous extracorporeal membrane oxygenation
3. Veno-arterial (VA) ECMO for cardiac or respiratory failure
4. ECMO in the ambulatory patient

There are several forms of ECMO, the two most common of which are veno-arterial (VA) and veno-venous (VV). In both modalities, blood drained from the venous system is oxygenated outside of the body. In VA ECMO, this blood is returned to the arterial system and in VV ECMO the blood is returned to the venous system. In VV ECMO, no cardiac support is provided.

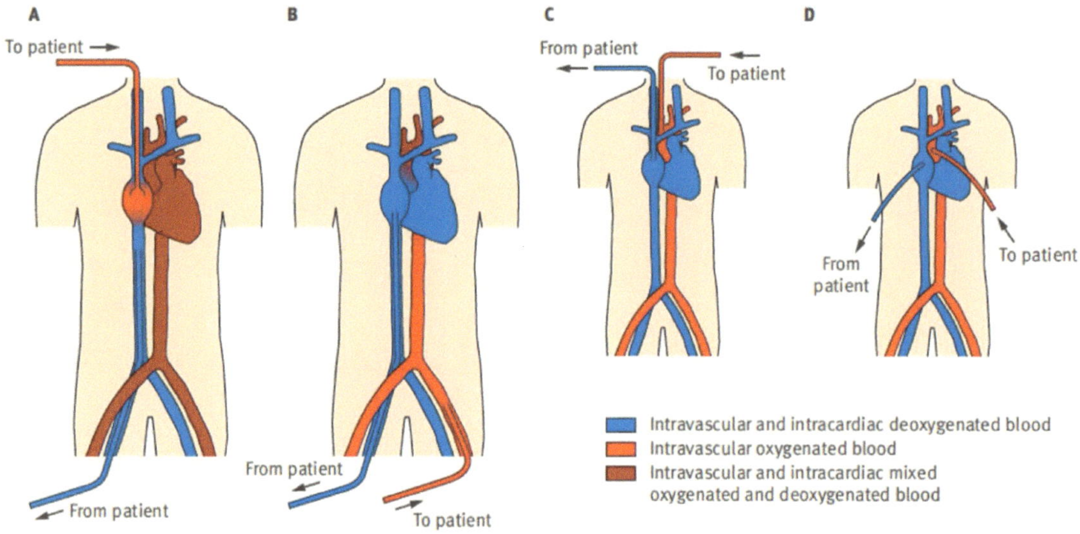

Fig.29.2 Extra Corporeal Membrane Oxygenation (ECMO) Support in Critically Ill Patients

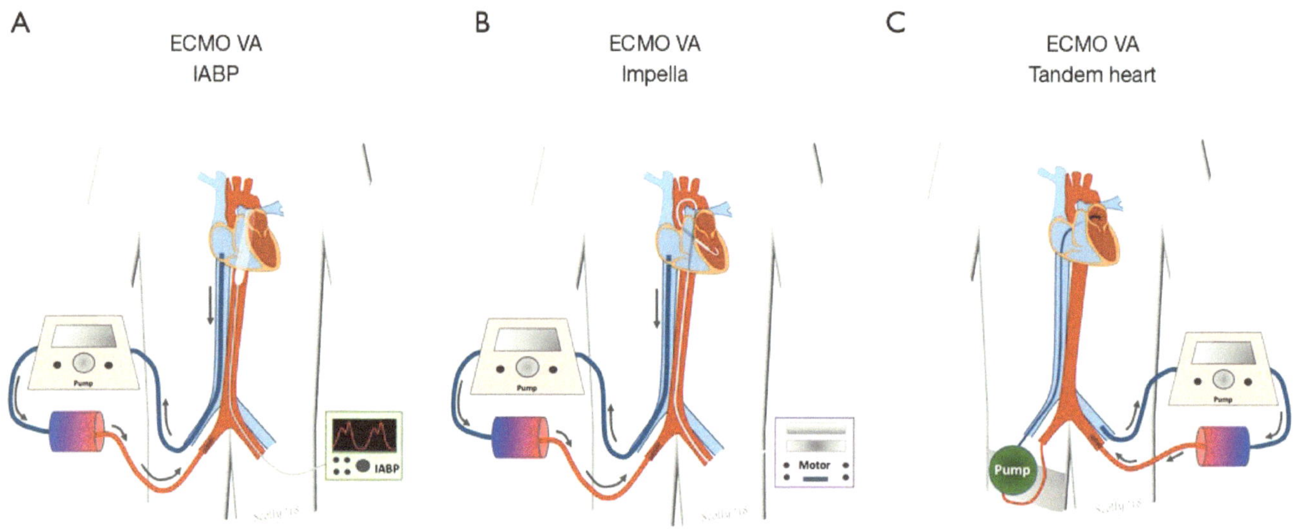

Fig.29.3 Percutaneous mechanical circulatory support devices, such as intra-aortic balloon counterpulsation (IABP) (A), Impella (B) or Tandem-Heart (C), in combination with veno-arterial ECMO. ECMO, extracorporeal membrane oxygenation; VA, veno-arterial.

Veno-arterial (VA)

In veno-arterial ECMO-a venous cannula is usually placed in the right common femoral vein for extraction and an arterial cannula is usually placed into the right femoral artery for infusion The tip of the femoral venous cannula should be maintained near the junction of the inferior vena cava and right atrium, while the tip of the femoral arterial cannula is maintained in the iliac artery. In adults accessing the femoral artery is preferred because the insertion is simpler.

Veno-venous (VV)

In Veno-venous ECMO - venous cannulae are usually placed in the right common femoral vein for drainage and right internal jugular vein for infusion.

INDICATIONS FOR ECMO

Patients with the following 2 major neonatal diagnoses require the use of ECMO:

- Primary diagnoses associated with primary pulmonary hypertension of the newborn (PPHN), including idiopathic PPHN, meconium aspiration syndrome, respiratory distress syndrome, group B streptococcal sepsis, and asphyxia (Fig. 26.6).
- Congenital diaphragmatic hernia (CDH)

Selection criteria for neonates include the following:

- Gestational age of 34 weeks or more
- Birth weight of 2000 g or higher
- No significant coagulopathy or uncontrolled bleeding
- No major intracranial hemorrhage (grade 1 intracranial hemorrhage)
- Mechanical ventilation for 10–14 days or less
- Reversible lung injury
- No lethal malformations
- No major untreatable cardiac malformation
- Failure of maximal medical therapy
- Failure to meet these criteria is a relative contraindication for ECMO.

Qualifying patient criteria for ECMO are applied only when the infant has reached maximal ventilatory support of 100% oxygen (fraction of inspired oxygen [FiO_2] equals with peak inspiratory pressures (PIP) often as high as 35 cm water. They include the alveolar-arterial gradient, the oxygenation index, and acute deterioration.

The alveolar-arterial (A-a) gradient of 600–624 mm Hg for 4–12 hours at sea level may be computed as follows (where 47=partial pressure of water vapor):

Pediatric ECMO is indicated or considered in the following situations:

- Low cardiac output resulting from right, left, and biventricular failure following repair of congenital heart defect

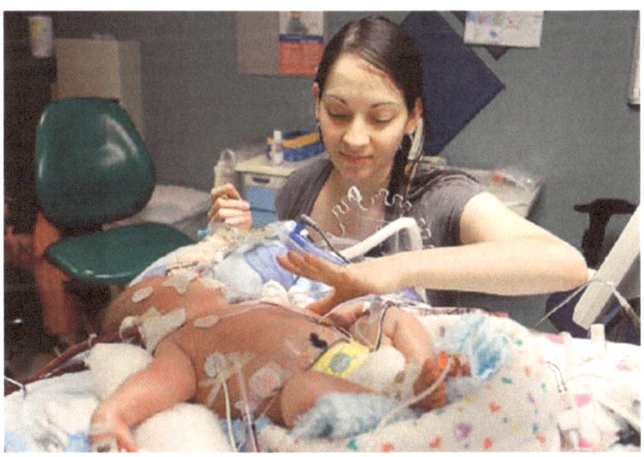

Fig. 29.4 : A New born baby with cardiorespiratory failure is being treated with ECMO in neonatal ICU.

- Pulmonary vasoreactive crisis following repair of congenital heart defect leading to severe hypoxemia, low cardiac output, or both
- Rarely, as a bridge to cardiac surgery in patients with serious end-organ damage resulting from profound low cardiac output related to congenital heart disease
- As a bridge to cardiac transplant
- Possibly, as a bridge to recovery in temporary cardiomyopathy secondary to renal failure, myocarditis, and burns.

Today, other indications or less strict selection of patients in certain institutions have made the use of this technology more diverse, not only in acute cardiac problems but also in primary pulmonary diseases.

The clinical outcomes of patients undergoing ECMO can be categorized according to the indication for the ECMO: severe acute respiratory failure or cardiac failure.

Acute Respiratory Failure

With acute respiratory failure use of ECMO has been shown to improve survival rates. Survival rates from 50–70 percenthave been reported in observational and uncontrolled clinical trials. The survival rates reported are better than historical survival rates.

Cardiac Failure

Venoarterial (VA) ECMO can provide acute support in cardiogenic shock or cardiac arrest in adults. Assuming that the brain function is normal or only minimally impaired, ECMO is provided until the patient recovers or receives a long-term ventricular assist device as a bridge to cardiac transplantation.

INDICATIONS OF ECMO IN ADOLESCENTS

VA-ECMO is indicated in patients with refractory cardiogenic shock who have an underlying potentially reversible heart condition, although it can also be used as a bridge to a ventricular assist device or cardiac transplantation. VA-ECMO can also be used as a salvage technique during cardiac arrest, and the current data support its use after 10 min of adequate but unsuccessful Advanced Life Support (ALS)

In-hospital survival rate of patients with VA-ECMO varies from 30 to 50% according to the cause of the cardiac dysfunction. VA-ECMO can be considered in patients with systolic arterial pressure lower than 85 mm Hg, cardiac index lower than 1.2 litre min-1 m-2, despite adequate preload, more than two inotropes in use, intra-aortic balloon counterpulsation, and systemic signs of low cardiac output. The paucity of data in the literature makes it difficult to determine which patients will benefit from VA-ECMO and when ECMO support will be futile. Thus, it is strongly recommended to discuss all possible cases with the nearest ECMO centre in these circumstances.

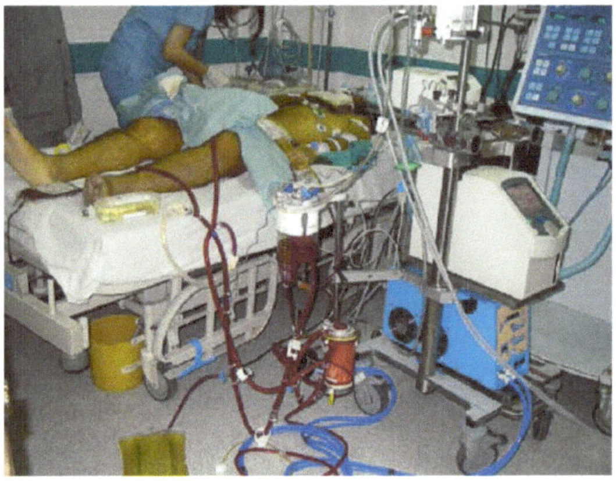

Fig. 29 5 : Adolescent patient with refractory cardiogenic shock is being treated with ECMO system in ICU.

The aim of VV-ECMO in adult patients is to provide oxygenation and rest the lungs, decreasing the insult caused by mechanical ventilation. Hence, VV-ECMO should be considered as an alternative to conventional therapy for adults with ARDS and patients with graft dysfunction after lung transplantation. VV-ECMO has a lower risk of thromboembolic complications and lung perfusion allows endocrine pulmonary function in comparison with VA-ECMO. It is sometimes necessary to use VA-ECMO if significant haemodynamic compromise becomes apparent or if oxygenation that is provided is not sufficient; this may require changes of the cannulae position.

ECMO is associated with significant inherent risks, and benefit compared with conventional therapies is still unclear. ECMO gained popularity during the H1N1/2009 pandemic, when clinicians were confronted with severe, refractory, and rapidly progressive hypoxaemia in young and fit patients. It made clinical sense to use the new generation of safer ECMO circuits in this situation. This was substantiated by the release of the Cesar trial results and no doubt catalysed by the media, influencing political choices. The Cesar trial is the third randomized controlled trial evaluating the benefits of ECMO in ARDS. The endpoint of the trial was to compare the survival at 6 months in the absence of severe disability, in patients who had developed ARDS and been randomized to be treated either in their original centre or in the treatment centre. The trial demonstrated that patients transferred to a centre with ECMO available had a better outcome than those treated at the original hospital with conventional therapy, and that this approach was cost-effective.

Whether ECMO can really replace conventional treatment of adult ARDS is still unknown. Studies to determine the group that may benefit most are still lacking but patients mechanically ventilated for longer than 7 days or in multiorgan failure are considered poor candidates as underlying lung damage might then be irreversible, and ECMO is generally not offered.ECMO therapy in ARDS allows a decrease in the stress imposed on the lung by ventilation at high airway pressure that may eventually damage the lung, and should be offered to patients with refractory hypoxaemia or hypercapnia despite optimal ventilation.

The best survival rates are observed in patients with non-necrotizing viral pneumonia and associated respiratory failure, probably because (i) these are often younger patients, (ii) they have fewer co-morbidities, and (iii) the associated lung injury is often reversible.

AV-ECMO is particularly useful in patients with severe hypercapnia, respiratory acidosis, and moderate hypoxaemia. The absence of a pump makes this device simpler to use, but it means that cardiac function must be preserved for the blood to be effectively pumped. However, mortality has been reported to be high in patients with ARDS who had AV-ECMO, and some patients may require conversion from AV-ECMO to VV- or even VA-ECMO. It does allow however easier transportation than other ECMO modes as no source of energy is required and it is smaller in size and weight.

Techniques Employed in ECMO

ECMO currently comes in two varieties: venoarterial (VA), and venovenous (VV). VA ECMO takes deoxygenated blood from a central vein or the right atrium, pumps it past the oxygenator, and then returns the oxygenated blood, under pressure, to the arterial side of the circulation (typically to the aorta). This form of ECMO partially supports the cardiac output as the flow through the ECMO circuit is in addition to the normal cardiac output. VV ECMO takes blood from a large vein and returns oxygenated blood back to a large vein. VV ECMO does not support the circulation. VA ECMO helps support the cardiac output and delivers higher levels of oxygenation support than does VV ECMO. VA ECMO carries a higher risk of systemic emboli than does VV. VV ECMO systems

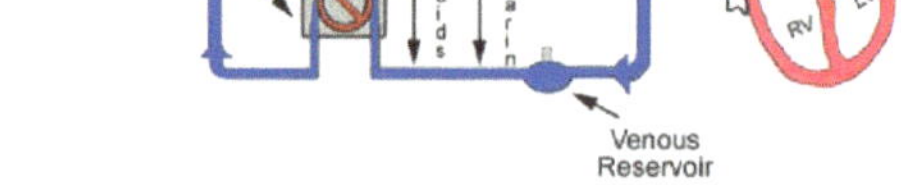

Fig. 29.6 : Showing extracorporeal membrane oxygenation (ECMO) system.

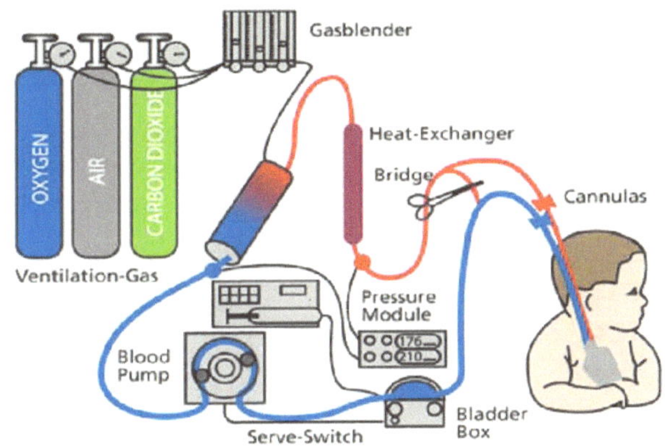

Fig.29.7: Application of ECMO in neonatal cardiorespiratory failure.

may actually recirculate previously oxygenated blood depending on the placement of the inflow and outflow catheters. Another variant of VV ECMO is extracorporeal CO_2 removal (ECCO2R). With this mode of support, oxygenation is provided by slow ventilation of the native lungs while CO_2 removal is accomplished by the ECMO circuit. In all forms of ECMO, CO_2 removal is more efficient than O_2 addition because of the solubility and diffusion properties of CO_2 relative to O_2. In fact, CO_2 normally has to be added to ECMO circuits to offset this efficiency at CO_2 removal. The flow through the ECMO circuit is typically on the order of 100 mL/kg/minute. This would be from 25–75% of the cardiac output. This high flow requires the placement of large catheters into the circulation. For adults, the intravascular catheters may be 20 Fr or larger while 14 Fr catheters might be used in infants. These are generally placed by cut-down. Current circuits require the use of systemic anticoagulation with heparin to keep the systems patent. This anticoagulation is, in large part, responsible for bleeding complications that can be seen with the use of ECMO. Bleeding may occur either at the site of catheter insertion or at remote sites such as intracranial or the gastrointestinal tract. Future catheters with inpregnated heparin may obviate the need for systemic anticoagulation and would be expected to reduce bleeding complications. Once blood leaves the patient, it comes in contact with a gas-permeable membrane that allows gas exchange to occur between the blood and the gasses (oxygen and carbon dioxide) that are run into the oxygenator. Carbon dioxide levels leaving the oxygenator can be adjusted about as low as the physician wants while oxygen levels typically reach the 400–500 mm Hg level. Note that CO_2 content varies fairly directly with partial pressure while O_2 content follows the shape of the oxyhemoglobin dissociation curve. Under normobaric conditions, this limits the amount of oxygen that can be loaded into blood. If you were to try to predict the final mixed arterial oxygen content or partial pressure during VA ECMO, you would need to know the pulmonary venous oxygen content, the ECMO effluent oxygen content, and the % of cardiac output flowing through the ECMO circuit:

$$CaO_2 = (EO \times EF + NO \times NF)/(EF + NF)$$

Where
EO = ECMO oxygen content
EF = ECMO flow
NO = non-ECMO oxygen content
NF = non-ECMO flow

Predicting final arterial content during VV ECMO is more complex and cannot be easily calculated. During VV ECMO, the lungs may actually excrete oxygen rather than remove it from the inspired gas. Once ECMO has been started, the ventilator is typically reduced to minimal settings to prevent atelectasis and barotrauma. The FIO_2 is

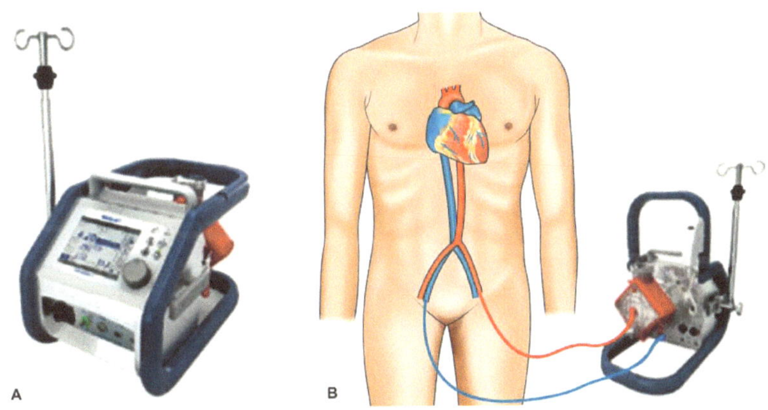

Fig. 29.8 : The device is compact and easily portable, with a total weight of only 9 kg. (A) Veno-arterial extracorporeal membrane oxygenation (ECMO) is established by cannulation of a femoral vein and artery using the Seldinger technique. To expedite interhospital transfer these vessels can be located with guidewires before arrival of the outreach team. The cannulas can then be inserted rapidly to begin ECMO before transport by air or ground ambulance. Images of the Cardiohelp®device courtesy of ©Maquet Cardiopulmonary AG.

lowered as much as possible, perhaps to room air. The ECMO flow rate is adjusted to the minimum needed to provide for adequate gas exchange and/or circulation support in the case of VA ECMO. ECMO is typically used for 7–12 days and is weaned when there is evidence of pulmonary improvement as indicated by compliance or radiologic appearance. ECMO can also be stopped if there are major complications or if the patient's condition is determined to be hopeless.

Types of Patient Selected for Application of ECMO

As mentioned previously, usual ECMO criteria include patients with a severe reversible process that would result in a very high predicted mortality with conventional ventilatory support. The best candidates are those without multi-system organ failure that are otherwise considered to be salvageable. It would be expected, that once ECMO becomes safer and more accepted by physicians, that these criteria would be revised to eliminate the requirement for a very high predicted pre-treatment mortality. There are several ways to evaluate patients to determine if they are 'sick enough' for ECMO. APACHE and other scoring sysztems could be used to predict mortality. More frequently, indexes to assess refractory hypoxemia are used. The a:A ratio or A-a gradient can be used, but the oxygenation index (OI) is currently in more common use: OI = (FIO2) (MAP) / PaO2 An OI greater than 0.40–0.55 is thought to predict an 80% predicted mortality. Unfortunately, mortality predictors have been notoriously pessimistic since they are derived by looking at retrospective data and tend to do a poor job of predicting prospective results.

Contraindications

Most contraindications are relative, balancing the risks of the procedure (including the risk of using valuable resources which could be used for others) *vs* the potential benefits. The relative contraindications are:

1. Conditions incompatible with normal life if the patient recovers
2. Preexisting conditions which affect the quality of life (CNS status, end stage malignancy, risk of systemic bleeding with anticoagulation)
3. Age and size of patient
4. *Futility:* patients who are too sick, have been on conventional therapy too long, or have a fatal diagnosis.

Maintenance

Once the initial respiratory and hemodynamic goals have been achieved, the blood flow is maintained at that rate. Frequent assessment and adjustments are facilitated by continuous venous oximetry, which directly measures the oxyhemoglobin saturation of the blood in the venous limb of the ECMO circuit.

Special Considerations

VV ECMO is typically used for respiratory failure, while VA ECMO is used for cardiac failure. There are unique considerations for each type of ECMO, which influence management.

Blood Flow

Near maximum flow rates are usually desired during VV ECMO to optimize oxygen delivery. In contrast, the flow rate used during VA ECMO must be high enough to provide adequate perfusion pressure and venous oxyhemoglobin saturation (measured on drainage blood), but low enough to provide sufficient preload to maintain left ventricular output.

Diuresis

Since most patients are fluid overloaded when ECMO is initiated, aggressive diuresis is warranted once the patient is stable on ECMO. Ultrafiltration can be easily added to the ECMO circuit if patients are unable to produce sufficient urine for diuresis.

Left Ventricular Monitoring

Left ventricular output is rigorously monitored during VA ECMO because left ventricular output can become worse.

Weaning and Discontinuing

For patients with respiratory failure, improvements in radiographic appearance, pulmonary compliance, and arterial oxyhemoglobin saturation indicate that the patient may be ready to be taken off of ECMO support. For patients with cardiac failure, enhanced aortic pulsatility correlates with improved left ventricular output and indicates that the patient may be ready to be taken off of ECMO support. Once the decision has been made to discontinue ECMO, the cannulae are removed.

Complications

ECMO complications are those associated with cannulation (pneumothorax, vascular disruptions, bleeding, infection, emboli), those associated with systemic anticoagulation (GI bleeding, intracranial bleeding etc.), and exsanguination resulting from circuit disruptions. These potential complications require that a trained ECMO technician be present at the bedside 24 hours per day in addition to the patient's usual nursing presence. As many as 30% of ECMO treated infants reported to the Extracorporeal Life Support Organization (ELSO) registry suffer some degree of CNS injury.

A common consequence in ECMO-treated adults is neurological injury, which may include subarachnoid hemorrhage, ischemic watershed infarctions, hypoxic-ischemic encephalopathy, unexplained coma, and brain death. Fatal sepsis may occur when the large catheters inserted in the neck provide fertile field for infectionAdditional risks include bleeding. In adults, ECMO survival rates are around 60%. ECMO has yet to have proven survival benefit in adults with acute respiratory distresssyndrome (ARDS). In VA ECMO, patients whose cardiac function does not recover sufficiently to be weaned from ECMO may be bridged to a ventricular assist device (VAD) or transplant.

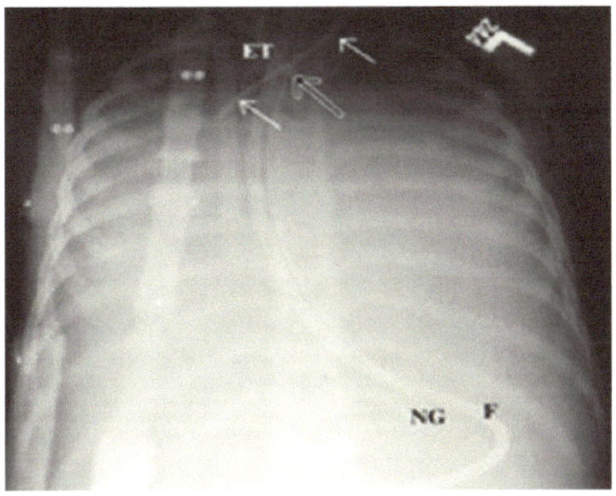

Fig. 29.9: Portable chest radiograph of a patient undergoing extracorporeal membrane oxygenation shows pulmonary edema in the lungs and the tubing ("d) going to the patient's right carotid artery and right jugular vein. Also seen are an endotracheal tube (ET), a right internal jugular vein catheter (black arrow), a left internal jugular vein catheter (white arrows), a nasogastric tube (NG), and a feeding tube (F).

In infants aged less than 34 weeks of gestation several physiologic systems are not well-developed, especially the cerebral vasculature and germinal matrix, resulting in high sensitivity to slight changes in pH, PaO2, and intracranial pressure. Preterm infants are at unacceptably high risk for intraventricular hemorrhage (IVH) if administered ECMO at a gestational age less than 32 weeks. Also later, given the risk of IVH, it has become standard practice to ultrasound the brain prior to administering ECMO.

Bleeding

Bleeding occurs in 30 to 40 percent of patients who receive ECMO and can be life threatening. It is due to both the necessary continuous heparin infusion and platelet dysfunction. Meticulous surgical technique, maintaining platelet counts greater than 100,000/mm^3, and maintaining the target ACT reduce the likelihood of bleeding.

Thromboembolism

Systemic thromboembolism due to thrombus formation within the extracorporeal circuit is an infrequent complication that can be devastating. Its impact is greater with VA ECMO than VV ECMO because infusion is into the systemic circulation. Heparin infusion that achieves its target ACT and vigilant observation of the circuit for signs of clot formation successfully prevents thromboembolism in most patients.

Cannulation-related

A variety of complications can occur during cannulation, including vessel perforation with hemorrhage, arterial dissection, distal ischemia, and incorrect location (e.g. venous cannula within the artery). These complications are rare (<5 percent). A skilled and experienced surgeon is important to avoid or address such complications.

Heparin-induced Thrombocytopenia

Heparin-induced thrombocytopenia (HIT) is increasingly common among patients receiving ECMO. When HIT is suspected, the heparin infusion is usually replaced by a non-heparin anticoagulant.

Veno-Arterial Specific Complications

Pulmonary Hemorrhage

Pulmonary hemorrhage can occur in patients who receive VA ECMO.

Cardiac Thrombosis

There is retrograde blood flow in the ascending aorta whenever the femoral artery and vein are used for VA ECMO. Stasis of the blood can occur if left ventricular output is not maintained, which may result in thrombosis.

Coronary or Cerebral Hypoxia

During VA ECMO, fully saturated blood infused into the femoral artery from the ECMO circuit will preferentially perfuse the lower extremities and the abdominal viscera. Blood ejected from the heart will selectively perfuse the heart, brain, and upper extremities.

Future

Applications for ECMO may expand in the future to include percutaneous temporary left ventricular assistance and low flow ECMO for CO2 removal (ECOOR)]. In addition, new technologies will improve the simplicity and safety of ECMO, including new oxygenators, pumps, and surface coatings.

Other Uses

ECMO use on cadavers can increase the viability rate of transplanted organs.

BIBLIOGRAPHY AND ACKNOWLEDGEMENT

- Abrams D, Brodie D, Combes A. What is new in extracorporeal membrane oxygenation for ARDS in adults? Intensive Care Med 2013;39:2028–2030.
- Barth E, Durand M, Heylbroeck C, et al. Extracorporeal life support as a bridge to high-urgency heart transplantation. Clin Transplant 2012;26:484–488.

- Bermudez CA, Rocha RV, Toyoda Y, et al. Extracorporeal membrane oxygenation for advanced refractory shock in acute and chronic cardiomyopathy. Ann Thorac Surg 2011;92: 2125–2131.
- Brogan TV, Thiagarajan RR, Rycus PT, Bartlett RH, Bratton SL (2009). Extracorporeal membrane oxygenation in adults with severe respiratory failure: a multi-center database. Intensive Care Med 2009;35(12):2105–14.
- Cave DM, Gazmuri RJ, Otto CW, et al. Part 7: CPR techniques and devices: 2010 American Heart Association guidelines for cardiopulmonary resuscitation and emergency cardiovascular care. Circulation 2010;122:S720–S728.
- Chen YS, Lin JW, Yu HY, et al. Cardiopulmonary resuscitation with assisted extracorporeal life-support versus conventional cardiopulmonary resuscitation in adults with in-hospital cardiac arrest: an observational study and propensity analysis. Lancet 2008;372:554–561.
- Cheng R, Hachamovitch R, Kittleson M, et al. Complications of extracorporeal membrane oxygenation for treatment of cardiogenic shock and cardiac arrest: a meta-analysis of 1,866 adult patients. Ann Thorac Surg 2014;97:610–616.
- Chung JC, Tsai PR, Chou NK, Chi NH, Wang SS, Ko WJ; Extracorporeal membrane oxygenation bridge to adult heart transplantation. Clin Transplant 2010;24:375–380.
- Cohen G, Permut L. Decision making for mechanical cardiac assist in pediatric cardiac surgery. Seminars in Thoracic and Cardiovascular Surgery. Pediatric Cardiac Surgery Annual: 2005;41–50.
- Cornell T, Wyrick P, Fleming G, Pasko D, Han Y, Custer J et al. A case series describing the use of argatroban in patients on extracorporeal circulation. ASAIO J 2007;53 (4): 460–3.
- D'Alessandro C, Aubert S, Golmard JL, et al. Extra-corporeal membrane oxygenation temporary support for early graft failure after cardiac transplantation. Eur J Cardiothorac Surg 2010;37:343–349.
- D'Alessandro C, Golmard JL, Barreda E, et al. Predictive risk factors for primary graft failure requiring temporary extracorporeal membrane oxygenation support after cardiac transplantation in adults. Eur J Cardiothorac Surg 2011; 40:962–969.
- Doll N, Kiaii B, Borger M, et al. Five-year results of 219 consecutive patients treated with extracorporeal membrane oxygenation for refractory postoperative cardiogenic shock. Ann Thorac Surg 2004;77:151–157.
- Groopman, Jerome. How Doctors Think. Houghton Mifflin Harcourt 2007. ISBN 978-0-618-61003-7.
- Haley MJ, Fisher JC, Ruiz-Elizalde AR, Stolar CJ, Morrissey NJ, Middlesworth W. Percutaneous distal perfusion of the lower extremity after femoral cannulation for venoarterial extracorporeal membrane oxygenation in a small child. J Pediatr Surg. 2009;44:437–440.
- Heilmann C, Geisen U, Beyersdorf F, et al. Acquired von Willebrand syndrome in patients with extracorporeal life support ECLS. Intensive Care Med 2012;38:62–68.
- Hemmila MR, Rowe SA, Boules TN, Miskulin J, McGillicuddy JW, Schuerer DJ, et al. Extracorporeal life support for severe acute respiratory distress syndrome in adults. Ann Surg 2004;240(4):595–605;.
- Jackson KW, Timpa J, McIlwain RB, et al. Side-arm grafts for femoral extracorporeal membrane oxygenation cannulation. Ann Thorac Surg 2012;94:e111–e112.
- Johnson SM, Itoga N, Garnett GM, Kilcommons M, Puapong DP, Woo RK. Increased risk of cardiovascular perforation during ECMO with a bicaval, wire-reinforced cannula. J Pediatr Surg 2014;49:46–50.
- Kagawa E, Dote K, Kato M, et al. Should we emergently revascularize occluded coronaries for cardiac arrest? Rapidresponse extracorporeal membrane oxygenation and intraarrest percutaneous coronary intervention. Circulation 2012;126:1605–1613.
- Kolla S, Awad SS, Rich PB, Schreiner RJ, Hirschl RB, Bartlett RH. Extracorporeal life support for 100 adult patients with severe respiratory failure. Ann Surg 1997;226(4): 544–64.
- Lebreton G, Nicolescu M, Leger P, Leprince P. Implantation of left ventricular support under extracorporeal membrane oxygenation. Eur J Cardiothorac Surg 2011;40:e165–e167.
- Lewandowski K, Rossaint R, Pappert D, Gerlach H, Slama KJ, Weidemann H, et al. High survival rate in 122 ARDS patients managed according to a clinical algorithm including extracorporeal membrane oxygenation. Intensive Care Med 1997;23(8):819–35.
- Madershahian N, Nagib R, Wippermann J, Strauch J, Wahlers T (2006). A simple technique of distal limb perfusion during prolonged femoro-femoral cannulation. J Card Surg 2006; 21(2):168–9.
- Maekawa K, Tanno K, Hase M, Mori K, Asai Y. Extracorporeal cardiopulmonary resuscitation for patients with out-ofhospital cardiac arrest of cardiac origin: a propensitymatched study and predictor analysis. Crit Care Med 2013;41:1186–1196.
- Maggio P, Hemmila M, Haft J, Bartlett R. Extracorporeal life support for massive pulmonary embolism. J Trauma 2007;62:570–576.
- Marasco SF, Vale M, Pellegrino V, et al. Extracorporeal membrane oxygenation in primary graft failure after heart transplantation. Ann Thorac Surg 2010;90:1541–1546.
- Mateen FJ, Muralidharan R, Shinohara RT, et al. Neurological Injury in Adults Treated With Extracorporeal Membrane Oxygenation Archives of Neurology 2011.
- Munakata R, Yamamoto T, Hosokawa Y, et al. Massive pulmonary embolism requiring extracorporeal life support treated with catheter-based interventions. International heart journal 2012;53:370–374.

- Peek GJ, Moore HM, Moore N, Sosnowski AW, Firmin RK. Extracorporeal membrane oxygenation for adult respiratory failure. Chest 1997;112(3):759–64.
- Rahimi RA, Skrzat J, Reddy DR, et al. Physical rehabilitation of patients in the intensive care unit requiring extracorporeal membrane oxygenation: a small case series. Phys Ther 2013;93:248–255.
- Rastan AJ, Dege A, Mohr M, et al. Early and late outcomes of 517 consecutive adult patients treated with extracorporeal membrane oxygenation for refractory postcardiotomy cardiogenic shock. J Thorac Cardiovasc Surg 2010;139: 302–311.
- Rehder KJ, Turner DA, Hartwig MG, et al. Active rehabilitation during extracorporeal membrane oxygenation as a bridge to lung transplantation. Respir Care 2013;58:1291– 1298.
- Rich PB, Awad SS, Kolla S, Annich G, Schreiner RJ, Hirschl RB et al. An approach to the treatment of severe adult respiratory failure. J Crit Care 1998;13(1):26–36.
- Rosenzweig E, Brodie D, Abrams D, Agerstrand C, Bacchetta M. Extracorporeal membrane oxygenation as a novel bridging strategy for acute right heart failure in group 1 PAH. ASAIO J 2014;60:129–133. 67
- Russo CF, Cannata A, Lanfranconi M, et al. Veno-arterial extracorporeal membrane oxygenation using Levitronix centrifugal pump as bridge to decision for refractory cardiogenic shock. J Thorac Cardiovasc Surg 2010;140:1416–1421.
- Schmidt M, Brechot N, Hariri S, et al. Nosocomial infections in adult cardiogenic shock patients supported by venoarterial extracorporeal membrane oxygenation. Clin Infect Dis 2012;55:1633–1641.
- Shin TG, Jo IJ, Sim MS, et al. Two-year survival and neurological outcome of in-hospital cardiac arrest patients rescued by extracorporeal cardiopulmonary resuscitation. Int J Cardiol 2013;168:3424-3430
- Takayama H, Naka Y, Kodali SK, et al. A novel approach to percutaneous right-ventricular mechanical support. Eur J Cardiothorac Surg 2012;41:423–426.
- Takayama H, Truby L, Koekort M, et al. Clinical outcome of mechanical circulatory support for refractory cardiogenic shock in the current era. J Heart Lung Transplant 2013;32: 106–111.
- Turner DA, Cheifetz IM, Rehder KJ, et al. Active rehabilitation and physical therapy during extracorporeal membrane oxygenation while awaiting lung transplantation: a practical approach. Crit Care Med 2011;39:2593–2598.
- Ullrich R, Lorber C, Röder G, Urak G, Faryniak B, Sladen RN et al. Controlled airway pressure therapy, nitric oxide inhalation, prone position, and extracorporeal membrane oxygenation (ECMO) as components of an integrated approach to ARDS. Anesthesiology 1999;91(6):1577–86.
- Van Meurs, K, Lally, KP, Peek, G, Zwischenberger, JB. ECMO: Extracorporeal Cardiopulmonary Support in critical care, Extracorporeal Life Support Organization, Ann Arbor 2005.
- Vural KM. Ventricular assist device applications. Anadolu Kardiyoloji Dergisi: AKD=the Anatolian Journal of Cardiology 2008;8(Suppl 2):117–30.
- Wang D, Zhou X, Liu X, Sidor B, Lynch J, Zwischenberger JB. Wang-Zwische double lumen cannula-toward a percutaneous and ambulatory paracorporeal artificial lung. ASAIO J 2008;54(6):606–11.

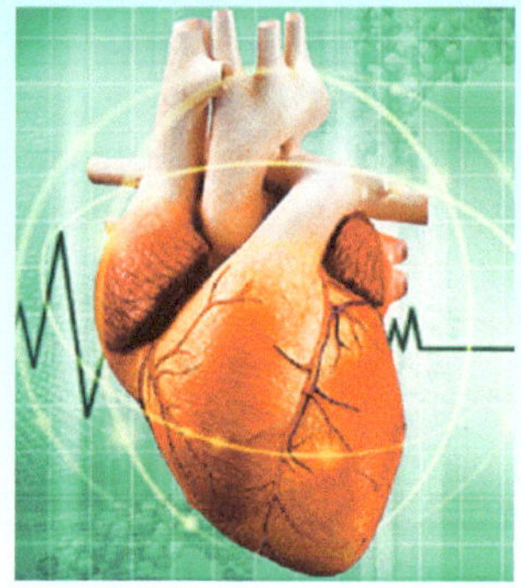

30 Fetal Cardiac Emergent Interventions. Over View

The potential benefits of fetal cardiac intervention (FCI) have been realized for many years. In 1975, Eibschitz et al. reported intrapartum treatment of fetal ventricular tachycardia by administering propranolol to the mother, and as early as 1986, in-utero pacing was attempted for complete heart block in a human fetus. Recently, however, interest in FCI has accelerated. As with other fetal interventions, FCI can only become a highly useful clinical tool if it is applied to conditions in which a feasible mode of therapy is available and either the fetus is at risk for demise as a result of the condition or intervention may alter the evolution of the condition such that the severity of the postnatal disease is substantially reduced. For conditions in which the fetus is at high risk for prenatal or neonatal death, the rationale for FCI is obvious, to improve survival. If death is not imminent but the disease is likely to have major life-long morbidity, the rationale is that FCI will modify the course of cardiac growth, function, and/or development in-utero sufficiently to alter postnatal outcome and justify the potential risks of the procedure. Prenatal intervention may also allow the fetus to recover in the supportive in-utero environment, during a developmental period when there is enhanced wound healing and the capacity for myocyte proliferation.

This construct rightfully emphasizes death or significant morbidity as therapeutic targets. FCI can entail substantial short-term risk to the fetus, uncertain long-term risk to the fetus and child, and at least some risk to the mother. There are no known medical benefits to the mother. With that risk profile, FCI will not be embraced by the maternal-fetal medicine and cardiology communities unless it is used to treat serious conditions in which the potential benefits to the fetus are high and can be achieved in a reasonable percentage of cases.

Although many recent publications have dealt with closed, 'minimally invasive' FCI, there is a considerable body of evidence regarding pharmacological and surgical FCI as well. This review will touch on all of these topics, with a focus on the most recent literature.

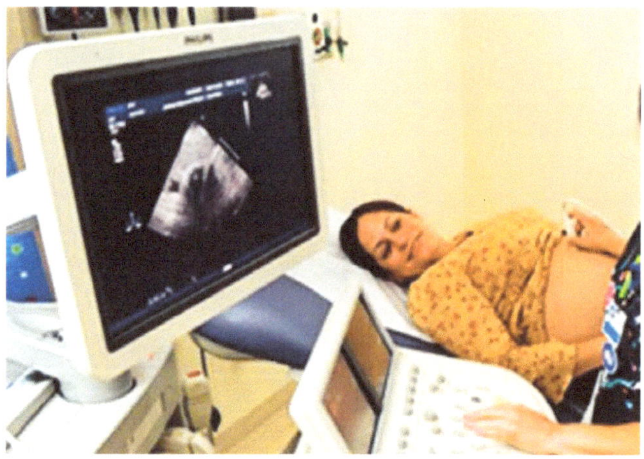

Fig. 30.1: Doctor performing foetal echocardiography

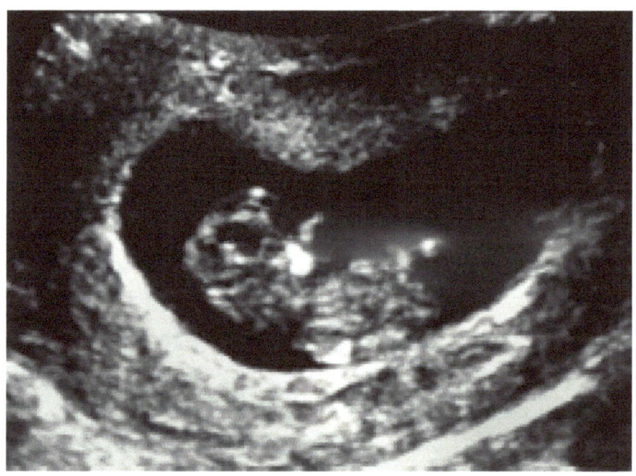

Fig. 30.2: Abdominal ultrasound showing viable intrauterine 10 weeks old foetus

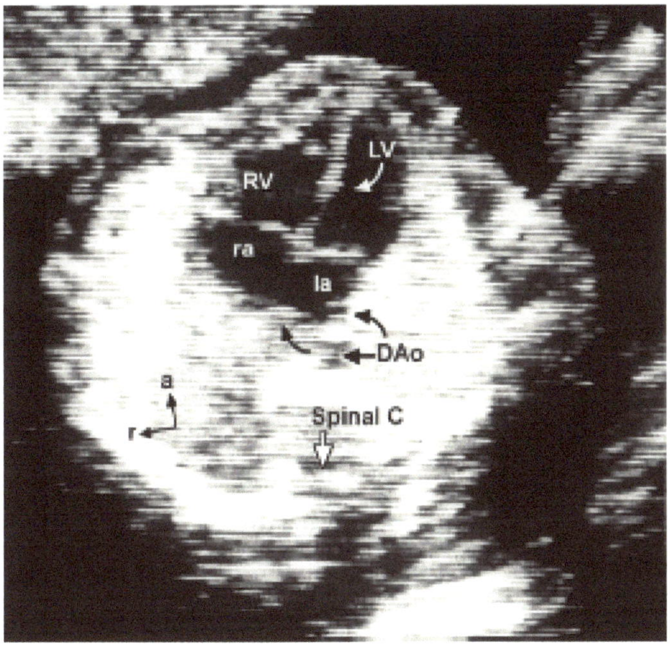

Fig. 30.3: Fetal echocardiography showing well formed four chambers of the heart with concordant AñV valves communicating through their respective chambers

FETOSCOPIC AND ULTRASONOGRAPHIC TECHNIQUES IN FCI

These are useful not only in diagnosis of congenital heart defects in-utero but also helps in the management of critical cardiovascular disorders.

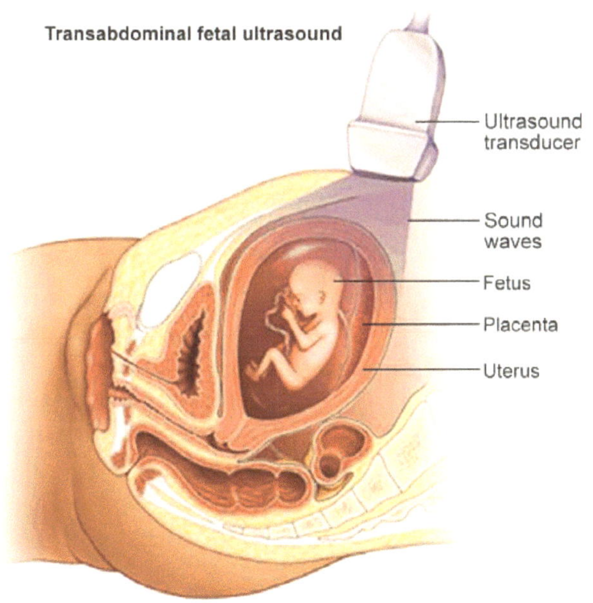

Fig. 30.4: Ultrasound beam striking at different parts of fetus for their identification and perfomance of selected percutaneous intervention

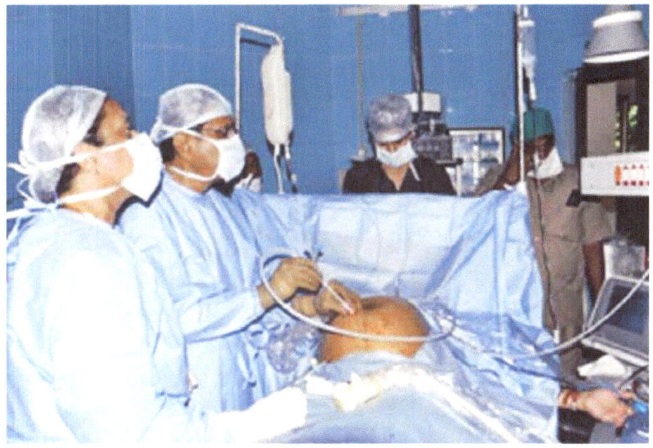

Fig. 30.5: A team of doctors performing fetoscopy procedure on a pregnant woman for assessment of fetal health

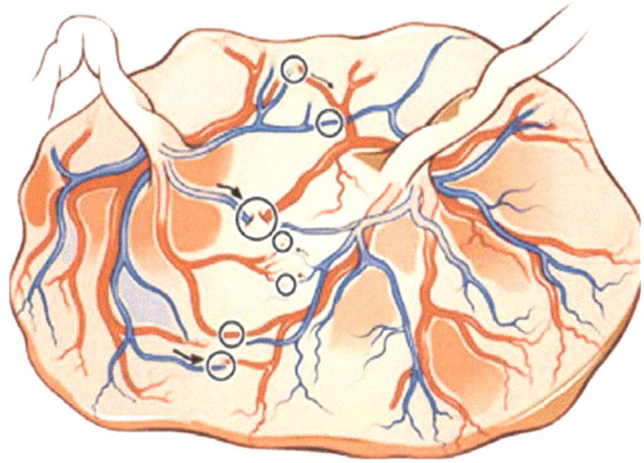

Fig. 30.6: Drawing of the shared placenta in twin-to-twin transfusion syndrome. Multiple vessels connect both fetuses over what is called ëanastomosesí (open circles). These anastomoses are the subject of laser coagulation

FETAL ULTRASONOGRAPHY IN DIAGNOSIS AND MANAGEMENT OF CONGENITAL DISORDERS

Fetal visualization By Ultrasound

Ultrasound is a noninvasive procedure for imaging fetal anatomy. It is harmless to both the fetus and the mother. Ultrasound can evaluate gestational age, as well as identify twins; fetal position; placental location; fetal growth, development, and movement; and any structural birth defects. It also can assess amniotic fluid volume.

Many fetal organ systems and anatomical lesions, including some genitourinary, gastrointestinal, skeletal, and central nervous system abnormalities and congenital cardiopathies, can be visualized by ultrasound between 16–20 weeks' gestation. Using ultrasound, Romain et al. carried out prenatal detection of congenital cataract in an unborn fetus with trisomy. Aslan et al. carried out prenatal diagnosis of Neu-Laxova syndrome at 38 weeks' gestation.

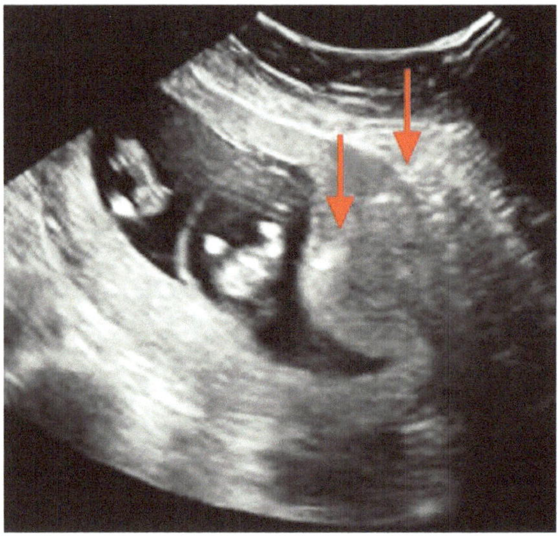

Fig. 30.7: Fetal skin biopsy is the optimal way to evaluate ambiguity that occasionally arises in the interpretation of amniocentesis data. These biopsies are performed without a hospital stay, and under ultrasound guidance

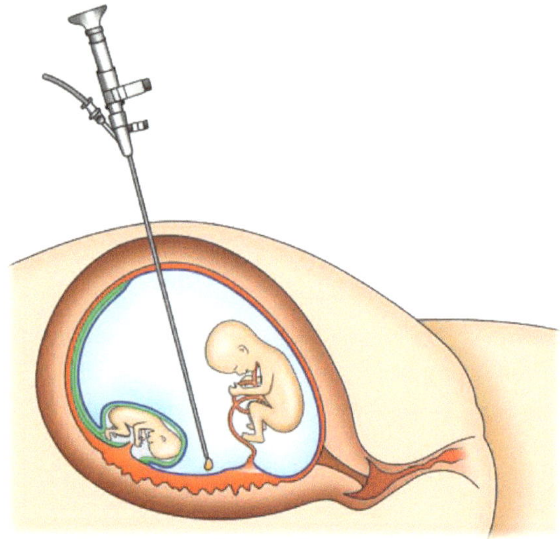

Fig. 30.9: A fetoscopic laser treatment. A cannula has been placed through the abdominal wall, through which a scope and laser beam has been passed. The connecting vessels are identified and subsequently destroyed

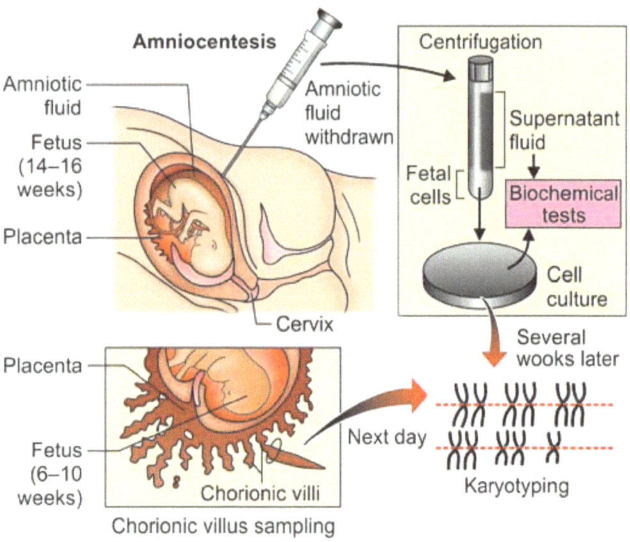

Fig. 30.8: The technique of amniocentesis for identification fetal genetic disorders

Ultrasound also is used to guide invasive sampling, such as amniocentesis, CVS, cordocentesis, and various fetal biopsies.

Bernard et al. found that spina bifida may be detected early in pregnancy with biparietal diameter (BPD) on ultrasound. BPD is lower in spina bifida babies. Half of the deformities could be detected by this modality.

Fetal visualization ByFetal echocardiography

Fetal echocardiography can be performed at 15 weeks' gestation and beyond. When this technique is used with duplex or color flow Doppler, it can identify a number of major structural cardiac defects and rhythm disturbances. By fetal echocardiography, Saygili et al. diagnosed absent pulmonary valve syndrome in a male infant prenatally at 22 weeks' gestation. Fetal echocardiography is recommended in cases where cardiac defects are suspected, including the following:

- Identification of an extracardiac malformation on routine ultrasound
- Abnormality of another major organ system
- Suspected genetic disease or fetal chromosome abnormality associated with heart defects
- Exposure to potentially teratogenic agents
- Family history of congenital heart defects, particularly in a parent or sibling
- Maternal diseases, such as diabetes or phenylketonuria associated with fetal structural heart defects, in particular heart blocks, such as lupus or other immune disorders
- Alcohol or drug consumption by mother during pregnancy
- Maternal rubella infection during pregnancy

PHARMACOLOGICAL FCI

The first reported and most entrenched mode of FCI is pharmacological therapy, most often for fetal arrhythmia or heart block. Pharmacological FCI typically consists of medication taken orally by the mother with transplacental passage to the fetus, but it may be provided directly through the umbilical vein or by fetal intramuscular or intravascular injection

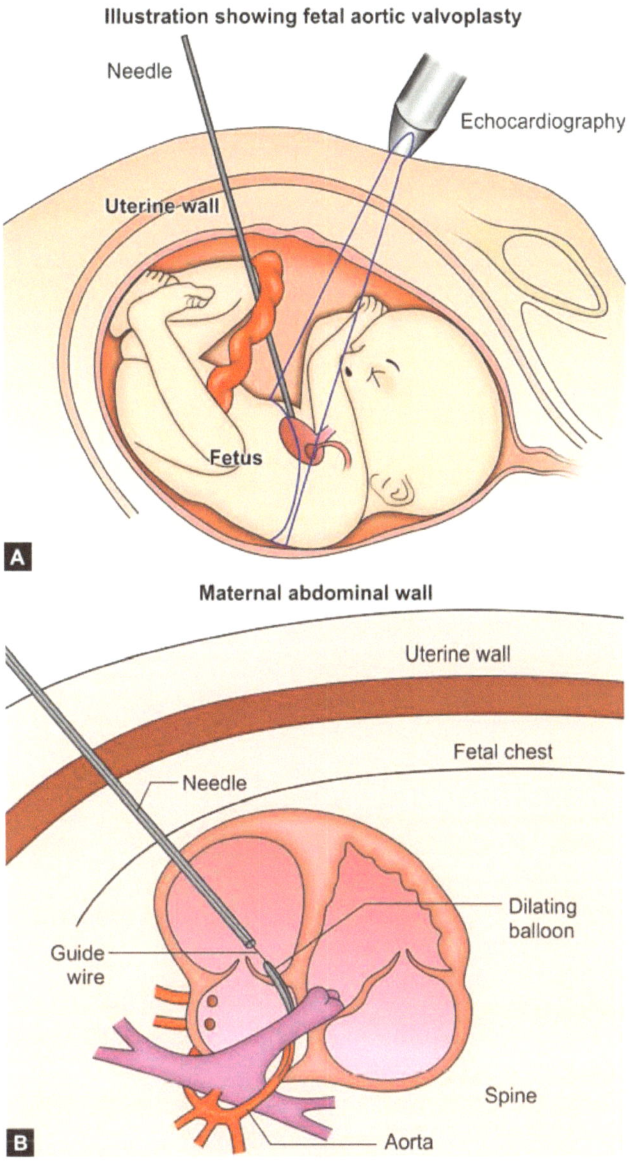

Fig. 30.10: (A and B) Deal fetal position and cannula course. Fetal left chest is anterior, and pathway from maternal abdomen to LV apex is unobstructed. This pathway, which corresponds to cannula course, continues from LV apex to aortic valve

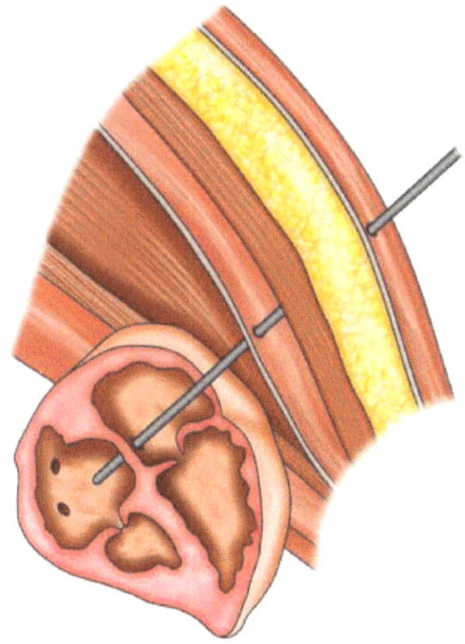

Fig. 30.11: Optimal fetal position and needle trajectory for atrial septoplasty. The right atrium is punctured through the fetal chest and the needle advanced through the atrial septum, which is thickened and bows tensely into the right atrium

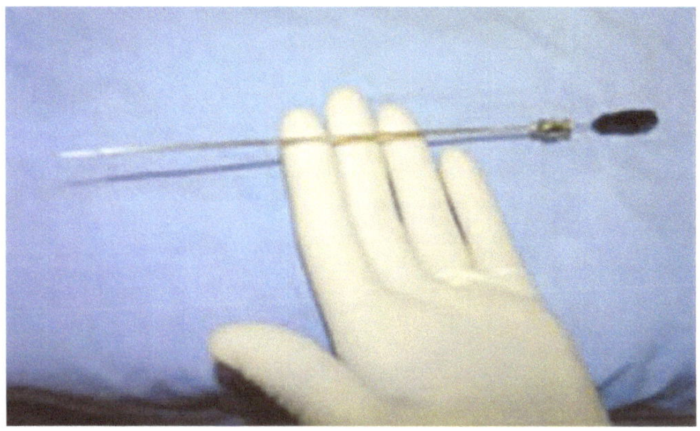

Fig. 30.12: Chiba needle used for fetal invasive procedures

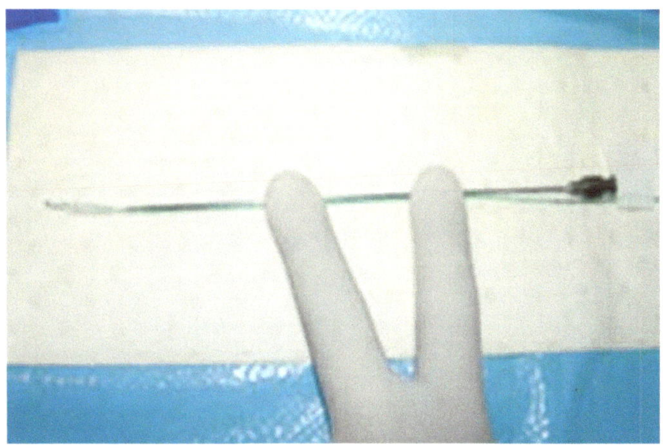

Fig. 30.13: Balloon angioplasty preassembled on guide that will be introduced through the needle Chiba to dilate the aortic valve

FETAL TACHYARRHYTHMIAS

Pharmacological FCI was first described by Eibschitz et al. who treated fetal tachycardia with propranolol in 1975.Maternal digoxin was first used to treat fetal supraventricular tachycardia several years later. Fetal supraventricular tachycardia, most often atrioventricular (AV) re-entry or atrial flutter, probably remains the most common indication for pharmacological FCI. Over the years, most antiarrhythmic agents have been used to treat fetal supraventricular tachycardia. Digoxin has been a mainstay of therapy; other agents have come io more common use recently, including sotalol, darone, and

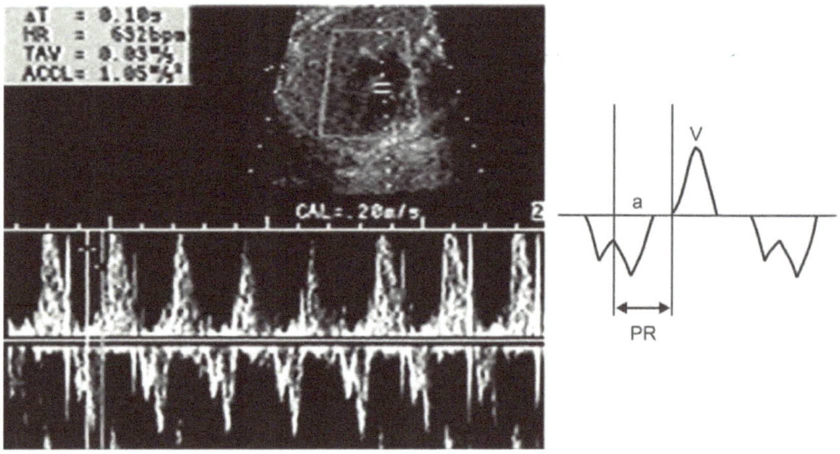

Fig. 30.14: Mitral valve and aortic valve Doppler in a 20-week fetus. Calculation of the PR interval to assess for first degree heart block is made measuring from the onset of the mitral a wave to the onset of the aortic outflow wave (a=mitral a wave, V=aortic outflow)

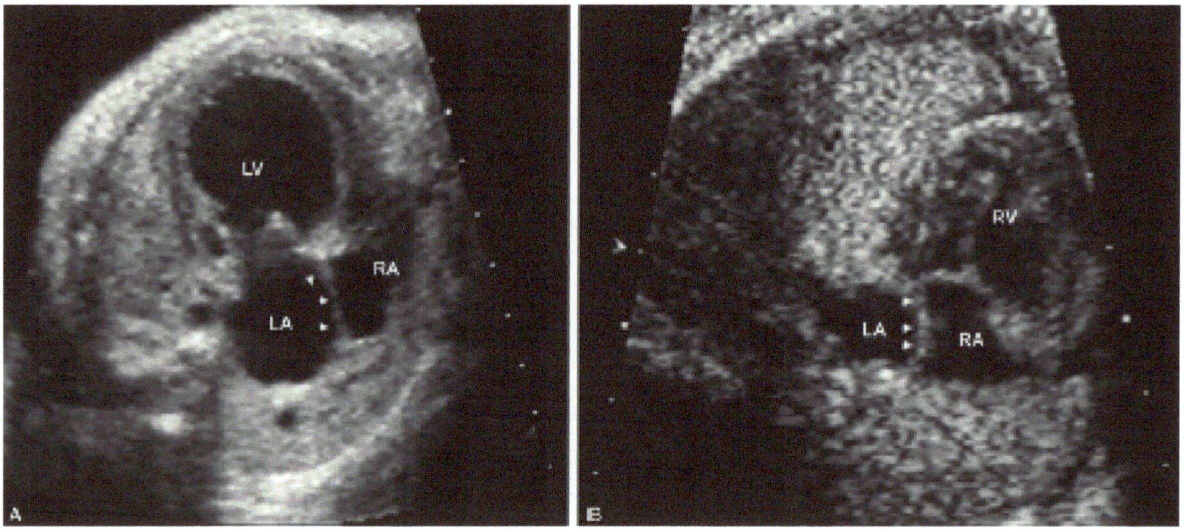

Fig. 30.15: Fetal echocardiographic apical view of the heart in a fetus with foramen ovale closure and ductus arteriosus closure and transposition of the great arteries (A) and in a fetus with foramen ovale closure and hypoplastic left heart syndrome (B) (RA=right atrium, RV=right ventricle, LA=left atrium, LV=left ventricle, arrows demarcate the atrial septum)

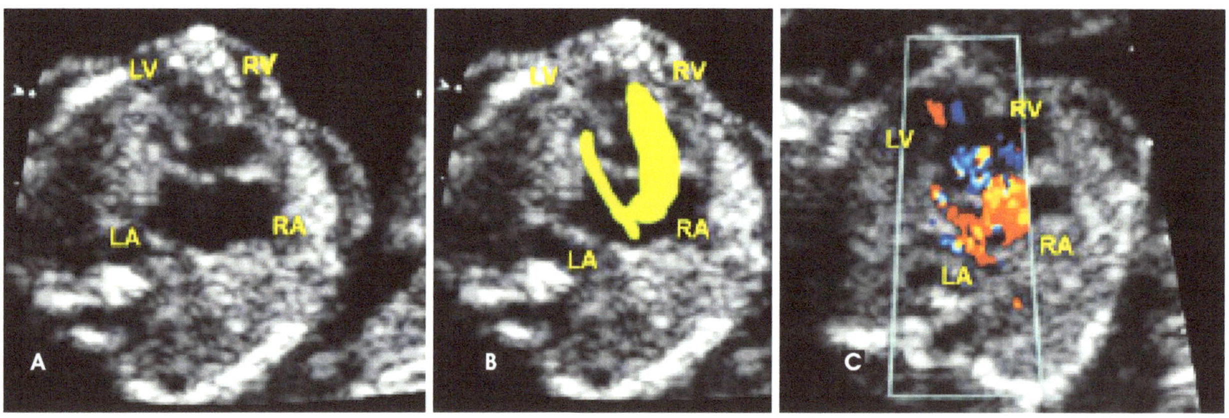

Fig. 30.16: (A and B) Hypoplastic left heart syndromeóthe left ventricle diminutive, with color doppler, (C) there is an asymmetric color perfusion of the chambers

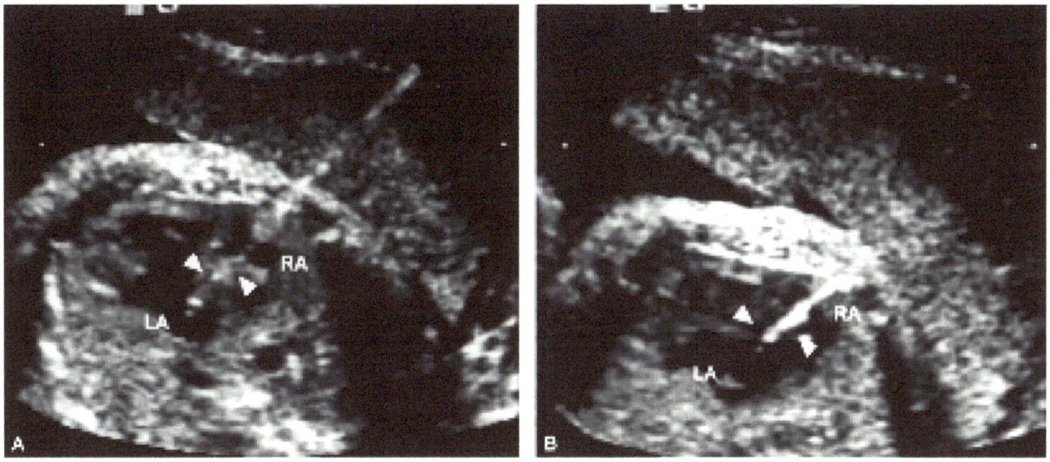

Fig. 30.17: Fetal echocardiographic views of aortic balloon dilation in fetuses with aortic stenosis. (A) Note the needle approaching the left ventricular apex. (B) Note the wire crossing the left ventricular outflow tract. Note the balloon being inflated at the level of the aortic valve (RV=right ventricle, LV=left ventricle, arrows demarcate needle, wire, or balloon during the procedure. Images courtesy of Dr Wayne Tworetsky from Boston Children's Hospital)

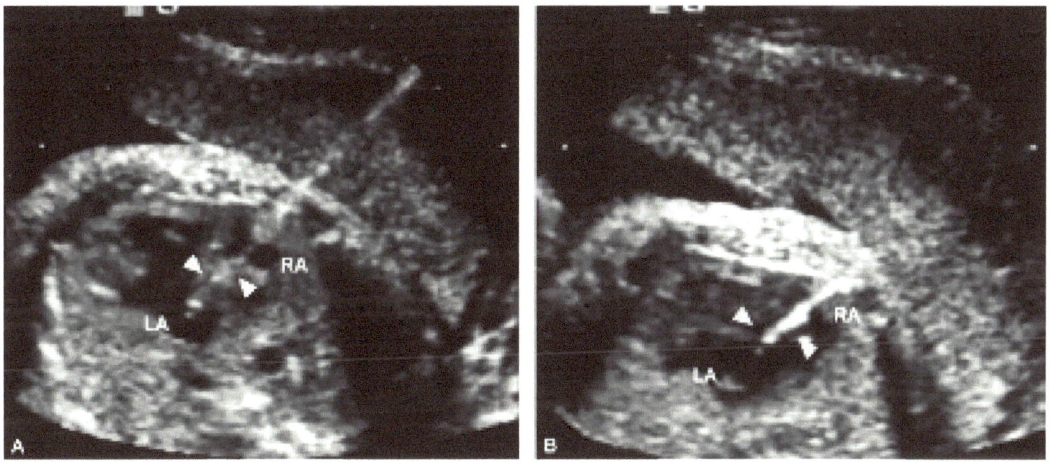

Fig. 30.18 : Fetal echocardiographic views of an atrial septal dilation in a fetus with hypoplastic left heart syndrome and an intact atrial septum. (A) Note the needle crossing the atrial septum. (B) Note the balloon crossing the atrial septum (RA=right atrium, LA=left atrium, arrows demarcate the needle or balloon for the procedure)

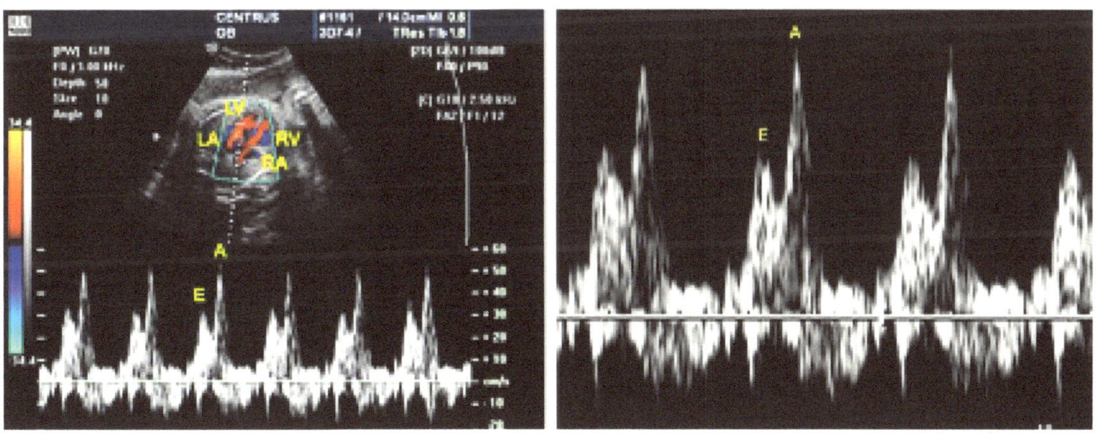

Fig. 30.19: Low velocity waveform across the tricuspid valve at 28 weeks of gestation (left) (E-wave=early ventricular filling and A-wave=atrial ventricular filling)

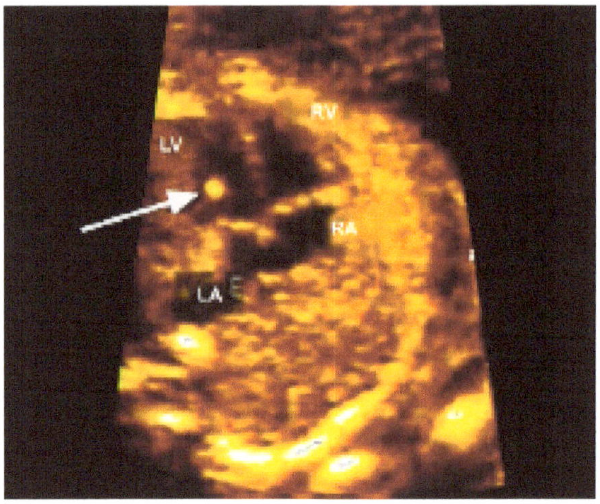

Fig. 30.20: Four-chamber view. Note the white arrow pointing the echogenic foci in the left ventricule. Echogenic foci are usually of no pathological significance and in more than 90% of cases the resolve by the third trimester or during pregnancy. However they are sometimes associated with cardiac defects and chromosomal abnormalities. For isolated hyperechogenic foci the risk for trisomy 21 may be 3 times the background maternal age and gestation related risk

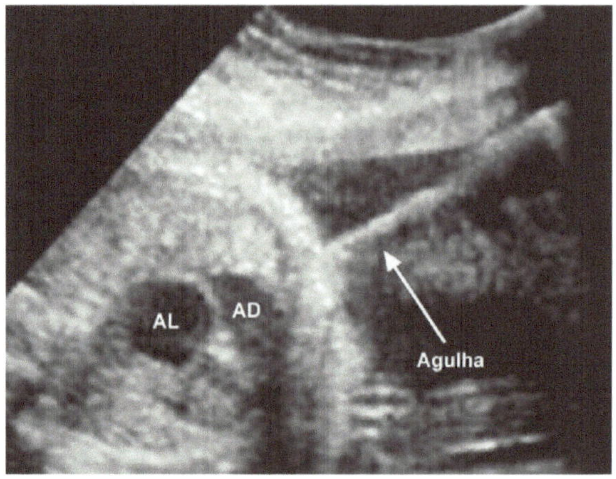

Fig. 30.22: Ultrasound image of fetal atrioseptostomy. The balloon is being inflated at the atrial level. Note the interatrial septum tense and bulging into the right atrium due to left atrial hypertension. AD=right atrium; AE=left atrium

flecainide. Transplacental therapy with first-line agents is usually effective in nonhydropic fetuses, but outcomes remain suboptimal, with fetal death in 10% of cases overall and a higher percentage of fetuses with hydrops.

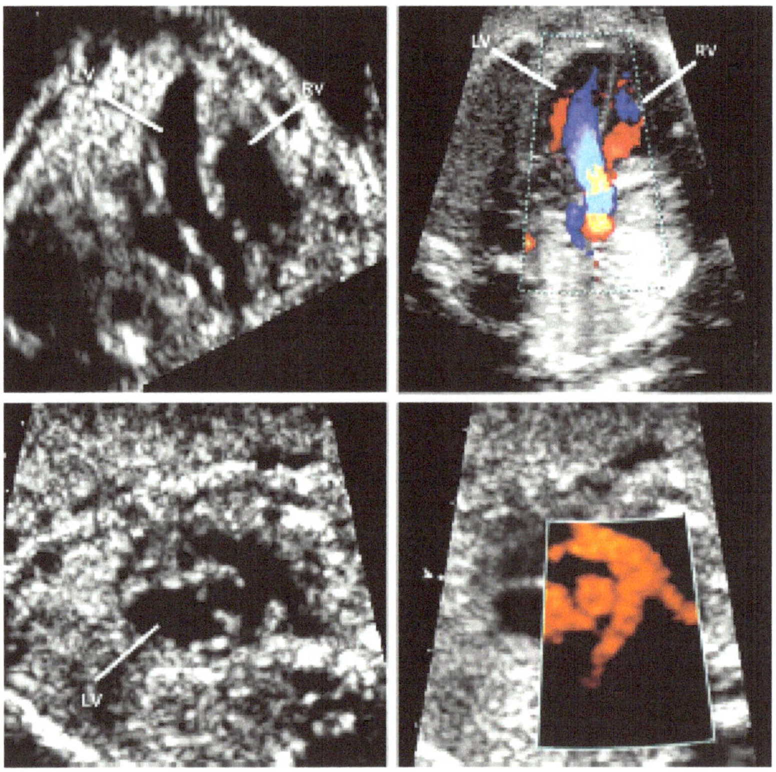

Fig. 30.21: Five-chamber view of the fetal heart with superimposed color-Doppler showing the aorta (blue) originating from the left ventricle (top). Short-axis view of the fetal heart with superimposed color-Doppler showing the pulmonary artery originating from the right ventricle (bottom)

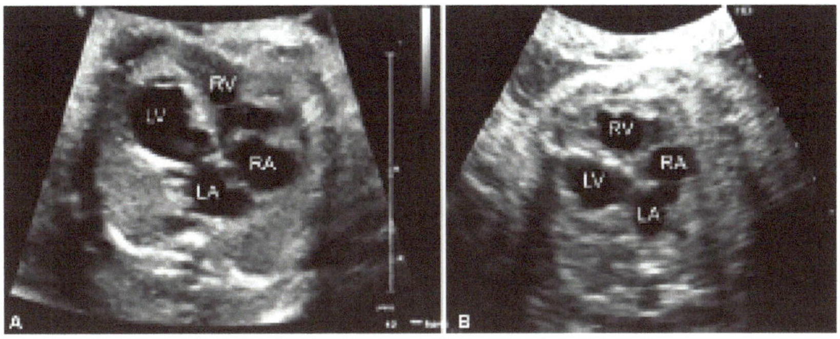

Fig. 30.23: Fetal echocardiogram fetus with critical aortic valve stenosis. (A) The left ventricle is dilated with signs of diffuse endocardial fibroelastosis, and we note a mild pericardial effusion. (B) After the valvuloplasty note a significant improvement in left ventricular dilatation has observed 3 days after the procedure. RA=right atrium; LA=left atrium; RV=right ventricle

The optimal therapeutic strategy for fetal supraventricular tachycardia has not been determined in a standardized trial, and practice varies. The indications for therapy may depend on fetal age and disease severity. When hydrops is present, pharmacological FCI may help as a bridge to delivery and postnatal treatment. In preterm fetuses, sustained tachycardia should probably be treated regardless of cardiac dysfunction or hydrops, because these sequelae can develop rapidly. For intermittent tachycardia, treatment is generally unnecessary, unless hydrops or

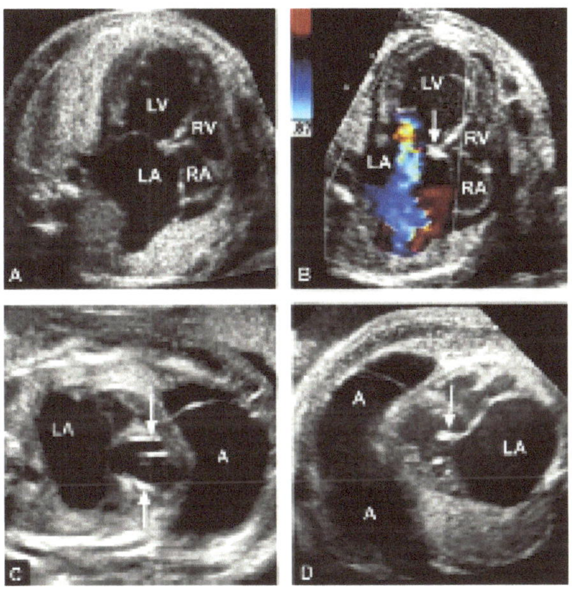

Fig. 30.24: Fetal echocardiogram images. (A) Fetal echocardiogram in a four-chamber view, demonstrating severe left atrial (LA) enlargement, with bowing of the atrial septum (*) into the right atrium (RA) and partial obstruction of the tricuspid valve. The right ventricle (RV) is compressed by a dilated left ventricle (LV). (B) Doppler color flow image in a four-chamber view from the same fetus demonstrating severe LA and LV enlargement, severe mitral regurgitation, and an anatomically abnormal mitral valve with an echogenic anterior leaflet (**arrow**). There is significant compression of the RA and RV (C and D) These oblique transverse images from a different fetus demonstrate severe LA enlargement, ascites (A), and moderate to severe LV endocardial fibroelastosis (**arrows**). In D, the anterior leaflet of the mitral valve (**arrow**) is bright and immobile

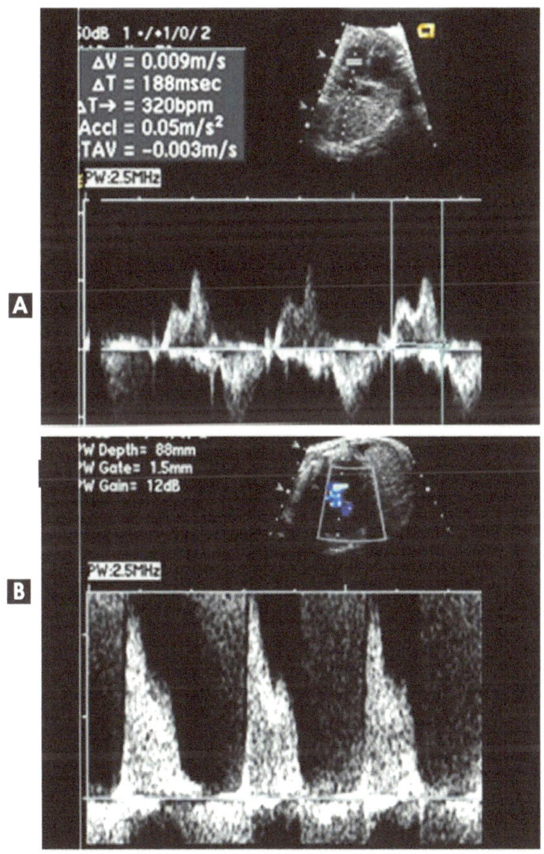

Fig.30.25 A and B: Mitral and tricuspid valve Doppler inflow patterns. (A) Normal mitral valve Doppler. (B) Abnormal Doppler with a partially fused mitral valve inflow pattern

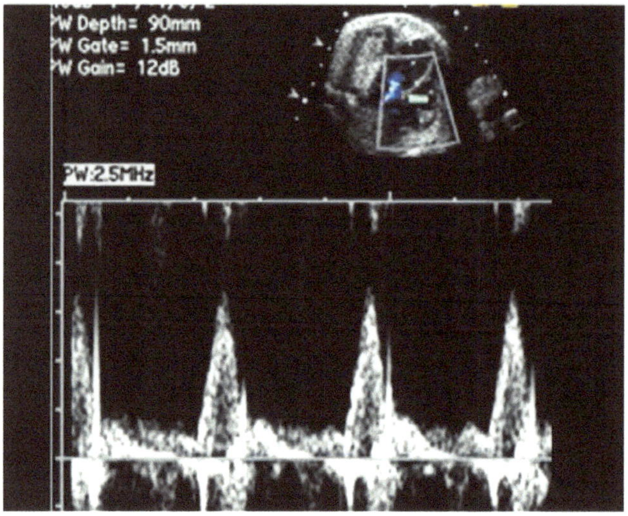

Fig. 30.25 C: Mitral and tricuspid valve Doppler inflow patternsó tricuspid valve monophasic Doppler pattern

cardiac dysfunction is evident. Transplacental delivery of some drugs is impaired in the setting of hydrops, and supraventricular tachycardia may be refractory for other reasons as well. In such circumstances, intravascular administration and/or oral agents with better placental uptake kinetics may be indicated. Direct administration, usually by percutaneous umbilical venous injection, introduces the risks of cordocentesis and is reserved for high-acuity refractory cases.

FETAL BRADYCARDIA

Sustained fetal bradycardia may be caused by sinus node dysfunction, long-QT syndrome, AV block, or fetal distress with acidosis. The most common fetal bradyarrhythmia and the primary indication for FCI is high-grade AV block. The potential consequences of fetal AV block are cardiomyopathy and hydrops. AV block in the fetus generally occurs in association with either maternal autoimmune disease, malformation syndromes such as heterotaxy, or L-loop transposition of the great arteries.

Autoimmune fetal AV block can be treated with maternal administration of dexamethasone and/or sympathomimetic agents. Several recent multicenter studies found that transplacental dexamethasone did not reverse high-grade block, although it may have prevented the progression of first-degree block to second- or third-degree block, and it was associated with a higher risk of

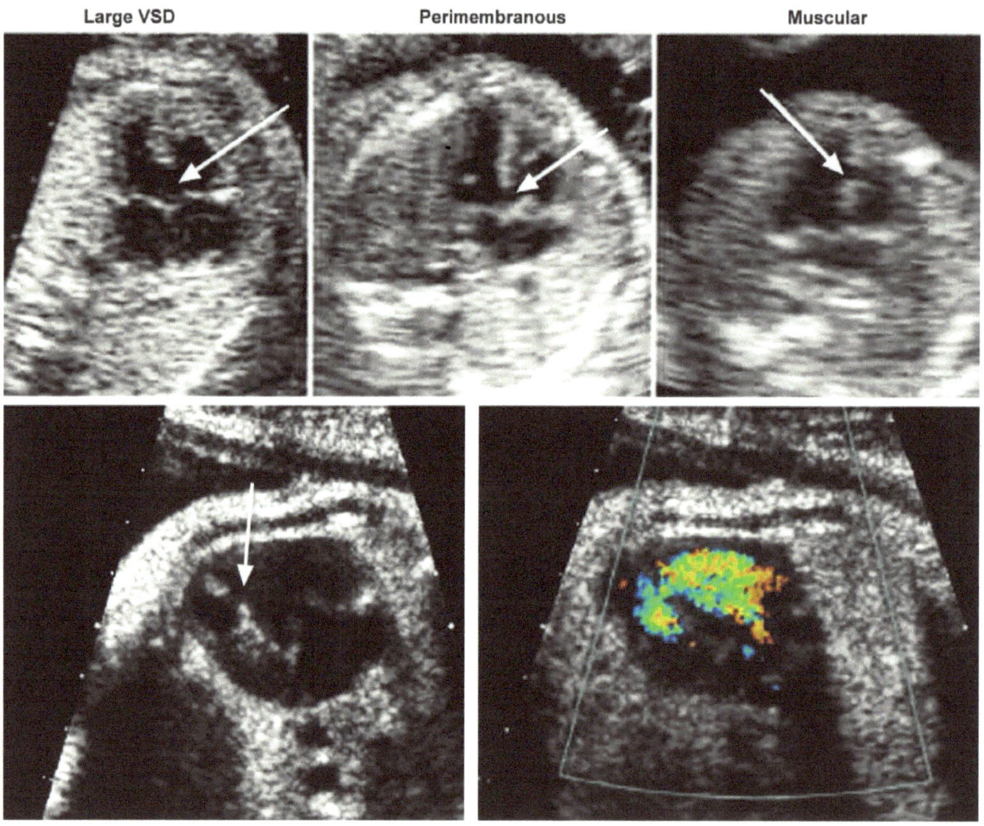

Fig. 30.26: Foetal echocardiogram showing different types of VSD

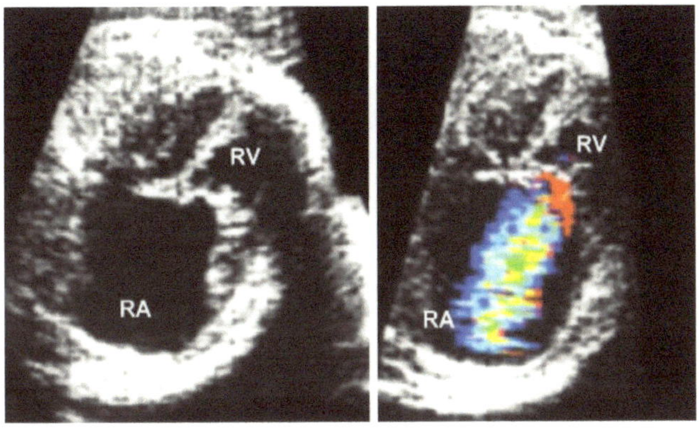

Fig. 30.27: Foetal echocardiogram showing tricuspid valve dysplasia with severe tricuspid insufficiency and cardiomegaly. Retrograde flow from the right ventricle (RV) to the right atrium (RA) is seen in blue and turbulence is coded by green pixels

premature birth and growth restriction. Other studies reported that dexamethasone, typically in association with β-adrenergic agonists when significant bradycardia was present, improved the overall prognosis in fetuses with autoimmune AV block. Sympathomimetic agents may increase the heart rate in fetuses with bradycardia due to AV block or sinus node dysfunction, but they do not restore AV synchrony. It is unclear whether in utero β-adrenergic stimulation improves outcome, because the postnatal management of AV block associated with complex congenital heart disease is challenging under any circumstances.

FETAL HYDROPS DUE TO OTHER CARDIAC CAUSES

Transplacental treatment with digoxin has also been described for fetal hydrops resulting from other conditions, including structural anomalies (e.g. Ebstein's anomaly, absent pulmonary valve syndrome), right heart dysfunction

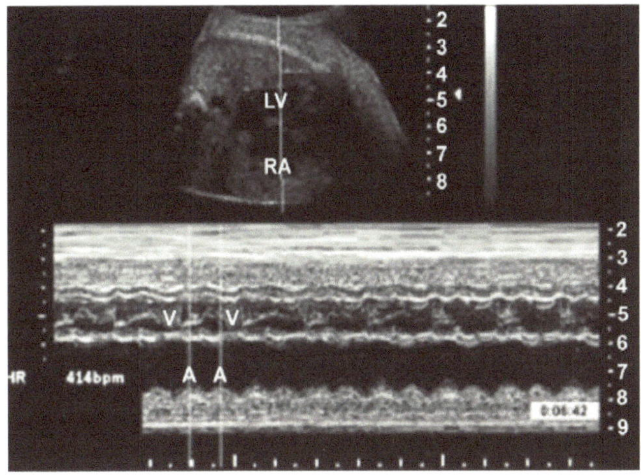

Fig. 30.29 : M-mode tracing using a four-chamber view to demonstrate atrial (A) and ventricular (V) wall motions. The M-mode is directed simultaneously through the left ventricle (LV) and right atrium (RA). There is atrial flutter with an atrial rate of 414 beats/min (bpm), functional 2:1 atrioventricular block, and a regular ventricular rate of 207 bpm

from left heart disease, premature closure of the ductus arteriosus, intrauterine myocardial infarction, cardiac tumor, cardiomyopathy, and others. These are uncommon conditions, with published reports limited to individual cases, so the efficacy of digoxin in their management is unknown.

Maternal Hyperoxia

Maternal hyperoxia, which affects fetal vascular function and hemodynamics, has been used to assess placental function and treat intrauterine growth retardation, but its benefits have not been established. Recently, Szwast et al. reported using maternal hyperoxia to assess pulmonary vasoreactivity in fetuses with hypoplastic left heart

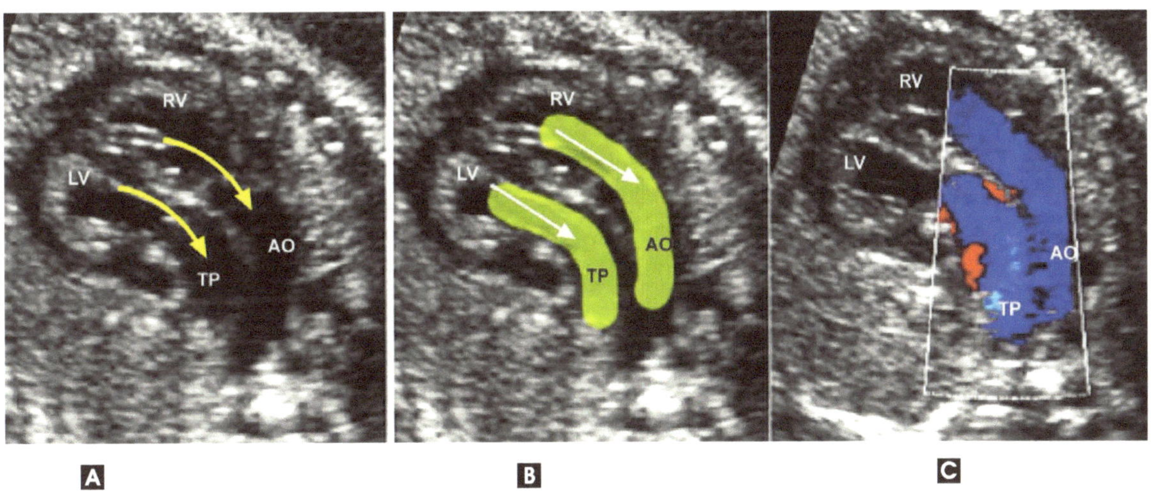

Fig. 30.28: (A to C) Fetal echocardiogram showing transposition of the great arteries demonstrating the abnormal connection of the right ventricle (RV) with the aorta (AO) and the left ventricle (LV) with the pulmonary trunk (TP). Both great arteries show a parallel course associated with tricuspid atresia

Table 30.1: Pharmacological interventions in fetal arrhythmias

Condition and drug	Dose range	Therapeutic level and effect	Adverse effects
Atrial flutter			
Digoxin	LD 1,200 µg per 24 h IV in 3 divided doses; MD 375–750 µg daily PO in two equal daily doses	0.7–2.0 ng/mL Mild nausea, fatigue and sinus bradycardia, first-degree atrioventricular block, rare noctumal Wenchebach atrioventricular block	Severe nausea and/or vomiting, severe sinus bradycardia or atrioventricular block, maternal and fetal proarrhythmia
Sotalol	160–480 mg daily in two equal daily doses or every 8 h PO	NA Improved survival, bradycardia, first-degree atrioventricular block, P and QRS widening, QT prolongation	Nausea and/or vomiting, dizziness, fatigue, bundle branch block, maternal and/or fetal proarrhythmia
*Supraventricular tachycardia**			
Flecainide‡	100–300 mg daily in equal doses given every 8 h PO	0.2–1.0 µg/mL Mild IVCD, headache, QT prolongation	Visual and central nervous system symptoms, bundle branch block, QT prolongation, fetal or neonatal proarrhythmia
Amiodarone‡	LD 1,800–2,400 mg daily in equal doses given every 6 h for 48 h; MD 200–600 mg daily PO	0.7–2.8 µg/mL Maternal and/or fetal sinus bradycardia, cardia, first-degree atrioventricular block, P and QRS widening, QT prolongation	Nausea and/or vomiting, maternal and/or fetal thyroid dysfunction, photosensitivity rash, thrombocytopenia, bundle branch block, proarrhythmia, torsades de pointes in fetuses with long QT syndrome
Procainamide‡	LD 500–600 mg over 20 min IV; MD 2–6 mg/min IV initially 1,250 mg, followed in 1 h by 750 mg, then 250–1,000 mg every 3–6 h PO	4–10 µg/mL Uterine irritability, QT prolongation	Nausea and/or vomiting, hypotension, proarrhythmia, blood dyscrasias

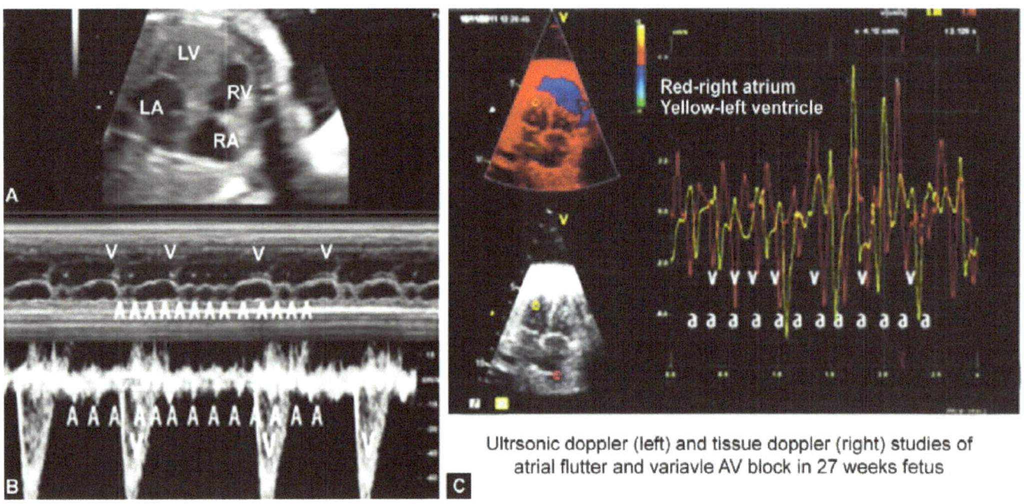

Fig. 30.30: Assessment of a 27-week fetus with atrial flutter and variable A-V conduction. (A) M-mode tracings demonstrate the timing of atrial A and ventricular V contractions. (B) Simultaneous superior vena cava and ascending aortic pulsed Doppler spectra show timing of a wave reversal in atrial systole in the superior vena cava A and forward flow in the aorta during ventricular systole V.(C) Tissue color-Doppler tracings also demonstrate the temporal relationship between atrial A and ventricular V contractions by changes in myocardial velocities. The atrial rate (A-atrial contraction or systolic flow) is roughly 300 bpm whereas the ventricular rates (V-ventricular contraction or systolic flow) range from 100ñ200 bpm. A-atrial

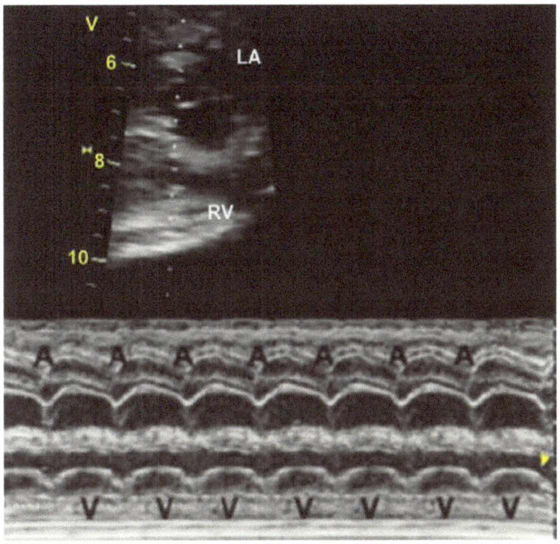

Fig. 30.31: SVT with a heart rate of 240 bpm. M-mode tracing through the right atrium (bottom) and the right ventricle (top). There is 1:1 AV-conduction with a short AV-interval

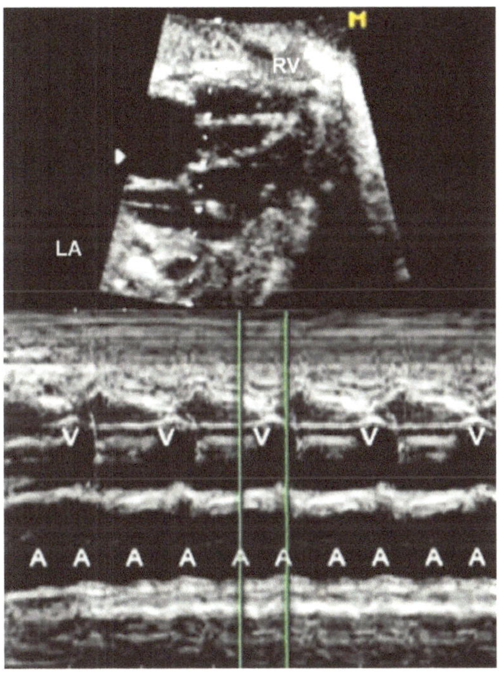

Fig. 30.32: Atrial flutter. Simultaneous M-mode tracing to record the RV and LA freewall movements during the cardiac cycles. The atrial rate is very fast and regular at 462 bpm while the ventricular rate is 231 bpm suggesting 2:1 AV conduction

syndrome (HLHS) and found diminution of the normal pulmonary arterial flow response to predict fetuses at high risk for critical atrial septal restriction after birth. Although not therapeutic, maternal hyperoxia in this application is a form of pharmacological transplacental FCI that may have implications for postnatal intervention and other methods of prenatal intervention.

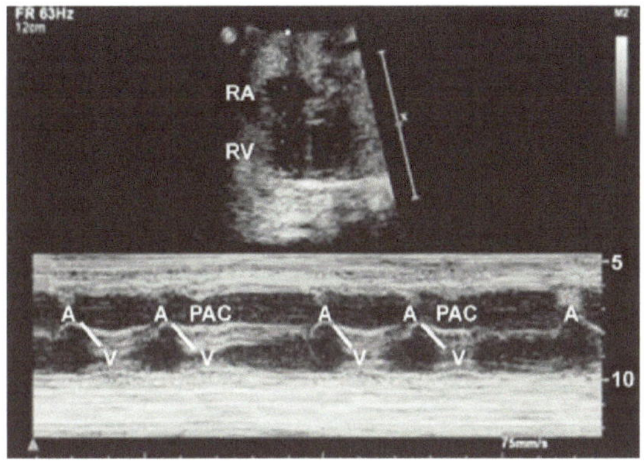

Fig. 30.33: Blocked PAC. M-Mode tracing from a four-chamber view with the transducer beam through the RA and the RV. There are blocked PAC's in a trigeminy pattern. Only the normal atrial contractions (A) are followed by a ventricular contraction (V)

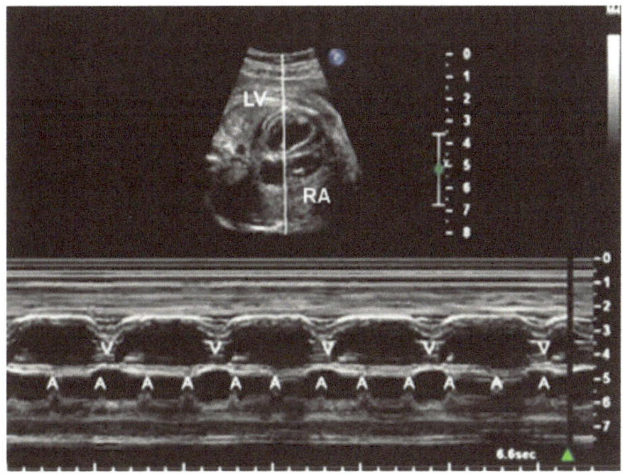

Fig. 30.34: Complete heart block. M-Mode tracing from a four chamber view with the transducer beam through the RA and the LV. There are regular atrial contractions (A) with a normal heart rate of 125 bpm and independent ventricular contractions (V) with a heart rate of 50 bpm

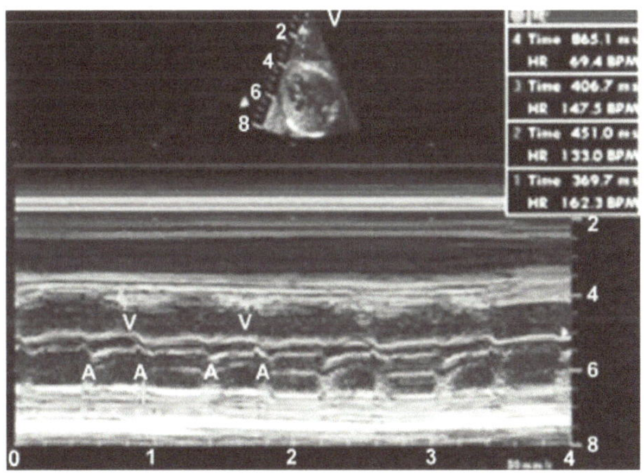

Fig. 30.35: M-mode echocardiography at 20 weeks showing significant fetal bradycardia (VñV: 67 beats/min) related to atrial bigeminy. There is atrial beat-to-beat variation with the premature atrial beats (AñA interval: 370 ms) being blocked and the normal atrial impulses (450 ms) being conducted. A repeat echocardiogram showed normal cardiac rhythm 1 week later

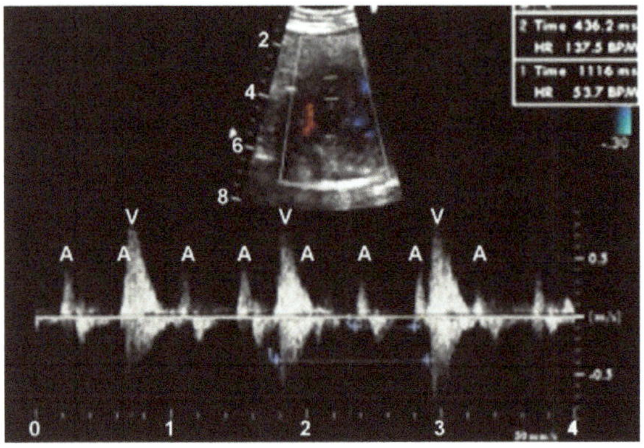

Fig. 30.36: Simultaneous Doppler of the aorta and superior vena cava showing complete atrioventricular block. The atrial (A-A) rate was 138 beats/min (bpm) and the ventricular (V-V) rate was 54 bpm, with complete atrioventricular dissociation

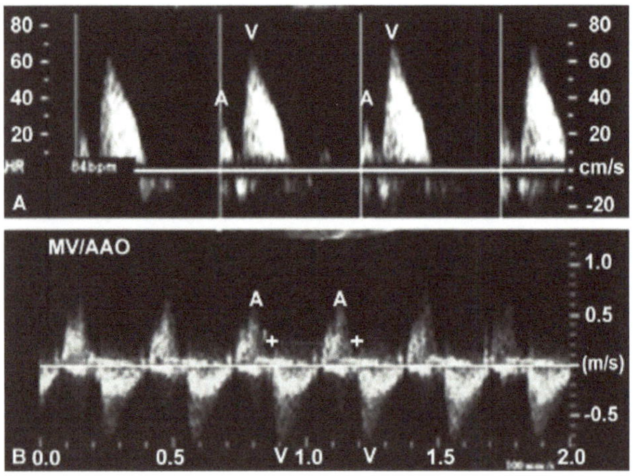

Fig. 30.37: Pulsed Doppler flow modalities. (A) Simultaneous ascending aorta (V) and superior vena cava (A). Doppler flow recording at 20 weeks of gestation showing sinus bradycardia with normal 1:1 atrioventricular conduction. (B) Simultaneous inflow/outflow Doppler of a 19-week fetus with long ventriculo-atrial tachycardia of 190 beats/min due to fetal thyrotoxicosis. The mother had a medical history of Graves' disease for which she had been treated with propylthiouracil and radioactive iodine

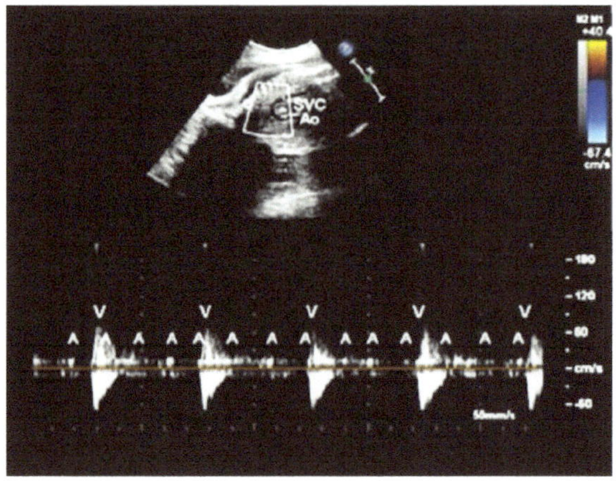

Fig. 30.38: Simultaneous pulse wave Doppler of the aorta and vena cava superior of a fetus with complete heart block showing backflow following atrial contractions (A) in the superior vena cava with an atrial rate of 140/min (A) and in the same direction aortic outflow following ventricular contractions (V) which are independent with a regular rate of 60/min

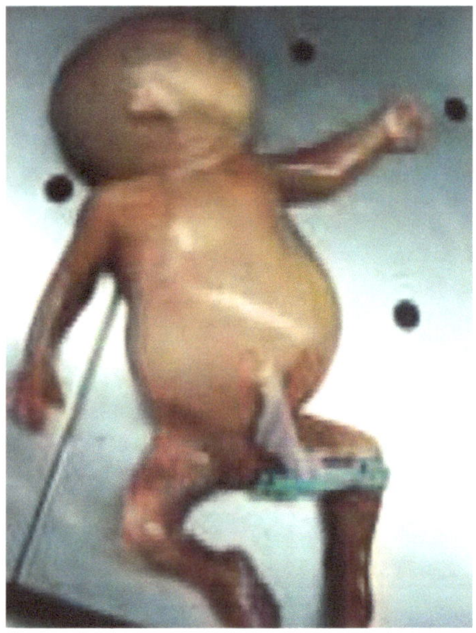

Fig.30.39: A 22 weeks of gestation fetus with generalized hydropic aspect. Subcutaneous edema and abdominal distention secondary to ascites

Open Fetal Cardiac Intervention

For the present review, 'open FCI' denotes any intervention in which the uterus is opened surgically or accessed through a surgical trochar $\geq$3 mm in diameter, which includes most fetoscopic techniques. This delineation is based on reports that preterm labor occurs in 80% of fetal surgical procedures in which a single 10F (3.3 mm) port is used and almost universally with larger ports or incisions

Experimental Fetal Cardiac Surgery

Research on fetal cardiac surgery has been performed for more than 25 years. The major focus of investigation has been the pathophysiology of extracorporeal circulatory bypass, which is likely to be necessary for fetal cardiac surgery. In early studies, it was shown that a 1–1.5 kg lamb fetus could be placed on and separated from cardiac bypass reproducibly, but that post-bypass fetal demise was imminent. Further work in sheep, goats, and primates has furthered our knowledge of the pathophysiology of fetal cardiac bypass and the feasibility of fetal cardiac surgery. Survival to term can now be achieved in a high percentage of cases.

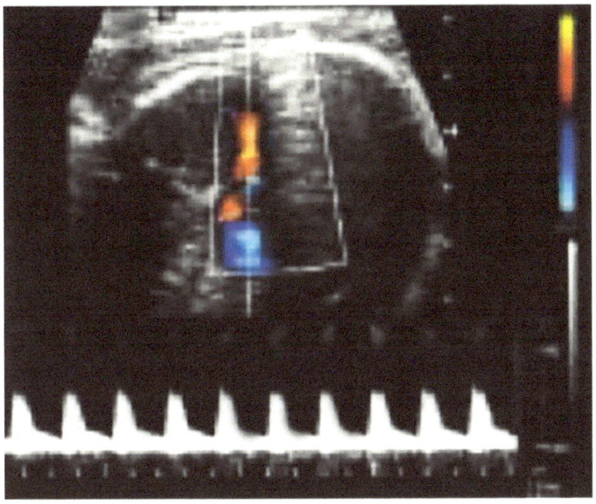

Fig. 30.40: Hydrops. During diagnostic evaluation a meticulous ultrasound must be performed in order to detect fetal or placental malformations and to exclude fetal anemia by Doppler study of the peak systolic velocity of the middle cerebral artery

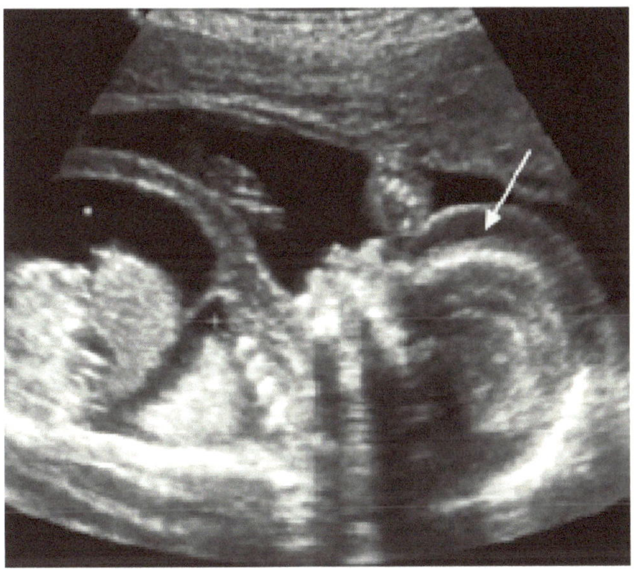

Fig. 30.41: Hydrops. Severe ascites (*), pleural effusion (+) subcutaneous edema (**white arrow**)

Cardiovascular and Placental Response to Extracorporeal Circulation

The most significant response to fetal bypass when the placenta is incorporated as the oxygenator is severe placental dysfunction characterized by increased vascular resistance, reduced blood flow, and consequent impairment in fetal gas exchange, with fetal acidosis rapidly ensuing during and after bypass. The pathophysiology of post-bypass placental dysfunction is multifactorial and includes bypass-induced production of prostanoids, endothelial dysfunction, leukocyte and complement activation, and other endogenous vasoactive and inflammatory pathways. Fetal cardiac bypass and surgery may also lead to changes

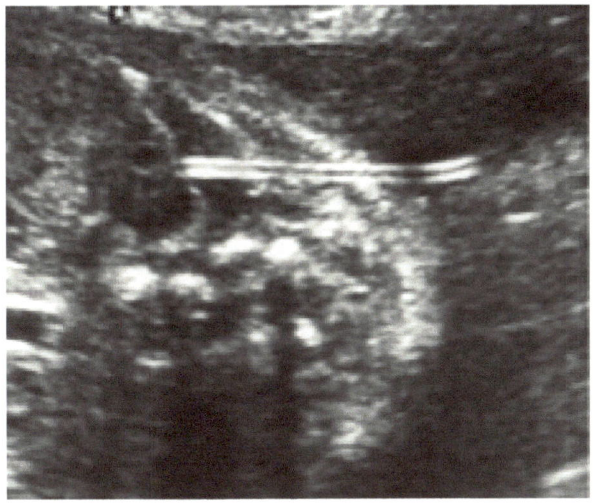

Fig. 30.42: Placement of a catheter in one of the cysts connecting with the amniotic cavity

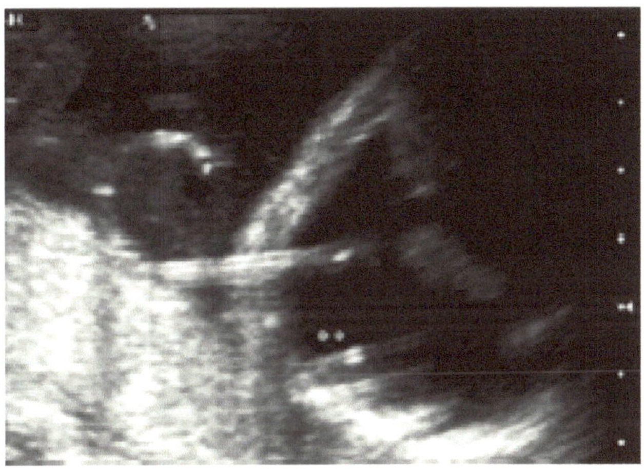

Fig. 30.43: Left pleural effusion. Pleuroamniotic shunting (pig tail). One of the ends is within the amniotic cavity (*) the other (**) in the pleural cavity. It allows to drain the effusion, decompress the lung and prevent pulmonary hypoplasia

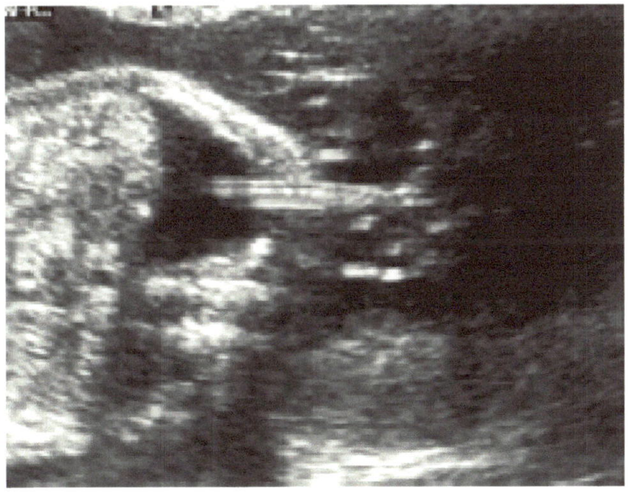

Fig. 30.44 A: Thoracoamniotic shunt.

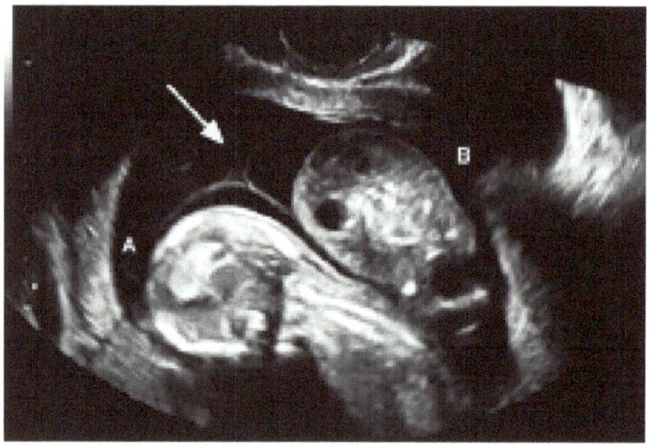

Fig.30.44 B: Two-dimensional cross section at 12 postmenstrual weeks showing monochorionic-diamniotic twins. The arrow points to the dividing membranes. Note the pump twin A, on the left and the grossly abnormal acardiac twin B, on the right with absence of the head and heart

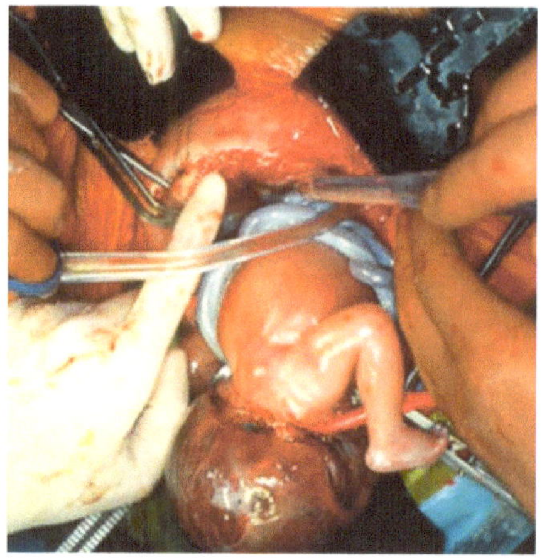

Fig.30.44 C: The first prenatal resection of SCT for fetal hydrops was performed, and despite successful resection of the mass and resolution of fetal hydrops, fetus could not survive

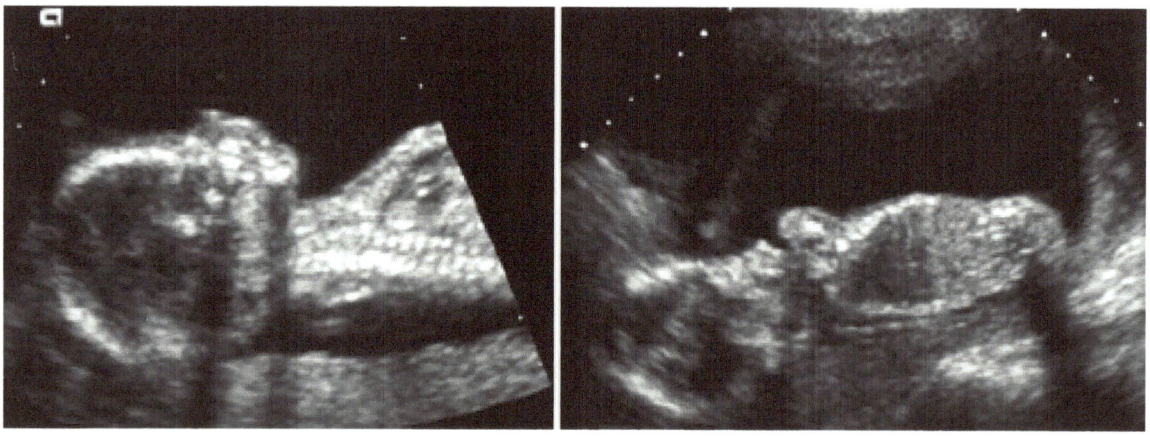

Fig. 30.45: Amniotic fluid volume alters imaging. The large baby on the left (recipient) has increased amniotic fluid, so a clear profile and clear imaging are obtained. The donor, on the right, is tightly wrapped in his membrane and imaging is very indistinct

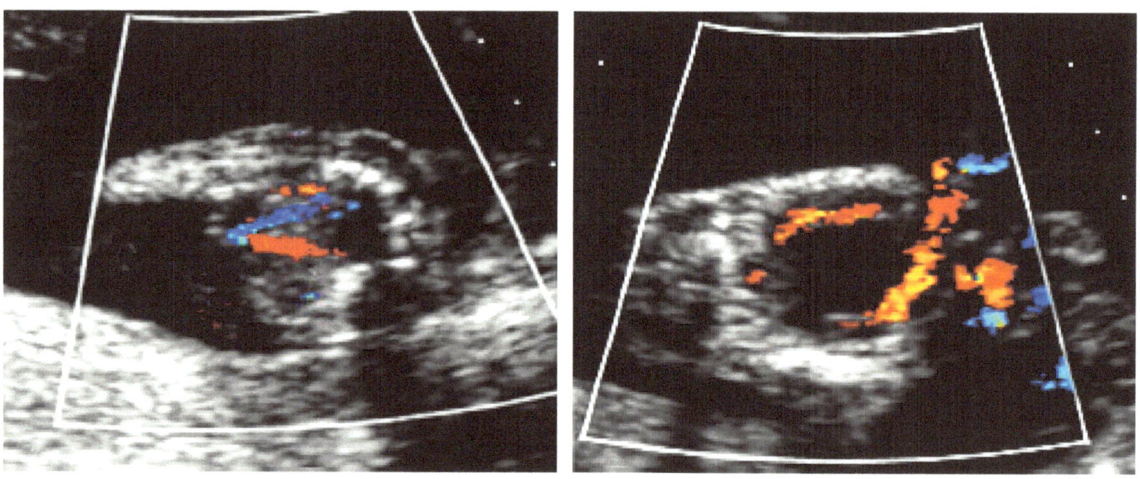

Fig. 30.46: The donor on the left has no visible bladder (the colored lines represent umbilical arteries, one on each side of the bladder, which is empty). The recipient on the right has a continuously over-filled bladder (the black circle in between the two arteries)

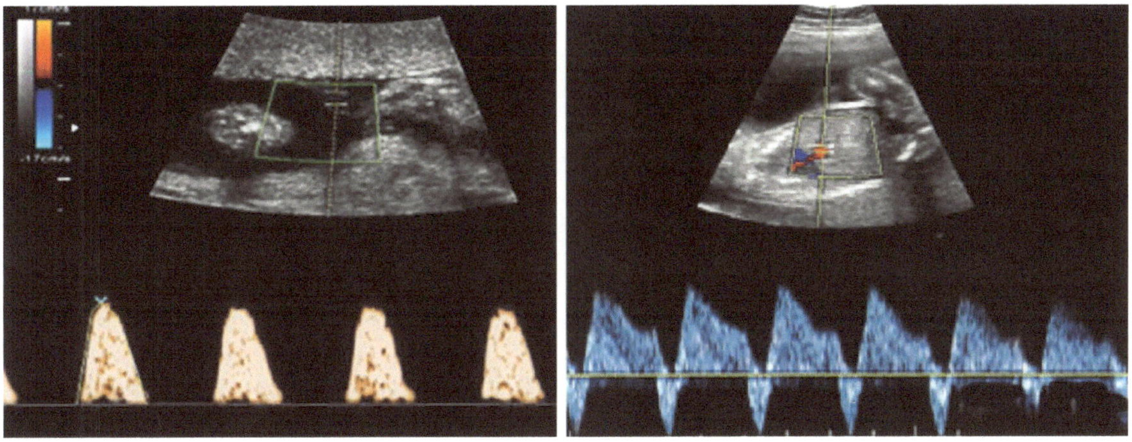

Fig. 30.47: Each baby has circulatory problems as TTTS progresses. On the left, the donor has severe placental resistance and very low blood flow to the placenta. On the right, the recipient is struggling with heart failure, with blood running backward during the cardiac cycle

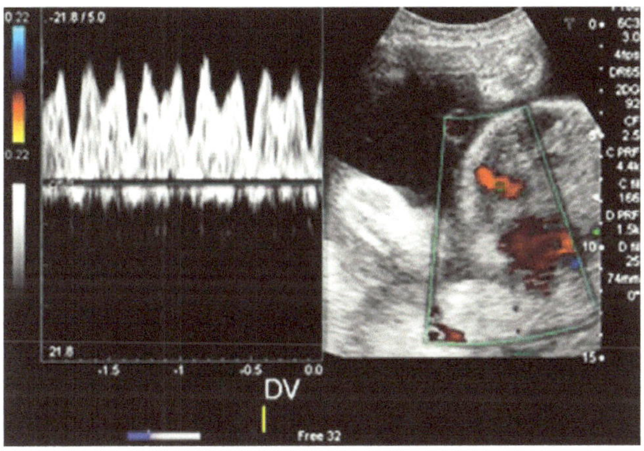

Fig. 30.48: Twin-twin transfusion syndrome. The ductus venosus flow in the recipient twin is still within acceptable limits, though the atrial contraction ëaí wave is almost reaching the baseline. Such a flow pattern needs to be monitored closely

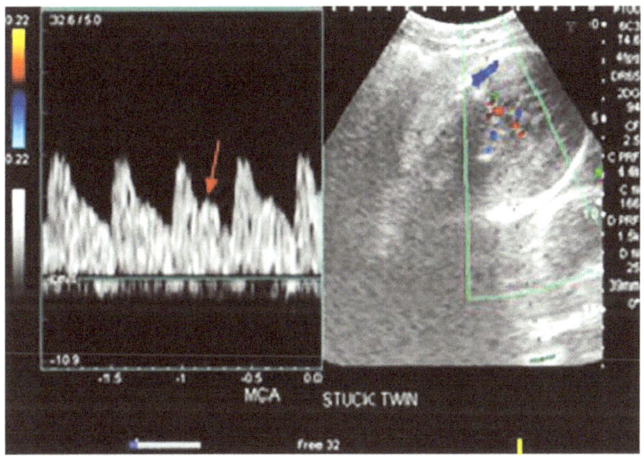

Fig. 30.50: Twin-twin transfusion syndrome. Middle cerebral artery Doppler of the donor (stuck) twin shows high diastolic flow (arrow), suggesting a brain-favoring effect and fetal adaptation to hypoxemia

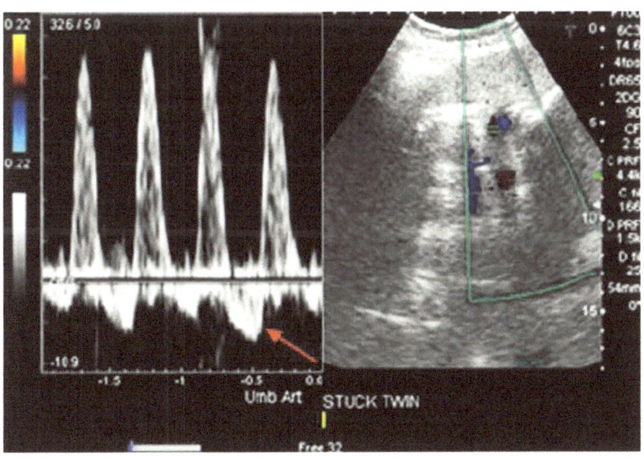

Fig. 30.49: Twin-twin transfusion syndrome. Umbilical artery Doppler of the donor (stuck) twin shows diastolic reversal (arrow). This is a predictor of poor outcome

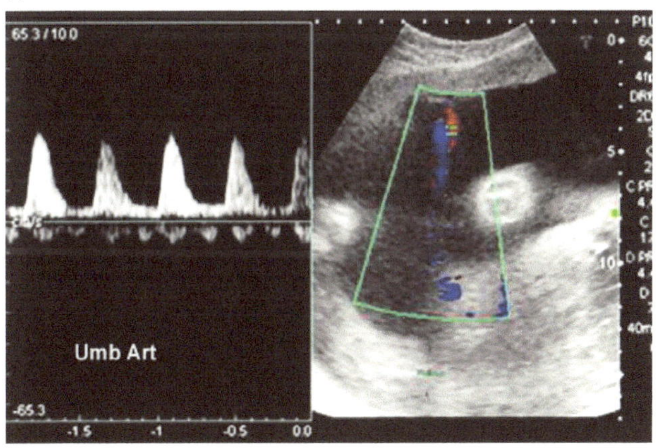

Fig. 30.51: Twin-twin transfusion syndrome. Umbilical artery Doppler in the recipient twin. The flow pattern is unidirectional, but the diastolic flow is very low. This is an indicator of a poor prognosis

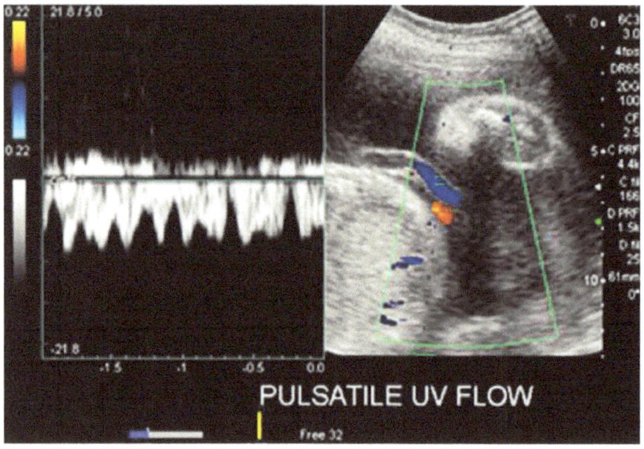

Fig. 30.52: Twin-twin transfusion syndrome. Pulsatile umbilical venous flow in the recipient twin suggests a critically ill fetus. Normal umbilical venous flow is continuous and nonpulsatile, with phasic/respiratory variations at times

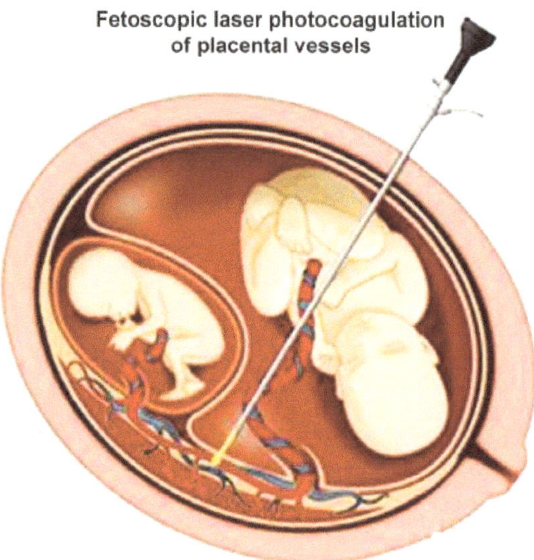

Fig. 30.53: Illustration shows placental vessels supply in twin to twin transfusion syndrome and applicabitity of radiofrequency ablation in coagulation of blood supply to the weeker fetus in order to save the other fetus.

on the maternal side of the placenta, with reduction in uterine arterial flow and consequent impairment of fetoplacental gas exchange.

Fetal Cardiac Function and the Fetal Stress Response

Fetal cardiac bypass and surgery induce a significant stress response that has important effects on fetal hemodynamics independent of the placental dysfunction discussed above. The stress response stimulates a rise in endogenous fetal catecholamines, which increases total vascular resistance and cardiac afterload. Because the contractile apparatus of the fetal myocardium is immature, the heart tolerates increased afterload poorly. In ovine fetal bypass studies, survival to term was first achieved with spinal anesthesia to blunt the stress response and indomethacin to block prostaglandin synthesis. More recently, it was shown that

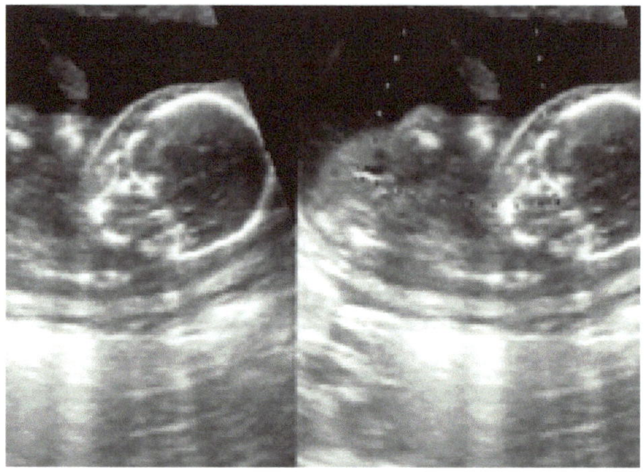

Fig. 30.54: Absent blood flow in the umbilical cord of the second twin after radiofrequency cord ablation

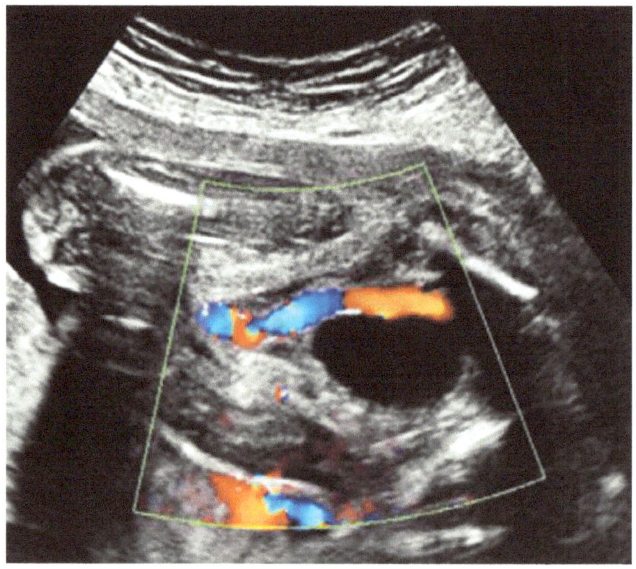

Fig. 30.55: Color-Doppler image of single umbilical artery around the fetal bladder.

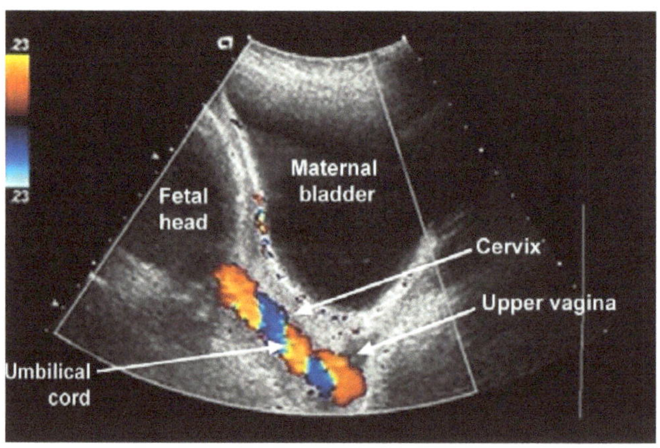

Fig. 30.56: Fetal color-Doppler echocardiography shows umbilical-cord prolapse at 29 weeksí gestation

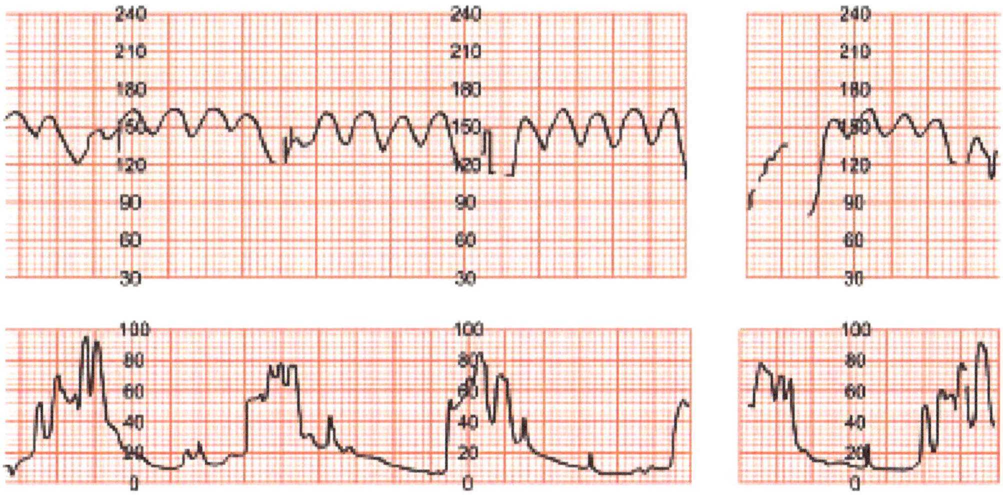

Fig. 30.57: Intrapartum cardiotocograph tracing (term gestation) in a patient with placental abruption revealing a sinusoidal fetal heart rate pattern just before delivery

Table 30.2: Congenital cardiovascular anomalies potentially amenable to FCI

Indication for intervention and condition	Actual or possible FCI
MR indicates mitral regurgitation	
Risk of fetal or early neonatal death	
Fetal tachycardia with hydrops	Maternal antiarrhythmic pharmacotherapy
Structural anomalies causing hydrops	Maternal digoxin
Congenital heart block	Pacemaker; maternal antiarrhythmic and/or b-adrenergic pharmacotherapy
Severe Ebstein malformation	Tricuspid valve repair; tricuspid valve occlusion
Severe congenital MR with AS and intact atrial septum	Balloon or surgical aortic valvuloplasty; creation of atrial septal defect
HLHS with intact atrial septum	Creation of atrial septal defect
Obstructed, totally anomalous pulmonary venous return	Stenting of obstructed vertical vein/ductus venosus; surgical repair
Risk of primary anomaly evolving into more severe condition	
Fetal AS with evolving HLHS	Balloon or surgical aortic valvuloplasty; resection of endocardial fibroelastosis
PA/IVS with evolving hypoplastic right heart	Percutaneous or open pulmonary valve perforation and dilation
Premature closure of ductus arteriosus with evolving pulmonary hypertension	Ductal stenting
Absent pulmonary valve syndrome with evolving bronchomalacia	Pulmonary arterioplasty and/or valvuloplasty

fetal bypass leads to cardiac injury, reflected in troponin elevation and increased plasma natriuretic peptides. Calcium-handling properties of the fetal myocardium differ from the more mature state, and recent studies have started to define strategies for myocardial protection during fetal open heart surgery.

Technical Considerations for Fetal Cardiac Surgery

In experimental fetal cardiac bypass, surgical exposure, intervention, and cardiac bypass have proven technically feasible. Nevertheless, successful fetal bypass requires consideration of several technical adaptations.

Placental function during fetal bypass is altered by inclusion or exclusion of the placenta in the bypass circuit. Placental inclusion obviates the need for an extracorporeal oxygenator, which decreases contact activation of inflammatory and vasoactive mediators. On the other hand, inclusion of the high-capacitance, low-resistance placenta in the circuit requires high flow rates, which can be limited by cannula size. Placental perfusion during bypass also

A

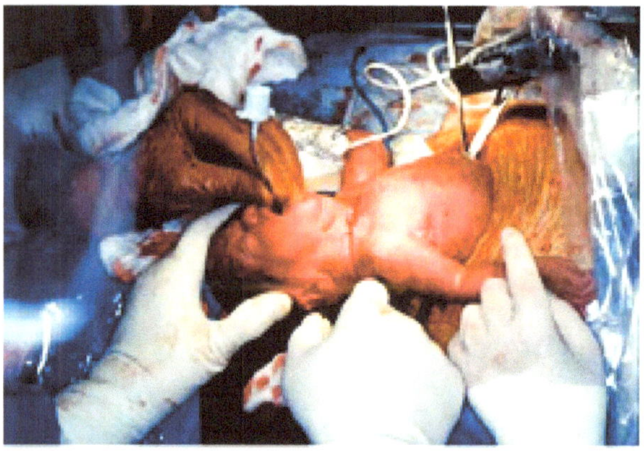

B

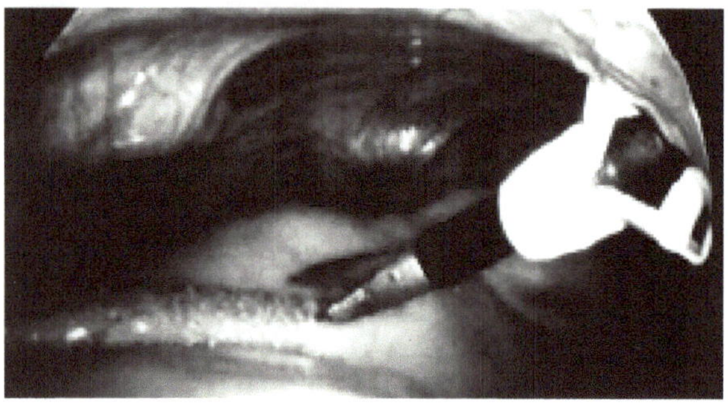

Fig. 30.58: (A and B) Fetus undergoing ex-utero intrapartum treatment

causes placental endothelial damage and dysfunction, although these effects may be mitigated when bypass is performed with pulsatile rather than continuous flow, possibly owing to preserved nitric oxide production during the former.

The systemic effects of postnatal cardiopulmonary bypass are known to result in part from blood contact with artificial surfaces in the bypass circuit. Thus, miniaturization of the fetal bypass circuit has been a technical priority. For example, in fetuses undergoing cardiac bypass with a modified bypass circuit that uses an in-line axial flow pump and no maternal blood prime, placental function was preserved relative to control fetuses in which a conventional circuit was used. Despite these difficulties, models of congenital heart disease created in-utero confirm the feasibility of operating on the heart of the lamb fetus with survival to full term.

Fetoscopic and Adjunctive Forms of Closed FCI

Fetoscopic access has been investigated as an approach to FCI and fetal monitoring during cardiac and noncardiac interventions. Although the relative risks of percutaneous and fetoscopic access have not been assessed, port-access uterine entry for fetoscopic FCI may carry a higher risk of premature labor than percutaneous access.

Open FCI in Humans

The first reported open FCI procedure in a human fetus was pacemaker placement for complete AV block. Subsequently, animal models were developed to evaluate pacing for fetal AV block, but this has not become a clinically viable treatment strategy, isolated human cases not withstanding. Human FCI aided by fetoscopy and cardioscopy has also been reported, with technical success and fetal survival in several cases. We are aware of 1 open heart surgery performed in a third-trimester human fetus with tricuspid valve dysplasia, severe tricuspid regurgitation, and hydrops by Dr Frank Hanley in 2003 (personal communication, June 6, 2009). Cardiopulmonary bypass was initiated and the tricuspid valve repaired successfully, but separation from bypass was prevented by anatomic pulmonary atresia (thought to be functional atresia before surgery), and the fetus died.

Closed Fetal Cardiac Intervention

In the present review, 'closed FCI' indicates mechanical interventions in which the uterus is not opened or accessed with a port $\geq$3 mm in diameter . In practice, closed FCI consists primarily of percutaneous interventions in which an 18- to 19-gauge needle is used to gain uterine and fetal access. The first reported case of closed FCI was a balloon aortic valvuloplasty performed in 1989. Since then, FCI has been reported in human fetuses with aortic stenosis (AS), HLHS with atrial septal restriction, pulmonary atresia or stenosis, and AV block. In 2000, a program for FCI,was started, initially to treat fetal AS with evolving HLHS, then expanding to include HLHS with an intact or highly restrictive atrial septum, pulmonary atresia with an intact ventricular septum (PA/IVS) and evolving hypoplastic right heart syndrome, and structural anomalies causing hydrops.

Typically, FCI is performed,using a percutaneous ultrasound-guided approach with maternal and fetal anesthesia; in a minority of cases, laparotomy without hysterotomy is used to facilitate fetal imaging or access. All of the procedures we perform consist of opening an atretic or restrictive valve or septum, and instrumentation is limited and simple, with an access cannula, a guidewire,

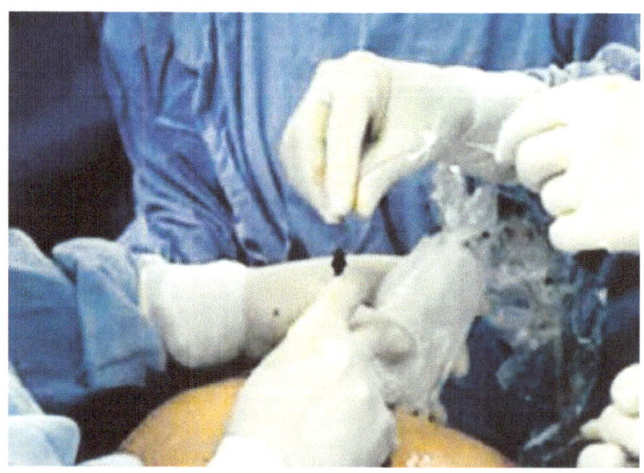

Fig. 30.59: Experts performing aortic valvoplasty with premounted balloon in the needle that is positioned below the aortic valve with the help of maternal transabdominal ultrasound monitoring

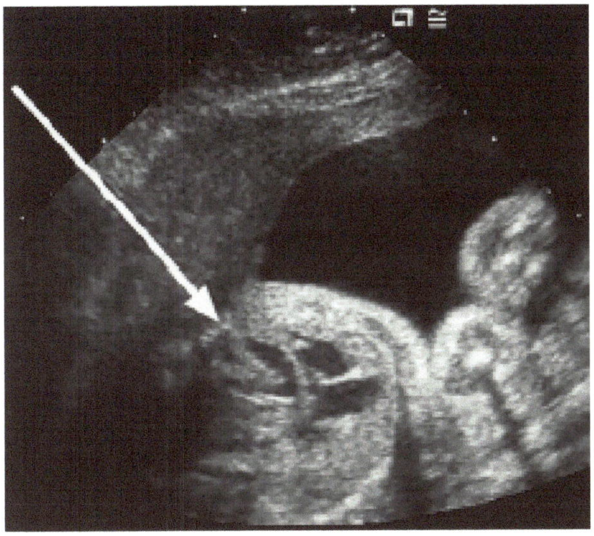

Fig. 30.60: Fetal aortic stenosis, intraoperative image illustrating the needle trajectory that will afford access to the left ventricle and aortic valve. The initial needle course must be precise, as very little manipulation is possible once the device has punctured the left ventricle

an angioplasty balloon and/or stent, and sometimes an additional needle to enter the heart or perforate an atretic valve or septum. With the exception of an 18-gauge curved-tip cannula that was developed specifically for FCI.

FETAL AORTIC VALVULOPLASTY

The most common closed FCI procedure is aortic valvuloplasty, and the primary indication for fetal aortic valvuloplasty is to alter the in utero natural history of midgestation fetal AS with evolving HLHS. Some patients with HLHS are diagnosed during the second trimester with valvar AS and a normal-sized or dilated left ventricle (LV) and evolve to HLHS over the course of gestation. In other fetuses diagnosed with AS in midgestation, left heart growth and function will remain sufficient for a biventricular outcome. Several abnormal physiological features are associated with progression to HLHS. Retrograde flow in the transverse aortic arch, severe LV dysfunction, monophasic and short mitral valve inflow, and left-to-right flow across the foramen ovale. Thus, one can reliably predict which midgestation fetuses with AS will evolve to HLHS. The potential benefit of FCI for

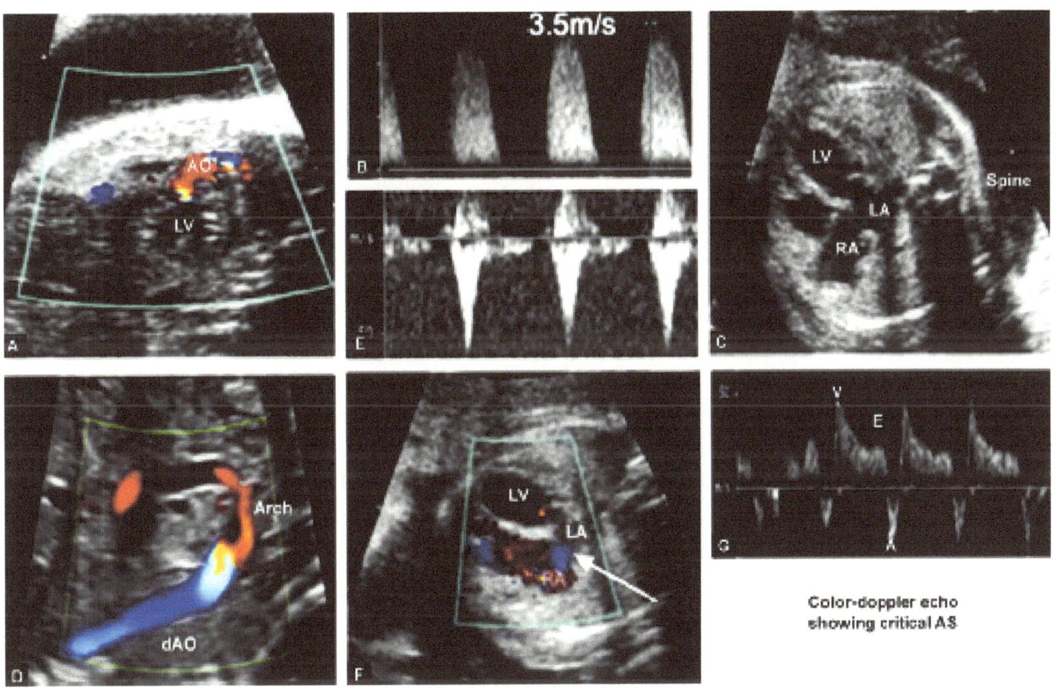

Fig. 30.61: Critical AS encountered in a mid trimester fetus. (A) Early in gestation the left ventricle was hypertrophied and there was turbulent forward flow by color-Doppler through the aortic valve. (B) CW Doppler interrogation suggested the peak aortic valve was 30–35 mmHg. As the obstruction worsened. (C) The LV became dilated with reduced systolic function and (D) eventually retrograde flow was observed through the distal arch. (E) In addition to systolic dysfunction, a uniphasic rather than biphasic Doppler inflow pattern was observed suggesting reduced LV diastolic function, a feature associated with progressive LV hypoplasia. (F) Increased LV filling pressure resulted in left to right atrial level shunting (arrow). (G) As a consequence of increased left atrial pressure, there was reversal of flow during atrial systole in the pulmonary veins (A=flow in atrial systole; V=flow in ventricular systole; E=flow through the pulmonary veins in early ventricular diastole; LV=left ventricle; RA=right atrium; LA=left atrium; Ao=aorta; dAo=descending aorta)

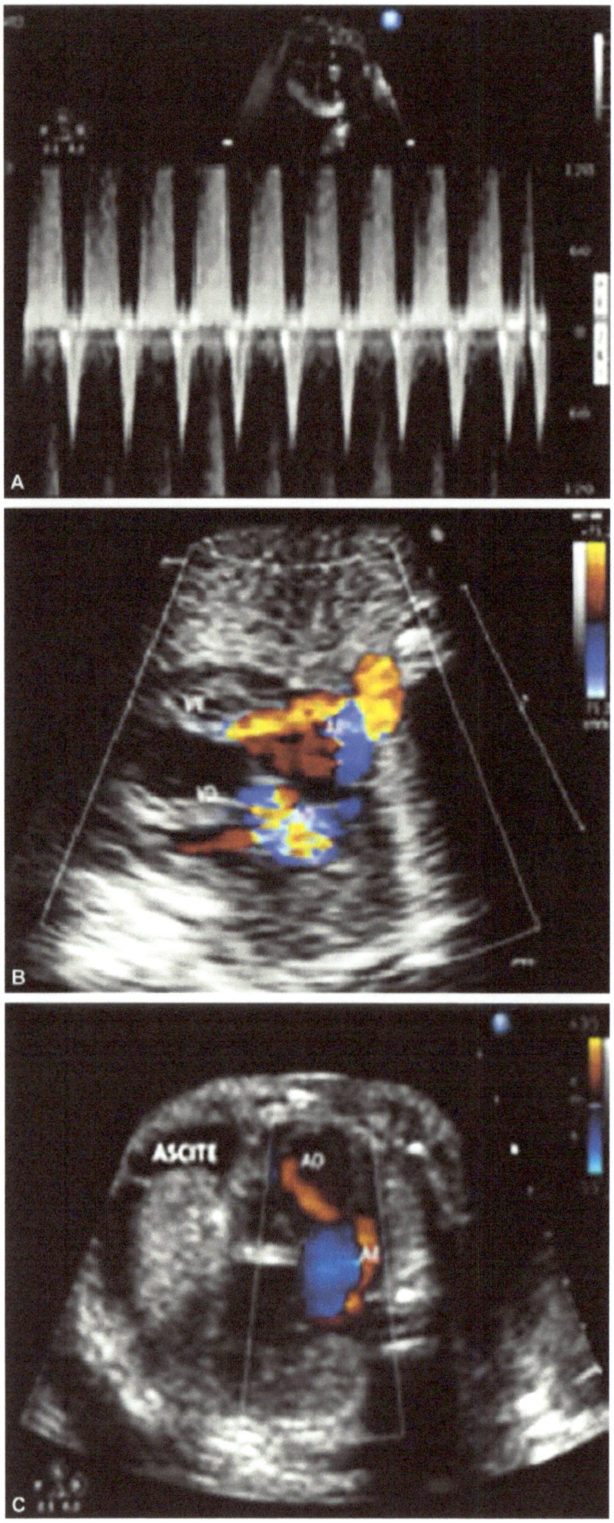

Fig. 30.62: Echocardiographic images of fetus with aortic stenosis with parameters indicative of progression to left ventricular hypoplasia. (A) Color Doppler of the mitral valve demonstrating single-phase left ventricular filling and mitral insufficiency important. (B) Reverse flow in the ascending aorta. (C) Left-right flow through the atrial septum

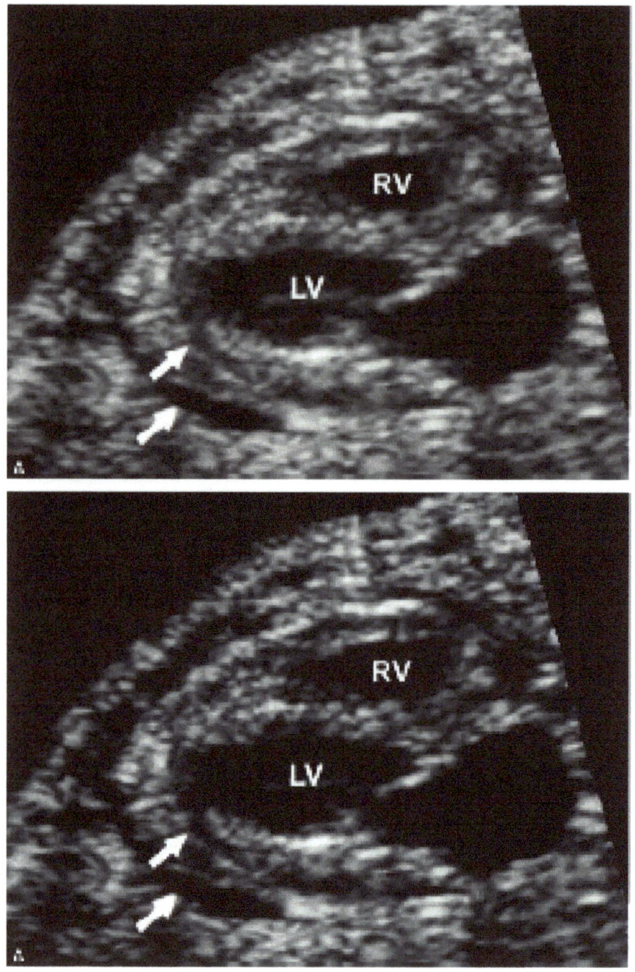

Fig. 30.63: Long-axis echocardiograms demonstrating a partially coagulated hemopericardium after transventricular fetal aortic valvuloplasty (A) and drainage of a hemopericardium (B). (A) The pericardial space has echolucent regions consistent with liquid blood and echogenic areas consistent with thrombus; arrows demarcate the epicardial surface of the LV and the pericardium. (B) The arrow is positioned over the hemopericardium and indicates the tip of the pericardiocentesis needle

evolving HLHS is that decreasing LV afterload or promoting flow through the left heart may help prevent progressive left heart dysfunction and hypoplasia over the subsequent course of gestation and, in the process, prevent evolution to HLHS.

The first known fetal aortic valvuloplasty was performed in 1989. Kohl et al. reviewed the published experience with this procedure in 2000. From 1989 to 1997, 12 cases were performed in third-trimester fetuses with AS or atresia (not midgestation AS with evolving HLHS) at 6 centers. A balloon was passed across the valve and expanded in 7 of the 12 fetuses, but only 1 of these 7 survived beyond the newborn period. This early experience highlighted several important issues, including the technical feasibility of third-trimester closed FCI, the importance of delivering the

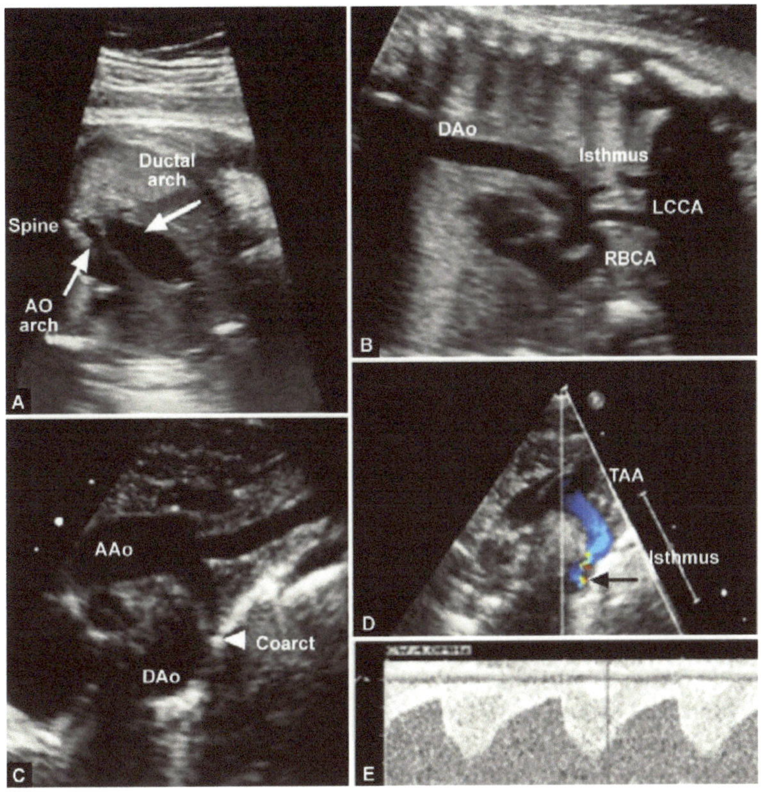

Fig. 30.64: Images obtained from a 35-week fetus with gastroschisis and postnatal coarctation. The only cardiac finding before birth was (A) a discrepancy in the aortic and ductal arches shown in a cross-sectional view through the fetal chest and (B) mild transverse and distal arch hypoplasia. With ductus arteriosus constriction after birth there was progressive severe discrete distal arch obstruction with (C) a very small lumen (arrow) and high velocity continuous flow by (D) color and (E) CW Doppler (systolic gradient 64 mmHg) prompting surgical intervention (AO=aortic; DAo=descending aorta; RBCA=right brachiocephalic artery; LCCA=left common carotid artery; TAA=transverse aortic arch; AAo=ascending aorta; DAo=descending aorta)

valvuloplasty balloon through an access cannula without a sharp edge, and the risk and potential consequences of fetal bradycardia.

After an initial learning curve, technical success has been achieved consistently in 75–80% of procedures. When the valve is dilated, there is immediate improvement in flow across the aortic valve, and there may be an obvious decrease in LV size. Moderate or severe postdilation aortic regurgitation (AR) occurs in nearly 40% of technically successful procedures. As with postnatal aortic valvuloplasty, the larger the balloon–annulus diameter ratio, the higher the likelihood of significant AR, but in contrast to neonatal aortic valvuloplasty, the target ratio is 1.1 to 1.2 instead of 0.9.

After successful fetal aortic valvuloplasty, in-utero aortic and mitral valve growth are improved relative to control fetuses, but there is no difference in LV short- or long-axis growth velocity. In contrast to the modest changes in left heart growth, there are clear beneficial changes in left heart physiology after fetal aortic valvuloplasty, as reported previously. Namely, after successful FCI, the left heart physiological parameters reported by Makikallio et al. to predict progression to HLHS were improved in a large majority of successfully treated fetuses but not in controls that were similar before intervention. In summary, there is solid evidence that balloon dilation of the aortic valve in fetuses with AS and evolving HLHS improves left heart physiology and leads to improved growth of the aortic and mitral valves but has no apparent effect on LV growth per se.

Ultimately, the goal of FCI for AS with evolving HLHS is to alter left heart physiology and growth sufficiently to allow postnatal survival with a healthy biventricular circulation. In recently published experience, just over 30% of patients who underwent technically successful FCI for this indication had a biventricular circulation from birth, and another 8% were converted to a biventricular circulation after initial univentricular palliation. Patients with larger LV size and higher LV pressure at the time of intervention are more likely to have a biventricular outcome. Using multivariable analysis, identification of a cohort of patients with essentially no chance of biventricular outcome was done and modified the selection criteria to exclude patients who fall below a defined threshold score. It has become

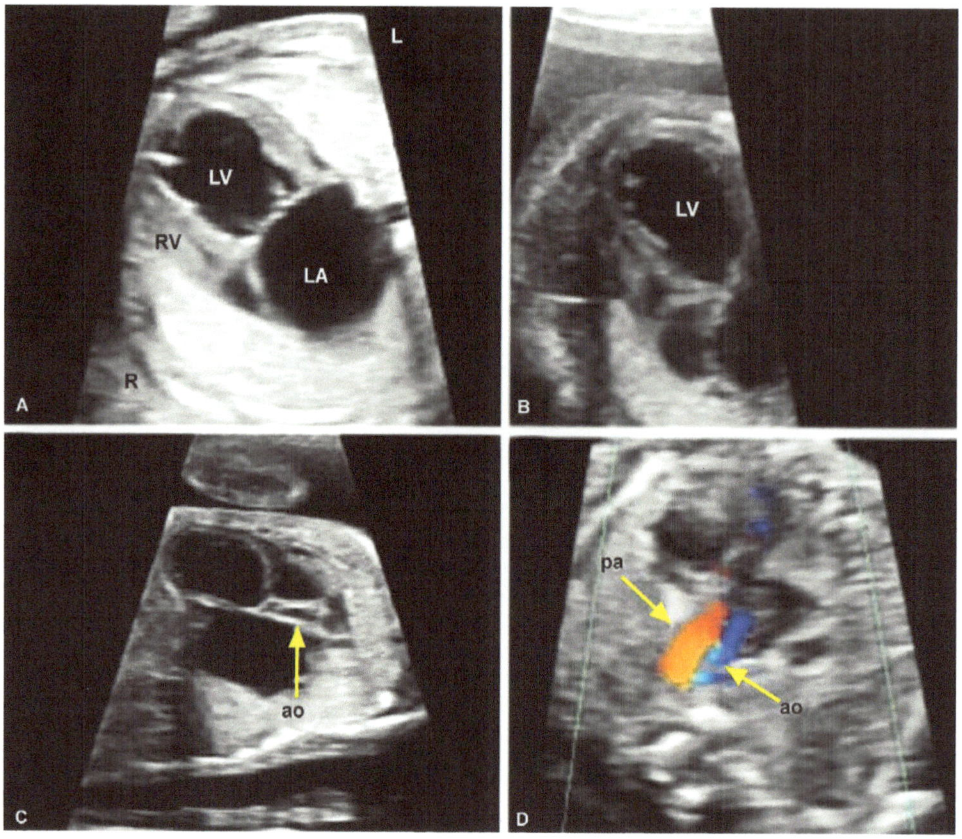

Fig. 30.65: Echocardiographic images. (A and B) Dilated left ventricle, left atrium and compressed right ventricle, (C) critical aortic stenosis, (D) in the three-vessel and tracheal view, the aortic diameter is much smaller than the pulmonary artery with reversed flow in the aortic arch

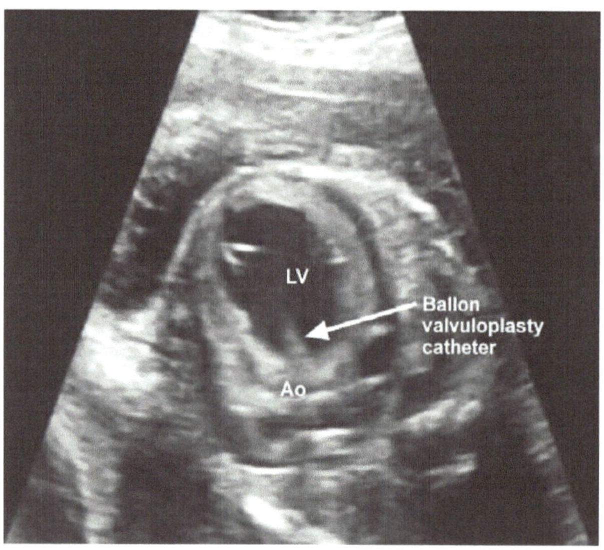

Fig. 30.66: Echocardiographic image showing introducer cannula and balloon catheter inflation in the aortic valve

clear that prenatal intervention is not a standalone intervention. In all cases that have gone on to biventricular outcome postnatally, postnatal interventions have been required, including repeat aortic valvuloplasty in most cases, temporary left atrial decompression, and frequently surgical intervention such as coarctation repair, resection of endocardial fibroelastosis, and mitral valvuloplasty.

Almost half of fetuses undergoing prenatal aortic valvuloplasty experience a combination of bradycardia and right ventricular dysfunction of variable severity. Fetal hemodynamic instability occurs almost exclusively in fetuses undergoing ventricular puncture (as opposed to atrial access) and may become evident either before the balloon is introduced into the ventricle, during dilation, or even after removal of equipment from the fetal heart. In early experience, these were treated with intramuscular or intracardiac epinephrine, but currently use a prophylactic approach, introducing epinephrine and bicarbonate through the balloon catheter at the time of intervention, regardless of whether bradycardia and right ventricular dysfunction have been identified. If subsequent treatment

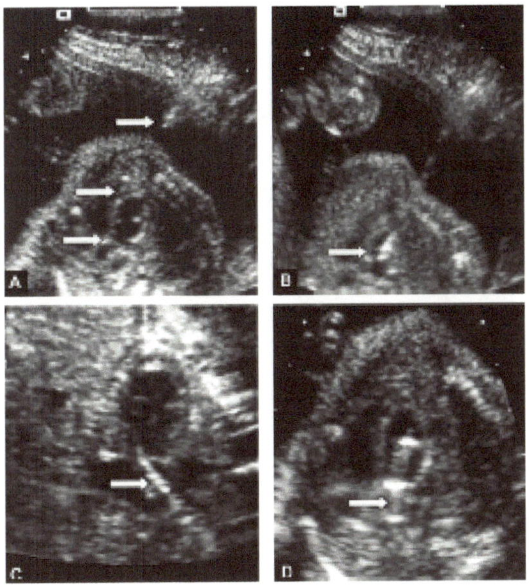

Fig. 30.67: Ultrasound images of technically successful percutaneous in-utero aortic valvuloplasty. (A) LV before intervention. Four-chamber view demonstrating echogenic LV, apex-forming RV, and alignment of needle (arrow), LV apex (arrow), aortic valve, and ascending aorta (arrow). (B) Cannula in LV. After LV puncture with cannula, LV appears smaller. Cannula can be seen as echo-bright line in LV, with its tip directed at aortic valve (arrow). (C) Guidewire across aortic valve in ascending aorta (arrow). (D) Balloon across valve. Correct position of balloon across aortic valve is confirmed by external measurements of catheter and by ultrasound imaging. Balloon inflation appears as movement of bright reflection along line of LV outflow track and across level of valve (arrow)

is necessary, intracardiac or intramuscular medication is given as well. In addition to fetal hemodynamic instability, hemopericardium is also common and may be accompanied by bradycardia. The hemopericardium is frequently small (less than 1—2 mm) but may be substantially larger, in which case percutaneous drainage is attempted, usually with successful removal of fluid. In fetuses that develop hemodynamic instability or hemopericardium, treatment generally results in restoration of an adequate circulation. The pathophysiology and inciting factors for hemodynamic instability are not entirely clear but are likely the result of some combination of fetal hypoxemia and autonomic or direct response to ventricular compression and puncture. The foundation for FCI in fetuses with AS and evolving HLHS is the belief that a biventricular circulation is superior to a univentricular circulation. Of course, this is not a simple dichotomous calculus, because all univentricular or biventricular circulations are not of equal functional quality. Although this determination is central to the debate about the practice of FCI, the details are beyond the scope of this review. Another potential benefit of FCI for AS, in the event that a biventricular circulation is not achieved, is a greater contribution of the left side of the heart to the functionally univentricular circulation, which may improve its efficiency and/or durability.

The risks of fetal aortic valvuloplasty for AS with evolving HLHS have not been defined completely.

In the final analysis, the risk-benefit analysis of FCI for evolving HLHS depends to a large extent on individual opinions about the importance of biventricular versus univentricular physiology, and it must take into account both the chronic morbidity and mortality risks of a functionally univentricular circulation and the unknown longer-term risks of a biventricular circulation after FCI. The robustness and health of a biventricular circulation can vary, and the presence of multilevel left heart disease may significantly impact the health of a biventricular circulation. Thus, any risk-benefit analysis before FCI is necessarily speculative and based on the limited available data, as well as being situated in the context of evolving management options and outcomes in patients with both univentricular and biventricular heart disease.

FETAL HLHS WITH INTACT OR HIGHLY RESTRICTIVE ATRIAL SEPTUM

Although neonatal survival in infants with HLHS continues to improve, outcomes among certain subsets of patients remain poor; one of the strongest risk factors for early mortality is an intact or highly restrictive atrial septum. Although limited pulmonary venous egress may be well tolerated in utero, neonates with major septal restriction are at substantially higher risk of death than those without. There are two primary problems associated with this condition—(1) profound hypoxemia after birth due to restricted outflow from the pulmonary veins, which results in little effective pulmonary blood flow, and (2) chronic pulmonary venous hypertension in-utero due to restriction to left atrial outflow, which results in

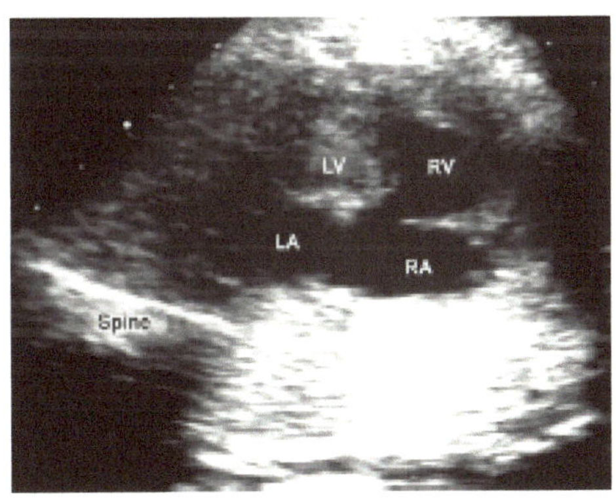

Fig. 30.68: Ultrasonography showing small sized left atrium, hypoplastic heart forming the apex and atresic mitral valve in an unborn baby with hypoplastic left heart syndrome

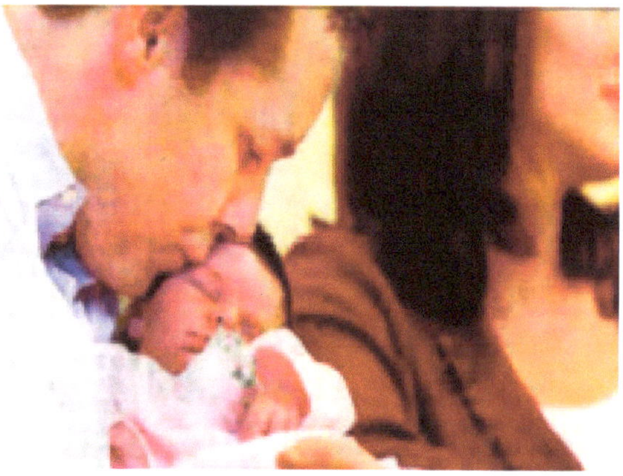

Fig. 30.69: Photograph of a newborn baby. Grace out of US National couple with mother Angela VanDer-werken of Virginia who became worlds first baby to receive intrauterine stent for the treatment of hypoplastic left heart syndrome when this baby was 7 months old in the womb of the mother. This surgery was performed by the team of experts under chief surgeon Dr James Lock, at children hospital Boston and Brigham and women hospital, Boston

pulmonary venous thickening and perioperative morbidity and mortality. Thus, even if postnatal opening of the atrial septum is rapid and effective, damage to the pulmonary vasculature may contribute to further mortality in the first few weeks or months of life.

In fetuses with HLHS and an intact atrial septum, FCI may improve both of the major problems posed by the restriction of pulmonary venous outflow. If the left atrium can be decompressed before birth, the profound perinatal hypoxemia and acidosis and their associated morbidities may be prevented. If left atrial decompression can be achieved sufficiently early in gestation, adverse pulmonary venous remodeling may also be prevented. Physiologically, the earliest possible treatment of left atrial hypertension on diagnosis of atrial septal restriction should maximize

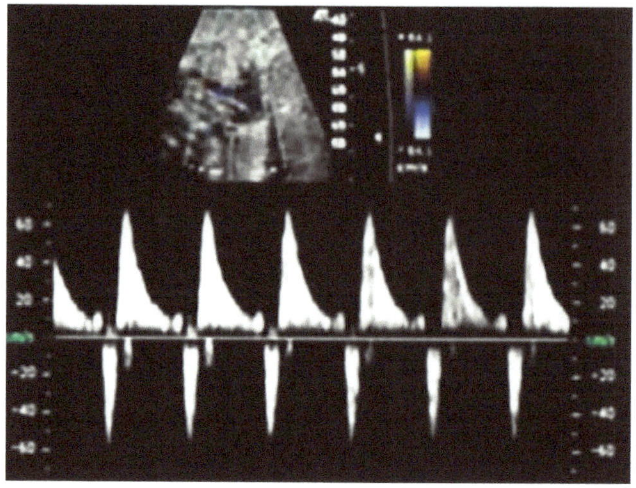

Fig. 30.71: Pulmonary vein Doppler of fetal carrier syndrome showing hypoplasia of the left heart with critically restrictive foramen ovale. Note that the flow is bidirectional wave at the expense of the reverse flow

the benefit of normalizing the developmental conditions for the pulmonary vasculature.

Recently some workers have reported their experience with FCI in 21 fetuses with HLHS and an intact or highly restrictive atrial septum. Prenatal atrial septoplasty for this condition has also been reported by others with various monitoring and interventional approaches. The atrial septum is crossed and an interatrial communication created in all cases, either with balloon dilation or placement of a stent. Among neonates delivered after FCI for HLHS with significant atrial septal restriction, surgical survival remains quite poor (58%); however, in-utero creation of an atrial septal defect does appear to have some benefit in terms of preoperative management, because neonates with an interatrial defect <3 mm after FCI had higher oxygen saturation at birth and are less likely to need urgent postnatal

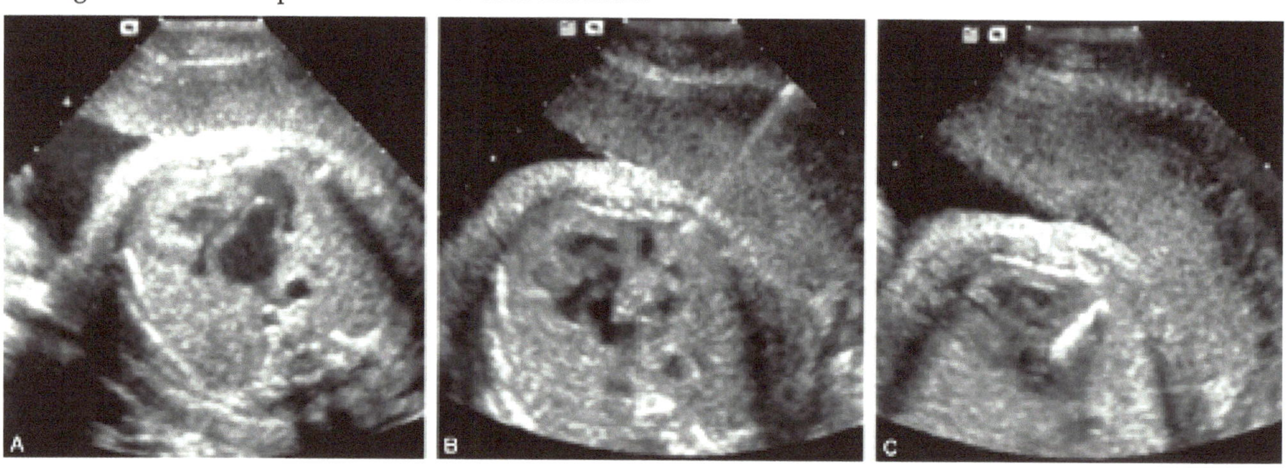

Fig. 30.70: Creation of an atrial septal defect in utero for fetuses with hypoplastic left heart syndrome and intact or highly restrictive atrial septum. Transabdominal ultrasound image of heart in 1 fetus with dilated left atrium and thin, bulging atrial septum before atrial septal puncture (A), during septal puncture with Chiba needle (B), and during dilation with 3 mm coronary angioplasty balloon (C)

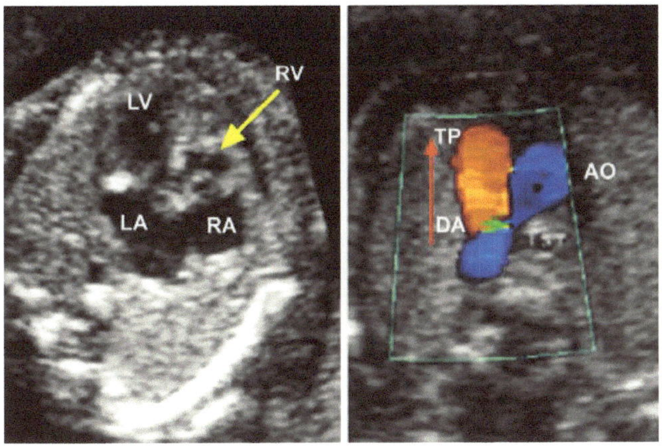

Fig. 30.72: Hypoplastic right ventricle (**arrow**) in a fetus with pulmonary atresia and intact ventricular septum (A). Color-Doppler of the four chamber view with asymmetric flow between the left heart and right heart. Pulmonary valve atresia can be diagnosed using color-Doppler by visualizing the great vessels vews aorta (Ao) and pulmonary trunk (TP)—in the upper thorax and demonstrating the retrograde flow from the descending aorta across the ductus arteriosus toward the pulmonary valve

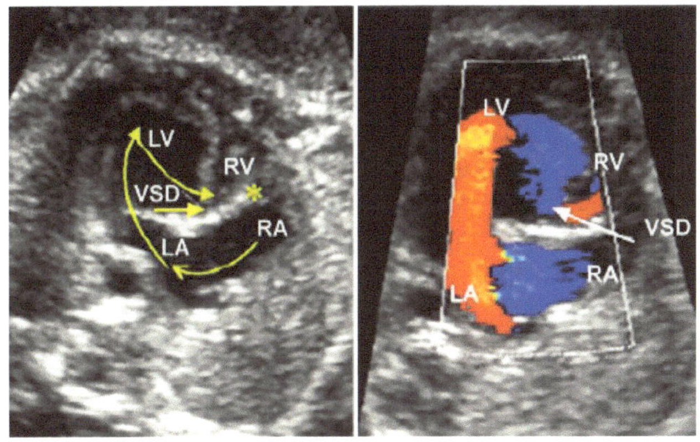

Fig. 30.73: Tricuspid atresia (*) and ventricular septal defect (VSD). Arrows show the direction of flow; due to the atresia of the tricuspid valve, blood entering the right atrium cannot enter directly into the right ventricle and it flows to the left atrium, left ventricle and across the VSD to the hypoplastic right ventricle (**Right**)

left atrial decompression. Although assessment of any postnatal survival benefit of FCI in patients with HLHS and an intact atrial septum will require more extensive experience, the potential to avert immediate postnatal deterioration has been demonstrated, and FCI indicated for the comprehensive management of these high-risk fetuses.

RIGHT SIDED FETAL CARDIAC LESIONS

Fetal pulmonary atresia with evolving hypoplastic right heart

Fetal intervention for severe right ventricular outflow obstruction via transthoracic per-ventricular balloon pulmonary valvuloplasty has also been attempted. The role of intervention is to promote right heart functional development and to improve the possibility of postnatal biventricular circulation.

Fetal pulmonary atresia with intact ventricular septum. Right ventricle is small and hypertrophied at 27 weeks, with tricuspid valve size 3 standard deviations below normal for gestational age. This would represent borderline candidate for fetal procedure, as success with postnatal therapy alone is likely.

Isolated case reports and one series have described this procedure. In a series of 10 affected fetuses, a group from Boston reported technical success in 60% of fetuses along with subsequent in-utero growth of right heart structures, 40% of whom were able to achieve biventricular circulation after birth.

Identification of potential candidates is generally based on the risk of progression to univentricular circulation if left untreated, though this risk is less well defined for fetuses with right heart obstruction than for those with aortic valve obstruction.

Reviews of the evolution of severe pulmonary outflow tract obstruction have shown that a preprocedure tricuspid valve annulus dimension of more than 3 standard deviations below gestational age-based normal values and diminutive size of the pulmonary valve and the outflow are more likely to be associated with evolution of right heart hypoplasia sufficient to preclude biventricular circulation at birth despite aggressive postnatal intervention. This should guide future attempts at fetal pulmonary valvuloplasty.

Therefore, although technical success is possible for fetal aortic and pulmonary valvuloplasty and atrial septoplasty, further work is needed before these techniques are widely adopted, in part because of the rarity of the lesions for which intervention would be warranted.

For instance, of all cases of HLHS encountered in one large referral center over several years, only 1.6% involved a dilated left heart and suspected critical aortic stenosis at initial prenatal diagnosis. Fewer than one-quarter of infants with left-side hypoplasia have been observed to have some degree of clinically important atrial septal restriction, and many of these infants may have sufficient decompression in the preoperative period.

Ideally, randomized multicenter trials that include long-term follow-up of patients who have undergone these procedures will provide the most definitive conclusions as to efficacy, safety, and superiority over current palliative pathways that include only postnatal interventions.

FETAL COMPLETE HEART BLOCK

Complete heart block in the fetus can be a life-threatening emergency that may present without warning. Diagnosis relies on fetal M-mode and Doppler ultrasonography to relate atrial and ventricular mechanical events. Heart block in the fetus may be associated with structural heart disease, may result from maternal autoimmune disease, or may be idiopathic.

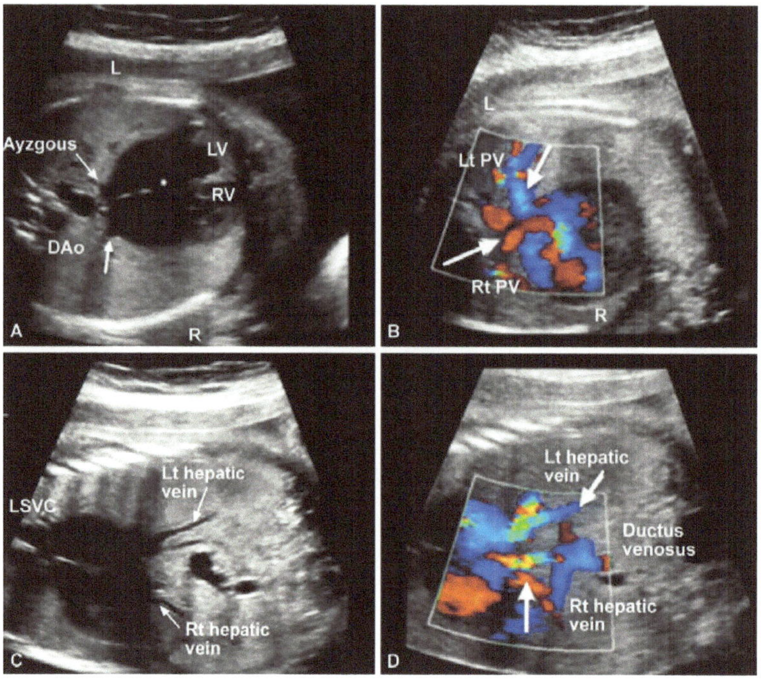

Fig. 30.74: Images from a 30-week fetus with left atrial isomerism, mesocardia and anomalous systemic and pulmonary venous connections. Left and right pulmonary veins (**A and B, arrows**) and left and right hepatic veins (**C and D, arrows**) can be seen connecting on either side of the atrial septum by 2D and color flow map imaging. A coronary sinoseptal defect was identified (*). The dilated azygous vein connected with a left superior vena cava that drained into the left sided atrium. Surgical repair with intra-atrial baffling of systemic and pulmonary veins was used to correct this lesion at 9 months. L=left; R=right; Lt=left; Rt=right; DAo=descending aorta; RV=right ventricle; LV=left ventricle; PV=pulmonary vein; LSVC=left superior vena cava

In most cases associated with a structurally normal heart, maternal autoantibodies are present in the maternal serum. The mothers may not show clinically apparent symptoms of lupus or Sjögren syndrome; however, in both, transplacental passage of the antibodies can potentially cause inflammation and fibrosis at the atrioventricular (AV) node in particular.

Although some success has been reported with administration of corticosteroids to the mother of a fetus with first- or second-degree AV block, pharmacologically effective options are available for treatment of third-degree or complete heart block, and fetuses with low intrinsic ventricular rates are at risk for significant morbidity and mortality. Administration of beta-mimetics to increase fetal heart rate have somewhat improved fetal survival.

A few isolated investigators over the past two decades have attempted treatment to increase ventricular rates in the face of hydrops and imminent demise of the fetus in the form of implantation of fetal pacemakers. The results appeared mixed, with some reporting initial good results, with complete resolution of hydrops and achievement of normal heart rates.

Theoretically, this approach should provide relief in the gestational period wherein the insult is the most severe, prolonging pregnancy and promoting feasibility of early postnatal permanent pacemaker implantation. However, to date, no survivors following institution of fetal pacing have been reported.

Previous approaches have relied on the placement of an epicardial pacing lead on the fetal heart with an extrauterine pulse generator implanted in the maternal abdomen, with failure attributed to lead dislodgment due to fetal movement. Owing to a lack of information regarding successful performance of this procedure, this approach is not discussed further in this article.

FETAL PULMONARY ATRESIA WITH INTACT VENTRICULAR SEPTUM (PA/IVS)

It occurs as a spectrum of hypoplastic right heart disease, with cases at the mild end of the spectrum amenable to biventricular repair and those with more severe right heart hypoplasia managed with univentricular palliation or transplantation. In newborns with PA/IVS, the likelihood of a biventricular outcome can be estimated from the Z-score of the tricuspid valve annulus, with a Z-score above 3 associated with biventricular outcome and below 3 with univentricular palliation.

The potential role of FCI in fetuses with PA/IVS is to promote right heart growth and functional development and increase the chance of a biventricular circulation

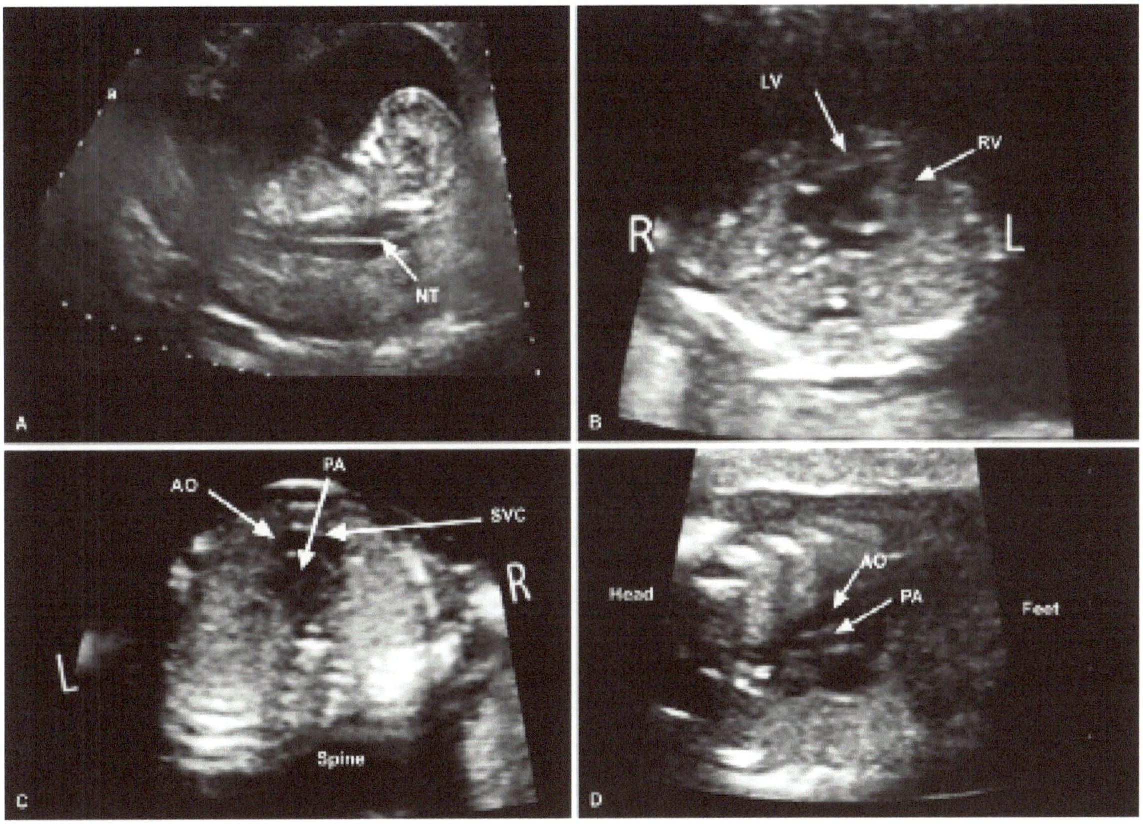

Fig. 30.75: 12 and 37 weeks gestational age fetus with (A) a 7 mm nuchal translucency (NT). (B) On further assessment, the four-chamber revealed levocardia inverted ventricles and a mildly foreshortened left sided right ventricle. At 14 weeks, the presence of L-transposition (ëcorrected transpositioní) of the great arteries demonstrated by (C) an abnormal 3 vessel view with an anterior and leftward aorta arising from the right ventricle and posterior pulmonary artery from the left ventricle and (D) parallel arrangement of the great arteries (L=left; R=right; AO=ascending aorta; PA=pulmonary artery; LV=left ventricle; RV=right ventricle; SVC=superior vena cava

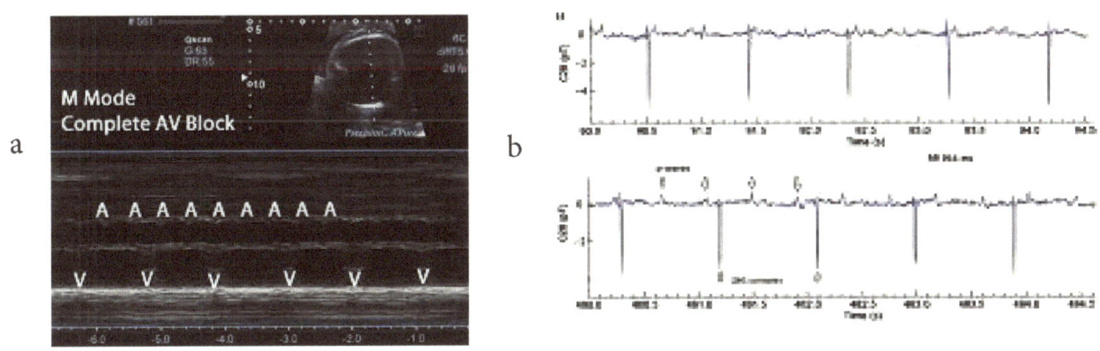

Fig. 30.76: Fetal M-Mode Echo (a) and ECG (b) of complete atrioventricular block before pacemaker implantation

after birth. Identification of potential candidates for FCI for PA/IVS should be based on the risk of progression to a functionally univentricular circulation postnatally without FCI and the possibility of altering that progression prenatally. There is limited information about predictors of postnatal outcomes in fetuses with PA/IVS. Both anatomic and physiological characteristics are likely to be important, but many patients are in the middle of the severity spectrum, and postnatal management strategy plays an important role in the ultimate outcome.

On the basis of this limited experience, it appears that prenatal pulmonary valve perforation and dilation may be performed successfully in midgestation fetuses, with maintenance of valvar patency throughout gestation and apparently improved growth of right heart structures. The effects of this strategy on right heart functional development and postnatal outcome remain to be determined. Because postnatal outcomes for the majority

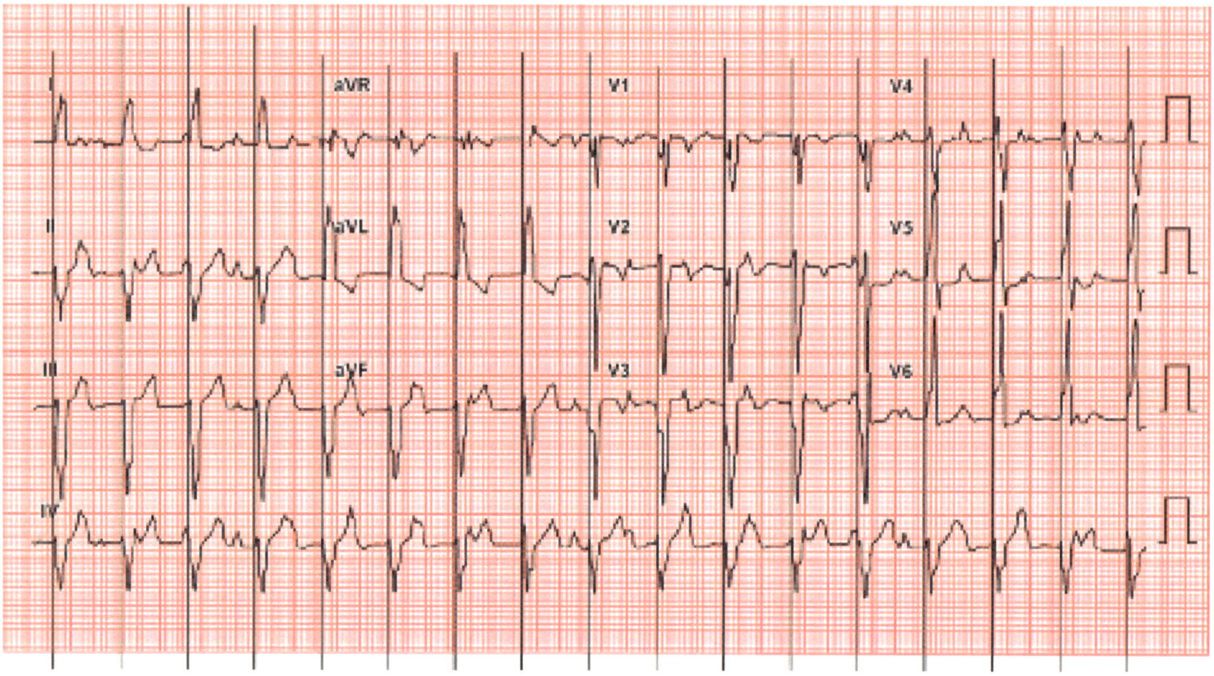

Fig. 30.77: Electrocardiography: regular ventricular pacing rhythm after pacemaker implantation

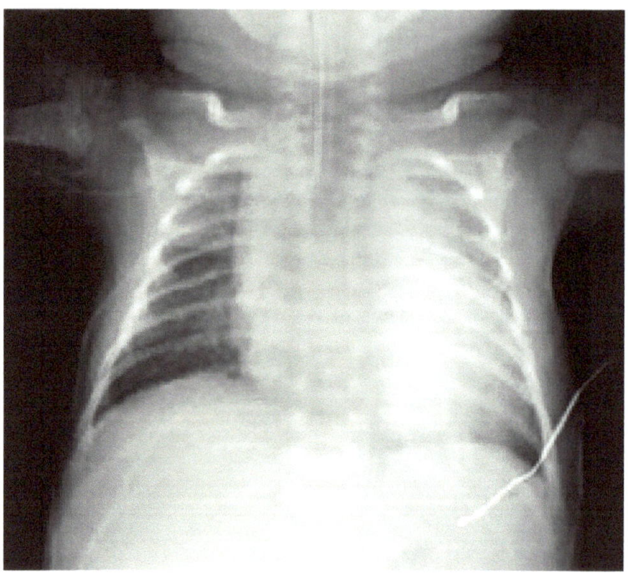

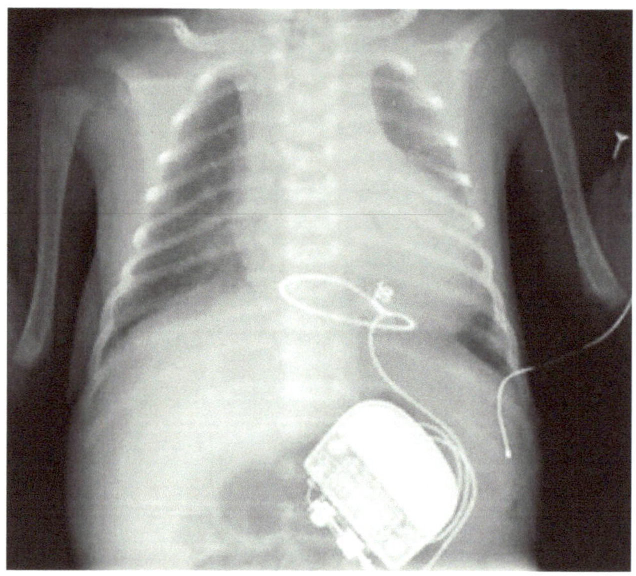

Fig. 30.78: (A) Chest X-rayócardiomegaly and impending congestive heart failure before pacemaker implantation. (B) Chest X-ray: normal heart size after pacemaker implantation

of patients with PA/IVS are usually favorable, it may be more of a challenge to appropriately select patients and demonstrate effectiveness than for the previously discussed anomalies.

Twin-to-twin Transfusion Syndrome

Most pregnancies result in one baby. In about one in 80 pregnancies, twins are conceived. This can occur in one of two ways.

The more common way (which accounts for two-thirds of cases) is for the two different sperm to fertilize two different eggs, resulting in what is called a dizygotic (DZ) twin gestation. These twins are often called fraternal twins. In this type of twinning each twin has its own sac of amniotic fluid and its own placenta (afterbirth). Dizygotic twins have two sets of membranes surrounding their amniotic fluid sacs (one inner amnion layer and one outer chorion layer), and therefore they are known as diamniotic, dichorionic.

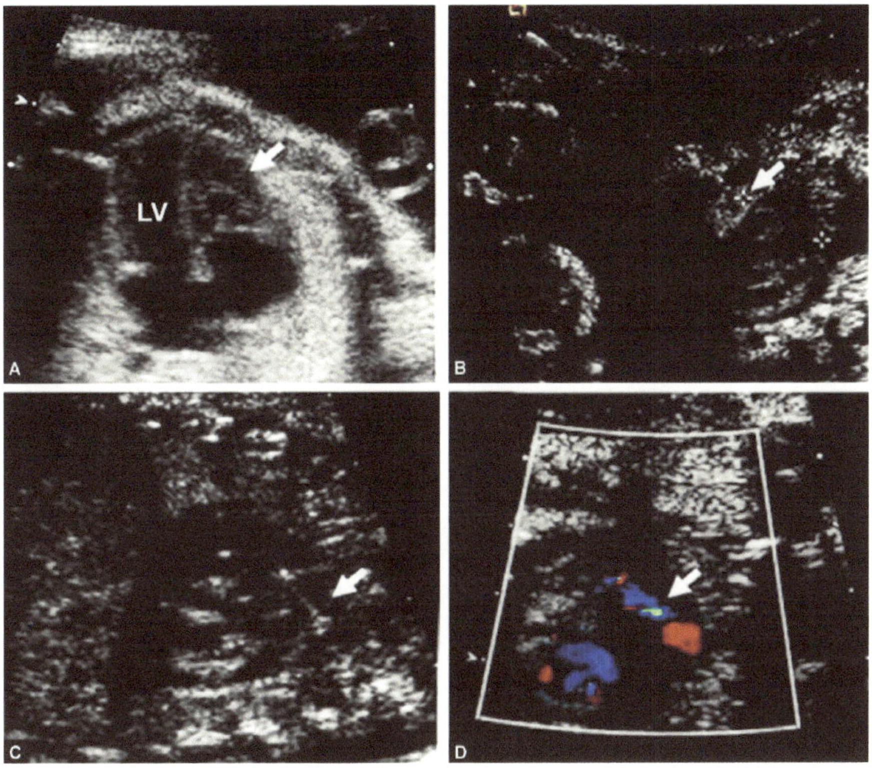

Fig. 30.79: Echocardiographic images obtained during the intervention for patient. (A) This four-chamber view demonstrates a hypoplastic RV (**arrow**). (B) In this oblique projection, the 19-gauge cannula can be seen passing through the uterus, amniotic cavity, and chest wall of the fetus and approaching the RV outflow tract (**arrow**). (C) This short-axis image demonstrates the tip of the Chiba needle in the pulmonary artery (**arrow**). (D) After successful valvuloplasty, color-Doppler ultrasound flow imaging demonstrates an antegrade jet of flow across the patent PV (**arrow**)

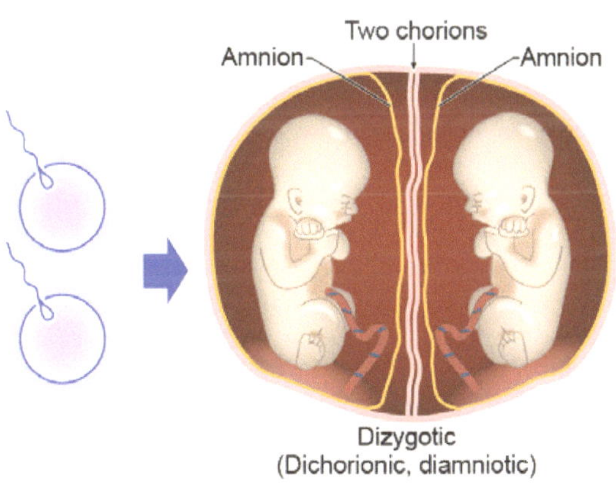

Fig. 30.80: Dizygotic (dichorionic and diamniotic fetuses

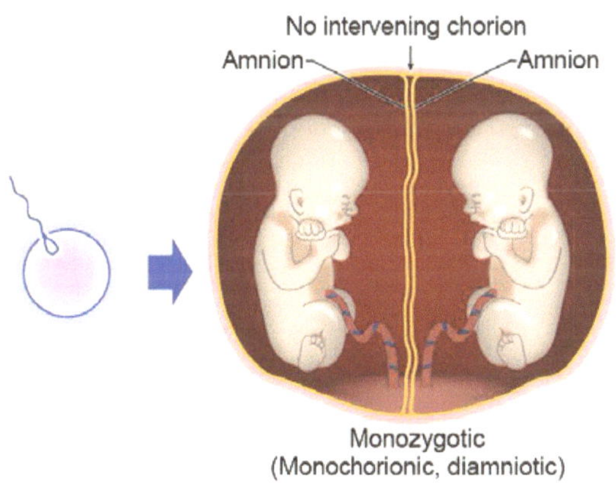

Fig. 30.81: Monozygotic (monochorionic and diamniotic fetuses

In about one-third of twin pregnancies, one sperm fertilizes one egg, but this splits into two embryos resulting in what is known as monozygotic (MZ) twins. These twins are often referred to as identical twins since they have the same genetic material. Approximately one-third of MZ twins look just like fraternal twins on prenatal ultrasound since there are two separate amniotic sacs and two separate placentas. However, in two-thirds of identical twins, each twin has its own amniotic sac but shares a common placenta. This type of MZ twinning is called monochorionic,

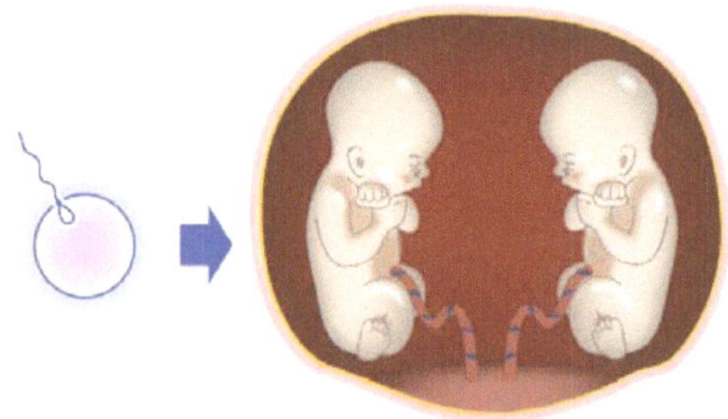

Fig. 30.82: Monozygotic (monochorionic and monoamniotic fetuses

diamniotic since there is an inner layer surrounding the amniotic sac of each twin, but there is only one common outer layer (chorion) surrounding both of the sacs. This type of twinning occurs in approximately one in 360 pregnancies. Monochorionic twins are at higher risk for complications since they share a common placenta. Less than 1% of identical twins (about one in 2,400 pregnancies) will have one amniotic sac and one placenta for both twins. This type of twinning is referred to as monchorionic, monoamniotic twinning. These twins are at very high risk for loss of the pregnancy due to entangled umbilical cords.

What is Twin-twin Transfusion Syndrome and How Does One Get it?

This condition occurs only in those identical twins that are monochorionic, diamniotic (one-third of all identical or monozygotic twins). In almost all of these pregnancies, the single placenta contains blood vessel connections between the twins. For reasons that are not clear, in 15%–20% of monochorionic, diamniotic twins, the blood flow through these blood vessel connections becomes unbalanced, resulting in a condition known as twin-twin transfusion syndrome (TTTS). This is not an inherited or genetic condition. It is not caused by something that a mother or father has done or not done.

In TTTS, the smaller twin (often called the donor twin) does not get enough blood while the larger twin (often called the recipient twin) becomes overloaded with too much blood.

In an attempt to reduce its blood volume, the recipient twin will increase the urine it makes. This will eventually result in the twin having a very large bladder on ultrasound, as well as too much amniotic fluid around this twin. This is known as polyhydramnios.

At the same time, the donor twin will produce less than the usual amount of urine. The amniotic fluid around the donor twin will become very low or absent. This is known as oligohydramnios.

As the disease progresses, the donor will produce so little urine that its bladder may not be seen on ultrasound. The twin will become wrapped by its amniotic membrane (known as a 'stuck' twin). Often the polyhydramnios of the recipient twin is the first thing noticed by the patient due a sudden increase in the size of the uterus. Clothes may become tight fitting over a short period of time. At other times the differences in the amniotic fluid volumes between the twins is only noted at the time of a routine ultrasound.

How is Twin-twin Transfusion Syndrome Diagnosed?

The diagnosis of TTTS is made with an ultrasound evaluation that shows a twin pregnancy with one placenta, twins of the same sex in separate amniotic sacs, and polyhydramnios in the recipient's sac and oligohydramnios in the donor's sac. Amniotic fluid volume is measured with ultrasound by determining the deepest pocket measurement from the patient's skin to her back. This measurement is known as the maximum vertical pocket (MVP) (Fig. 36.83).

What are the Twin-twin Transfusion Syndrome Five Stages of Classification?

Quinterol has proposed five stages of TTTS based on ultrasound findings

- **Stage I:** This is the initial way that TTTS is seen on ultrasound. In stage I, there is oligohydramnios in the donor's sac with an MVP of two centimeters or less (three-quarters of an inch) and polyhydramnios in the recipient's sac with a maximum vertical pocket of fluid of 8 cm or more (just over 3-inch). The bladder of the donor baby is still seen.
- **Stage II:** As defined above, there is polyhydramnios and oligohydramnios, but the bladder is no longer seen in the donor twin during the ultrasound evaluation.
- **Stage III:** Blood flow in the fetus can be measured with a special type of ultrasound called Doppler. In addition to the findings of Stages I and II, careful study of the blood flow in the umbilical cord and fetal ductus venosus (the large blood vessel in the fetus that returns blood to the heart from the placenta) reveals abnormal patterns in stage III. These patterns can occur in either or both fetuses.

In the umbilical cord, the diastolic flow can be either absent or reversed in the umbilical artery. This pattern is usually seen in the donor twin. In the ductus venosus, the diastolic flow can either be absent or reversed. This

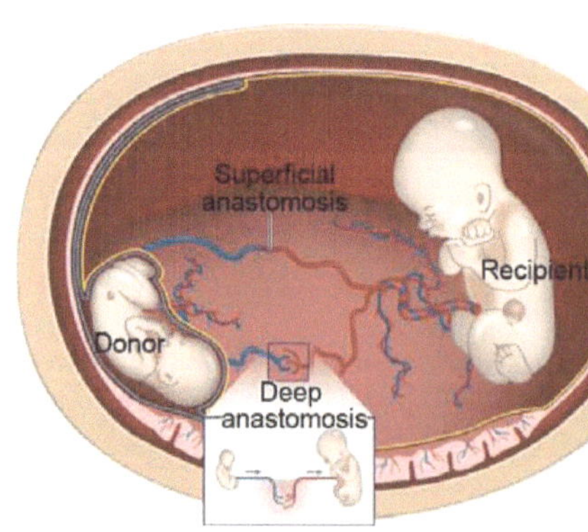

Fig. 30.83: Anastomosis in twin-twin transfusion syndrome

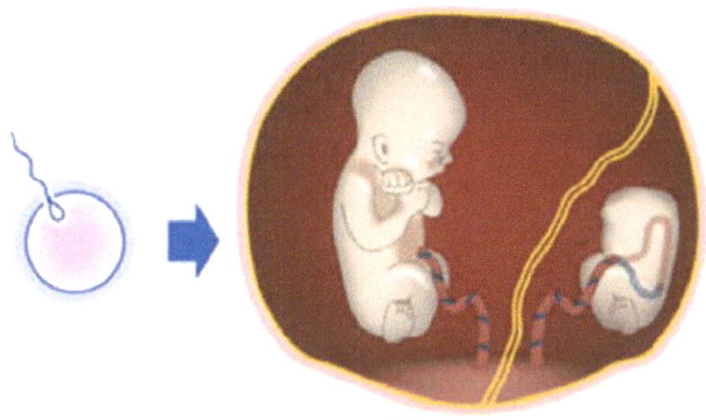

Fig. 30.84: Trap sequence (twin-reversed arterial perfusion sequence) in twin-twin transfusion syndrome

pattern is usually see in the recipient twin due to early heart failure. The recipient twin can also exhibit leakage across the main valve on the right side of the heart, this is known as tricuspid regurgitation.

- **Stage IV:** One or both babies shows signs of hydrops. This means there is excess fluid in parts of the baby such as swelling of the skin around the head (scalp edema), fluid in the abdomen (ascites), fluid around the lungs (pleural effusions) or fluid around the heart (pericardial effusion). These findings are evidence of heart failure and are typically seen in the recipient twin.
- **Stage V:** One or both babies have died. The survival of the twins is poorer when there is progression to a higher stage over time. It has been estimated that half of patients will progress to a higher stage, 30% will remain at the same stage and 20% will improve to a lower stage.

What is an Acardiac Twin or Twin Reversed Arterial Perfusion (TRAP) Syndrome?

An usual form of TTTS occurs in about one in 15,000 pregnancies. In these monochorionic twins, one twin develops normally while the other twin fails to develop a heart as well as other body structures. The abnormal twin is called an acardiac twin. In these pregnancies, the umbilical cord from the acardiac twin branches directly from the umbilical cord of the normal twin. Blood flow to the acardiac twin comes from the normal twin, which is also known as a pump twin. This blood flow is reversed from the normal direction leading to the name for this condition—twin reversed arterial perfusion syndrome or TRAP. In some cases the blood flow from the pump twin to the acardiac twin stops on its own and the acardiac twin stops growing. In other cases, the flow continues and the acardiac twin continues to increase in size. This eventually leads to heart failure and polyhydramnios in the pump twin. Without treatment, more than 50% of cases of TRAP will result in the death of the pump twin.

What is the Outcome for Twin-twin Transfusion Syndrome (TTTS)?

There are a number of ways to treat TTTS, any of which many be the correct method depending on ultrasound findings, the gestational age of the pregnancy and a couple's specific needs.

Left untreated, TTTS prior to 24 weeks' gestation (6 months of pregnancy), 80–90% of cases are associated with the loss of one or both twins. If one of the twins should die, the blood vessel connections in the placenta can place the surviving twin at risk for long-term brain damage in as many as one-third of cases. In general, more advanced stages of TTTS have a worse prognosis than the earlier stages. When severe TTTS occurs at a very early gestational age (prior to 16 weeks or the fourth month of pregnancy), the option of termination of the pregnancy can be considered due to the grim prognosis.

The various therapies that are available target either the unequal fluid between the twins' sacs or interrupt the blood vessel communications between the twins on the single placenta. The successful outcome of these treatments has been based on the number of babies that survive, as well as the number of babies who do not have brain damage. The treatments that are currently available are described below.

Treatments

Reduction amniocentesis

Serial amniocentesis involves the removal of the excessive amniotic fluid from the sac of the recipient twin using a needle that is passed through the maternal abdomen.

The amount of amniotic fluid removed will vary based on the initial volume in the recipient sac, the gestational age and the development of uterine contractions during the procedure. As a general rule no more than three liters (approximately two and one-half quarts) of amniotic fluid is removed at any one time. The procedure is usually completed within 30 minutes or less. The procedure may temporarily restore the balance in the amniotic fluid in both twins' sacs. This technique may be useful for milder cases of TTTS that occur later in pregnancy.

However, reduction amniocentesis usually requires repeat procedures to be undertaken every few days to weekly when the fluid returns to high levels. The procedure is generally not thought to be effective for more advanced stages of TTTS (stages III and IV).

Complications of repeated amniocenteses for the treatment of TTTS include premature labor with early delivery in 3% of cases, premature rupture of the membranes in 6% of cases, infection in about 1% of cases, and premature separation of the placenta from the wall of the womb (called an abruption) in 1% of cases.

Pregnancies managed with serial reduction amniocentesis on average deliver by 29–30 weeks of gestation (approximately ten weeks prior to the 'due date'). If there is progression of TTTS to a more advanced stage, serial amniocenteses will reduce the success rate for such procedures such as laser (see below). Reported survival rates have varied from 18–83%, with a recent study noting that just over half (56%) of severe TTTS cases managed with reduction amniocentesis will end with at least one infant without brain damage. Approximately, 20–25% of the TTTS survivors from pregnancies treated with reduction amniocentesis have been found to have long-term developmental delay.

Septostomy

Septostomy also known as microseptostomy) is the creation of a hole in the membrane between the babies' sacs using a needle. This causes fluid to move from the amniotic sac with excessive fluid (the recipient's sac) into the sac with absent or low fluid (donor's sac). Since septostomy is performed with a needle that is used to perform amniocentesis, complications of infection, premature labor and premature rupture of the membranes are rare. Septostomy carries the additional potential risk for the hole to become larger between the two sacs and could even allow the babies to share the same amniotic space if the entire separating membrane becomes disrupted. This has been reported to occur in 3% of septostomies. In the worst case scenario, the umbilical cords of the twins could become entangled, leading to the death of one or both fetuses. In one large series, survival to birth was 80% for at least one twin and was 60% for both twins. Patients undergoing septostomy typically require fewer procedures than those treated with amnioreduction. There is no data currently available regarding neurologic outcome in survivors of septostomy.

Selective Laser Ablation of the Placental Anastomotic Vessels

In more advanced stages of TTTS (stage II and higher) laser ablation of the communicating vessels on the placenta between the twin fetuses can be a curative procedure (Fig. 36.86).

The procedure is performed in an operating room. After the patient's abdomen has been washed with an antiseptic and covered with sterile paper drapes, an ultrasound is performed to determine the appropriate spot to enter the uterus. The skin is then injected with an anesthetic medication to 'numb' the area and deep tissues directly under the selected site. An anesthesiologist will also administer medications through an intravenous line to produce

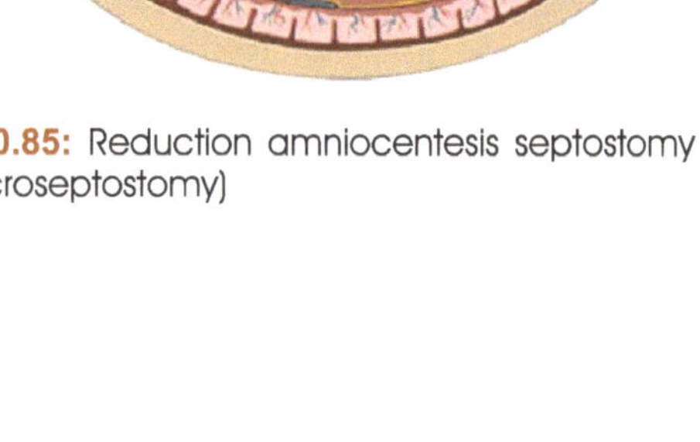

Fig. 30.85: Reduction amniocentesis septostomy (also known as microseptostomy)

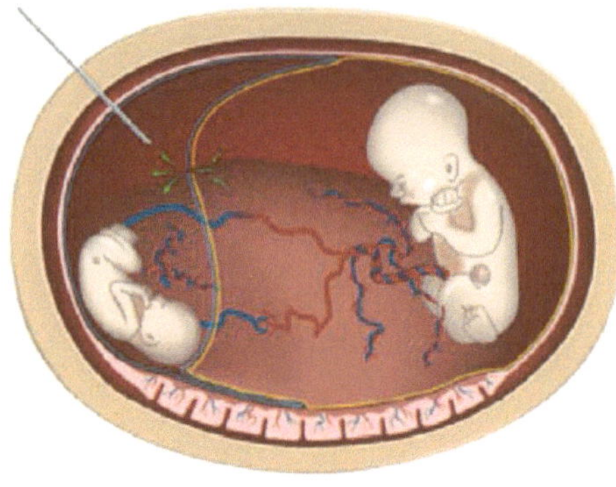

Fig. 30.86: Selective laser ablation of the placental anastomotic vessels

sedation. A small skin cut is made to allow the introduction of a thin hollow tube and needle. The instruments are inserted under ultrasound guidance into the amniotic sac of the recipient twin. The needle is removed and a telescope (fetoscope) with a thin fiber to carry the laser energy is then inserted through the hollow tube. The fetoscope is used to look directly at the blood vessels on the surface of the placenta. Vessels that are found to communicate between the twins are then closed using laser light energy. At the completion of the surgery, the extra-amniotic fluid in the recipient twin's sac is removed to achieve a normal volume. The procedure may take 45 minutes to 2 hours depending on the difficulty of the case.

Because the fetoscope requires a larger hole to be made into the amniotic cavity than would be the case with an amnioreduction or septostomy procedure, laser ablation is associated with a higher risk of complications such as premature contractions, premature rupture of the membranes (15–20% of cases), placental separation (2%) and infection. For this reason, special medications to prevent contractions and antibiotics to prevent infection will be given before and after the procedure. In addition, laser therapy may be associated with unique risks since the laser energy may cause certain areas of the placenta or blood vessels on the surface of the placenta to bleed.

Laser ablation has been shown to result in the survival of at least one twin in 70–80% of cases and both twins in one-third of cases. Should one fetus die after the procedure, the likelihood that the surviving fetus will develop complications is reduced from 35% to approximately 7%. This is because the babies are no longer sharing blood vessels between them. In one-third of cases, neither twin will survive. Studies to date have indicated that approximately 8% of survivors following laser ablation will have a long-term mental handicap. This is approximately half of the rate of problems seen in survivors treated with amnioreduction.

Selective Cord Coagulation

In some cases, a couple may make the difficult decision to proceed with the purposeful loss of one twin to save the

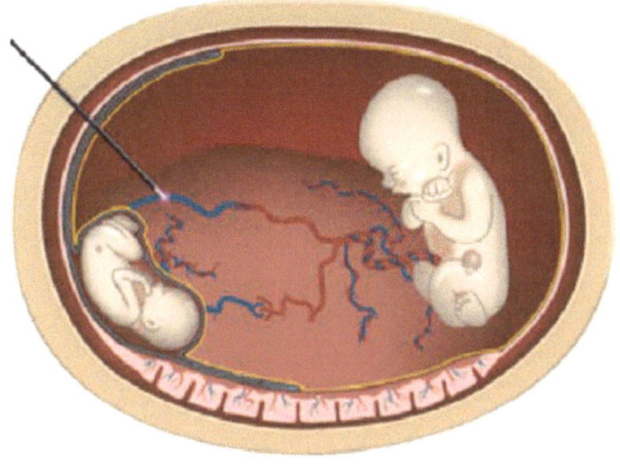

Fig. 30.87: Laser ablation of the placental anastomotic vessels selective cord coagulation

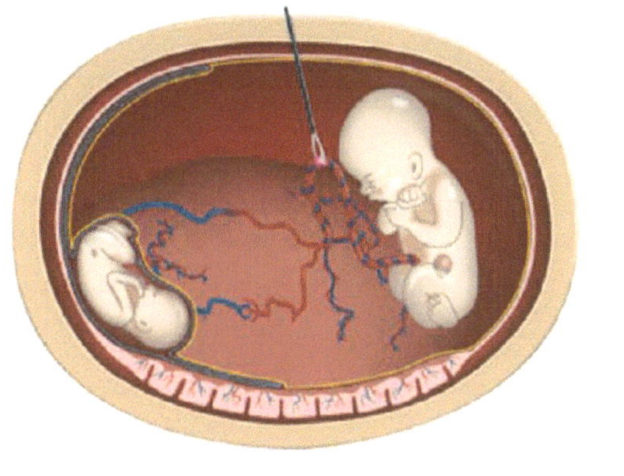

Fig. 30.88: Selective cord coagulation radiofrequency ablation

other twin. This procedure is used when laser ablation of the connecting vessels is not possible or if one of the twins is so close to death that laser ablation would likely not be successful. By stopping the flow in the cord of the dying twin, the other twin can be protected from the consequences of its sibling's death. The procedure is performed through the use of a special forceps that is placed into the amniotic sac of the recipient twin while watching with ultrasound. The umbilical cord is then grasped and electrical current is applied to burn (coagulate) the blood vessels in the cord so that the blood flow will stop to this fetus. The communication between the fetuses is definitively ended; however, this eliminates the chance of survival for one of the twins. Complications of this procedure include premature delivery and premature rupture of the membranes. Rupture of the membranes has been reported to occur in about 20% of cases. Survival of the one remaining fetus can be expected in 85% of cases.

Radiofrequency Ablation

This procedure is usually reserved for TRAP sequence. The umbilical cord of the acardiac fetus is usually very short and difficult to see on ultrasound (Fig. 36.88). As a result, it is often difficult to stop the blood flow into the acardiac fetus by coagulation of the umbilical cord. For this reason, a major blood vessel in the acardiac fetus is often targeted as the site for occlusion of blood flow. This can be accomplished through the use of a radiofrequency ablation catheter. In this procedure, a specialized needle is passed into the amniotic fluid and then into the body of the acardiac fetus. A special current is then applied to the needle to burn the area around the major blood vessel in the abnormal fetus. This will stop the blood flow and allow the pump twin (normal twin) to no longer have to send blood to the acardiac twin. Complications of infection, premature contractions and premature rupture of the membranes can occur as in any needle procedure. In one series, the risk for premature rupture of the membranes was 8%. In this same series, the chance for a successful live birth for the pump twin was 90%.

What Can I Expect After Surgery?

Following surgery, you will be taken to the recovery room in labor and delivery or a labor room where you and your fetus or fetuses will be closely monitored. Your abdomen will be a little tender or sore once the local anesthetic wears off. You may be given medications after surgery to relax the uterus and stop any contractions. The pain and discomfort after surgery is usually minimal. If needed, pain relief medicine is available. Your spouse or other support person may remain with you in your room. Following surgery, you may have food as tolerated. You will be admitted to the hospital for an overnight stay. That night, activity is restricted to bathroom privileges only, but this depends upon your specific condition. You will undergo an ultrasound the day after surgery to determine how the babies are doing.

What Can I Expect After I am Discharged Home?

You will then be discharged home to the care of your primary obstetrician and/or your referring maternal-fetal medicine specialist. Your instructions will include bed rest with bathroom privileges for 7 days after the surgery, with a gradual increase in activity. We will also ask that you get a thermometer and take your temperature 3 times per day. You should notify your primary obstetrician for any increase above 100.4°F of an oral temperature. The site of the surgery can get wet in a shower within 24 hours of the procedure. You can remove the steri-strips over the incision yourself 1 week after the surgery.

After 4 weeks you can resume normal activity based on your pregnancy condition and the comfort level of your primary obstetrician. Weekly ultrasounds are recommended for the next month. After that time, if all is going well, ultrasounds are performed as directed by your doctor.

Although you are returning home, we will continue to follow your pregnancy closely through our care coordinator. Please make arrangements with your doctor to forward your ultrasound reports and any other pertinent information to us. We also ask that you inform your obstetrician and labor nurse that we would like to have your placenta sent back to us after you delivery. This information is useful to further our knowledge and will assist in the future treatment of patients with TTTS.

Social services and pastoral care are available for all our patients and their families. If you would like to see them at any time, you need only to request it and they can be contacted. We are sensitive to the psychological, social and spiritual needs of our families. We will provide any support that is necessary. Please contact us if you have any questions, concerns or special requests. For our out of town patients, we realize that traveling may be difficult or stressful and want you to know that we will do everything we can to accommodate your special needs and schedule.

Future Directions

There is much that remains to be learned about the benefits and potential adverse effects of FCI. Although pharmacological FCI is well established in the management of fetal arrhythmias and heart block, there is room for improvement nonetheless. In addition, novel pharmacological strategies, such as maternal hyperoxia, and the prospect of other agents for other conditions will inevitably emerge. On the basis of the experimental evidence, open FCI appears feasible, although the indications for and establishment of open FCI in humans must be explored critically. There are severe congenital cardiac anomalies for which more complex interventions may be beneficial, such as severe Ebstein's malformation with fetal hydrops.

Ultimately, the utility of FCI will depend on a variety of clinical and technological factors, including more frequent, earlier diagnosis of congenital heart disease in-utero, characterization of prognostic features in fetuses with congenital heart disease, better understanding of the capacity and optimal gestational windows for cardiovascular remodeling after FCI, and improved and focused technology. Advances in imaging and instrumentation should facilitate greater precision and effectiveness of intervention and may open the door to procedures for more complex indications. More sophisticated image-guided or robotic interventional approaches to closed FCI are being explored and may help improve precision and success, potentially shifting the gestational horizon to allow safe intervention in younger fetuses. At the same time, as experience with FCI accumulates, risk profiles can be expected to improve, which may facilitate FCI for less severe conditions if such procedures can be expected to improve outcomes.

BIBLIOGRAPHY AND ACKNOWLEDGEMENT

- Ahuja P, Sdek P, MacLellan WR. Cardiac myocyte cell cycle control in development, disease, and regeneration. Physiol Rev 2007;87:521–44.
- Arzt W, Tulzer G, Aigner M, Mair R, Hafner E. Invasive intrauterine treatment of pulmonary atresia/intact ventricular septum with heart failure. Ultrasound Obstet Gynecol 2003; 21:186–8.
- Battaglia C, Artini PG, D'Ambrogio G, Bencini S, Galli PA, Genazzani AR. Maternal hyperoxygenation in the treatment of mild intrauterine growth retardation: a pilot study. Ultrasound Obstet Gynecol 1994;4:472–5.
- Carpenter R, Strasburger JF, Garson A, Smith RT, Deter RL, Englehardt H. Fetal ventricular pacing for hydrops secondary to complete atrioventricular block. J Am Coll Cardiol 1986;8:1434–6.
- Cortes RA, Farmer DL. Recent advances in fetal surgery. Semin Perinatol 2004;28:199–211.
- Dickinson JE, Evans SF. The progression of disease stage in twin-twin transfusion syndrome. J Matern Fetal Neonatal Med 2004;16:95–101.
- Eibschitz I, Abinader EG, Klein A, Sharf M. Intrauterine diagnosis and control of fetal ventricular arrhythmia during labor. Am J Obstet Gynecol 1975;122:597–600.
- Fenton KM, Heinemann MK, Hanley FL. Exclusion of the placenta during fetal cardiac bypass allows improved systemic perfusion and provides important information about the mechanism of placental injury. J Thorac Cardiovasc Surg 1993;105:502–12
- Fenton KN, Heinemann MK, Klautz RJM, Liddicoat JR, Hanley FL. Inhibition of fetal stress response improves cardiac output and gas exchange after fetal cardiac bypass. J Thorac Cardiovasc Surg 1994;107:1416–22.
- Fenton KN, Zinn HE, Heinemann MK, Liddicoat JR, Hanley FL. Long-term survivors of fetal cardiac bypass in lambs. J Thorac Cardiovasc Surg 1994;107:1423–7.
- Fesslova V, Vignati G, Brucato A, De Sanctis M, Butera G, Pisoni MP, Chiappa E, Acaia B, Meroni PL. The impact of treatment of the fetus by maternal therapy on the fetal and postnatal outcomes for fetuses diagnosed with isolated complete atrioventricular block. Cardiol Young 2009;19:282–90.
- Friedman DM, Kim MY, Copel JA, Llanos C, Davis C, Buyon JP. Prospective evaluation of fetuses with autoimmune- associated congenital heart block followed in the PR Interval and Dexamethasone Evaluation (PRIDE) Study. Am J Cardiol 2009;103:1102–6.
- Galindo A, Gutierrez-Larraya F, Velasco JM, de la Fuente P. Pulmonary balloon valvuloplasty in a fetus with critical pulmonary stenosis/atresia with intact ventricular septum and heart failure. Fetal Diagn Ther 2006;21:100–4.
- Gurtner GC, Werner S, Barrandon Y, Longaker MT. Wound repair and regeneration. Nature 2008;453:314–21.
- Hecher K, Plath H, Bregenzer T, Hansmann M, Hackeloer BJ. Endoscopic laser surgery versus serial amniocenteses in the treatment of severe twin-twin transfusion syndrome. Am J Obstet Gynecol 1999;180:717–24.
- Jaeggi ET, Fouron JC, Silverman ED, Ryan G, Smallhorn J, Hornberger LK. Transplacental fetal treatment improves the outcome of prenatally diagnosed complete atrioventricular block without structural heart disease. Circulation 2004;110: 1542–8.

- Kleinman CS, Donnerstein RL, DeVore GR, Jaffe CC, Lynch DC, Berkowitz RL, Talner NS, Hobbins JC. Fetal echocardiography for evaluation of in utero congestive heart failure. N Engl J Med 1982;306:568–75.
- Kohl T, Breuer J, Heep A, Wenningmann I, Weinbach J, Gembruch U. Fetal transesophageal echocardiography during balloon valvuloplasty for severe aortic valve stenosis at 28+6 weeks of gestation. J Thorac Cardiovasc Surg 2007; 134:256–7.
- Kohl T, Müller A, Tchatcheva K, Achenbach S, Gembruch U. Fetal transesophageal echocardiography: clinical introduction as a monitoring tool during cardiac intervention in a human fetus. Ultrasound Obstet Gynecol 2005;26:780–5.
- Kohl T, Sharland G, Allan LD, Gembruch U, Chaoui R, Lopes LM, Zielinsky P, Huhta J, Silverman NH. World experience of percutaneous ultrasound-guided balloon valvuloplasty in human fetuses with severe aortic valve obstruction. Am J Cardiol 2000;85:1230–3.
- Kunisaki SM, Jennings RW. Fetal surgery. J Intensive Care Med 2008;23:33–51.
- Lee H, Wagner A, Bobert B, et al. Radiofrequency ablation for TRAP sequence. Am J Obstet Gynecol 2005;191:S18.
- Maeno Y, Himeno W, Saito A, Hiraishi S, Hirose O, Ikuma M, Inamura N, Kawataki M, Mizukami A, Ota M, Shiraishi H, Satomi G, Kato H. Clinical course of fetal congenital atrioventricular block in the Japanese population: a multi-centre experience. Heart 2005;91:1075–9.
- Mari G, Roberts A, Detti L, et al. Perinatal morbidity and mortality rates in severe twin-twin transfusion syndrome: results of the International Amnioreduction Registry. Am J Obstet Gynecol 2001;185:708–15.
- Marshall AC, Levine J, Morash D, Silva V, Lock JE, Benson CB, Wilkins-Haug LE, McElhinney DB, Tworetzky W. Results of in utero atrial septoplasty in fetuses with hypoplastic left heart syndrome. Prenat Diagn 2008;28:1023–8.
- Marshall AC, van der Velde ME, Tworetzky W, Gomez CA, Wilkins-Haug L, Benson CB, Jennings RW, Lock JE. Creation of an atrial septal defect in utero for fetuses with hypoplastic left heart syndrome and intact or highly restrictive atrial septum. Circulation 2004;110:253–8.
- McElhinney DB, Marshall AC, Wilkins-Haug LE, Brown DW, Benson CB, Silva V, Marx GR, Mizrahi-Arnaud A, Lock JE, Tworetzky W. Predictors of technical success and postnatal biventricular outcome after in utero aortic valvuloplasty for aortic stenosis with evolving hypoplastic left heart syndrome. Circulation 2009;120:1482–90.
- Mizrahi-Arnaud A, Tworetzky W, Bulich LA, Wilkins-Haug LE, Marshall AC, Benson CB, Lock JE, McElhinney DB. Pathophysiology, management, and outcomes of fetal hemodynamic instability during prenatal cardiac intervention. Pediatr Res. 2007;62:325–30.
- Moise KJ, Jr., Dorman K, Lamvu G, et al. A randomized trial of amnioreduction versus septostomy in the treatment of twin-twin transfusion syndrome. Am J Obstet Gynecol 2005; 193:701–7.
- Newburger JW, Keane JF. Intrauterine supraventricular tachycardia. J Pediatr 1979;95:780–6.
- Oudijk MA, Michon MM, Kleinman CS, Kapusta L, Stoutenbeek P, Visser GH, Meijboom EJ. Sotalol in the treatment of fetal dysrhythmias. Circulation 2000;101: 2721–6.
- Parry AJ, Petrossian E, McElhinney DB, Reddy VM, Hanley FL. Neutrophil degranulation and complement activation during fetal cardiac bypass. Ann Thorac Surg 2000;70: 582–9.
- Patel D, Cuneo B, Viesca R, Rassanan J, Leshko J, Huhta J. Digoxin for the treatment of fetal congestive heart failure with sinus rhythm assessed by cardiovascular profile score. J Matern Fetal Neonatal Med 2008;21:477–82.
- Pomini F, Noia G, Mancuso S. Hypothetical role of prosta-glandins in the onset of preterm labor after fetal surgery. Fetal Diagn Ther 2007;22:94–9.
- Quintero RA, Dickinson JE, Morales WJ, et al. Stage-based treatment of twin-twin transfusion syndrome. Am J Obstet Gynecol 2003;188:1333–40.
- Quintero RA, Huhta J, Suh E, Chmait R, Romero R, Angel J. In utero cardiac fetal surgery: laser atrial septotomy in the treatment of hypoplastic left heart syndrome with intact atrial septum. Am J Obstet Gynecol 2005;193:1424–8.
- Quintero RA, Morales WJ, Allen MH, Bornick PW, Johnson PK, Kruger M. Staging of twin-twin transfusion syndrome. J Perinatol 1999;19:550–5.
- Reddy VM, Liddicoat JR, Klein JR, McElhinney DB, Wampler RK, Hanley FL. Fetal cardiac bypass using an in-line axial flow pump to minimize extracorporeal surface and avoid priming volume. Ann Thorac Surg 1996;62:393–400.
- Reddy VM, Liddicoat JR, Klein JR, Wampler RK, Hanley FL. Long-term fetal outcome after fetal cardiac bypass: fetal survival to full term and organ abnormalities. J Thorac Cardiovasc Surg 1996;111:536–44.
- Richter RC, Slate RK, Rudolph AM, Turley K. Fetal blood flow during hypothermic cardiopulmonary bypass in utero. J Cardiovasc Surg 1985;26:86.
- Sabik JF, Assad RS, Hanley FL. Prostaglandin synthesis inhibition prevents placental dysfunction after fetal cardiac bypass. J Thorac Cardiovasc Surg 1992;103:733–42.
- Selamet Tierney ES, Wald RM, McElhinney DB, Marshall AC, Benson CB, Marcus EN, Marx GR, Levine JC, Wilkins-Haug L, Lock JE, Tworetzky W. Changes in left heart hemodynamics after technically successful in utero aortic valvuloplasty. Ultrasound Obstet Gynecol 2007;30:715–20.
- Strasburger JF, Cuneo BF, Michon MM, Gotteiner NL, Deal BJ, McGregor SN, Oudijk MA, Meijboom EJ, Feinkind L, Hussey M, Parilla BV. Amiodarone therapy for drugrefractory fetal tachycardia. Circulation 2004;109:375–9.

31 Robotic Assisted Cardiac Interventions

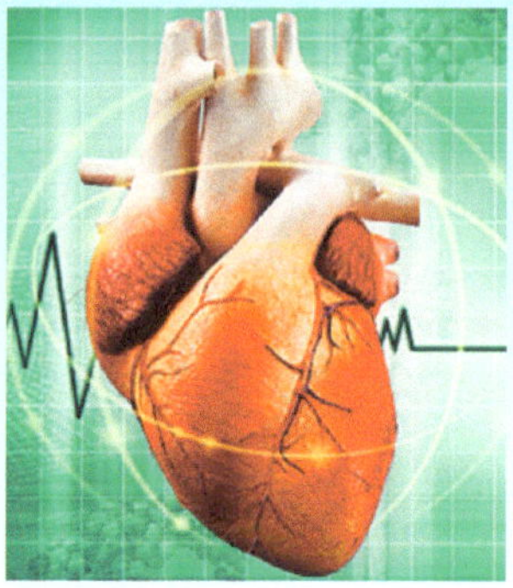

The Minimally Invasive Cardiac Surgery was invented by Francis Duhaylongsod, a Filipino heart surgeon in Hawaii. The first minimally invasive heart cardiac surgery was performed in the United States on January 21, 2005 at The Heart Institute at Staten Island University Hospital in Staten Island, New York by a team led by Dr. Joseph T. McGinn. This technique is an off-pump coronary artery bypass surgery. The procedure is much less invasive than traditional bypass surgery because it's performed through three small incisions rather than the traditional sternotomy. Since its first procedure, over 600 MICS CABG procedures have been performed at The Heart Institute amongst many more around the world.

Minimally invasive heart surgery (also called keyhole surgery) is performed through small incisions, sometimes using specialized surgical instruments. The incision used for minimally invasive heart surgery is about 3 to 4 inches instead of the 6- to 8-inch incision required for traditional surgery.

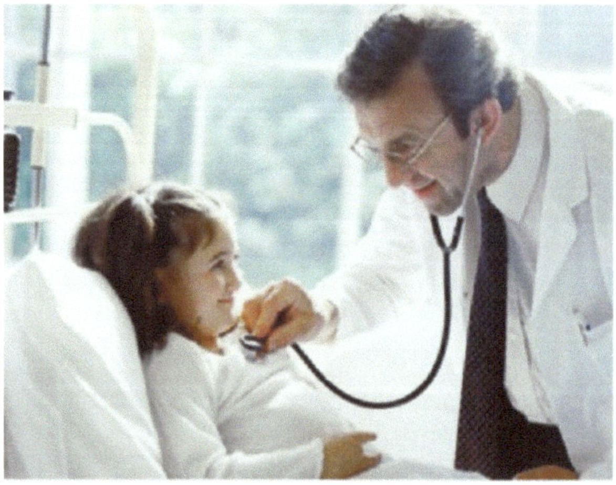

Fig. 31.1: *A young child is being examined by the cardiac surgeon for cardiovascular fitness prior to Robotic heart surgery*

Selection of Patients for Minimally Invasive or Robotic Surgery

Your surgeon will review the results of your diagnostic tests before your scheduled surgery to determine if you are a candidate for a minimally invasive or robotic surgery technique. The surgical team will carefully compare the advantages and disadvantages of these techniques with those of traditional surgery.

The type of treatment recommended for your condition depends on several factors, including the type and severity of heart disease, age, medical history and lifestyle.

The Procedure

MICS CABG is performed through one window incision that stretches 5–7 cm in the 4th intercostal space (ICS). In some cases the thoractomy may be necessary in the 5th ICS instead. A soft tissue refractor is used to allow for greater visibility and access.

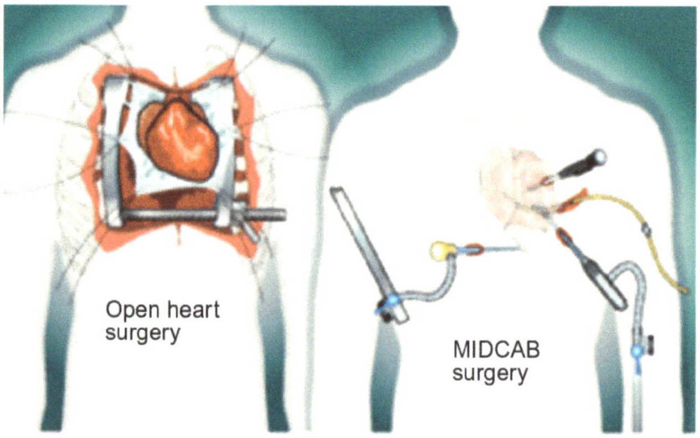

Fig. 31. 2: *Cardiac surgeons are operating on the heart through tiny openings in the chest, eliminating the need for sternotomy--a large incision through the breastbone (sternum). This method of surgery, called minimally invasive cardiac surgery, is a remarkable improvement over traditional, open-chest procedures.*

Two access incisions are also made at the 6th intercostal space and xphoid process to allow for operative Medtronic® instruments to pass through.

The McGinn Technique (Proximal Anastomoses)

The McGinn Proximal Technique is performed with blood pressure lowered to 90–100 systolic which reduces stress to the aorta, reducing the risk of damage. A series of tools are used to position and stabilize vessels. The technique uses devices developed by Medtronic® to support the surrounding heart tissues while vital surgery takes place. The devices are managed externally and access the heart through small incisions between the ribs.

Pump-Assisted Beating Heart Bypass

A cannula with a pump and vacuum action is fed up through an artery in the groin to reduce the stress on the heart so that it may still function during the operation. This pump flows at 2–3L per minute to support circulation and eliminates the need for a heart-lung bypass machine.

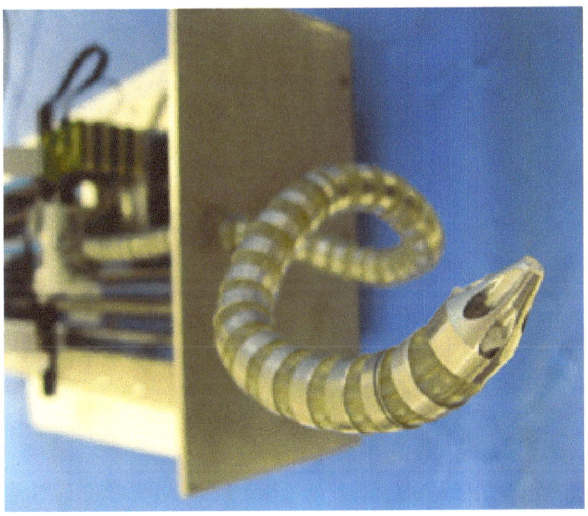

Fig. 31.3: *Serpentine Robots in Heart Surgery. Robotic Probe (HARP) to enter the thorax through a subxiphoid port and reach regions of the pericardium that are inaccessible with traditional techniques. It is believed that HARP's functionality will eventually lead to application such as multiple intrapericardial therapies (e.g. cell transplantation by intramyocardial injection, epicardial ablation, epicardial lead placement for resynchronization, etc)."*

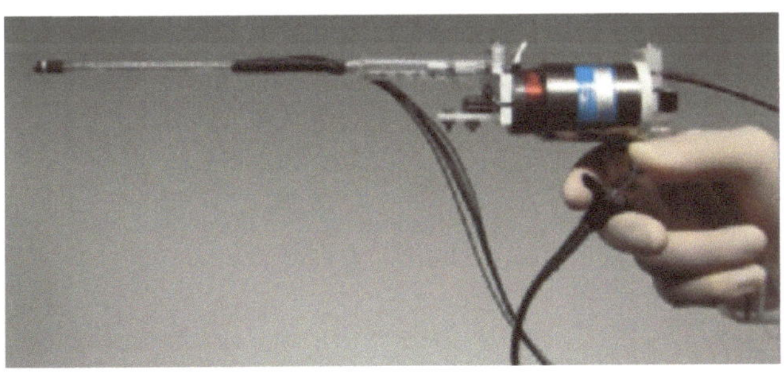

Fig. 31.4: *Biorobotics and its role in minimal-invasion cardia surgery (Image courtesy of Harvard SEAS)*

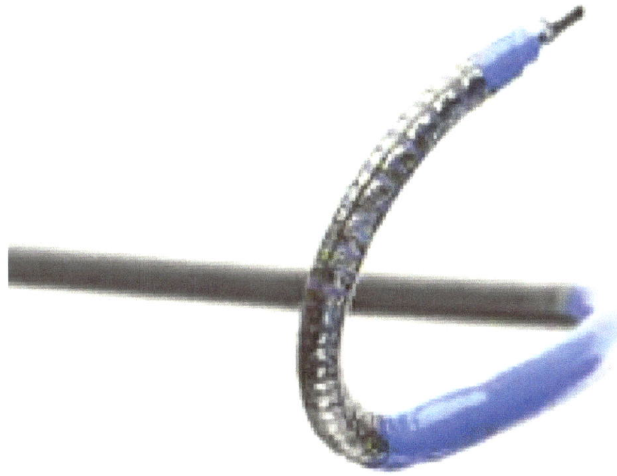

Fig. 31.5: *Hansen Medical's Robotic Catheter Control System for EP Study*

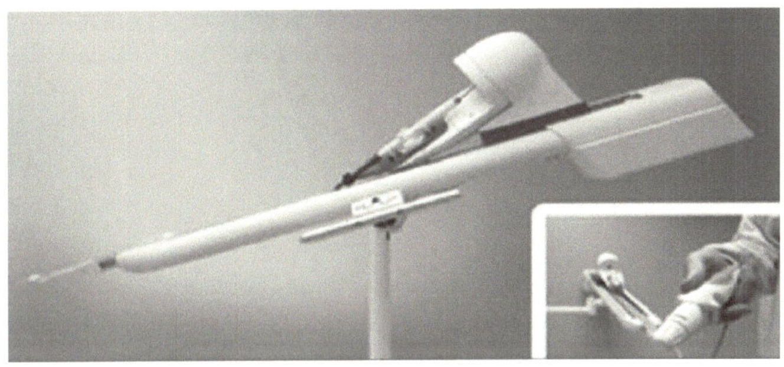

Fig. 31.6: *World's first remote heart rhythm treatment procedure using a Robotic Arm. The world's first remote robotic heart rhythm treatment procedure was conducted at the University Hospitals of Leicester. It was performed using the Catheter Robotics Remote Catheter Manipulation System. A patient with atrial fibrillation had a catheter ablation controlled by a robotic arm, while the cardiologist- sitting in a separate room - used remote control to steer the catheter endovascularly into the heart*

ROBOTICALLY ASSISTED HEART SURGERY

Robotically assisted heart surgery, also called closed-chest heart surgery, is a type of minimally invasive surgery. The cardiac surgeon uses a specially designed computer console to control surgical instruments on thin robotic arms. Robotically assisted technology allows surgeons to perform certain types of complex heart surgeries with smaller incisions and precise motion control, offering patients excellent outcomes. In robotic surgery, small incisions—less than 2 inches—are used, compared with the 3- to 4-inch incision used in traditional minimally invasive heart surgery.

Types of Robotically assisted Heart Surgeries

1. Robotic assisted CABG

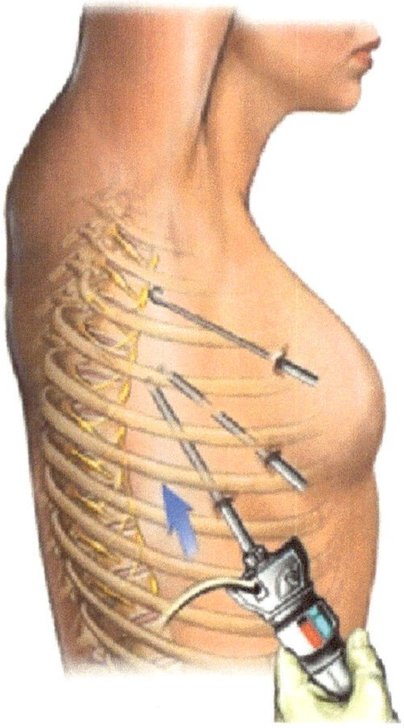

Fig. 31.7: *Sites of incisions endoscopes practiced in a operation theatre in conducting Robotic valve heart surgery*

2. Robotic assisted coronary angioplasty
3. Mitral valve repair and replacement surgery
4. Tricuspid valve repair and replacement surgery
5. Combined mitral and tricuspid valve surgery
6. Ablation of atrial fibrillation
7. Atrial septal defect (ASD) and PFO repair
8. Removal of cardiac tumors
9. Lead placement
10. Robot implant

Benefits of Minimally Invasive Surgical Techniques

The benefits of minimally invasive and robotic heart surgery techniques include:

1. Small incisions
2. Small scars
3. *Shorter hospital stay after surgery:* The average stay is 3 to 5 days after minimally invasive surgery, while the average stay after traditional heart surgery is 7 to 10 days
4. Low risk of infection
5. Low risk of bleeding and blood transfusion
6. Shorter recovery time and faster return to normal activities/work:

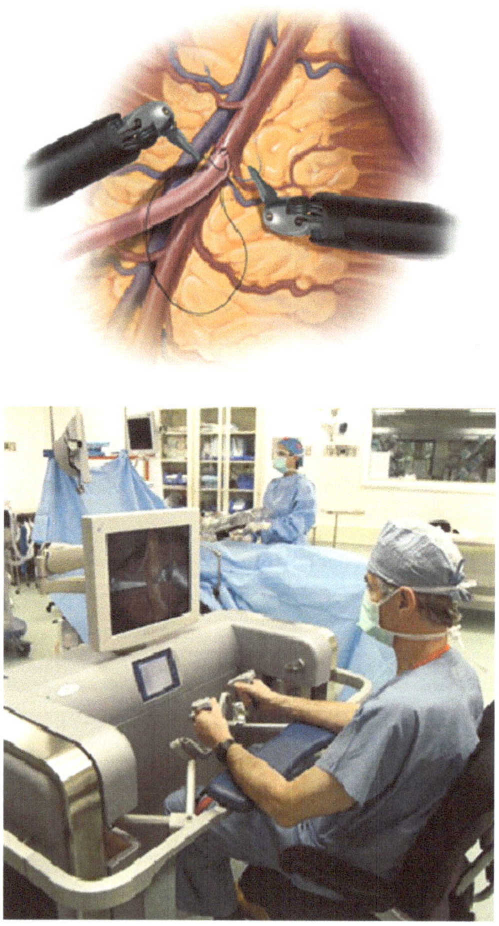

Fig. 31.8: *Robotic arms are performing coronary bypass with robot-assisted heart surgery, In this procedure a surgeon controls small surgical instruments attached to robotic arms*

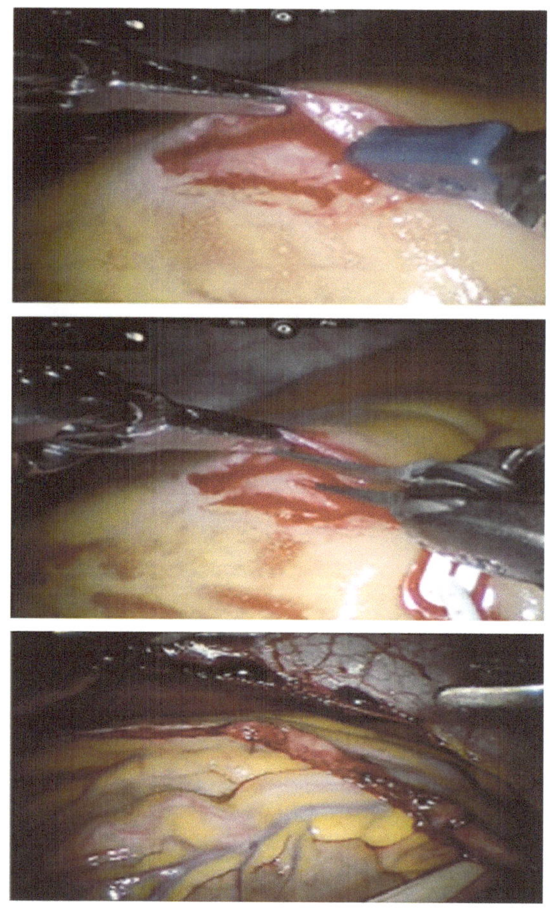

Fig. 31.9: *A. Opening of coronary with endoscopic knife. B. Coronary arteriotomy with endoscopic Pott scissors. C. Final result.in robotic coronary bypass surgery*

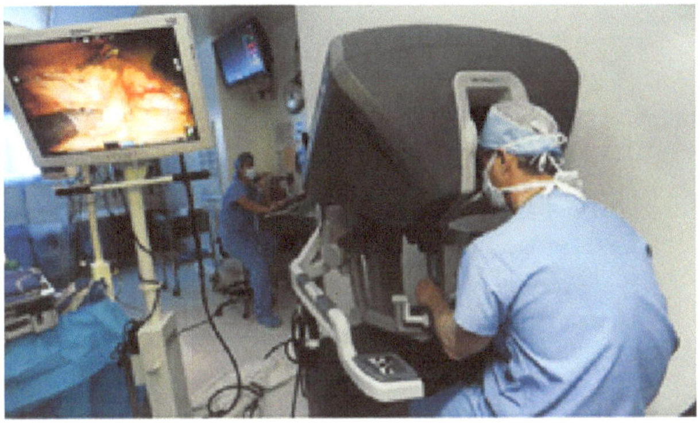

Fig. 31.10: *Surgeon is operating on patient with the help of the da Vinci's arms through the system's console (right)*

The average recovery time after minimally invasive surgery is 1 to 4 weeks, while the average recovery time after traditional heart surgery is 6 to 8 weeks. The recovery time and return to regular activities is shorter for patients who undergo robotically assisted heart surgery.

Division of the breastbone is not needed for robotically assisted heart surgery.

Important note: Not everyone is a candidate for these surgical techniques. Your surgeon will review the results of your diagnostic tests before your scheduled procedure to determine if you are a candidate for minimally invasive surgery. The surgical team will carefully compare the advantages and disadvantages of minimally invasive techniques versus traditional surgery techniques.

Types of Minimally Invasive Heart Surgeries

Minimally Invasive Valve Surgery

Valve surgeries, including valve repairs and valve replacements, are the most common type of minimally invasive surgery, accounting for 87 percent of all minimally invasive cardiac surgeries performed at Cleveland Clinic.

Minimally Invasive CABG Surgery

Minimally invasive direct coronary artery bypass graft (MIDCABG) surgery is an option for some patients who require a left internal mammary artery bypass graft to the left anterior descending artery.

Saphenous (leg) vein harvest also may be performed using small incisions.

Several techniques for minimally invasive CABG surgery are being explored at Cleveland Clinic, including surgeries performed on a beating (off-pump) or non-beating (on-pump) heart.

Off-pump/beating heart bypass surgery allows surgeons to perform surgery on the heart while it is still beating. A medication may be given to slow the heart during surgery, but the heart keeps beating during the procedure. This type of surgery may be an option for patients with single-vessel disease (such as disease of the left anterior descending artery or right coronary artery).

Traditionally, CABG surgery is performed using a heart-lung bypass machine. This machine allows the heart's beating to be stopped, so the surgeon can operate on a surface that is blood-free and still. The heart-lung bypass machine maintains life despite the lack of a heartbeat, removing carbon dioxide from the blood and replacing it with oxygen before pumping it around the body.

During off-pump/beating heart surgery, the heart-lung machine is not used. The surgeon uses advanced operating equipment to stabilize (hold) portions of the heart and bypass the blocked artery in a highly controlled operative environment. Meanwhile, the rest of the heart keeps pumping and circulating blood to the body.

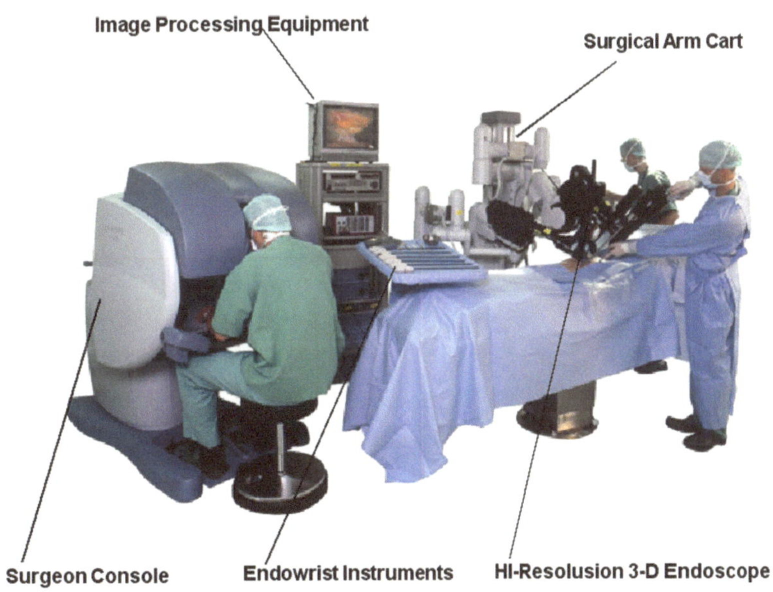

Fig. 31.11: *Different equipments in a operation theatre utilized in conducting Robotic heart surgery*

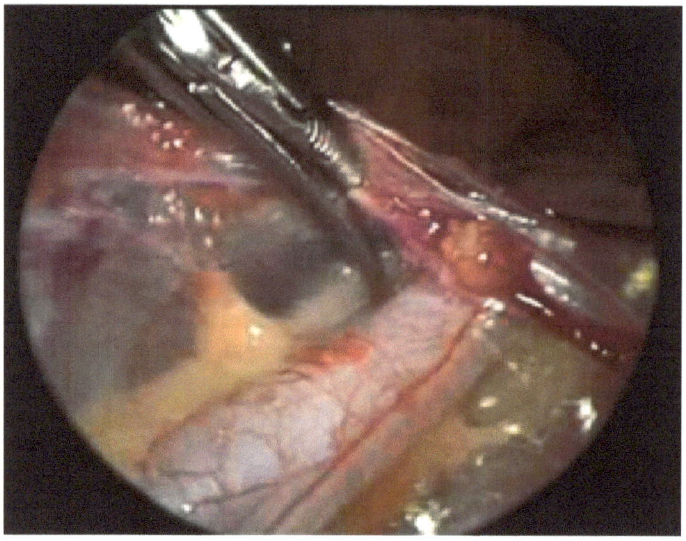

Fig. 31.12: *Videoscopic photograph taken from one of the patients undergoing Robotic heart surgery*

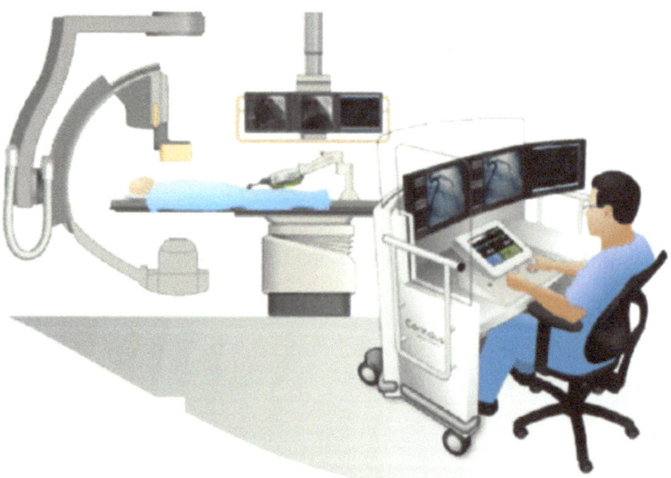

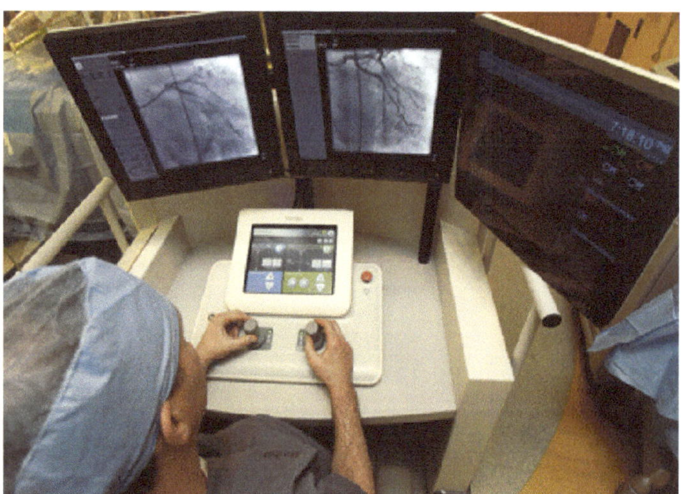

Fig. 31.13: *The method of performing robot-assisted coronary angioplasty*

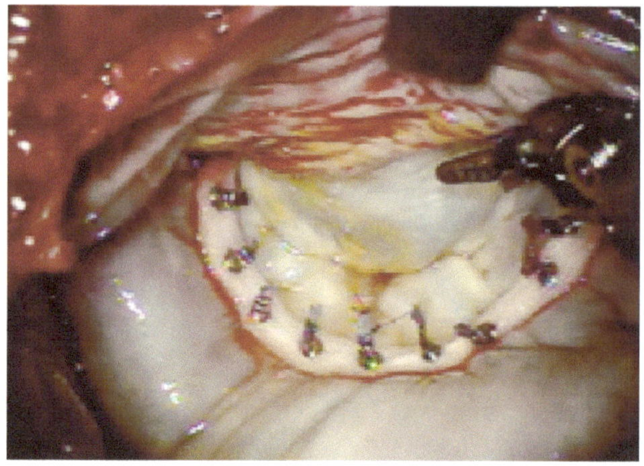

Fig. 31.14: *Intraoperative view of a competent mitral valve repaired using robotic assistance*

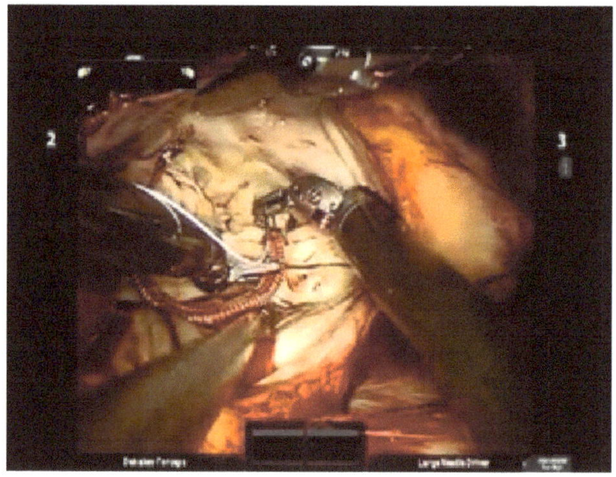

Fig. 31.15: *Robotic assisted mitral and tricuspid valve repair*

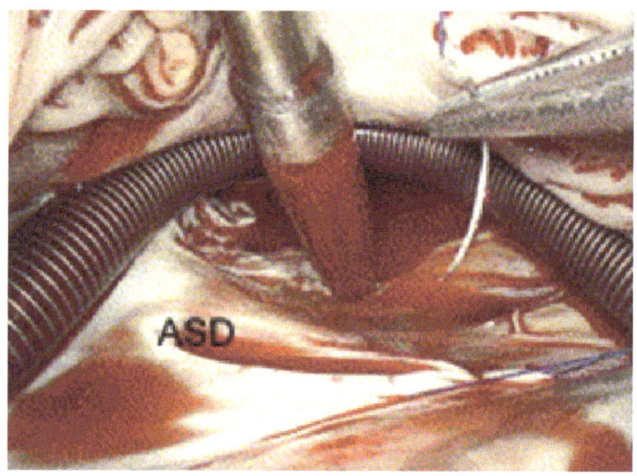

Fig. 31.16: *An intraoperative view of atrial septal defect (ASD that was closed by sutures?*

Types of Robotically Assisted Heart Surgeries

Robotically Assisted CABG Surgery

Robotically assisted CABG surgery can be performed without opening the sternum (breastbone). Robotically

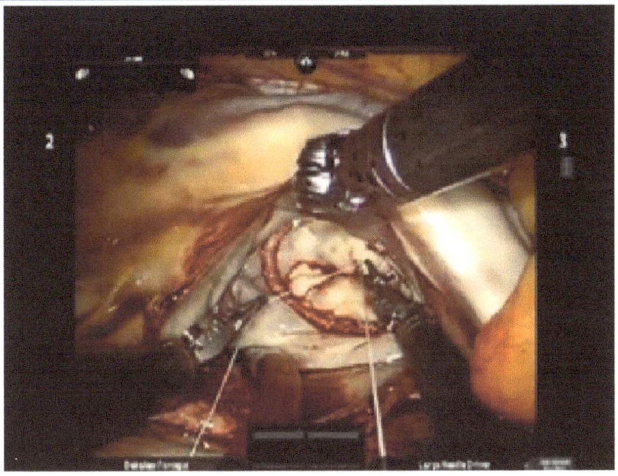

Fig. 31.17: *Robotic repair of mitral valve and PFO closure*

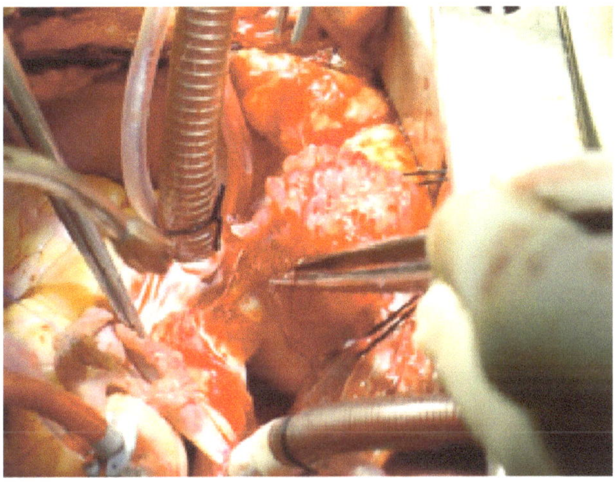

Fig. 31.18: *Intraoperative robotic surgery showing LA Myxoma on stalk*

assisted CABG surgery also can be performed "off pump," which means the surgery can be performed on a beating heart, without using the heart-lung bypass machine.

Robotically Assisted Valve Surgery

Robotically assisted mitral valve repair can be used to treat mitral valve regurgitation. Tricuspid valve surgery also can be performed using the robotically assisted surgical technique.

Robotically Assisted ASD and PFO Repair

Robotically assisted atrial septal defect (ASD) and patent foramen ovale (PFO) repair surgeries can be performed using a robotically assisted approach. Robotic instruments are used to harvest a small patch of pericardial tissue (the sac that surrounds the heart). The patch is then sutured (sewn) over the defect.

Robotically Assisted Removal of Cardiac Tumors

The most common benign tumor of the heart is a myxoma, which most frequently occurs in the left atrium. This type of tumor increases the risk of stroke. Removal of these tumors almost always cures the problem and greatly reduces the risk of stroke. During the robotically assisted tumor removal procedure, the surgeon's hands control the movement and placement of the endoscopic instruments through small incisions in the chest wall, and the instruments are used to remove the tumor.

Robotically assisted heart surgery is performed through a small working incision and three small incisions (ports) that are made in the spaces between the ribs . The surgical instruments (attached to the robotic arms) and one tiny camera are placed through these ports. Motion sensors are attached to the robotic "wrist," so the surgeon can control the movement and placement of the surgical instruments to perform the procedure

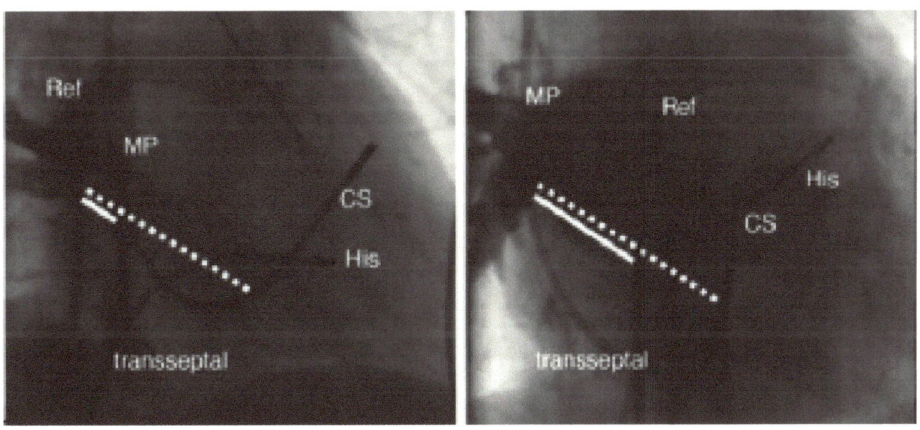

Fig. 31.19: *Remote Robotic Navigation and Electroanatomical Mapping for Ablation of Atrial FibrillationSelective angiographies of the RIPV (RAO 30°). The distance between the anterior border of the RPV ostium and the coronary sinus catheter (dCS, dotted line) and the transseptal puncture site (dTS, full line) were measured. The left panel shows a patient with a posterior transseptal puncture (ratio dCS:dTS, 0.12). The right panel shows a patient with an antero-medial transseptal puncture (ratio dCS:dTS, 0.68). CS indicates coronary sinus catheter; His, multipolar catheter at the His bundle; Ref, Reference catheter on the back of the patient; MP, multi-purpose catheter for angiography*

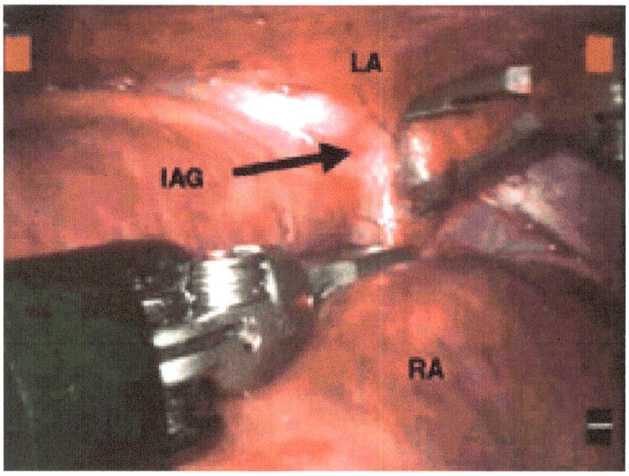

Fig. 31.20: *Atrial fibrillation. Robot-assisted ablation of the PVs Opening of the transverse and oblique sinus was performed robotically. Opening of the pericardial reflections between the superior right PV and the superior caval vein, and between the inferior right PV and the inferior caval vein, and development of the inter-atrial groove were also performed robotically.*

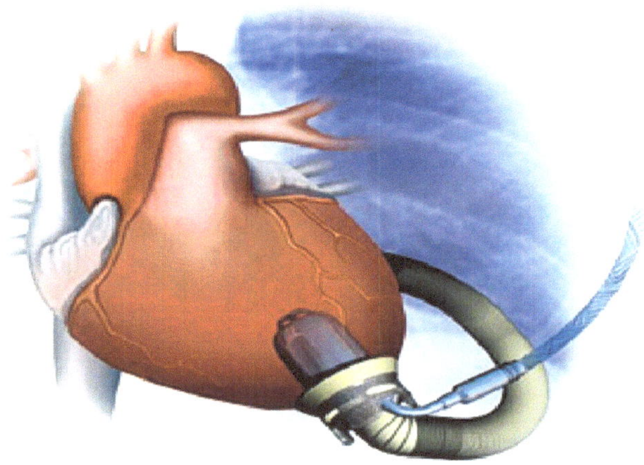

Fig. 31.21: *This type of Robot implant is to be used on a permanent basis rather than a more common temporary artificial heart*

During robotically assisted surgery, the sternum (breastbone) does not need to be opened to perform the procedure. Depending on the technique, the surgeon may choose to perform surgery on a "beating heart," in which case the patient is not placed on the heart-lung bypass machine (this is called"off-pump" surgery).

In comparison, traditional valve and CABG surgery involve using the heart-lung bypass machine to circulate the patient's oxygenated blood during surgery and stopping the heart in order to stabilize the blood vessels; creating a 6- to 8-inch incision through the sternum; and spreading the ribs to view the heart.

Robotically Assisted Atrial Fibrillation Surgery

During the robotically assisted ablation procedure for atrial fibrillation (an irregular heart rhythm that begins in the upper chambers of the heart), the surgeon's hands control the movement and placement of the endoscopic instruments to open the pericardium (thin sac that surrounds the heart). The instruments are used to precisely place the catheter for ablation, in which energy is applied to correct the abnormal heart rhythm

Robotically Assisted Device Implant for Heart Failure

During the robotically assisted biventricular pacemaker or defibrillator implant procedure, the surgeon's hands control the movement and placement of the endoscopic instruments through small incisions in the chest wall. This surgical technique can be used to place leads on the surface of the left ventricle. The leads then are attached to the biventricular device (defibrillator or pacemaker) to "resynchronize" the heartbeat and improve heart failure symptoms.

Patient's Health after Surgery

You may feel some discomfort at the incision site after surgery. You can take medications to help relieve this discomfort. Ask your doctor which medication you should take for pain relief. If you have discomfort in your chest

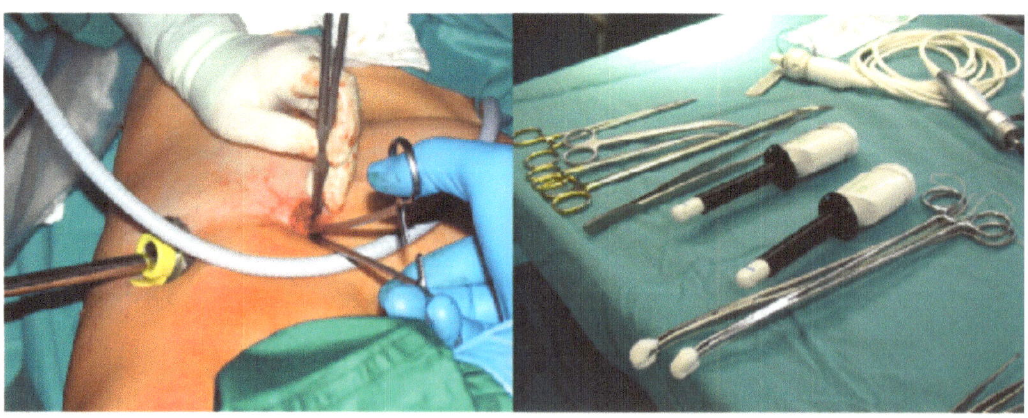

Fig. 31.22: *Instruments for epicardial lead implantation using the VATS two ports techniqueas done in resynchronization therapy in chronic heart failure*

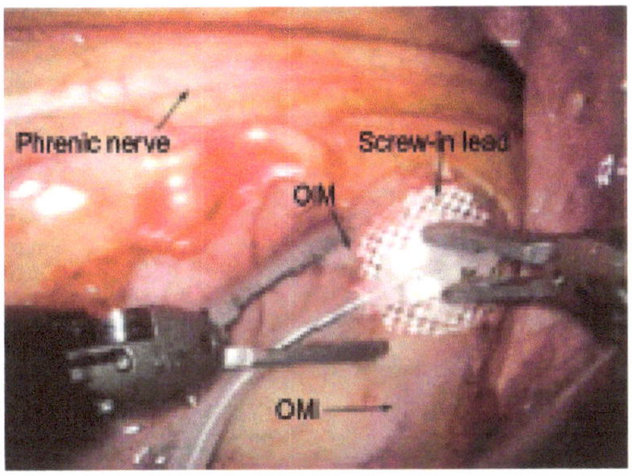

Fig. 31.23: *Robot-enhanced thoracoscopic approach may provide greater maneuverability in placement of an LV pacing lead on the lateral wall through small chest wall incisions*

that is similar to the symptoms you had before your surgery, call your doctor.

Recovery of Patient after Surgery

Patients who have minimally invasive or robotic surgery may be able to go home 2 to 5 days after surgery. Your healthcare team will follow your progress and help you recover as quickly as possible.

Your healthcare team will provide specific instructions for your recovery and return to work, including guidelines for activity, driving, incision care and diet.

Recovery after Minimally Invasive Heart Surgery

In general, you may be able to return to work (if you have a sedentary job), resume driving and participate in most non-strenuous activities within 1 to 4 weeks after traditional minimally invasive heart surgery. You can resume heavy lifting and other more strenuous activities within 5 to 8 weeks after surgery. Your healthcare team will provide specific guidelines based on your rate of recovery.

Recovery after Robotically assisted Heart Surgery

The recovery time after robotically assisted heart surgery is shorter than traditional minimally invasive heart surgery. Most patients can resume normal activities, drive and return to work as soon as they feel up to it—usually within 2 to four weeks after surgery. Your healthcare team will provide specific guidelines based on your rate of recovery.

Recovery for All Patients after Heart Surgery

To maintain your cardiovascular health after surgery, we strongly encourage you to make lifestyle changes and take your medications as prescribed. Heart-healthy lifestyle changes that are important to your recovery include:

- Quitting smoking
- Treating high cholesterol
- Managing high blood pressure and diabetes
- Exercising regularly

BIBLIOGRAPHY AND ACKNOWLEDGEMENT

- Argenziano M, Katz M, Bonatti J, et al. Results of the prospective multicenter trial of robotically assisted totally endoscopic coronary artery bypass grafting. Ann Thorac Surg. 2006;81(5):1666–1675. [PubMed]
- Aris A, Cámara ML, Montiel J, Delgado LJ, Galán J, Litvan H. Ministernotomy versus median sternotomy for aortic valve replacement: a prospective, randomized study. Ann Thorac Surg. 1999;67(6):1583–1588.
- Bonatti J, Schachner T, Bernecker O, et al. Robotic totally endoscopic coronary artery bypass: program development and learning curve issues. J Thorac Cardiovasc Surg. 2004;127(2):504–510.
- Bonatti J, Schachner T, Bonaros N, et al. How to improve performance of robotic totally endoscopic coronary artery bypass grafting. Am J Surg. 2008;195(5):711–716.
- Bonatti J, Schachner T, Bonaros N, et al. Robotic totally endoscopic double-vessel bypass grafting: a further step toward closed-chest surgical treatment of multivessel coronary artery disease. Heart Surg Forum. 2007;10:E239– E242.
- Brinkman WT, Hoffman W, Dewey TM, et al. Aortic valve replacement surgery: comparison of outcomes in matched sternotomy and PORT ACCESS groups. Ann Thorac Surg. 2010;90(1):131–135.
- Carpentier A, Loulmet D, Aupècle B, et al. Computer assisted open heart surgery First case operated on with success. CR Acad Sci III. 1998;321:437– 42.
- Carpentier A, Loulmet D, Carpentier A, et al. Open heart operation under videosurgery and minithoracotomy First case (mitral valvuloplasty) operated with success. CR Acad Sci. 1996;319(3):219–223
- Casselman FP, Van Slycke S, Wellens F, et al. Mitral valve surgery can now routinely be performed endoscopically. Circulation. 2003;108(Suppl 1):II48–II54.
- Chitwood WR, Jr, Elbeery JR, Chapman WH, et al. Videoassisted minimally invasive mitral valve surgery: the 'micromitral' operation. J Thorac Cardiovasc Surg. 1997;113(2):413– 414.
- Chitwood WR, Jr, Elbeery JR, Moran JF. Minimally invasive mitral valve repair: using a minithoracotomy and transthoracic aortic occlusion. Ann Thorac Surg. 1997;63:1477–1479.
- Chitwood WR., Jr Current status of endoscopic and robotic mitral valve surgery. Ann Thorac Surg. 2005;79(6):S2248–S2253
- Cohn LH, Adams DH, Couper GS, Bichell DP. Minimally invasive aortic valve replacement. Semin Thorac Cardiovasc Surg. 1997;9(4):331–336.

- Cohn LH, Adams DH, Couper GS, et al. Minimally invasive cardiac valve surgery improves patient satisfaction while reducing costs of cardiac valve replacement and repair. Ann Surg. 1997;226(4):421 428. [PMC free article].
- Cohn LH. Fifty years of open-heart surgery. Circulation. 2003;107(17):2168–2170.
- Cohn WE. Advances in surgical treatment of acute and chronic coronary artery disease. Tex Heart Inst J. 2010;37(3):328–330.
- Corbi P, Rahmati M, Donal E, et al. Prospective comparison of minimally invasive and standard techniques for aortic valve replacement: initial experience in the first hundred patients. J Card Surg. 2003;18(2):133–139.
- Cosgrove DM, 3rd, Sabik JF, Navia JL. Minimally invasive valve operations. Ann Thorac Surg. 1998;65(6):1535–1538.
- Cosgrove DM, 3rd, Sabik JF. Minimally invasive approach for aortic valve operations. Ann Thorac Surg. 1996;62(2):596–597.
- de Canniere D, Wimmer-Greinecker G, Cichon R, et al. Feasibility, safety, and efficacy of totally endoscopic coronary artery bypass grafting: Multicenter European experience. J Thorac Cardiovasc Surg. 2007;134:710–716.
- de Vaumas C, Philip I, Daccache G, et al. Comparison of minithoracotomy and conventional sternotomy approaches for valve surgery. J Cardiothorac Vasc Anesth. 2003;17(3):325–328.
- Detter C, Reichenspurner H, Boehm DH, et al. Minimally invasive direct coronary artery bypass grafting (MIDCAB) and off-pump coronary artery bypass grafting (OPCAB), two techniques for beating heart surgery. Heart Surg Forum. 2002;5:157–162.
- Estrera AL, Reardon MJ. Current approaches to minimally invasive aortic valve surgery. Curr Opin Cardiol. 2000;15(2):91–95.
- Falk V, Walther T, Autschbach R, Diegeler A, Battellini R, Mohr FW. Robot-assisted minimally invasive solo mitral valve operation. J Thorac Cardiovasc Surg. 1998;115(2):470–471.
- Farhat F, Lu Z, Lefevre M, et al. Prospective comparison between total sternotomy and ministernotomy for aortic valve replacement. J Card Surg. 2003;18(5):396–402.
- Galloway AC, Schwartz CF, Ribakove GH, et al. A decade of minimally invasive mitral repair: long-term outcomes. Ann Thorac Surg. 2009;88:1180–1184.
- Gammie JS, Bartlett ST, Griffith BP. Small-incision mitral valve repair: safe, durable, and approaching perfection. Ann Surg. 2009;250(3):409–415.
- Gammie JS, Zhao Y, Peterson ED, O'Brien SM, Rankin JS, Griffith BP. Less-invasive mitral valve operations trends and outcomes from the society of thoracic surgeons adult cardiac surgery database. Ann Thorac Surg. 2010;90:1401–1410.
- Gaudiani VA, Grunkemeier GL, Castro LJ, Fisher AL, Wu Y. Mitral valve operations through standard and smaller incisions. Heart Surg Forum. 2004;7(4):E337–E342.
- Greenspun HG, Adourian UA, Fonger JD, Fan JS. Minimally invasive direct coronary artery bypass (MIDCAB), surgical techniques and anesthetic considerations. J Cardiothorac Vasc Anesth. 1996;10:507–509.
- Grossi EA, Galloway AC. Minimally invasive mitral valve surgery: a 6-year experience with 714 patients. Ann Thorac Surg. 2002;74(3):660–664
- Grossi EA, LaPietra A, Ribakove GH, et al. Minimally invasive versus sternotomy approaches for mitral reconstruction: comparison of intermediate-term results. J Thorac Cardiovasc Surg. 2001;121(4):708–713.
- Holzhey DM, Jacobs S, Mochalski M, et al. Seven-year followup after minimally invasive direct coronary artery bypass: experience with more than 1300 patients. Ann Thorac Surg. 2007;83(1):108–114.
- Iribarne A, Karpenko A, Russo MJ, et al. Eight-year experience with minimally invasive cardiothoracic surgery. World J Surg. 2010;34(4):611–615.
- Iribarne A, Russo MJ, Easterwood R, et al. Minimally invasive versus sternotomy approach for mitral valve surgery: a propensity analysis. Ann Thorac Surg. 2010;90(5):1471–1477.
- Iribarne A, Russo MJ, Moskowitz AJ, Ascheim DD, Brown LD, Gelijns AC. Assessing technological change in cardiothoracic surgery. Semin Thorac Cardiovasc Surg. 2009;21(1):28–34.
- Kiaii B, McClure RS, Stewart P, et al. Simultaneous integrated coronary artery revascularization with long-term angiographic follow-up. J Thorac Cardiovasc Surg. 2008;136:702–708
- Korach A, Shemin RJ, Hunter CT, Bao Y, Shapira OM. Minimally invasive versus conventional aortic valve replacement: a 10-year experience. J Cardiovasc Surg (Torino) 2010;51(3):417–421.
- Kronzon I, Matros TG. Intraoperative echocardiography in minimally invasive cardiac surgery and novel cardiovascular surgical techniques. Am Heart Hosp J. 2004;2(4):198–204.
- Lapierre H, Chan V, Ruel M. Off-pump coronary surgery through mini-incisions: is it reasonable? Curr Opin Cardiol. 2006;21(6):578–583..
- Loulmet DF, Carpentier A. Less invasive techniques for mitral valve surgery. J Thorac Cardiovasc Surg. 1998;115(4):772–779.
- Machler HE, Bergmann P. Minimally invasive versus conventional aortic valve operations: a prospective study in 120 patients. Ann Thorac Surg. 1999;67(4):1001–1005.
- Mathew JP, Parks R, Savino JS, et al. Atrial fibrillation following coronary artery bypass graft surgery: predictors, outcomes, and resource utilization MultiCenter Study of Perioperative Ischemia Research Group. JAMA. 1996;276:300–306.
- Mihaljevic T, Cohn LH, Unic D, Aranki SF, Couper GS, Byrne JG. One thousand minimally invasive valve operations: early and late results. Ann Surg. 2004;240(3):529–534.

- Mohr FW, Falk V, Diegeler A, Walther T, van Son JA, Autschbach R. Minimally invasive port-access mitral valve surgery. J Thorac Cardiovasc Surg. 1998;115(3):567–576.
- Morgan JA, Thornton BA, Peacock JC, et al. Does robotic technology make minimally invasive cardiac surgery too expensive? A hospital cost analysis of robotic and conventional techniques. J Card Surg. 2005;20(3):246–251.
- Morishita A, Shimakura T, Miyagishima M, et al. Minimally invasive direct redo coronary artery bypass grafting. Ann Thorac Cardiovasc Surg. 2002;8(4):209–212.
- Navia JL, Cosgrove DM. Minimally invasive mitral valve operations. Ann Thorac Surg. 1996;62:1542–1544.
- Novick RJ, Fox SA, Kiaii BB, et al. Analysis of the learning curve in telerobotic, beating heart coronary artery bypass grafting: a 90 patient experience. Ann Thorac Surg. 2003;76(3):749–753.
- Pascucci S, Gunkel L, Zietak T, et al. Use of MIDCAB procedure for redo coronary artery bypass. J Cardiovasc Surg. 2002;43(2):143–146
- Pisano GP, Bohmer RM. Organizational differences in rates of learning: evidence from the adoption of minimally invasive cardiac surgery. Manag Sci. 2001;47(6):752–768.
- Plass A, Scheffel H, Alkadhi H, et al. Aortic valve replacement through a minimally invasive approach: preoperative planning, surgical technique, and outcome. Ann Thorac Surg. 2009;88(6):1851–1856.
- Puskas J, Cheng D, Knight J, et al. Off-pump versus conventional coronary artery bypass grafting: a metaanalysis and consensus statement from the 2004 ISMICS consensus conference. Innovations. 2005;1(1):3–27
- Reichenspurner H, Boehm DH, Gulbins H, et al. Threedimensional video and robot-assisted port-access mitral valve operation. Ann Thorac Surg. 2000;69(4):1176–1181.
- Riess FC, Lower C, Bleese N. Prevention of potential complications after minimal access aortic valve replacement. Ann Thorac Surg. 1998;66(5):1866.
- Robicsek F. Robotic cardiac surgery: time told! J Thorac Cardiovasc Surg. 2008;135(2):243–246.
- Schmitto JD, Mokashi SA, Cohn LH. Minimally-invasive valve surgery. J Am Coll Cardiol. 2010;56(6):455–462.
- Schwartz DS, Ribakove GH, Grossi EA, et al. Minimally invasive mitral valve replacement: port-access technique, feasibility, and myocardial functional preservation. J Thorac Cardiovasc Surg. 1997;113(6):1022–1030.
- Sellke FW, Chu LM, Cohn WE. Current state of surgical myocardial revascularization. Circ J. 2010;74(6):1031–1037.
- Sellke FW, DiMaio JM, Caplan LR, et al. Comparing on-pump and off-pump coronary artery bypass grafting: numerous studies but few conclusions: a scientific statement from the American Heart Association council non cardiovascular surgery and anesthesia in collaboration with the interdisciplinary working group on quality of care and outcomes research. Circulation. 2005;111:2858–2864.
- Shapira OM, Natarajan V, Kaushik S, et al. Off-pump versus on-pump reoperative CABG via a left thoracotomy for circumflex coronary artery revascularization. J Cardiac Surg. 2004;19(2):113–118.
- Srivastava S, Gadasalli S, Agusala M, et al. Use of bilateral internal thoracic arteries in CABG through lateral thoracotomy with robotic assistance in 150 patients. Ann Thorac Surg. 2006;81:800–806.
- Srivastava SP, Patel KN, Skantharaja R, et al. Off-pump complete revascularization through a left lateral thoracotomy (ThoraCAB), the first 200 cases. Ann Thorac Surg. 2003;76(1):46–49.
- Stamou SC, Hill PC, Dangas G, et al. Stroke after coronary artery bypass: incidence, predictors, and clinical outcome. Stroke. 2001;32:1508–1513.
- Stevens JH, Burdon TA, Peters WS, et al. Port-access coronary artery bypass grafting: a proposed surgical method. J Thorac Cardiovasc Surg. 1996;111(3):567–573.
- Stover EP, Siegel LC, Parks R, et al. Variability in transfusion practice for coronary artery bypass surgery persists despite national consensus guidelines: a 24-institution study Institutions of the Multicenter Study of Perioperative Ischemia Research Group. Anesthesiology. 1998;88:327–333.
- Subramanian VA, Patel NU. Current status of MIDCAB procedure. Curr Opin Cardiol. 2001;16:268–270.
- Svensson LG, Atik FA, Cosgrove DM, et al. Minimally invasive versus conventional mitral valve surgery: a propensity-matched comparison. J Thorac Cardiovasc Surg. 2010;139(4):926–932.
- Svensson LG, D'Agostino RS. J incision minimal-access valve operations. Ann Thorac Surg. 1998;66(3):1110–1112.
- Vanermen H, Farhat F, Wellens F, et al. Minimally invasive video-assisted mitral valve surgery: from port-access towards a totally endoscopic procedure. J Card Surg. 2000;15:51–60.
- Vleissis AA, Bolling SF. Mini-reoperative mitral valve surgery. J Cardiac Surg. 1998;13(6):468–470.
- Walther T, Falk V, Metz S, et al. Pain and quality of life after minimally invasive versus conventional cardiac surgery. Ann Thorac Surg. 1999;67:1643–1647.
- Walther TS. Midterm results after stentless mitral valve replacement. Circulation. 2003;108(Suppl 1):II85–II89.
- Wang D, Wang Q. Mitral valve replacement through a minimal right vertical infra-axillary thoracotomy versus standard median sternotomy. Ann Thorac Surg. 2009;87(3):704–708.
- Wong MC, Clark DJ, Horrigan MC, Grube E, Matalanis G, Farouque HM. Advances in percutaneous treatment for adult valvular heart disease. Intern Med J. 2009;39(7):465–474.
- Yamada T, Ochiai R, Takeda J, Shin H, Yozu R. Comparison of early postoperative quality of life in minimally invasive versus conventional valve surgery. J Anesth. 2003;17(3):171–176

32

Cardio - Pulmonary Resuscitation (CPR) In Infants and Children

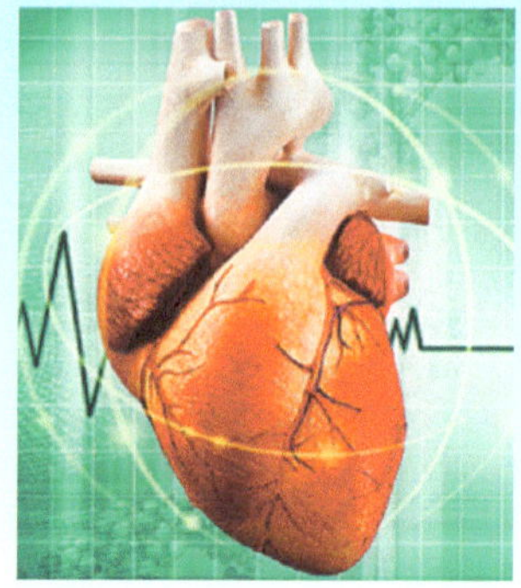

Cardio-pulmonary resuscitation from neonates to Infants

Birth asphyxia accounts for about 23% of the approximately 4 million neonatal deaths each year worldwide (Black et al., Lancet, 2010, 375(9730):1969-87). The majority of newborn infants require little assistance to undergo physiologic transition at birth and adapt to extrauterine life. Approximately 10% of infants require some assistance to establish regular respirations at birth. Less than 1% need extensive resuscitative measures such as chest compressions and approximately 0.06% require epinephrine (Wyllie et al. Resuscitation, 2010, 81 Suppl 1:e260–e287). Transition at birth is mediated by significant changes in circulatory and respiratory physiology. Ongoing research in the field of neonatal resuscitation has expanded our understanding of neonatal physiology enabling the implementation of improved recommendations and guidelines on how to best approach newborns in need for intervention at birth. Many of these recommendations are extrapolated from animal models and clinical trials in adults.

The key elements to a successful neonatal resuscitation include ventilation of the lungs while minimizing injury, the judicious use of oxygen to improve pulmonary blood flow, circulatory support with chest compressions, and vasopressors and volume that would hasten return of spontaneous circulation.

Key points

1.Cardiac arrest should be suspected in an infant or child who is unresponsive and not breathing normally — pulse check should not delay cardiopulmonary resuscitation (CPR)
2.CPR should be commenced if cardiac arrest is suspected
3.Ongoing management should be directed by the cardiac rhythm identified
4.Effective resuscitation relies on a coordinated team and good communication

Background

•The majority of arrests in children are due to hypoxia, hypotension and acidosis
• The most common dysrhythmias are severe bradycardia and asystole
• Ventricular fibrillation (VF) is the initial arrest rhythm in approximately 10%
• Traumatic cardiac arrest is a unique situation - the management is different to non-traumatic cardiac arrest and is not covered by this CPG
• Early allocation of roles can optimise resuscitation (if personnel available)

(1) Team leader
(2) Airway nurse and doctor
(3) Circulation nurse and doctor
(4) Cardiac compression personnel
(5) Defibrillator operator
(6) Assessment doctor
(7) Scribe + time keeper with stop watch

Resuscitation

Assess for signs of life or response; if they are absent commence CPR

A – Airway

1.Look, listen, feel for patency/added noises
2.Optimise head position
3.Consider simple airway manoeuvres (head-tilt chin-lift or jaw thrust)
4.Suction secretions/blood/vomit

B – Breathing

Look for chest rise and fall and auscultate

Commence artificial ventilation with self-inflating bag-valve-mask or anaesthetic t-piece using 100% oxygen

(a) Consider oro/nasopharyngeal airway for upper airway obstruction
(b) Consider 2-person technique for poor mask seal
(c) Intubation should be considered for persistent obstructed airway or at some stage during CPR *If available, continuous wave-form end-tidal CO2 monitoring, should be used to:

- Warn of accidental extubation during CPR
- Monitor for return of spontaneous circulation
- Ensure adequacy of ventilation

C - Circulation

If no signs of life continue CPR

•If signs of life assess pulse
•Palpate central pulse (brachial, femoral, carotid)
•Assessment of pulse can be difficult and inaccurate
•If no pulse, slow pulse (<60 in an infant) or unsure, continue CPR

Determine the cardiac rhythm: shockable or non-shockable

Technique

External cardiac compression

•CPR rate for all ages 100–120 bpm
•Ratio for CPR is 2 breaths : 15 compressions
•Once patient intubated compressions and breaths are independent of each other: compressions continue at rate 100–120 bpm and breaths at rate of 10 bpm
•Place the child on a firm surface. If on a bed, place the cardiac compression board under the patient, not under the mattress
•Perform external cardiac compressions to the lower half of the sternum in all patients including newborns
•Compress sternum 1/3 the depth of the chest
•Use the hand technique that allows you to achieve this:
For newborn infants the best technique is a two-handed hold in which both thumbs compress the sternum

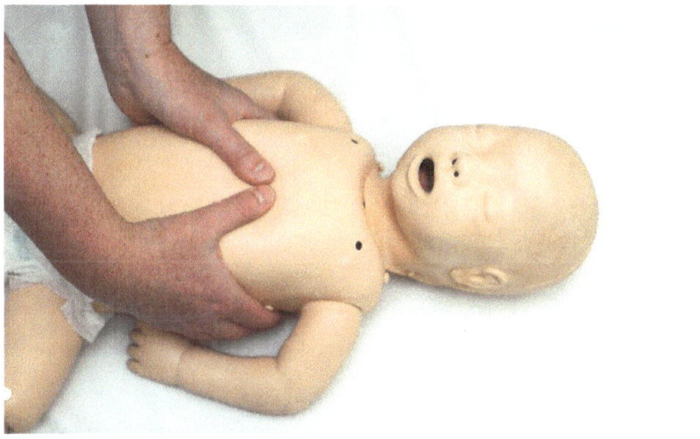

Fig.32.1 For newborn infants the best technique is a two-handed hold in which both thumbs compress the sternum

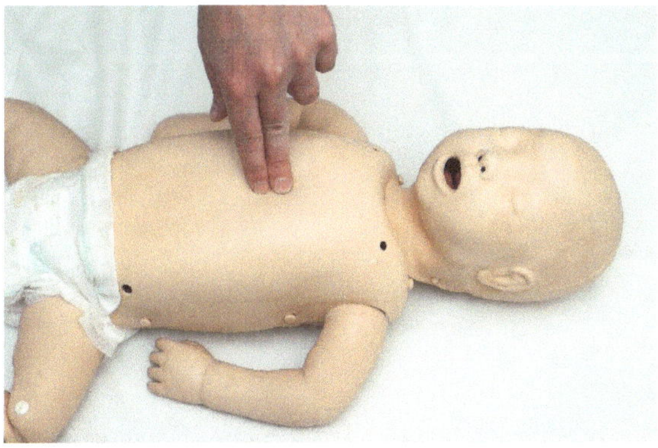

Fig.32.2 For infants two fingers may be used

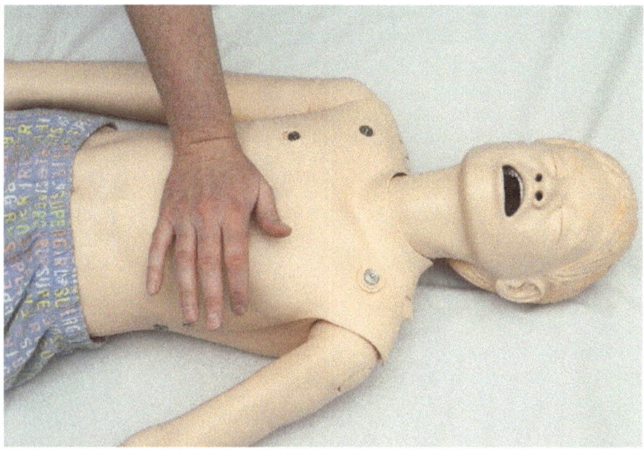

Fig.32.3 For small children use the heel of one hand

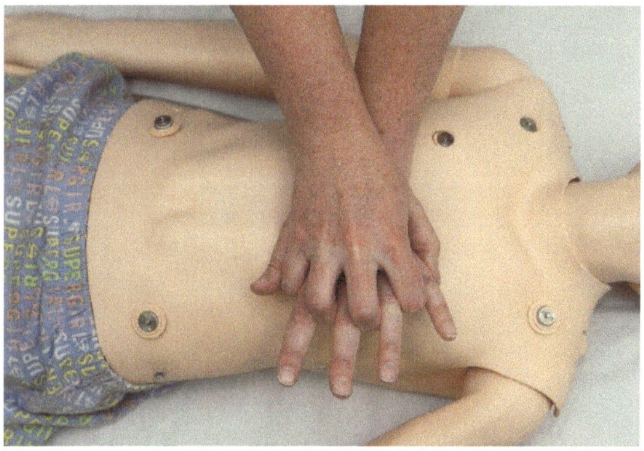

Fig.32.4 For larger children use the "heel" of one hand with the other superimposed

DO NOT interrupt CPR except for rhythm check or defibrillation
Defibrillator operator instructions:
"HANDS OFF" – pad placement or DC shock – "Continue CPR" "HANDS ON"
For rhythm check consider "COACHED"
•Continue CPR
•Oxygen •All clear
•Charge
•Hands off
•Evaluate rhythm
•Defibrillate or 'dump charge'

1. Frequent changes of cardiac compression personnel (every few minutes) is desirable
2.Continue CPR until the next designated rhythm check
3.Gain IV access as soon as possible
4.Consider intraosseous access early
5.If DC shock delivered, recommence CPR immediately for 2 minutes prior to rhythm check

During resuscitation

Correct treatable causes

•Hypoxaemia
•Hypovolaemia
• Hypo/hyperthermia
•Hypo/hyperkalaemia
•Tamponade

Table **32.1** Drugs for Resuscitation in Infants and Children

Medication	*Dose*	*Remarks*
Adenosine	0.1 mg/kg (maximum 6 mg) Repeat: 0.2 mg/kg (maximum 12 mg)	Monitor ECG Rapid IV/IO bolus
Amiodarone	5 mg/kg IV/IO; repeat up to 15 mg/kg Maximum: 300 mg	Monitor ECG and blood pressure Adjust administration rate to urgency (give more slowly when perfusing rhythm present) Use caution when administering with other drugs that prolong QT (consider expert consultation)
Atropine	0.02 mg/kg IV/IO 0.03 mg/kg ET* Repeat once if needed Minimum dose: 0.1 mg Maximum single dose Child 0.5 mg Adolescent 1 mg	Higher doses may be used with organophosphate poisoning
Calcium chloride (10%)	20 mg/kg IV/IO (0.2 mL/kg)	Slowly
Epinephrine	0.01 mg/kg (0.1 mL/kg 1:10 000) IV/IO 0.1 mg/kg (0.1/kg 1:1000) ET* Maximum dose: 1 mg IV/IO; 10 mg ET	Adult dose: 5–10 mL
Glucose	0.5–1 g/kg IV/IO	D10W: 5–10 mL/kg D25W: 2–4 mL/kg D50W: 1–2 mL/kg
Lidocaine	Bolus: 1 mg/kg IV/IO Maximum dose: 100 mg Infusion: 20–50 1/4 g/kg per minute ET*: 2–3 mg	
Magnesium sulfate	25–50 mg/kg IV/IO over 10–20 min faster in torsades Maximum dose: 2 g	
Naloxone	< 5 y or 20 kg: 0.1 mg/kg IV/IO/ET* 5 y or > 20 kg: 2 mg IV/IO/ET*	Use lower doses to reverse respiratory depression associated with therapeutic opioid use (1–15 1/4 g/kg)
Procainamide	15 mg/kg IV/IO over 30–60 min Adult dose: 20 mg/min IV infusion upto total maximum dose 17 mg/kg	Monitor ECG and blood pressure Use caution when administering with other drugs that prolong QT (consider expert consultation)
Sodium bicarbonate	1 mEq/kg per dose IV/IO slowly	After adequate ventilation

IV indicates intravenous; IO intraosseous; and ET, via endotracheal tube
*Flush with 5 mL of normal saline and follow with 5 ventilations

Amiodarone 5 mg/kg IV bolus can be given if defibrillation is unsuccessful after epinephrine. It may be repeated up to 2 times for refractory ventricular fibrillation (VF) or pulseless ventricular tachycardia (VT). If amiodarone is not available, lidocaine may be given at a loading dose of 1 mg/kg IV followed by a maintenance infusion of 20 to 50 mcg/kg/minute. Neither amiodarone nor lidocaine have been shown to improve survival to hospital discharge.

•Tension pneumothorax
•Toxins/poisons/drugs
•Thrombosis

Other considerations during resuscitation

(a) Aim for normal
(b) Aim for normal carbon dioxide (CO_2)
(c) Aim for normal temperature
(d) Toxin induced cardiac arrest requires urgent consultation with National Poisons Centre
(e) Resuscitation for toxin induced cardiac arrest and cardiac arrest following cold-water drowning may be prolonged

Extracorporeal Cardiopulmonary Resuscitation (ECPR)
ECPR is a procedure offered by specialised paediatric intensive care centres in Australia — eligibility should be discussed urgently with local retrieval service

Post resuscitation care - following return of spontaneous circulation

- Re-evaluate ABCD
- Ensure airway and breathing are managed effectively, including intubation if not already performed; do not extubate
- Titrate inspired to achieve normal saturations, avoid excessive oxygenation
- Ventilate to normal CO_2
- Perform CXR to confirm ETT in desired position and check for complications of CPR (pneumothorax, rib fractures, aspiration)
- Maintain normal blood pressure appropriate for age with use of inotropes as needed
- Perform 12 lead ECG
- Monitor for further arrhythmias and consider ongoing anti-arrhythmic medication
- Consider echocardiography to monitor contractility and exclude tamponade
- Check haemoglobin, pH, electrolytes and glucose and correct as necessary
- Aim for normal temperature (avoid hypo/hyperthermia)
- Use adequate sedation and analgesia

Withdrawal of CPR

The decision to withdraw CPR in children is difficult and must involve experienced senior clinicians who will consider the clinical context and the desires of patient and family

Family and staff support

Family members of patients undergoing resuscitation should be given the option to be present, ideally with an assigned support person. Most hospitals are likely to have a family presence policy and staff education strategy in place. Regardless of the outcome, resuscitation is stressful and can be psychologically traumatic to team members providing care. Debriefing and support should be offered to all involved staff who wish to attend

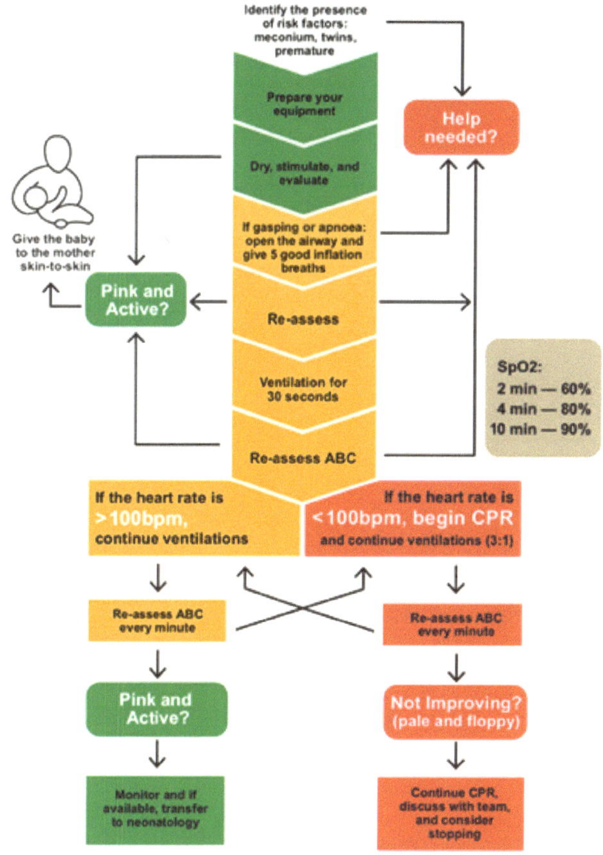

Fig.32.5 Algorithms of neonatal CPR

Administration of epinephrine or volume expansion

Drugs should not be routinely used and are considered a last resort. If, however, the heart rate remains below 60/min after consistent attempts at resuscitation, medication may be needed. Treat with epinephrine if the heart rate continues to be below 60/min. The easiest access route in an emergency situation is via the umbilical vein. Insert the cannula 2 to 4 cm deep. Even though there is little data on the effectiveness of epinephrine, it is widely used. Administer normal saline or a blood transfusion if blood loss is suspected. Intubation for meconium is no longer recommended.

Apgar scoring

Measure the Apgar score (developed by Virginia Apgar) at 1, 5, and 10 minutes. The scores are NOT used to guide resuscitation. They are, however, a good general marker of the success of a team's resuscitation attempts. The score is determined using 5 categories: heart rate, respiratory effort, muscle tone, reflex irritability, and color. The Apgar score predicts neonatal and infant death. The following general rules apply to Apgar scores: A score of 8 to 10 indicates a healthy infant with good cardiopulmonary adaptation. An infant with Apgar scores of 4 to 7 usually exhibits a need for resuscitation (as discussed before, this is not the initiator for resuscitation). An infant with Apgar scores of 0 to 3 almost definitely needs resuscitation, but again, Apgar scores are not the initiating factor for resuscitation.

Method 1 Assessing the Situation

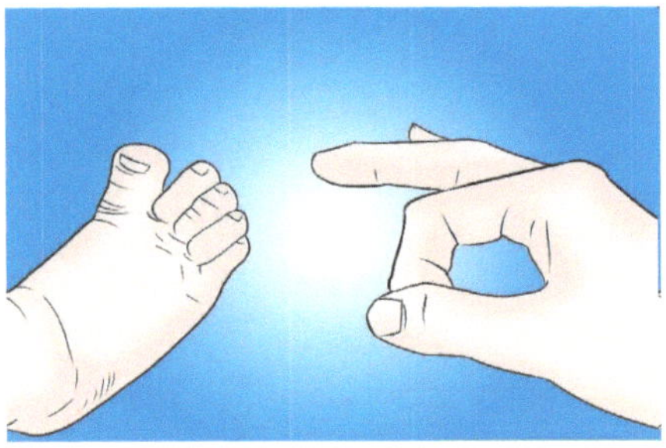

Fig 32.6. 1 Check if the baby is conscious. It's best to flick your fingers against the feet. If the baby doesn't respond, ask someone to call for emergency help while you go on to the next step. If you are alone with the baby, follow the steps below for 2 minutes (to provide immediate first aid) before calling emergency services.

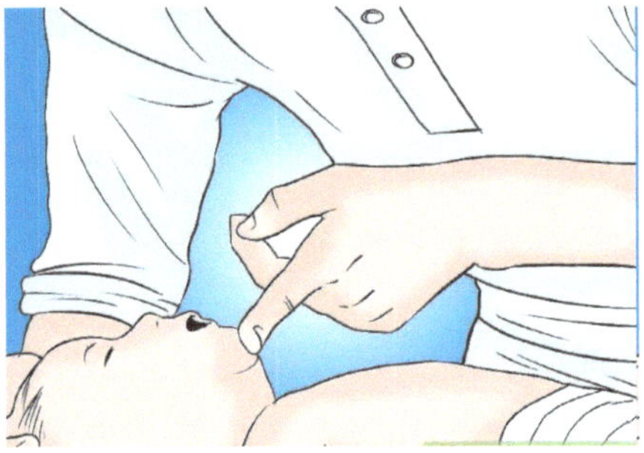

Fig 32.7 2 If the baby is conscious but choking, administer first aid before attempting CPR. Whether the baby is breathing should determine your course of action:

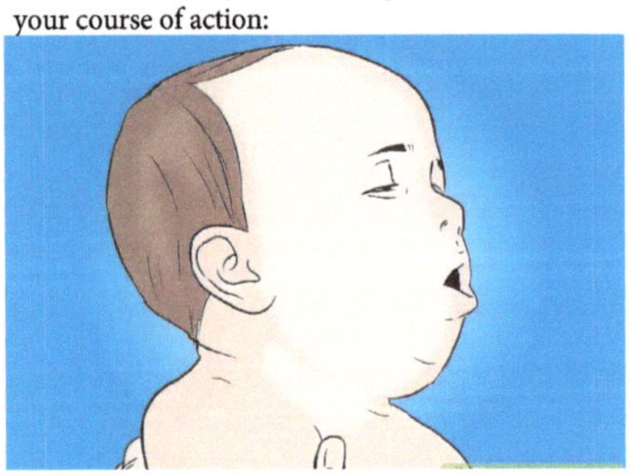

Fig 32.8 If the baby is coughing or gagging while choking, let her continue to cough and gag on her own. Coughing and gagging — a good sign — means that her airways are only partially blocked.

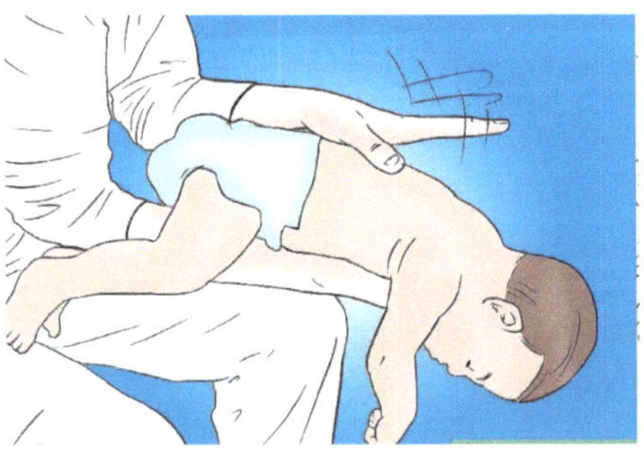

Fig 32.9 If the baby is not coughing then you'll need to be prepared to perform back blows and chest thrusts to dislodge whatever is blocking her airways.

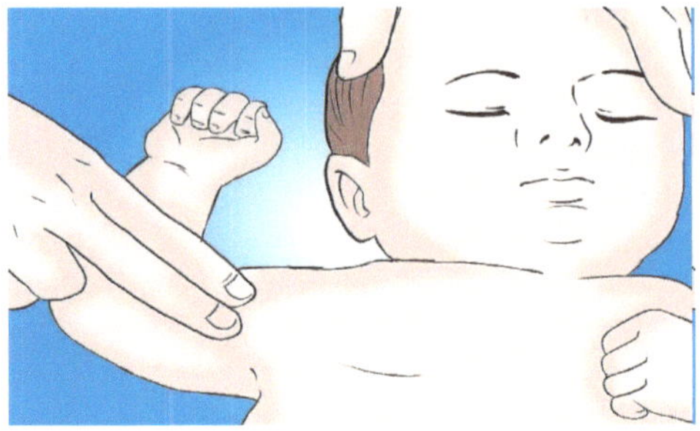

Fig 32.10 3 Check the baby's pulse. Check for breathing again, and this time place your index and middle fingers on the inside of the baby's arm, between the elbow and the shoulder.

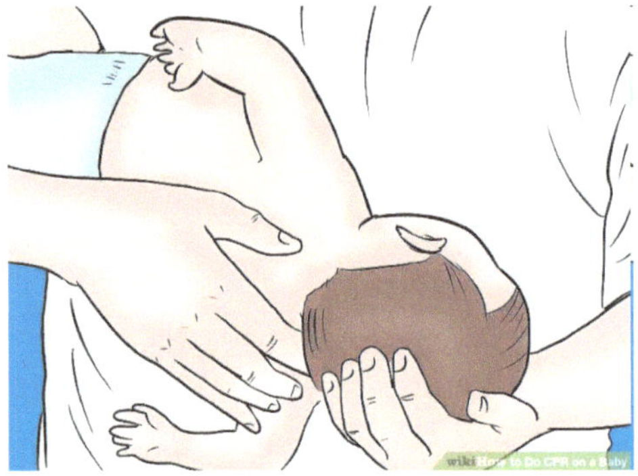

Fig 32.11 If the baby has a pulse and is breathing, put the body in the recovery position.

Method 2 Performing CPR

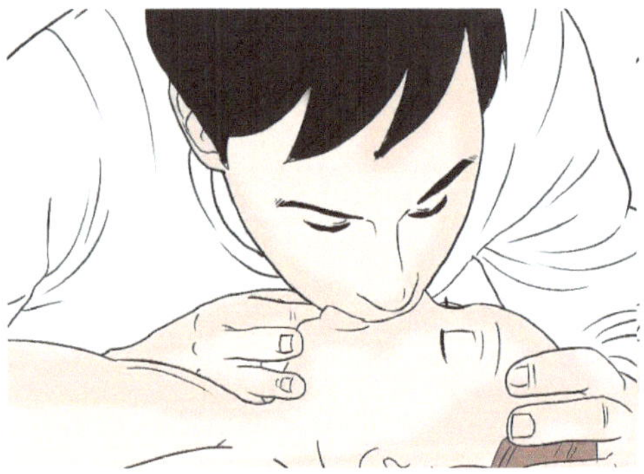

Fig 32.12 Two rescue breaths

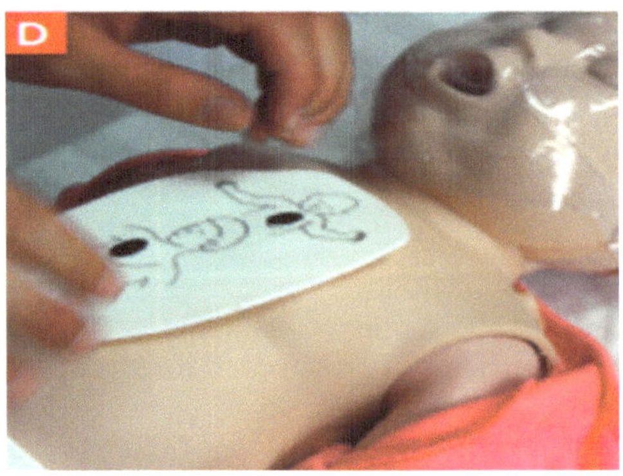

Fig 32.12 If no response to rescue breaths ,apply defibrillator

CPR in a Child (from age 1 to puberty)

Key points

1.Take an official course to learn real, hands-on CPR.

2.CPR involves both chest compressions and rescue breathing (mouth-to-mouth resuscitation).

Give 30 3.compressions and two rescue breaths; repeat this cycle until help arrives or your child recovers.

3..If your child is unresponsive and not breathing or only gasping despite stimulation, start CPR right away and have someone else call emergency number.

4.Once your child starts breathing, put them in the recovery position. This will keep their airway open.

What is CPR?

CPR stands for cardiopulmonary resuscitation. CPR is an emergency procedure that involves chest compressions (pushing hard down on the chest) and rescue breaths (mouth-to-mouth resuscitation). When given properly, CPR can help deliver oxygen to the brain and other organs until help arrives or until your child recovers.The method described on this page applies to children between one year of age and puberty. Once puberty has begun, children should receive CPR as adults

Giving CPR to your child

Check to see if your child is responsive by tapping them on the shoulder and asking loudly, "Are you OK?". If your child does not answer, follow these instructions depending on your situation:

1.If you are not alone, have someone else call 911 and get an AED (automated external defibrillator) right away, if available, while you are doing CPR.

2.If you are alone and have a cell phone, start CPR while calling 911 from your cell phone on speaker. After two minutes of CPR (five cycles), go get an AED if available.

3.If you are alone and have no cell phone, start CPR for two minutes (five cycles) and then call 911 from a landline and get an AED if available.

Step 1

Chest compressions: Push hard, push fast

Begin CPR by laying your child down on a firm, flat surface. Do not spend time trying to find a pulse. Place the heel of one or two hands over the lower third of your child's breastbone and give them 30 quick chest compressions (push fast). Be sure to push hard enough so their chest moves approximately 5 cm (2 inches) down (push hard).Count out loud. You should deliver about 100-120 compressions a minute. Wait for the chest to come all the way back to its initial position between compressions. This will get the blood flowing to your child's brain and other vital organs.

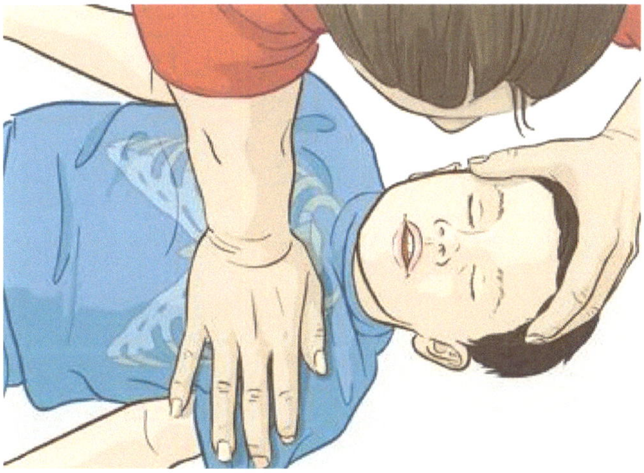

Fig.32.21 **Step 1. Chest compression .Push hard and fast**

Step 2

Rescue breaths: Open the airway

After the first 30 chest compressions, place the palm of your hand on your child's forehead. Place two fingers on the hard, bony tip of their chin and gently tilt their neck back. This will open your child's airway.

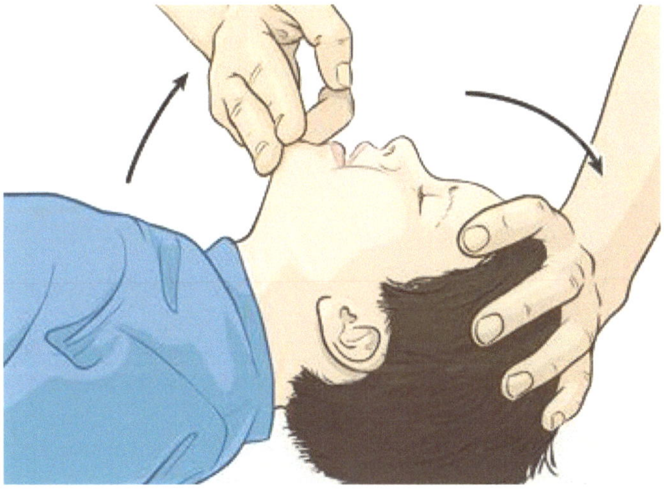

Fig.32.22 **Step 2. Rescue breaths: Open the airway**

Step 3

Two rescue breaths

Pinch your child's nose and place your mouth over their mouth and give two breaths. Each breath should be just enough to make your child's chest rise and should be no more than one second in length. Make sure you see your child's chest rise with each breath.

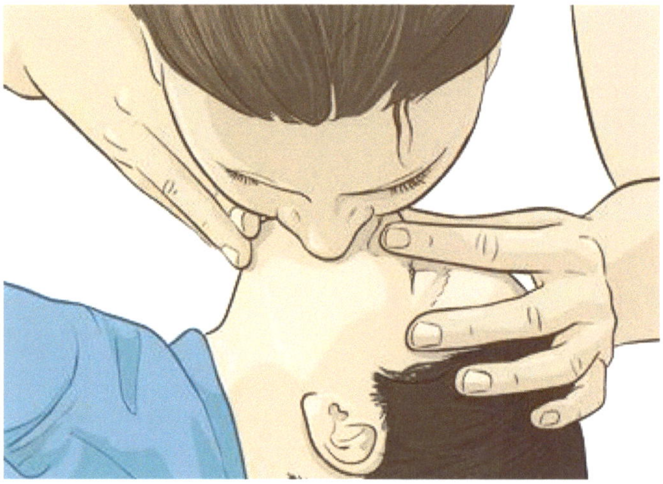

Fig. 32.23 **Step 3 Two rescue breaths**

Step 4

Repeat

Give cycles of 30 chest compressions and two breaths during two minutes and repeat until the ambulance arrives or your child starts breathing again. Two minutes usually allow for five cycles of 30 chest compressions and two breaths.A two-minute CPR cycle is usually tiring. If you are not alone, switch who is giving CPR every two minutes.

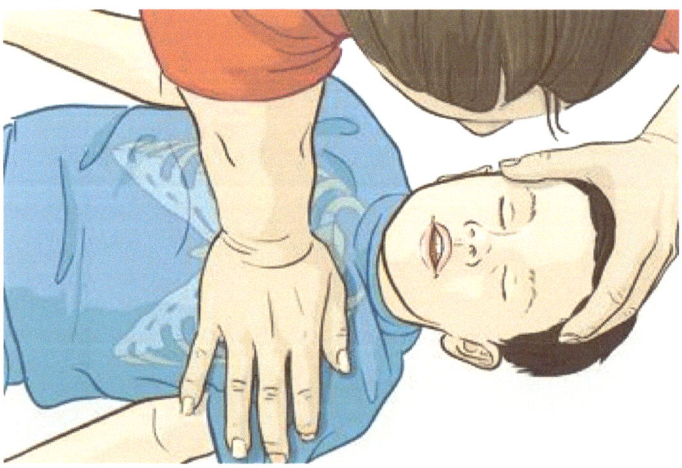

Fig. 32.24 **Step 4 Two rescue breaths**

Step 5

Recovery position

Once your child has recovered and started breathing again on their own, put them in the recovery position until help arrives. The recovery position will help keep your child's airway open and prevent them from choking on their own vomit. If your child vomits, wipe it away. Make sure nothing is blocking or covering their mouth and nose.

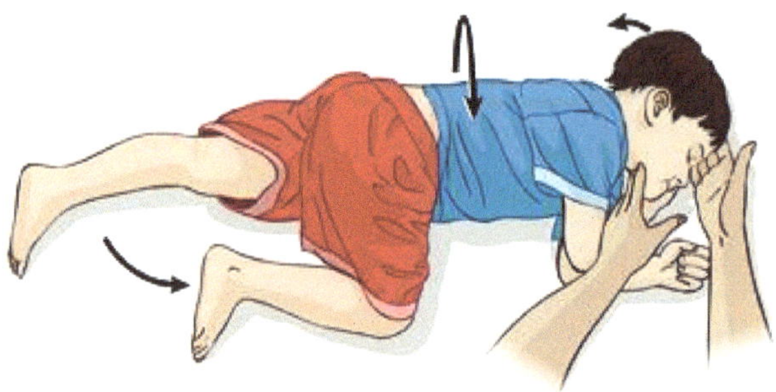

Fig.32.25 **Step 5 Recovery position**

Benefits of having an Automatic External Defibrillator(AED)

You can use a defibrillator whenever CPR is needed. A person needs CPR if they are unresponsive and not breathing normally. Remember, time is crucial. If someone is unresponsive and not breathing, call an ambulance on triple zero (000), start CPR and use a defibrillator as soon as possible.

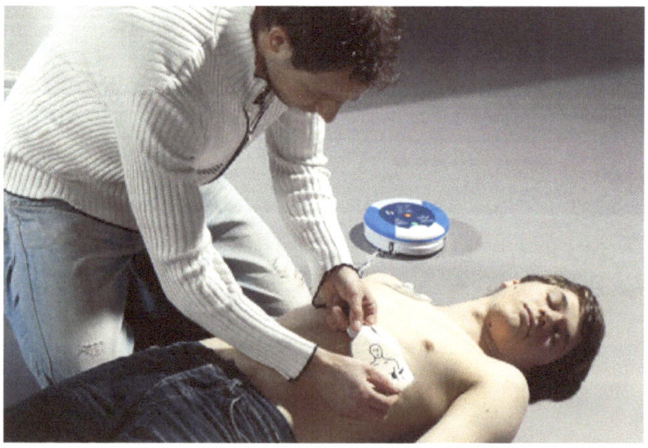

Fig. 32.26. **Use of AED when above measures of resuscitation fail to revive the patient.**

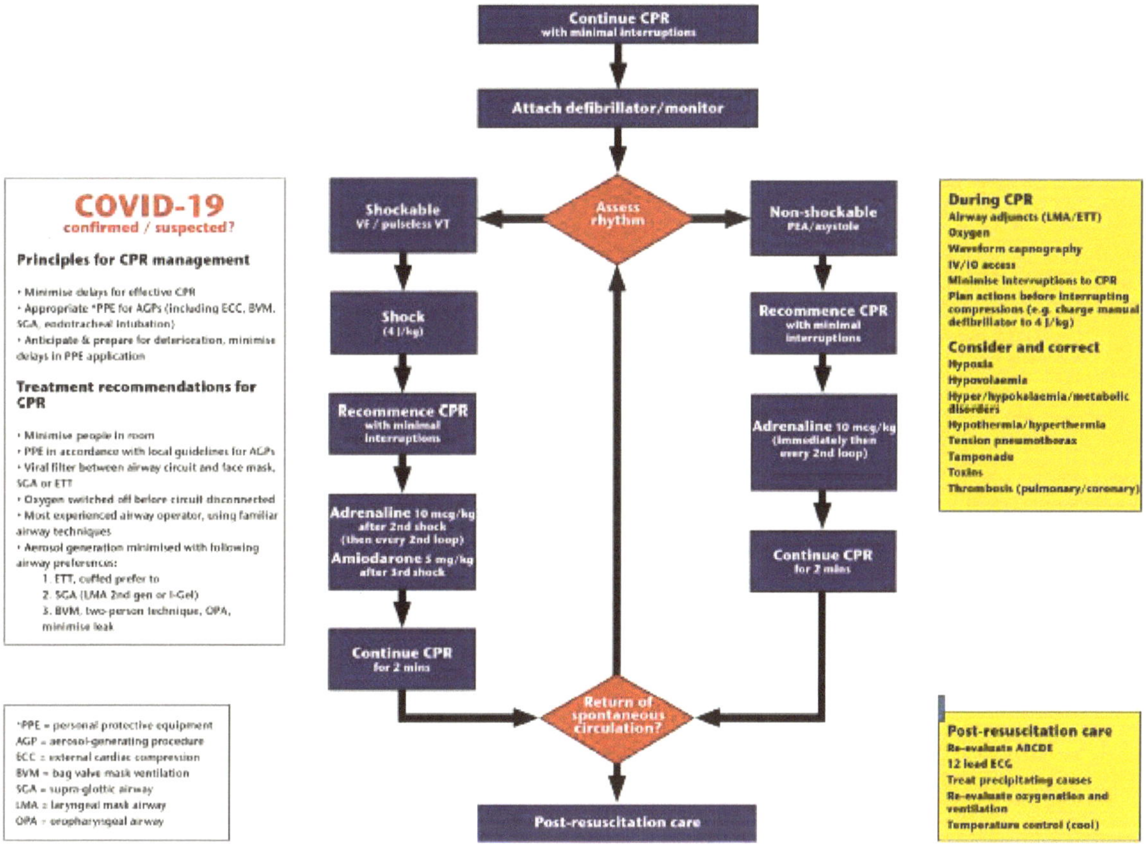

Fig. 32.21 Illustration showing Advanced Paediatric Life Support Algorithms - with COVID-19 considerations

BIBLIOGRAPHY AND ACKNOWLEDGEMENT

- Atkins DL, et al. 2019 American Heart Association focused update on pediatric basic life support: An update to the American Heart Association guidelines for cardiopulmonary resuscitation and emergency cardiovascular care. Circulation. 2019.
- Duff JP, et al. 2019 American Heart Association focused update on Pediatric Advanced Life Support: An update to the American Heart Association guidelines for cardiopulmonary resuscitation and emergency cardiovascular care. Circulation. 2019
- FAQ: Hands-only CPR. American Heart Association. https://cpr.heart.org/en/cpr-courses-and-kits/hands-only-cpr/hands-only-cpr-resources. Accessed Jan. 19, 2021.
- Highlights of the 2020 AHA guidelines update for CPR and ECC. American Heart Association. https://cpr.heart.org/en/resuscitation-science/cpr-and-ecc-guidelines. Accessed Jan. 28, 2021.
- Lokesh L, Kumar P, Murki S, Narang A. A randomized controlled trial of sodium bicarbonate in neonatal resuscitation-effect on immediate outcome. Resuscitation. 2004;60(2):219–223.
- Panchal AR, et al. Part 3: Adult basic and advanced life support: 2020 American Heart Association guidelines for cardiopulmonary resuscitation and emergency cardiovascular care. Circulation. 2020
- Pozner CN. Basic life support (BLS) in adults. https://www.uptodate.com/contents/search. Accessed Jan. 28, 2021
- Ralson ME. Pediatric basic life support (BLS) for health care providers. https://www.uptodate.com/contents/search. Accessed Jan. 28, 2021
- Salhab WA, Wyckoff MH, Laptook AR, Perlman JM. Initial hypoglycemia and neonatal brain injury in term infants with severe fetal acidemia. Pediatrics. 2004;114(2):361–366.
- Shankaran S, Laptook AR, Ehrenkranz RA, et al.; National Institute of Child Health and Human Development Neonatal Research Network. Whole-body hypothermia for neonates with hypoxic-ischemic encephalopathy. N Engl J Med. 2005;353(15):1574–1584.
- Topjian AA, et al. Part 4: Pediatric basic and advanced life support: 2020 American Heart Association guidelines for cardiopulmonary resuscitation and emergency cardiovascular care. Circulation. 202
- Vento M, Asensi M, Sastre J, García-Sala F, Pallardó FV, Viña J. Resuscitation with room air instead of 100% oxygen prevents oxidative stress in moderately asphyxiated term neonates. Pediatrics. 2001;107(4):642–647..
- Velaphi S, Vidyasagar D. Intrapartum and postdelivery management of infants born to mothers with meconium-stained amniotic fluid: evidence-based recommendations. Clin Perinatol. 2006;33(1):29–42.

33 Cardiovascular Disorders In Young Athletes

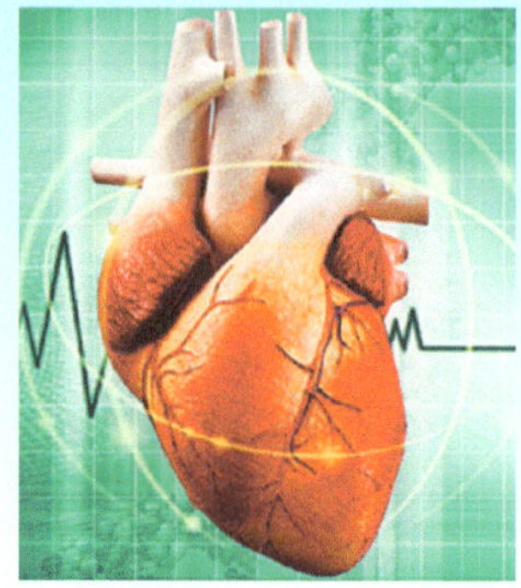

The majority of sudden deaths in young athletes occur in the context of underlying inherited or genetic cardiac disorders. The evaluation of every athlete regarding underlying cardiac disease is impractical and therefore needs to be targeted at those who are at a higher risk. A practical approach would be to channel efforts towards athletes with cardiac symptoms, those with a family history of inherited cardiac disease, and those with a family history of premature sudden death. There are potential pitfalls in the evaluation of young athletes using non-invasive tests when making the distinction between physiological adaptations to exercise and cardiac pathology. Physicians evaluating young athletes need to be aware of the spectrum of physiological adaptations and to be familiar with conditions responsible for sudden death in this population.

Athlete's heart is a constellation of structural and functional changes that occur in the heart of people who train for > 1 h most days.

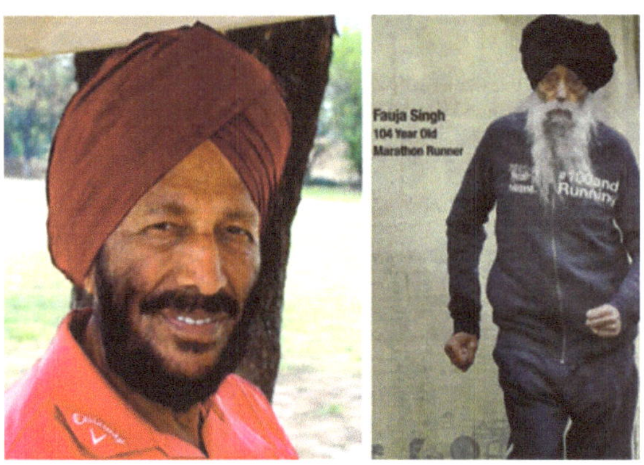

Fig. 33.1 Photograph of two India's athletics icons Milkha Singh (80 yrs, and S. Fauja singh (104 yrs) who are encouraging many indian young athletes to take part in differtent games. Playing games tones up your cardiovascular system and prolonges your life and one may remain drug and disease free even more than 100 years like these two living legendaries.

The changes are asymptomatic; signs include bradycardia, a systolic murmur, and extra heart sounds. ECG abnormalities are common. Diagnosis is clinical or by echocardiography. No treatment is necessary. Athlete's heart is significant because it must be distinguished from serious cardiac disorders. Intensive, prolonged endurance and strength training produces many physiologic adaptations. Volume and pressure loads in the left ventricle (LV) increase, which, over time, increase LV muscle mass, wall thickness, and chamber size. Maximal stroke volume and cardiac output increase, contributing to a lower resting heart rate and longer diastolic filling time. Lower heart rate results primarily from increased vagal tone, but decreased sympathetic activation and other non-autonomic factors that decrease intrinsic sinus node activity may play a role. Bradycardia decreases myocardial O_2 demand; at the same time, increases in total Hb and blood volume enhance O_2 transport. Despite these changes, systolic function and diastolic function remain normal. Structural changes in women are typically less than those in men of the same age, body size, and training. While the entity of athlete's heart has been recognized for over 100 years, only in the past two decades has the application of echocardiography and other non-invasive imaging techniques permitted definition with some precision of the alterations in cardiac dimensions associated with athletic (Figs. 33.1–33.5) conditioning.Echocardiography has demonstrated that long-term athletic training leads to an increase in left ventricular mass due to increases in left ventricular diastolic cavity dimension, wall thickness, or both. These changes in cardiac morphology are relatively mild in absolute terms, and the differences between athlete and non-athlete populations are statistically significant but generally small.Furthermore, cardiac alterations associated with training differ somewhat depending on the particular sport in which the individual athlete participates . In particular, the changes in left ventricular wall thickness, cavity dimension, or both

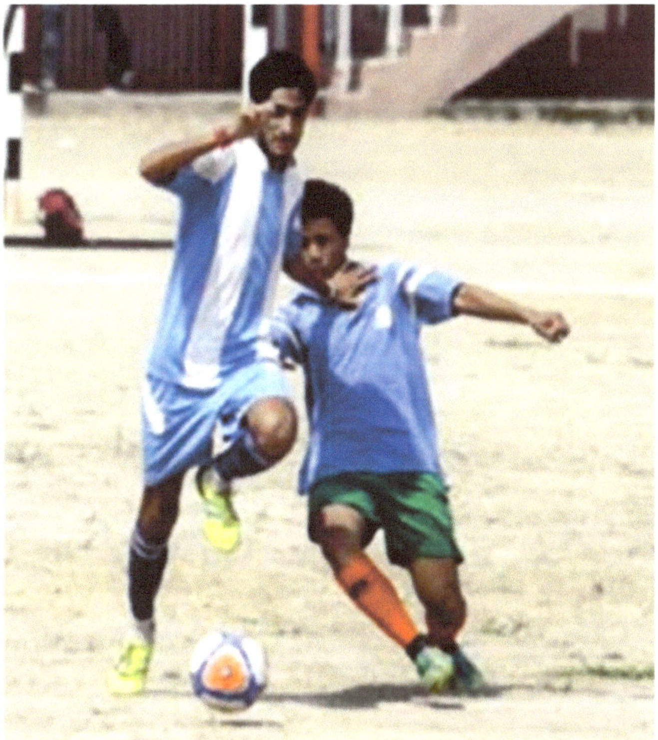

Fig. 33.2 Young footballers in dribbling and weaving tussle during Inter-School football match.

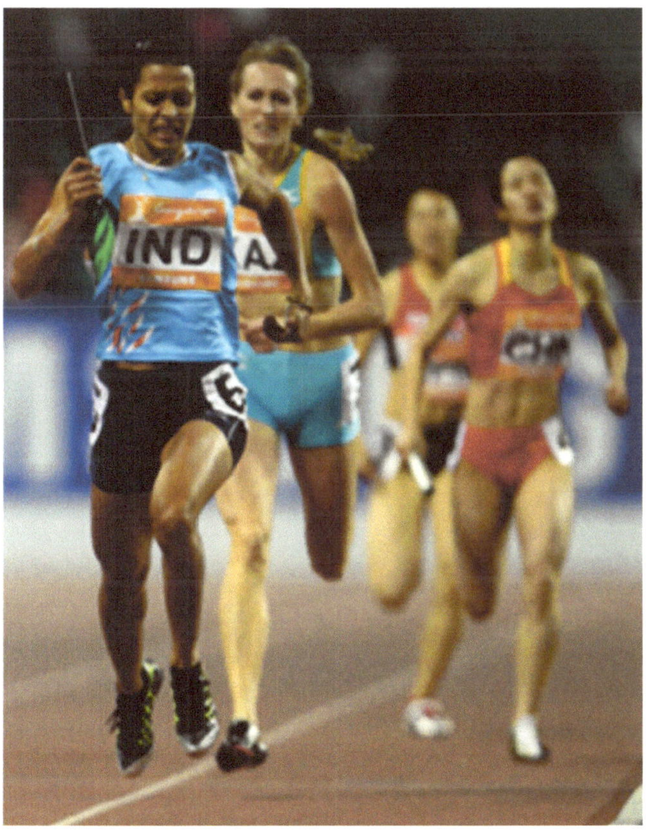

Fig. 33.3 Young International athletes including Indian taking part in running competition.

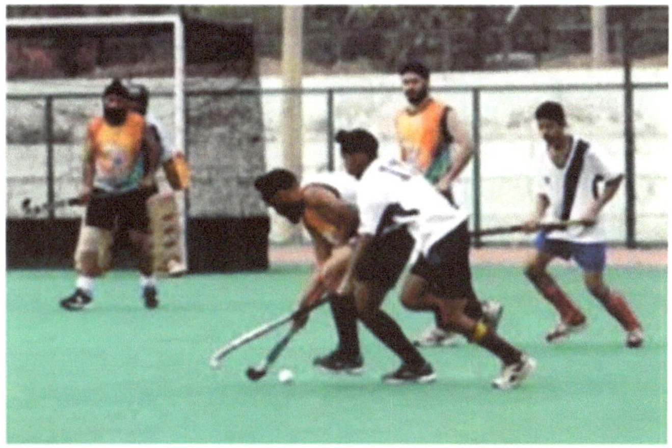

Fig. 33.4 Players in action during hockey match at KK Hakku Stadium, Jammu.

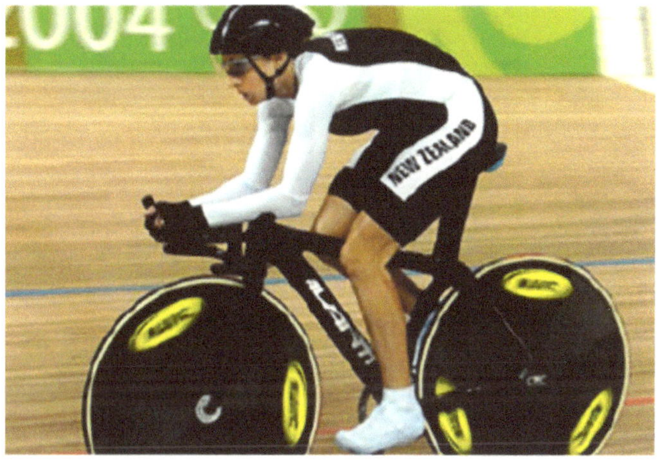

Fig. 33.5 A young athlete taking part in cycle race.

associated with long-term athletic training may be more striking in certain sports such as distance running, swimming, cycling, and rowing/canoeing. The differential diagnosis with cardiac disease is more likely to be raised in athletes training in such sports.

WHAT IS ATHLETES HEART?

Definition of Athletic Heart Syndrome

Athletic heart syndrome, (AHS) also known as athlete's heart, athletic bradycardia or exercise-induced cardiomegaly is a non-pathological condition commonly seen in sports medicine, in which the human heart is enlarged, and the resting heart rate is lower than normal.

Athletic Heart Historical Perspectives

The concept that the cardiovascular system of trained athletes differs structurally and functionally from others in the normal general population remarkably extends over a century. During that time, there has also been periodic controversy about the true nature of athlete's heart, *i.e.*, whether the findings are physiologically adapted, benign, and related only to training, or alternatively are potentially pathological and the harbinger of disease and disability.

The clinical entity of athlete's heart has been defined with increasing precision using a variety of techniques. Henschen is credited with the first description in 1899, using only a basic physical examination with careful percussion to recognize enlargement of the heart caused by athletic activity in cross-country skiers. Henschen concluded that both dilatation and hypertrophy were present, involving both the left and right sides of the heart, and that these changes were normal and favorable: "Skiing causes an enlargement of the heart which can perform more work than a normal heart."

Subsequent investigators used quantitative chest radiography to show that heart size was increased in athletes, particularly those engaged in endurance sports with large aerobic requirements. Some early observers even regarded the heart of the trained athlete to be weakened owing to the "strain" created by continuous and excessively strenuous training and believed that athletes were subject to deteriorating cardiac function and heart failure.

What is Athletic Heart Syndrome?

Athletic heart syndrome is a heart condition that may occur in people who exercise or train for more than an hour a day, most days of the week. Athletic heart syndrome isn't necessarily bad for you — if you're an athlete. And it's not what makes young athletes expire in mid-court. While it does lead to structural changes in the heart, a person with the condition usually doesn't notice any symptoms. Athletic heart syndrome doesn't require treatment and is important to diagnose only to rule out heart problems that are serious.

Like any other muscle, the heart gets stronger with exercise. Endurance exercises such as jogging, swimming, and cycling can make the organ bigger, allowing it to pump more blood with every beat. Short, intense workouts such as weight lifting further increase the pumping power by thickening the walls of the heart.

Just as body builders sculpt their abs and biceps into highly unusual shapes, many hard-core, competitive athletes develop extraordinary hearts. Not only is the heart extra large and thick, it also may produce some irregular rhythms (arrhythmia). A person with athletic heart syndrome may also have a markedly slow resting heart rate, in the range of 35 to 50 beats a minute. In addition, electrical impulses can take strange routes across the heart, causing abnormal readings on an electrocardiogram (ECG or EKG). Together, these changes produced by exercise are called athletic heart syndrome.

Physiology of Athletic Heart Syndrome

Cardiovascular adaptations to exercise have been systematically defined and differ with respect to the type of conditioning: endurance training (sometimes also described as dynamic, isotonic, or aerobic) such as long-distance running and swimming; and strength training (also referred to as static, isometric, power, or anaerobic) such as wrestling, weightlifting, or throwing heavy objects. Sports such as cycling and rowing are examples of combined endurance and strength exercise. Most athletic disciplines to some extent combine endurance and strength modes of physical conditioning, and training-related physiological alterations represent a complex set of central and peripheral mechanisms operating at structural, metabolic, and regulatory levels.

Acute responses to endurance exercise training include substantial increases in maximum oxygen consumption, cardiac output, stroke volume, and systolic blood pressure, associated with decreased peripheral vascular resistance. The immediate results of strength conditioning include only mildly increased oxygen consumption and cardiac output but substantial increases in blood pressure, peripheral vascular resistance, and heart rate.

Long-term cardiovascular adaptation to dynamic training produces increased maximal oxygen uptake due to increased cardiac output and arteriovenous oxygen difference. Strength exercise results in little or no increase in oxygen uptake. Thus, endurance exercise predominantly produces volume load on the left ventricle (LV), and strength exercise causes largely a pressure load.

Cardiac Enlargement: Pathology Versus Physiological Adaptation

The phenotypic overlap between exercise-induced cardiac remodeling and pathological structural heart disease is widely appreciated. Cardiac structural abnormality of unclear origin and significance may be detected during preparticipation cardiovascular disease screening, routine health examinations, or evaluation of the athlete with symptoms. Extreme cases of exercise-induced ventricular remodeling may be difficult to differentiate from mild forms of hypertrophic cardiomyopathy, familial or acquired dilated cardiomyopathy, and arrhythmogenic RV cardiomyopathy. The clinical task of differentiating marked exercise-induced remodeling from these important forms of disease remains important, with implications including sport restriction, pharmacological therapy, and placement of an implantable cardiac defibrillator. The overlap between features of the athlete's heart and characteristics of cardiomyopathy, specifically hypertrophic cardiomyopathy, that may affect young athletes has been coined the Maron gray zone. A valuable schema for approaching the athletic patient with LV hypertrophy of unclear origin has been presented, and remains useful in clinical practice. It is noteworthy that this diagnostic approach was developed at a time when non-invasive cardiovascular imaging was in its infancy and, for the most part, restricted to basic 2-dimensional echocardiography. Recent advances in cardiovascular diagnostics have proven to be useful additions to these original criteria. Functional myocardial echocardiography, including tissue Doppler and speckle-tracking imaging, permits detailed and accurate assessment of myocardial function. Tissue Doppler imaging permits assessment of myocardial relaxation and contraction velocity. Across numerous studies, early diastolic relaxation velocity has been shown to be normal or increased in athletes with LV hypertrophy resulting from exercise-induced remodeling. In contrast, pathological forms of LV hypertrophy are typically associated with reduced early diastolic relaxation velocity and peak systolic tissue velocity. Tissue strain and strain rate may also provide useful insight into the origin of LV hypertrophy in athletes.

Cardiac magnetic resonance imaging has similarly emerged as an invaluable tool for the evaluation of the athlete with indeterminate cardiac enlargement. Cardiac magnetic resonance allows highly accurate assessment of myocardial thickness, chamber volumes, tissue composition, extracardiac anatomy, and cardiac magnetic resonance–derived reference values in athletes have been published. Importantly, the use of gadolinium contrast with delayed imaging provides information about the presence and location of myocardial fibrosis. Recent data document myocardial fibrosis patterns that are relatively specific to certain cardiomyopathies and highlight the utility of cardiac magnetic resonance for the assessment of indeterminate cardiac enlargement in the athlete. At the present time, we use cardiac magnetic resonance in athletes with either indeterminate echocardiographic imaging or clinical features that suggest a diagnosis that may not be definitively assessed by echocardiography (*i.e.*, myocarditis). The interested reader is referred to a recently published comprehensive review on this topic. At the present time, there is no single diagnostic test with adequate accuracy for differentiating adaptive from pathological cardiomyopathy. Consequently, we encourage clinicians faced with this diagnostic dilemma to begin the assessment with an integrated consideration of personal and family medical history, 12-lead ECG, and echocardiography. In many cases, this relatively basic but informative triad will provide sufficient information for informed diagnostic decision making. In cases that remain unclear after this initial evaluation, further measures, including tissue Doppler echocardiography, speckle-tracking echocardiography, magnetic resonance imaging, cardiopulmonary exercise testing, prescribed detraining, and disease-specific genetic testing, may be considered.

The 'Athletic Heart Syndrome'. A Critical Review

Cardiological findings in athletes are often similar to those observed in clinical cases. Electrocardiographic and cardiac imaging abnormalities as well as physical findings may be the same in both of these groups. Bradycardia and rhythm disturbances are the most common abnormalities in athletes. Most athletes with abnormal electrocardiograms are asymptomatic and numerous investigators have failed to detect heart disease in association with such electrocardiograms.

In contrast to cardiac dysfunction observed in clinical cases, enhanced or normal ventricular systolic and diastolic function have been reported in athletes. In endurance athletes, this is associated with very high values for maximal aerobic power (VO_2max). Absolute and body size-normalised cardiac dimensions in most athletes do not approach values from chronic disease states, and may not exceed echocardiographic normal limits. In addition, pathological and physiological enlargement appear to be biochemically and functionally different. Myosin ATPase enzyme expression and calcium metabolism are different in rats with pathologically or physiologically induced enlargement. The reported biochemical differences underlie systolic and diastolic dysfunction in pathological enlargement. Conversely, trained rodents and humans have demonstrated enhanced systolic and diastolic function. It is important to

Table 33.1 Specific Athelete Characteristics Needed for Cardiovascular Testing

Portion of Examination	*Characteristics*
Personal history	• Exertional chest pain or discomfort • Unexplained syncope or near-syncope, assumed not vasovagal • History of hypertension • Excessive exertional and unexplained dyspnea/ fatigue • History of previously recognized heart murmur
Family history	• Sudden and unexpected premature death in at least one relative before age 50 years • Disability from heart disease in a close relative < 50 years old • Previously diagnosed inheritable heart disease in family members including, but not limited to, hypertrophic cardiomyopathy, dilated cardiomyopathy, congenital long QT syndrome or other ion channelopatheis, Marfan syndrome, or clinically important arrhythmias
Physical examination	• Heart murmur • Abnormal femoral pulses, suggestive of aortic coarctation • Physical stigmata of Marfan syndrome • Abnormal brachian artery blood pressure for age (taken in both arms in a sitting position)

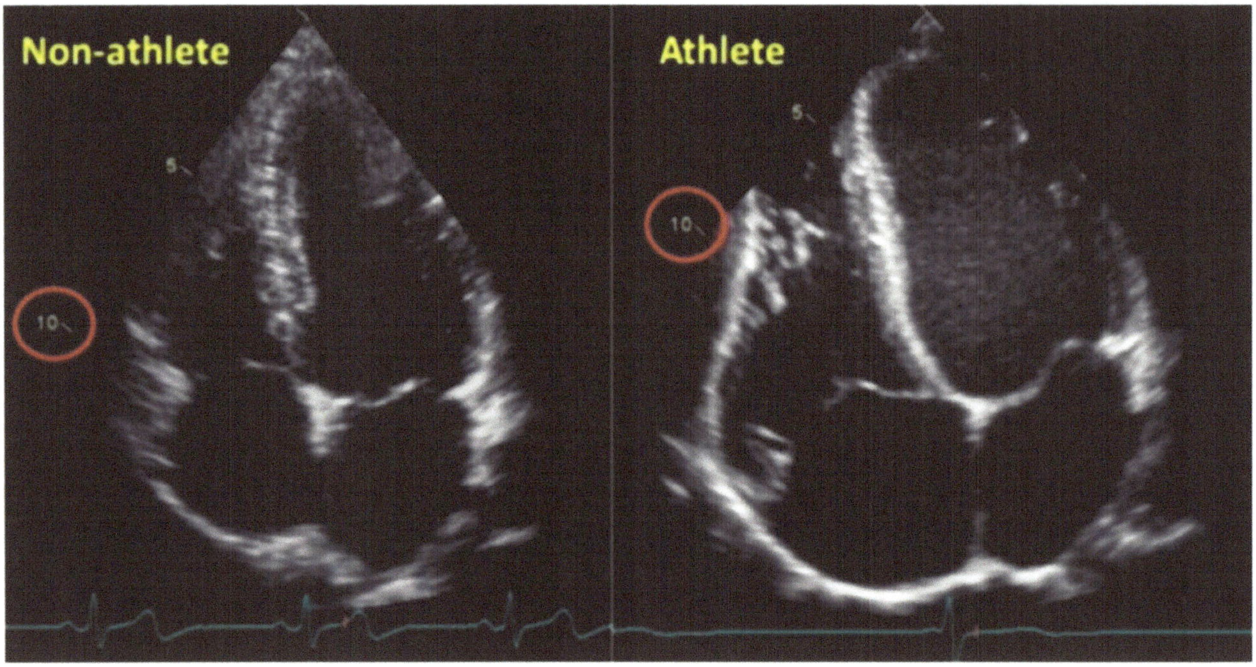

Fig. 33.6 Echo scans in 4C Apical views showing dilatation of athlete heart in comparision to normal heart.

note that cardiac enlargement observed in athletes is the result of normal adaptation to physical conditioning and/or hereditary influences. Conversely, pathological changes result from disease processes which can lead in turn to reduced function, morbidity and mortality. Since the mid 1970s echocardiography has been used to compare cardiac dimensions in male endurance- and resistance-trained athletes. A sport-specific profile of eccentric and concentric enlargement has been documented in endurance and resistance athletes, respectively. Subsequent studies of athletes have examined factors such as age, sex and degree of competitive success to determine their contribution to these sport-specific cardiac profiles. Unique athletic subgroups have also been analysed and have included ballet dancers, rowers, basketball players and triathletes. However, there is a paucity of data on cardiac dimensions in female athletes. Finally, physical conditioning studies have also examined echocardiographic dimensions before and after endurance and resistance training. Significant enlargement of internal dimensions, wall thickness or left ventricular mass have been reported but such increases are relatively small and by no means universal. Several conflicting explanations for enlarged cardiac dimensions appear in the literature. Chronic volume and pressure haemodynamic overloading during physical conditioning has been proposed to explain eccentric and concentric cardiac enlargement in endurance- and resistance-trained athletes respectively. However, twin studies suggest that hereditary factors may be important determinants of cardiac dimensions and/or the degree of cardiac adaptability to physical conditioning.

Diagnosis of Athletic Heart Syndrome

Athlete's heart is usually an incidental finding during a routine screening or during tests for other medical issues. An enlarged heart can be seen at echocardiography or sometimes on a chest X-ray. Similarities at presentation between athlete's heart and clinically relevant cardiac problems may prompt electrocardiography (ECG) and exercisecardiac stress tests.

The ECG can detect sinus bradycardia, a resting heart rate of fewer than 60 beats per minute. This is often accompanied by sinus arrhythmia. The pulse of a person with athlete's heart can sometimes be irregular while at rest, but usually returns to normal after exercise begins. **(Figs. 33.6 and Tables 33.1–33.2)**

Regarding differential diagnosis, left ventricular hypertrophy is usually indistinguishable from athlete's heart and at ECG, but can usually be discounted in the young and fit.

It is important to distinguish between athlete's heart and hypertrophic cardiomyopathy, a serious cardiovascular disease characterised by thickening of the heart's walls, which produces a similar ECG pattern at rest. This genetic disorder is found in 1 out of 500 Americans and is a leading cause of sudden cardiac death in young athletes (although only about 8% of all cases of sudden death are actually exercise-related).

Is Athletic Heart Syndrome Dangerous?

An enlarged heart, arrhythmia, and unusual ECG readings would all be signs of serious trouble for the average person. In fact, the rhythms and ECG readings associated with athletic heart syndrome often mimic life-threatening disorders. But

Table 33.2 Common ECG findings in atheletes. Training-related ECG alterations are common, physiological adaptations to regular exercise and are considered normal variants in atheletes.

Normal ECG findings
Sinus bradycia
Sinus arrhythmia
First-degree AV block
Incomplete RBBB
Early repolarisation
Isolated QRS voltage criteria for LVH

- "Isolated increase in QRS amplitude are common in trained athletes. However, QRS voltage criteria for LVH+ any non-voltage criteria for LVH (such as arterial enlargement, left axis deviation, a 'strain' pattern of repolarisation, ST-segment depression, T-wave inversion or pathological Q wave(s) are abnormal and require further evaluation.
- AV, atrioventricular, LVH, left ventricular hypertrophy; RBBB, right bundle branch block.

athletic heart syndrome itself is harmless. The "abnormal" changes in the athlete's heart are actually a testament to the body's ability to adapt.

If an athlete has symptoms of chest pain, reports irregular beats, or has passed out, he or she should get a medical exam to pinpoint the problem. Your doctor may want to run extra tests to determine whether the symptoms are a normal sign of your body's ability to adapt to training, or whether there's some abnormality in your heart. These tests may include an electrocardiogram, sonogram (a picture of the heart using sound waves), or another type of test.

Of course, some athletes really do have heart trouble. Occasionally, seemingly healthy young basketball or football players drop dead in the middle of a game or a practice. In almost every case, doctors trace the death to an unsuspected condition, such as congenital heart disease, but one that has nothing to do with athletic heart syndrome.

How is Athletic Heart Syndrome Treated?

Since athletic heart syndrome is harmless, there's no reason to treat it unless you experience regular light-headedness, chest pains, or you lose consciousness. If you really want a "normal" heart again, all you have to do is stop exercising. Soon, your heart, along with the rest of your body, will sag back into its former shape. But why not keep everything extra strong and healthy for a while? You should be proud of your athletic body, heart included.

EMERGENCY PLANNING

Cardiac emergencies are frightening events and can lead to chaos and confusion on the playing field. Proper emergency planning increases the likelihood of a coordinated, efficient response and a good outcome. Potential first responders to a cardiovascular emergency during training and competition should be identified. In US high schools, certified athletic trainers and coaches were the most likely first responders (47% and 33%, respectively) Additional personnel may include physiotherapists, strength and conditioning coaches, team physicians, officials and other staff or administrators. All personnel responsible for the care or training or athletes should be educated in the recognition of cardiac emergencies, CPR, AED use and have specific knowledge of the location of the nearest AED.

A communication system should be available at all venues to activate the local emergency medical system and any on-site response team. Transportation routes for emergency vehicles to access the specific location, as well as appropriate hospital facilities, should be predetermined.

Access to early defibrillation must be ensured through the strategic placement of AEDs. The chance of survival decreases approximately 10% with every minute defibrillation is delayed. The recommended time from collapse to first shock is less than 3 min.The number of AEDs and location, whether mounted or portable, is unique for every venue. AEDs should be registered with the local emergency medical system and checked regularly (per manufacturer recommendations) for maintenance or replacement of the device battery and leads. An extra set of pads should be available with every device in case the primary set is damaged or does not adequately adhere to the victim's chest. Supplies to remove clothing and improve adhesiveness of the pads should also be available and include a scissors, razor, towel and antiperspirant spray. Other emergency equipment is dependent on the level of training of the first responders and may include bag-valve masks, advanced airways, pulse oximetry, supplemental oxygen, sphygmomanometer, intravenous fluids and medications such as aspirin and nitroglycerin. A written emergency action plan should be developed for every sporting venue and organisation. The plan should be coordinated with the local emergency medical services system and any on-site safety or security officials. It should also include information on documenting and reporting a cardiac event after the initial resuscitation. Regular review and rehearsal of the plan (at least once annually) should be done with all potential responders.

EVALUATION OF ATHLETES HEALTH STATUS PRIOR TO PARTICIPATION IN COMPETITIVE GAMES.

Symptoms and Signs

There are no symptoms. Signs vary but may include bradycardia; an LV impulse that is laterally displaced, enlarged, and increased in amplitude; a systolic ejection (flow) murmur at the left lower sternal border; a 3rd heart sound (S3) due to early, rapid diastolic ventricular filling; a 4th heart sound (S4), heard best during resting bradycardia because diastolic filling time is increased; and hyperdynamic carotid pulses. These signs reflect structural cardiac changes that are adaptive for intense exercise.

Clinical Evaluation

Findings are typically detected during routine screening or during evaluation of unrelated symptoms. Most athletes do not require extensive testing, although ECG is often warranted. If symptoms suggest a cardiac disorder (e.g., palpitations, chest pain), ECG, echocardiography, and exercise stress testing are done.Athlete's heart is a diagnosis of exclusion; it must be distinguished from disorders that cause similar findings but are life threatening (*e.g.*, hypertrophic or dilated cardiomyopathies, ischemic heart disease, arrhythmogenic right ventricular dysplasia).

Electrocardiography (Figs. 33.7-33.26) and (Tables 33.3-33.5)

Numerous changes in rhythm and ECG morphology can occur; they correlate poorly with level of training and cardiovascular performance. The most common ECG finding is

Sinus Bradycardia

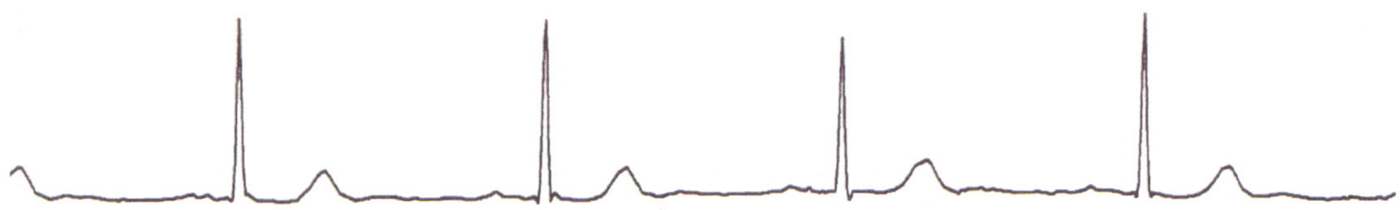

Fig. 33.7 ECG trace taken in one of the athletes showing sinus bradycardia

Rarely, heart rate is < 40 beats/min. Sinus arrhythmia often accompanies the slow heart rate. Resting bradycardia may also predispose to Atrial or ventricular ectopy (including couplets and bursts of non-sustained ventricular tachycardia); pauses after ectopic beats do not exceed 4 sec·

Wandering supraventricular pacemaker

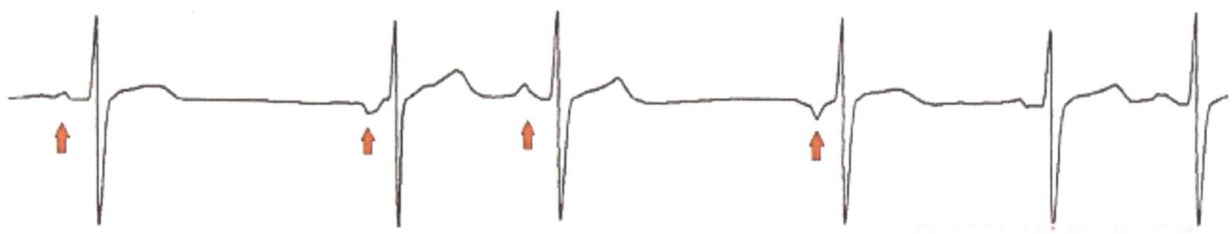

Fig. 33.8 Wandering atrial pacemaker is a benign rhythm change where the pacemaker site shifts from the sinus node into the atrial tissues. P-wave morphology varies with the pacemaker site.

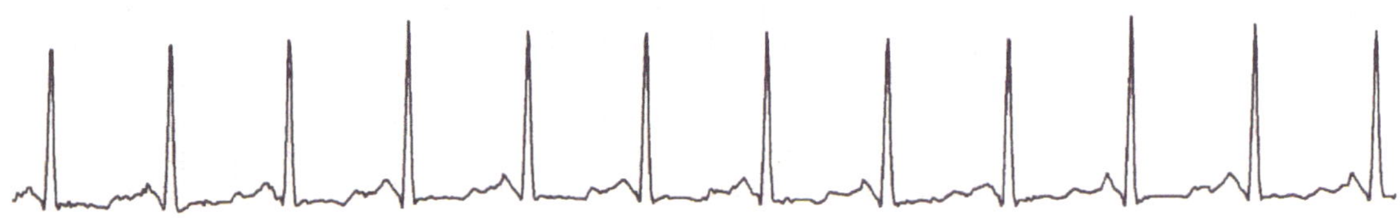

Fig. 33.9 ECG trace taken in one of the athletes showing sinus tachycardia.

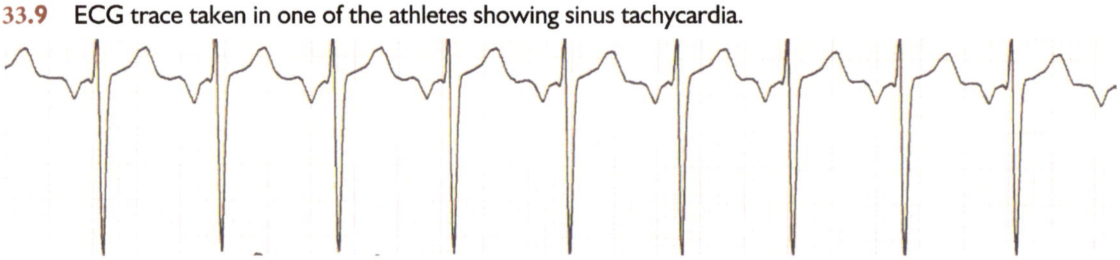

Fig. 33.10 ECG trace taken in one of the athletes showing Jjunctional tachycardia.

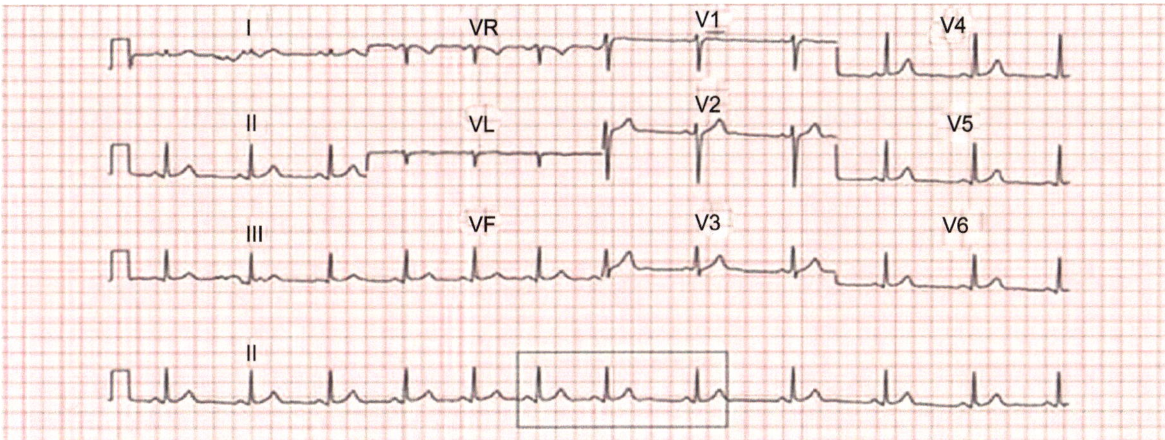

Fig. 33.11 Sinus arrhythmia. All P waves identical • Progressive shortening then lengthening of theR-R interval Identical P waves and irregular R-R interval.

Table 33.3 Classification of abnormalities of the athlete's electrocardiogram

Group 1: Common and training-related ECG changes	*Group 2: Uncommon and training-unrelated ECG changes*
Sinus bradycardia	T-wave inversion
First-degree AV block Incomplete RBBB	ST-segment depression Pathological Q-waves
Early repolarization Isolated QRS voltage criteria for left ventricular hypertrophy	Left atrial enlargement Left-axis deviation/left anterior hemiblock
	Right-axis deviation/left posterior hemiblock Right ventricular hypertrophy
	Ventricular pre-excitation Complete LBBB or RBBB
	Long-or short-QT interval Brugada-like early repolarization

RBBB, right bundle branch block; LBBB, left bundle branch block

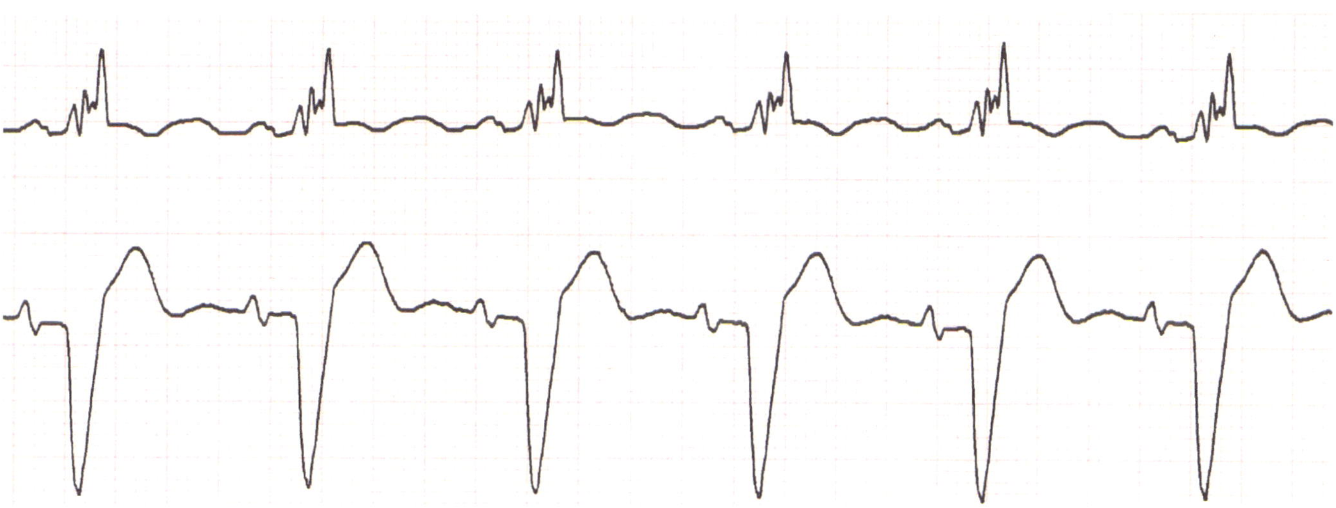

Fig. 33.12 ECG trace showing notched ,widened QRS complexs in leads 1, AVL V5, V6 and deep S waves in precordial leads V1—V4 in one of the athletes taking part in competitive games.

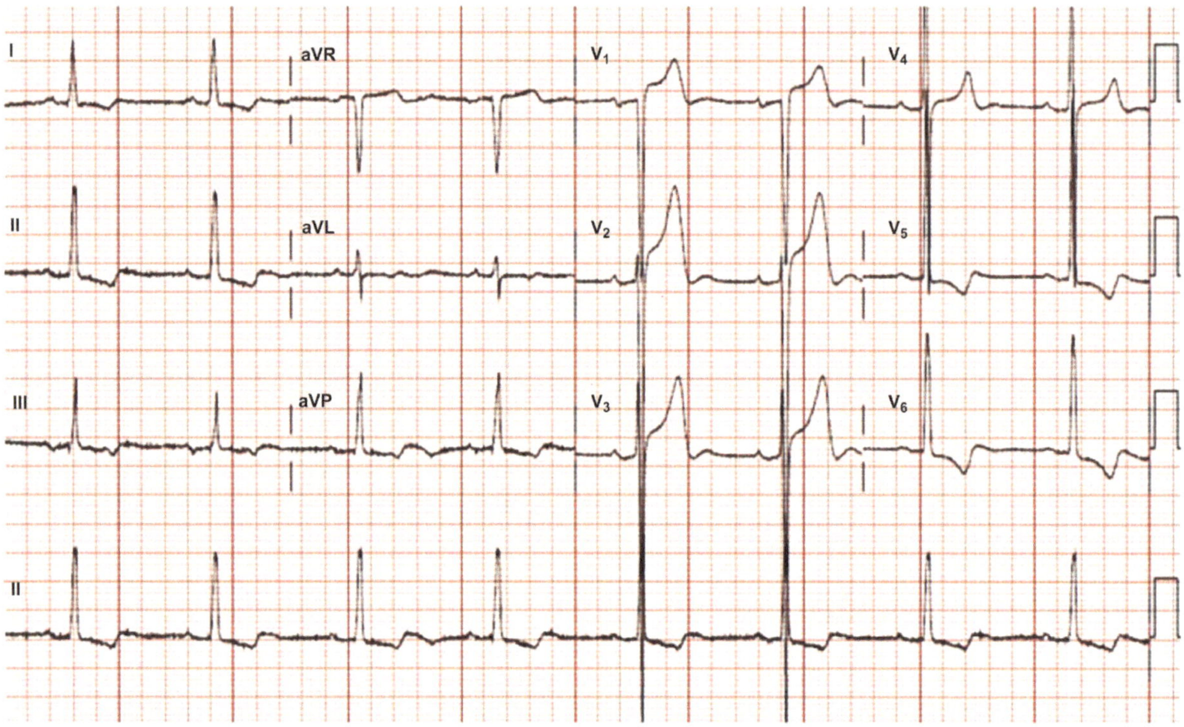

Fig. 33.13 ECG trace showing massively increased QRS voltages — the S waves in V3 are so deep they are literally falling off the page! The ST elevation in V1-3 is simply in proportion to the very deep S waves ("appropriate discordance"). The LV strain pattern is seen in all leads with a positive R wave ($V_{5\text{-}6}$, I, II, III, aVF).

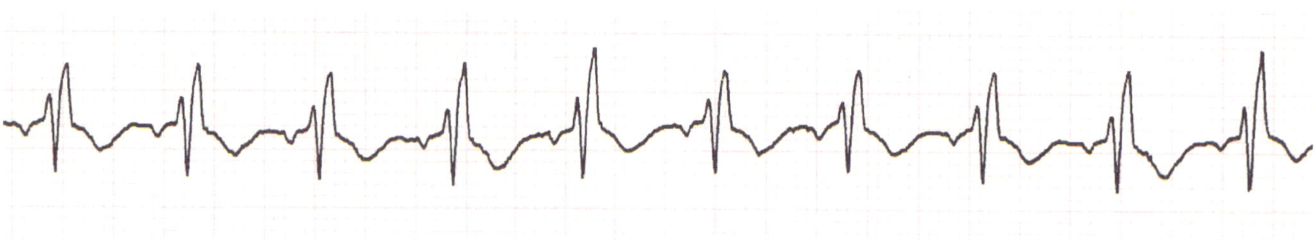

Fig.33.14 ECG trace showing right axis deviation (+150°) P pulmonale (P wave in lead II > 2.5 mm) Incomplete RBBB. Right ventricular strain pattern with T-wave inversion and ST depression in the right precordial (V1-3) and inferior (II, III, aVF) leads.

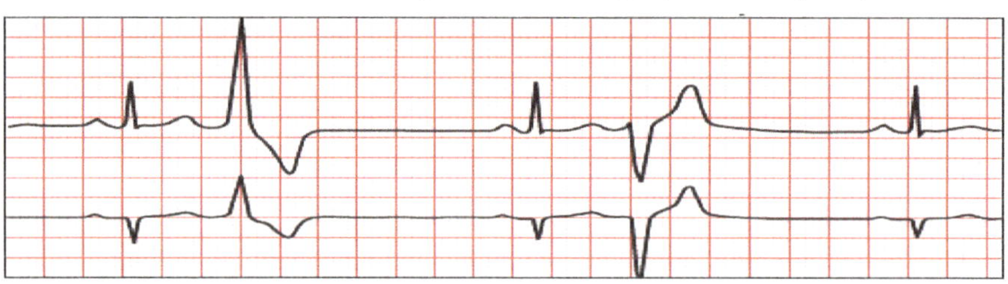

Fig. 33.15 ECG showing multifocal Ventricular contractions

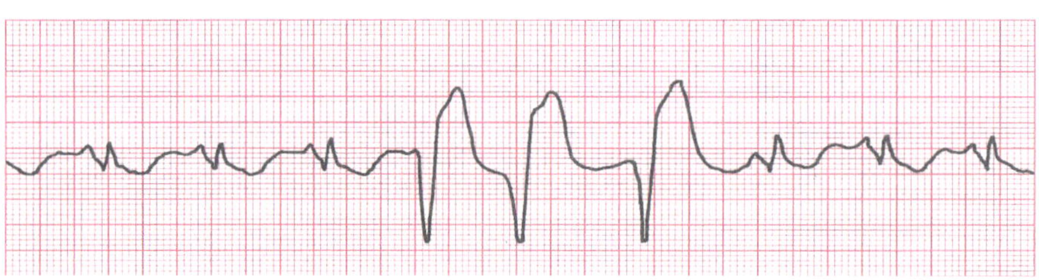

Fig. 33.16 ECG showing Example of run of PVC's

Table 33.4 Criteria for a positive 12-lead ECG in Atheletes

P-wave
Left atrial enlargement: negative portion of the P wave in lead V_1=0.1 mV in depth and =0.04 s in duration;
Right atrial enlargement: peaked P wave in leads II and III or V_1=0.25 mV in amplitude.
QRS complex
Frontal plane axis deviation: right = +120° or left -30° to -80°; Increased voltage: amplitude of R or S wave in a standard lead = 2mV, S wave In lead V_1 or V2=3 mV, or R wave in lead V5 or V6=3mV; Abnormal Q waves = 0.04 s in duration or =25% of the height of ensuing R wave or QS pattern in two or more leads; right or left bundle branch block with QRS duration =0.12 s; R or R' wave in lead V1=0.5 mV in amplitude and R/S ratio = 1.
ST-segment, T-waves, and QT interval
ST-segment depression or T-wave flattering or inversion in two or more lads:
Prolongation of heart rate corrected QT interval >0.44 s in makes and >0.46 s in females.
Rhythm and conduction abnormalities
Premature ventricular beats or more severe ventricular arrhythmias;
Supraventricular tachycardias, atrial flutter, or atrial fibrillation; short PR interval (<0.12s) with or without 'delta'wave;
Sinus bradycardia with resting heart rate = 40 beats/min;`
First (PR=0.21 s), second or third degree atrioventricular block.

[a]Increasing less than 100 beats/min during limited exercise test.
[b]Not shortening with hyperventilation or limited exercise test.
Modified from Corrado *et al.*

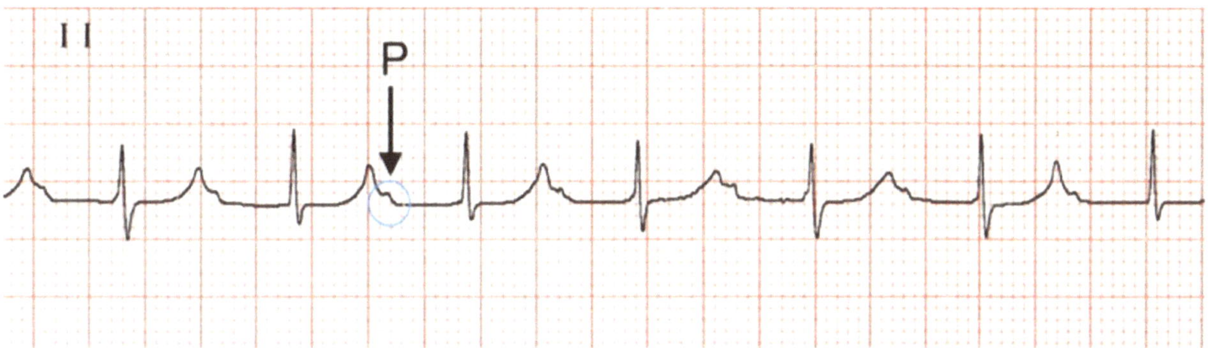

Fig. 33.17 ECG trace showing marked first degree heart block (PR interval > 300 ms, P waves are buried in the preceding T wave)

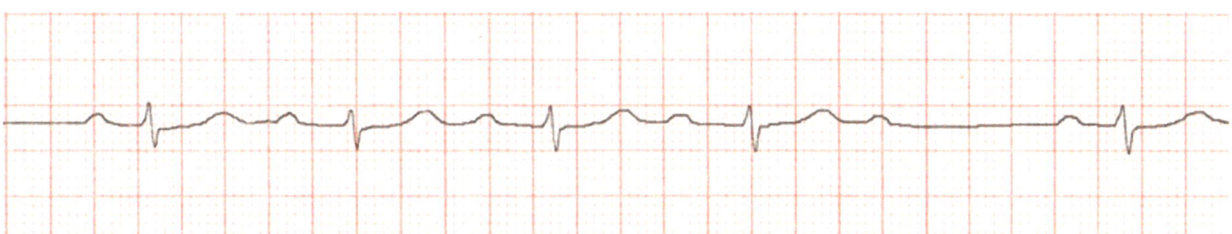

Fig. 33.18 ECG trace showing 1st degree AV block . Progressive prolongation of the PR interval culminating in a non-conducted P wave The PR interval is longest immediately before the dropped beat The PR interval is shortest immediately after the dropped beat

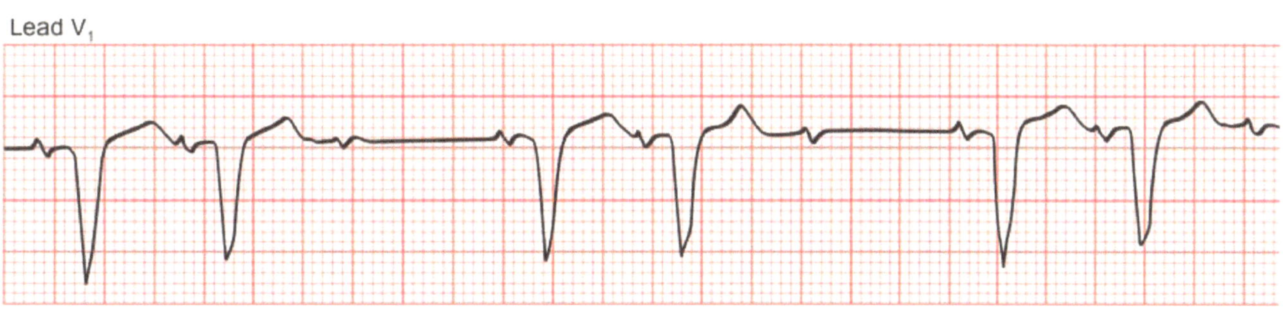

Fig. 33.19 ECG trace showing Type II (Mobitz)AV block the PR intervals are constant until a non-conducted P wave occurs. There must be two consecutive constant PR intervals to diagnose Type II AV block (I.e., if there is 2:1 AV block we can't be sure if its type I or II). The RR interval of the pause is equal to the two preceding RR intervals.

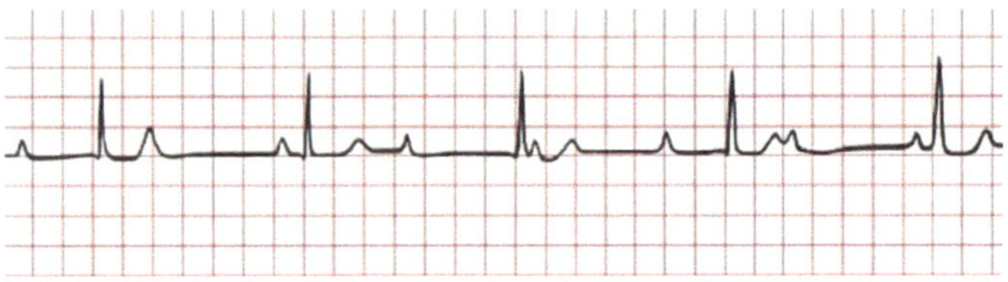

Fig. 33.20 ECG trace showing complete heart block, there is complete absence of AV conduction – none of the supraventricular impulses are conducted to the ventricles. Perfusing rhythm is maintained by a junctional or ventricular escape rhythm. Alternatively, the patient may suffer ventricular standstill leading to syncope (if self-terminating) or sudden cardiac death (if prolonged). Typically the patient will have severe bradycardia with independent atrial and ventricular rates, i.e. AV dissociation.

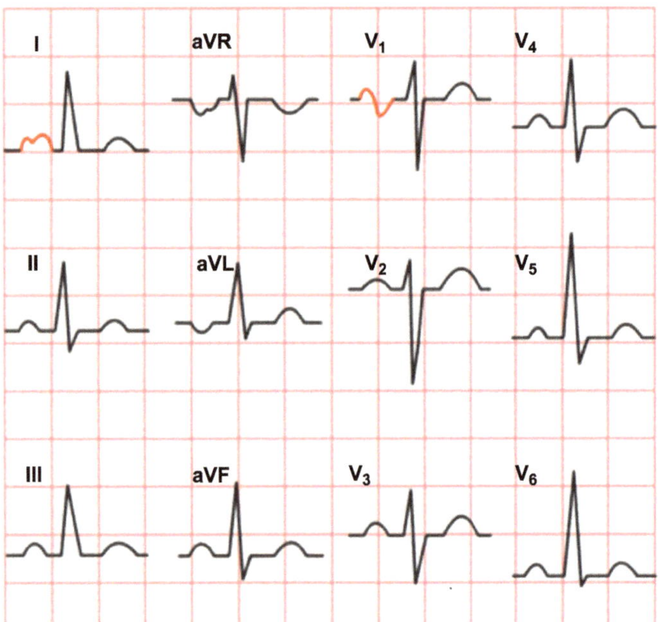

Fig. 33.21 ECG trace showing P wave with a broad (>0.04 sec or 1 small square) and deeply negative (>1 mm) terminal part in V1 P wave duration >0.12 sec in leads I and / or II.

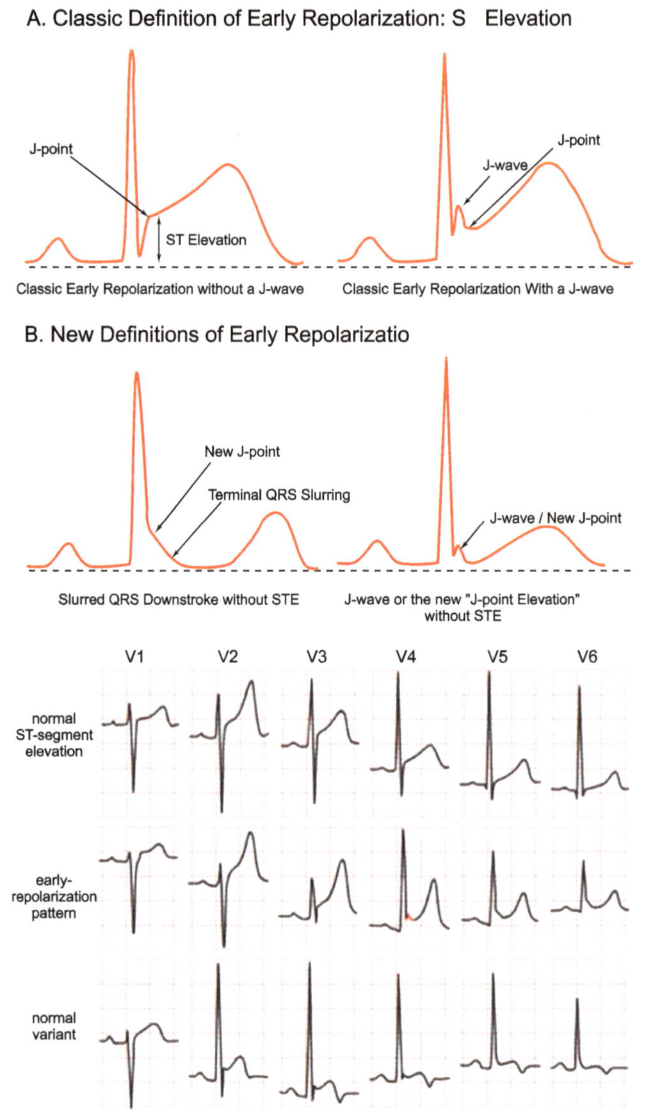

Fig 33.22 A,B (illustrations) and C A 12-lead electrocardiogram showing Type I (inferolateral) early repolarization pattern (ERP) (Red dot indicate J-wave elevation).

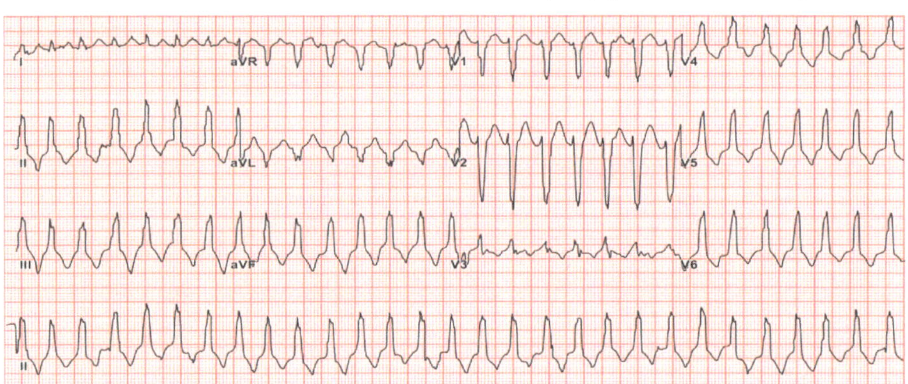

Fig. 33.23 Upper: 12 lead ECG showing the early repolarization pattern in the inferior leads (arrows) and the fractionated QRS with negative T wave in lead III (magnified view on the right side: the fractionation of the QRS was interpreted as a giant J wave). Lower: non-sustained ventricular fibrillation as recorded by the loop recorder (VS, ventricular sensed event by the device; FS, ventricular fibrillation sensing by the device, vertical values representing the instantaneous cycle length durations between successive ventricular events)

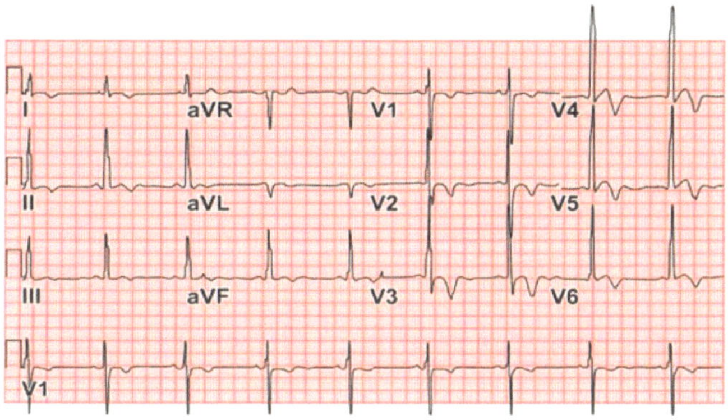

Fig. 33.24 ECG shows the typical pattern of apical HCM: Large precordial voltages. Giant T wave inversions in the precordial leads Inverted T waves are also seen in the inferior and lateral leads.

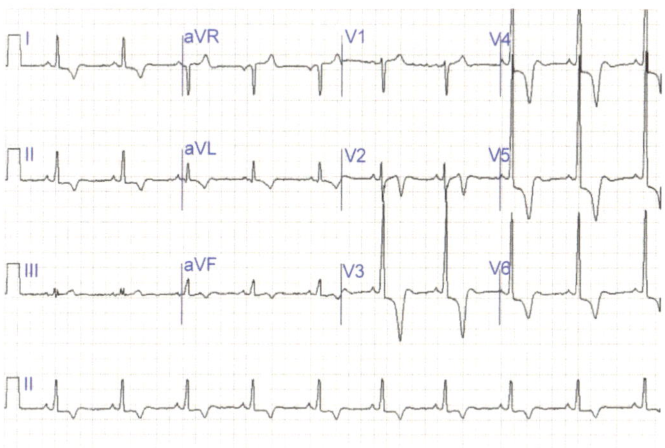

Fig. 33.25 Twelve-lead ECG of an asymptomatic athlete with HCM. The disease was suspected at pre-participation evaluation thanks to ECG abnormalities consisting of increased QRS voltages and inverted T-waves in lateral leads. HCM was diagnosed by echocardiography afterwards.

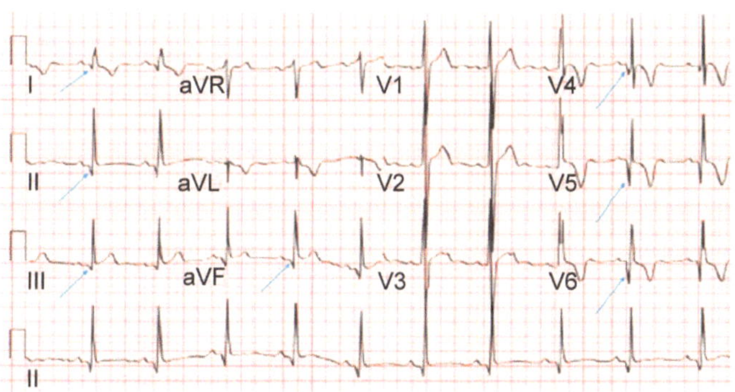

Fig.33.26 ECG shows Left ventricular hypertrophy results in increased precordial voltages and non-specific ST segment and T-wave abnormalities. Asymmetrical septal hypertrophy produces deep, narrow ("dagger-like") Q waves in the lateral (V5-6, I, aVL) and inferior (II, III, aVF) leads. These may mimic prior myocardial infarction, although the Q-wave morphology is different: infarction Q waves are typically > 40 ms duration while septal Q waves in HCM are < 40 ms. Lateral Q waves are more common than inferior Q waves in HCM. Left ventricular diastolic dysfunction may lead to compensatory left atrial hypertrophy, with signs of left atrial enlargement ("P mitrale") on the ECG.

There is an association between HCM and Wolff-Parkinson-White (WPW) syndrome: ECG features of WPW were seen in 33% of patients with HCM in one study. At least one genetic mutation has been identified that is associated with both conditions. Atrial fibrillation and supraventricular tachycardias are common. Ventricular dysrhythmias (*e.g.* VT) also occur and may be a cause of sudden death.

Table 33.5 Abnormal ECG criteria in athletes.

Abnormal ECG finding	Definition
T-wave inversion	>1 mm in depth from baseline in two or more adjacent leads not including aVR or V_1
St-segment depression	>1 mm in depth in two or more adjacent leads
Pathological Q waves	>3 mm in depth or >0.04 s in duration in two or more leads
Complete left bundle branch block	QRS>0.12 s, predominantly negative QRS complex in lead V1 (QS or rS), and upright monophasic R wave in leads I and V6
Complete right bundle branch block	QRS >0.12 s, terminal R wave in lead V1 (rsR') and wide terminal S wave in leads I and V6
Intraventricular conduction delay	Non-specific, QRS >0.12 s
Left atrial enlargement	Prolonged P wave duration of >0.12 s in leads I or II with negative portion of the P wave >1 mm in depth and >0.04 s in duration in lead V1
Left axis deviation	–30° to 90°
Right atrial enlargement	High/pointed P wave ≥2.5 mm in leads II and III or V
Right ventricular hypertrophy	Right axis deviation ≥120°, tall R wave in V1+persistent precordial S waves (R-V1+S–V5>10.5 mm)
Mobitz type II 2° AV block	Intermittently non-conducted P waves not preceded by PR prolongation and not followed by PR shortening
3° AV block	Complete heart block
Ventricular pre-excitation	PR inteval <0.12 s with a d wave (slurred upstroke in the QRS complex)
Long QT interval	QTc ≥0.47 s (99% men)
	QTc ≥0.48 s (99% women)
	(QTc ≥0.50 s (unequivocal LQTS)
Short QT interval	QTc ≤ 0.34 s
Brugada-like ECG pattern	High take-off and downslping ST-segment elevation in V_1-V_3
Epsilon wave	Small negative deflection just beyond the QRS in V_1 or V_2
Profound sinus bradycia	<30 BPM or sinus pauses ≥3s
Atrial tachyarrhythmias	Supraventricular tachycardia, atrioventricular nodal re-entrant tachycardia, atrial fibrillation, atrial flutter
Premature ventricular contractions	≥2 per tracing
Ventricular arhythmias	Couplets, triplets, non-sustained ventricular tachycardia

AV, atrioventriulcar, BPM, beats per minute; LQTS, long QT syndrome.

IMAGING STUDIES (FIGS. 10.27–10.32) AND (TABLE 10.6)

Echocardiography

Echocardiography can usually distinguish athlete's heart from cardiomyopathies but the distinction is not always clear because there is a continuum from physiologic to pathologic cardiac enlargement. The zone of overlap between the athlete's heart and cardiomyopathy is left ventricular septal thickness between 13 to 15 mm in men and 11 to 13 mm in women. In this overlap area, the presence of mitral valve systolic anterior motion strongly suggests hypertrophic cardiomyopathy. In general, echocardiographic changes correlate poorly with level of training and cardiovascular performance. Trace mitral regurgitation and tricuspid regurgitation are commonly detected.

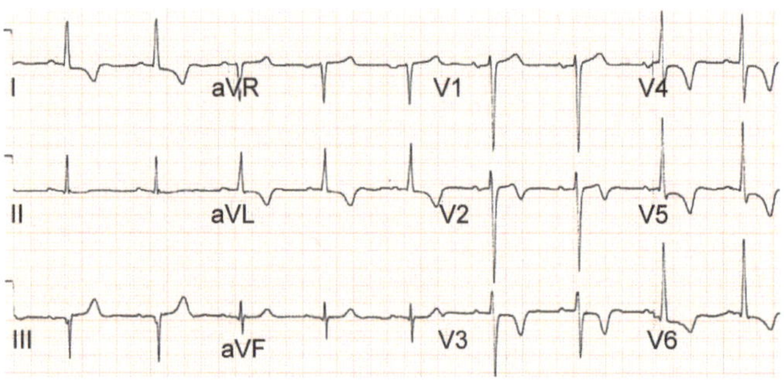

Fig. 33.27 Changes ECG from a patient with HCM demonstrating QRS voltage criteria for LVH in association with deep TWI and ST segment depression predominantly in the lateral leads (I, aVL, V4– V6), voltage criteria for left atrial and right atrial enlargement and left axis deviation. HCM, hypertrophic cardiomyopathy; LVH, left ventricular hypertrophy; TWI, T wave inversion.

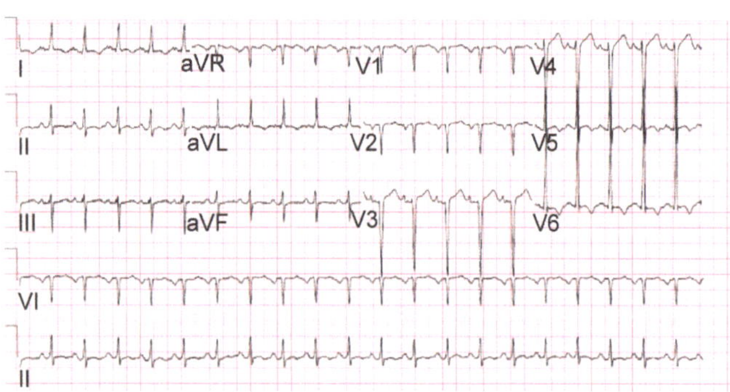

Fig.33.28 Reversible anabolic androgenic steroid-induced cardiomyopathy. EKG demonstrating sinus tachycardia with a rate of 125. Normal axis, PR, QRS, and QT intervals. Left ventricular hypertrophy, septal wall infarct of age undetermined age, and inverted T wave abnormality in V5-V6 which could signify lateral ischemia.

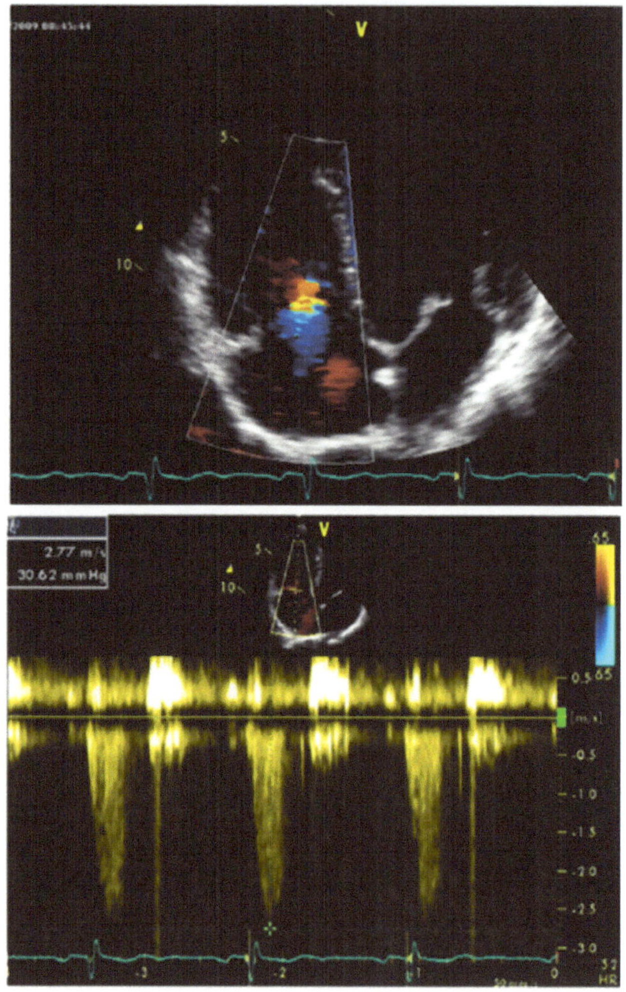

Fig. 33.29 Maximal tricuspid regurgitation peak velocity in an athlete, measured from the spectral profile of the tricuspid regurgitation jet in the apical four-chamber view.

Table 33.6 Showing differences between Atheletic heart syndrome and cardiomyopathy

Feature	*Athletic Heart Syndrome*	*Cardiomyopathy*
Left ventricular hypertrophy	<13 mm	>15 mm
Left ventricular end-diastolic diameter	< 60 mm	>70 mm
Diastolic function	Normal (E:A ratio > 1)	Abnormal (E:A ratio <1)
Septal hypertrophy	Symmetric	Asymmetric (in hypertrophic cardiomyopathy)
Family history	None	May be present
BP response to exercise	Normal	Normal or reduced systolic BP response
Deconditioning	Left ventricular hypertrophy regression	No left ventricular hypertrophy regression

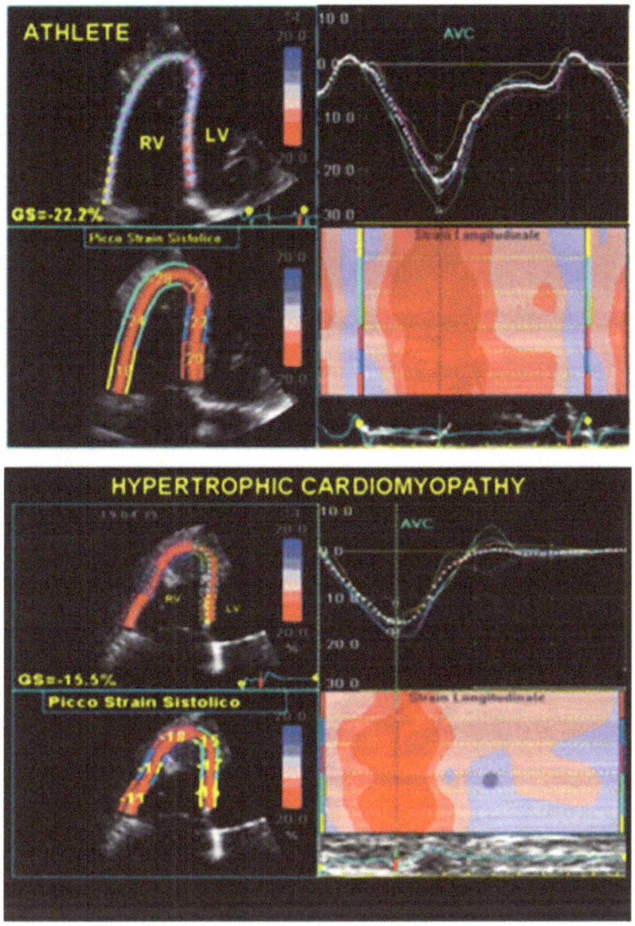

Fig. 33.30 Right ventricular two-dimensional speckle-tracking strain echocardiography pattern in an athlete an in a patient with hypertrophic cardiomyopathy (upper and lower panels, respectively).

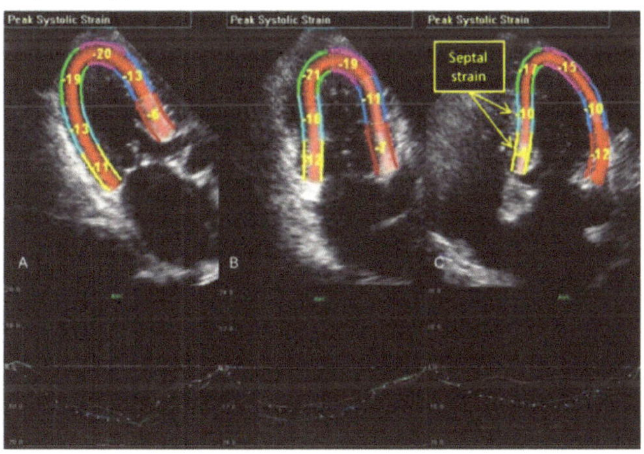

Fig.33.31 Longitudinal strain by speckle tracking echocardiography from a patient with obstructive HCM. (A) Apical short axis; (B) apical two-chamber; (C) apical four-chamber. Global longitudinal strain was obtained by averaging the maximum systolic shortening in a 16-segment model (6 basal, 6 mid, and 4 apical segments). Septal longitudinal strain was defined as mean of two septal segments (basal and mid segments from apical four-chamber view).

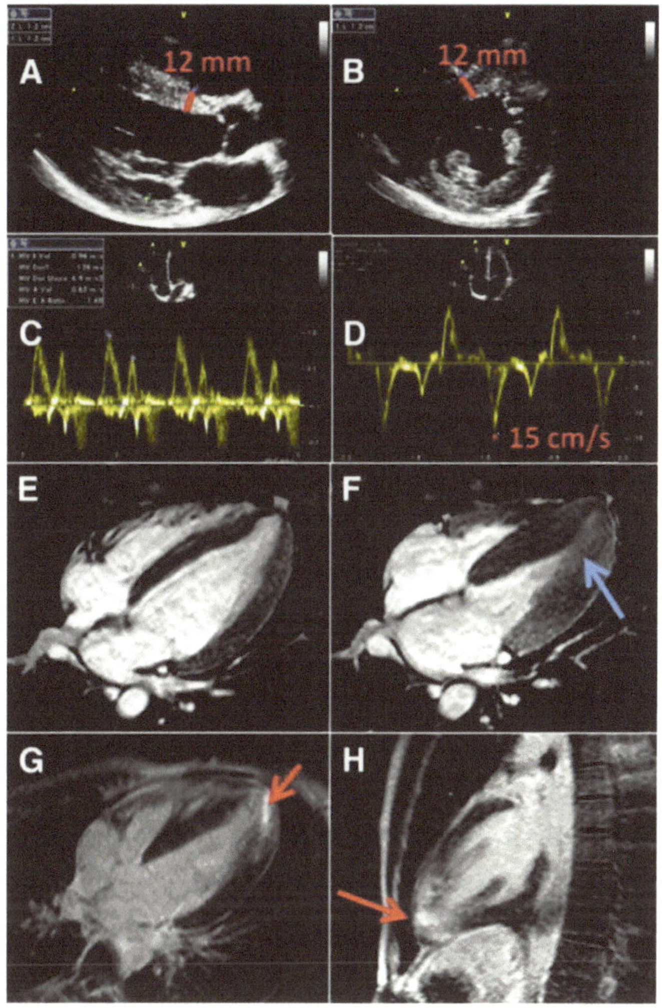

Fig.33.32 A young athlete with hypertrophic cardiomyopathy Example of the importance of CMR in diagnosing HCM in a young athlete who presented with aborted sudden cardiac death and in whom echocardiography was not diagnostic. Left ventricular wall thickness of 12 mm was within ranges accepted for his athletic training (A and B). Mitral inflow and early diastolic annular motion were normal (C and D). The concentric nature of the hypertrophy was atypical for an athlete (E = diastole, F = systole) resulting in intracavity obstruction (blue arrow). T1-weighted images after the administration of gadolinium contrast (G and H) demonstrate apical scarring(red arrows).

STRESS TESTING (FIGS. 33.33–33.41)

During exercise stress testing, heart rate remains lower than normal at submaximal stress and increases appropriately and comparably to non-athletes at maximal stress; it rapidly recovers after exercise. BP response is normal: Systolic BP increases, diastolic BP falls, and mean BP stays relatively constant. Many resting ECG changes decrease or disappear during exercise; this finding is unique to athlete's heart, distinguishing it from pathologic conditions. However, pseudonormalization of

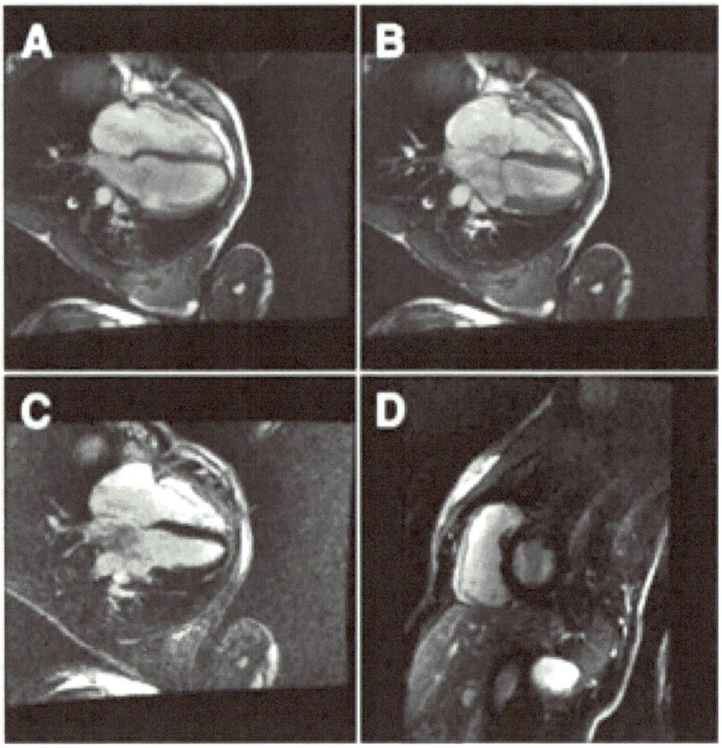

Fig. 33.33 An athlete with ventricular tachycardia and an abnormal right ventricle cardiovascular magnetic resonance study of an elite triathlete after sustained ventricular tachycardia. Cine images in diastole (A) and systole (B) demonstrate an enlarged right ventricle (RV) with reduced systolic function. Note also the septal shift in diastole suggesting significant volume loading. T1-weighted (late gadolinium enhancement) images (C and D) demonstrate increased signal (arrows) of uncertain significance given the spatial resolution constraints within the thin walled RV. A RV focus was identified on electrophysiology studies, which correlated with fibrosis on biopsy.

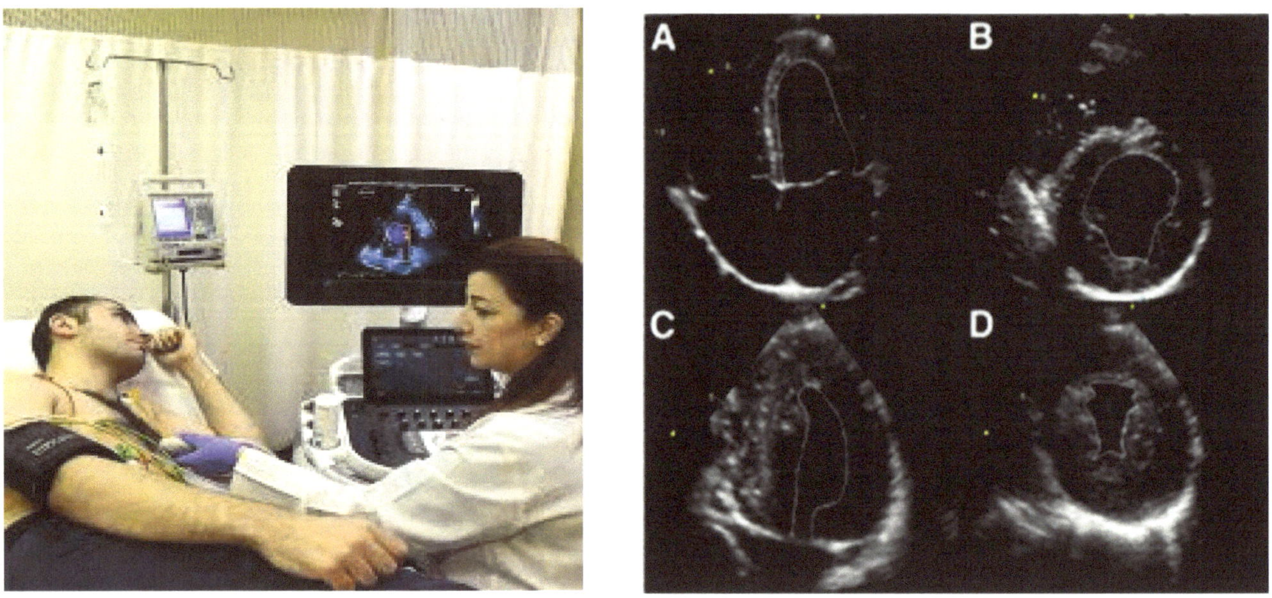

Fig. 33.34 Stress Echocardiography to exclude a Cardiomyopathy . Exercise can be used to differentiate low systolic function from a myopathic process. Imaging during exercise is critical in athletes and can be achieved using a recumbent ergometer (top panel). End systolic frames at rest (A and B) and peak exercise (C and D) demonstrate excellent augmentation of low-normal resting function.

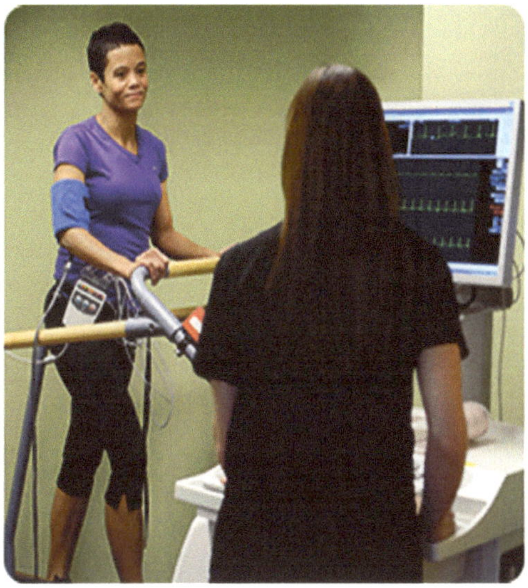

Fig. 33.35 Exercise Stress testing is being conducted for participation in atheletic events

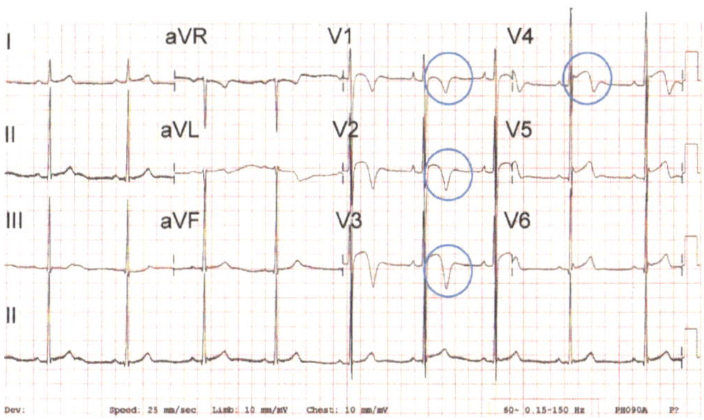

Fig. 33.36 Anterior Repolarization Changes in a Black Athlete Electrocardiogram from a black athlete demonstrating voltage criterion for left ventricular hypertrophy, J-point elevation, and convex ('domed') ST-segment elevation followed by T-wave inversion in V1 to V4 (circles). This is a normal repolarization pattern in black athletes.

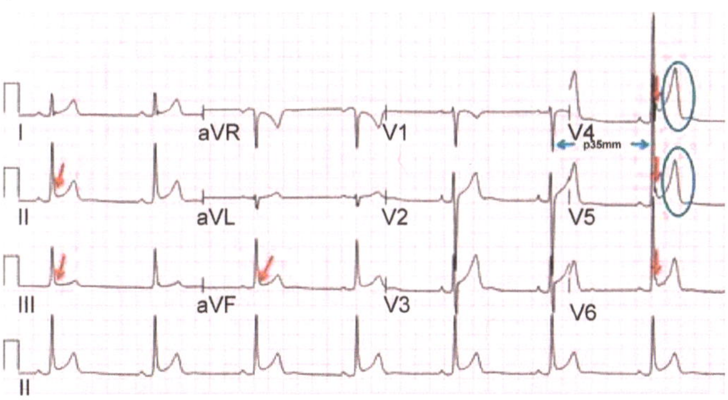

Fig. 33.37 Electrocardiogram of a 29-year-old male asymptomatic soccer player showing sinus bradycardia (44 beats/min), early repolarization in I, II, aVF, V2 to V6 (arrows), voltage criterion for left ventricular hypertrophy (S-V1 + R-V5 >35 mm), and tall, peaked T waves (circles). These are common, training related findings in athletes and do not require more evaluation.

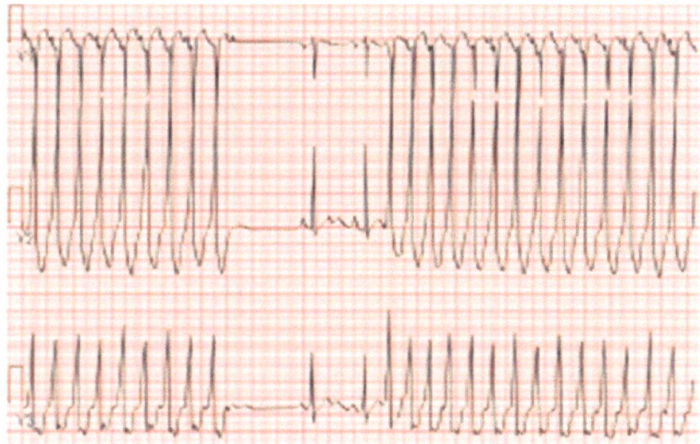

Fig. 33.38 Exercise-induced polymorphic ventricular tachycardia in a 20-year-old elite male swimmer.

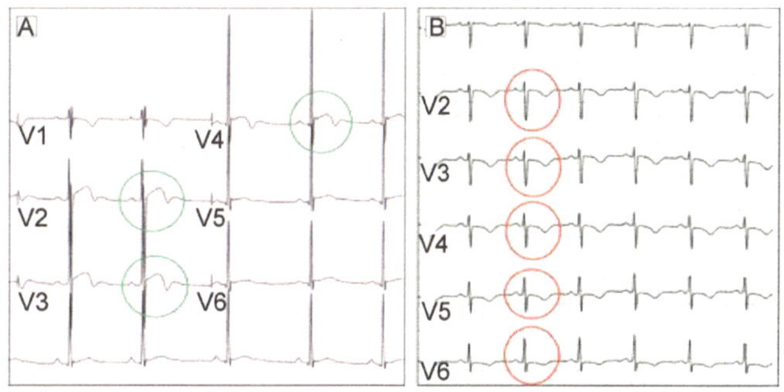

Fig. 33.39 Examples of Physiological and Pathological T-Wave Inversion(A) T-wave inversion in V1 to V4 preceded by J-point el-evation and convex 'domed' ST-segment elevation (green circles). This should not be confused with pathological T-wave inversion (B) which demonstrates T-wave inversion in V1 to V6 with absent J-point elevation and a downsloping ST-segment (red circles).

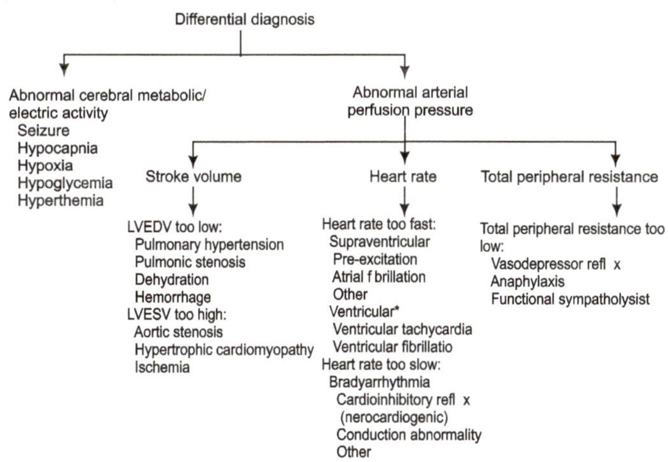

Fig. 33.40 Differential diagnosis of exercise-related syncope in young athletes. Arterial perfusion pressure is a function of the "triple product" of heart rate 3 stroke volume 3 total peripheral resistance. (LVEDV = left ventricular end diastolic volume; LVESV = left ventricular end systolic volume) Information from Levine BD, Buckey JC, Fritsch JM, Yancy CW Jr, Watenpaugh DE, Snell PG. Physical fitness and cardiovascular regulation: mechanisms of orthostatic intolerance. J Appl Physiol 1991;70:112-22.

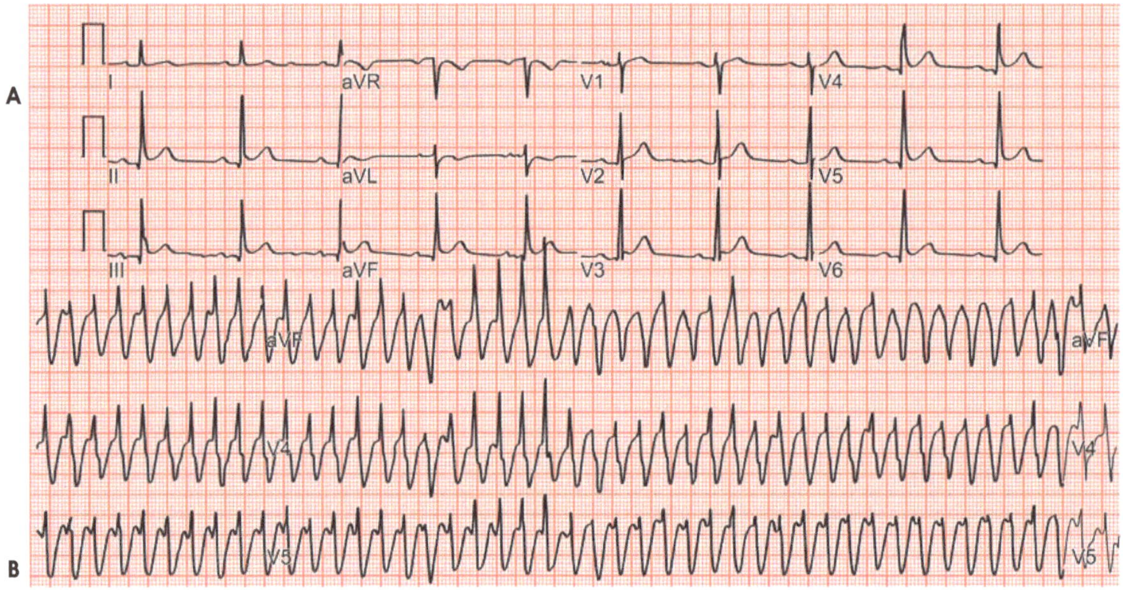

Fig. 33.41 Note the features of ERPV in the baseline ECG (A) recorded immediately before an exercise stress test (B) that resulted in Torsade de Pointe.

T-wave inversions could reflect myocardial ischemia and thus warrants further investigation in older athletes.

Differential Diagnosis between Athlete's Heart and Cardiovascular Disease (Figs. 33.42–33.50)

Dilated Cardiomyopathy: In an important minority of athlets, the increase in left ventricular diastolic cavity dimension that occurs with training overlaps with that characteristic of certain known pathological entities.

For example, while left ventricular end-diastolic cavity dimension in athletes is usually in the range of 53 to 58 mm, in some individuals it may extend into what may be regarded as the pathological range of >58 mm and thereby resemble dilated cardiomyopathy.However, the absence of left ventricular systolic dysfunction is usually sufficient to distinguish this physiological ventricular enlargement induced by training from that due to dilated cardiomyopathy.

Myocarditis: Myocarditis, a disorder associated with a heterogeneous clinical profile, has recently been incriminated as the possible cause of some highly publicized deaths in athletes. While myocarditis usually has an infectious origin, it can also be a consequence of drug abuse Sudden cardiac death

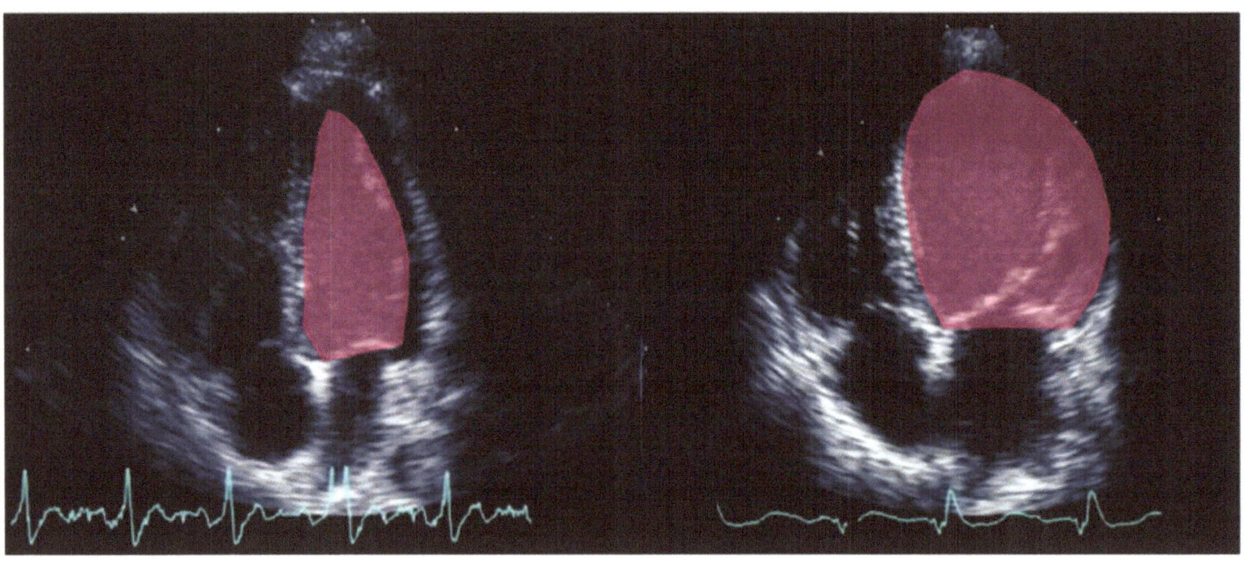

Fig. 33.42 Apical 4C views shows (Left) Normal scan (Right) dilated ,thin LV and LA with low LVEF

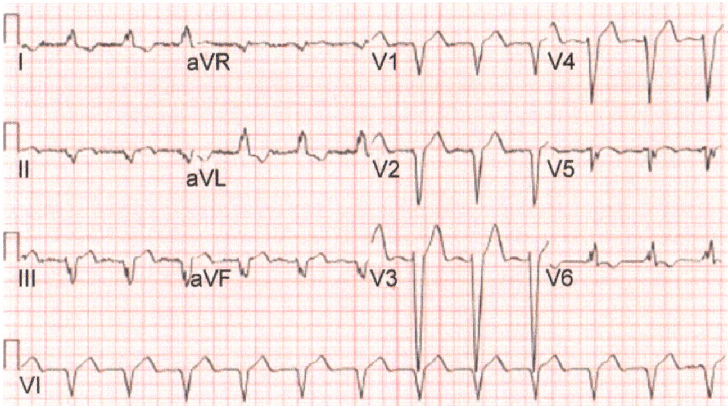

Fig. 33.43 ECG with complete LBBB demonstrating a QRS >120 ms, predominantly negative QRS complex in lead V1, upright R wave in leads I and V6, and ST segments and T waves in the opposite direction of the QRS. LBBB is always an abnormal finding in athletes and warrants a comprehensive evaluation to exclude myocardial disease. LBBB, left bundle branch block.

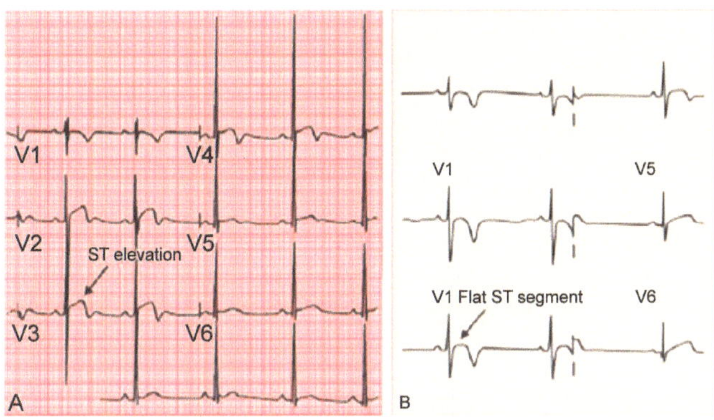

Fig. 33.44 (A) Normal variant repolarisation changes in a black/African athlete characterised by domed ST segment elevation and T wave inversion in V_1–V_4. (B) Pathological T wave inversion in V_1–V_3. Note the isoelectric ST segment. The absence of ST segment elevation prior to T wave inversion makes this ECG abnormal. Additional testing is required to rule out arrhythmogenic right ventricular cardiomyopathy. This figure is only reproduced in colour in the online version.

may occur in its active or healed phases as a consequence of complex arrhythmias that develop in the setting of an unstable myocardial electrical substrate. In an athlete with myocarditis, left ventricular cavity enlargement may be due to the disease, to athletic training, or to a combination of these, but the differential diagnosis with athlete's heart is usually resolved by the presence of clinically relevant and overt arrhythmias, cardiac symptoms such as syncope, presyncope and palpitations, or heart failure with systolic dysfunction. In some instances, the diagnosis may also be clarified by histological examination of myocardium obtained by endomyocardial biopsy.

Right Ventricular Dysplasia: Arrhythmogenic right ventricular dysplasia (or cardiomyopathy) is a heart muscle disorder of unknown cause that is characterized pathologically by fibrofatty replacement of the right ventricular myocardium. The clinical and phenotypic profile is variable but includes structural and functional abnormalities of the right ventricle, ventricular and supraventricular arrhythmias, familial occurrence, and the risk for sudden cardiac death. Indeed, it has been suggested that right ventricular dysplasia is an important cause of sudden death in the young, including competitive athletes, largely on the basis of reports from the north-eastern (Veneto) region of Italy.

Because highly trained athletes may demonstrate right ventricular enlargement and a variety of depolarization, repolarization, and conduction abnormalities on the ECG, the differential diagnosis between athlete's heart and right ventricular dysplasia may arise. Non-invasive identification of right vcntricular dysplasia by cchocardiography may bc difficult because of technical limitations in imaging right

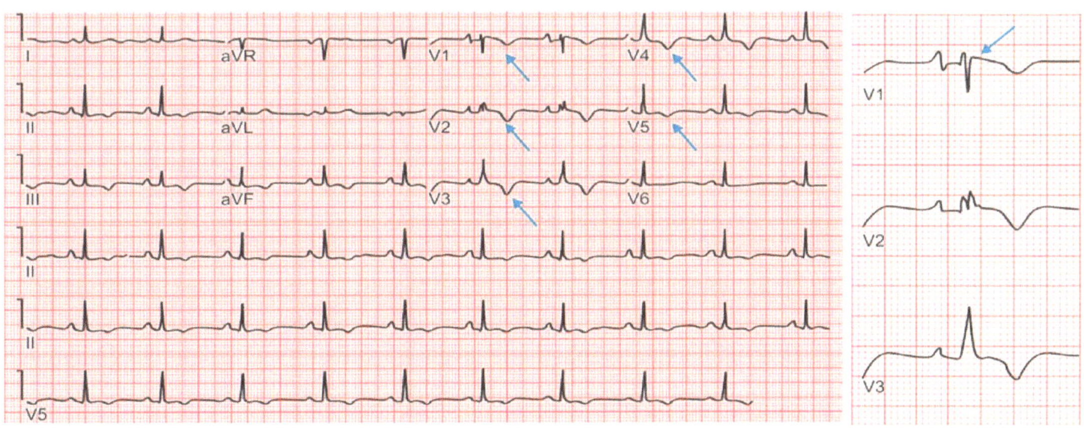

Fig. 33.45 ECG from a patient with arrhythmogenic right ventricular cardiomyopathy. (A) Inverted T waves in leads V_1–V_5. (B) A subtle epsilon wave with notching in V_1 at the terminal portion of the QRS complex.

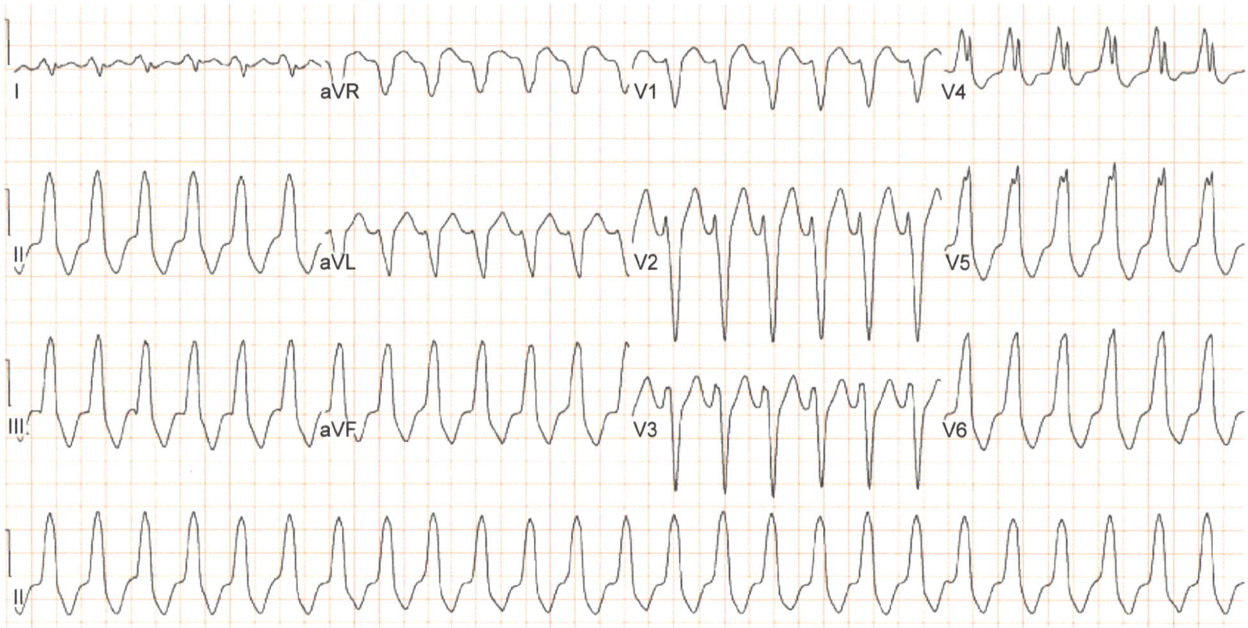

Fig. 33.46 ECG trace showing RVOT tachycardia: Broad complex tachycardia. LBBB-like morphology. Inferior axis (+ 90 degrees). due to right ventricular dysplasia.

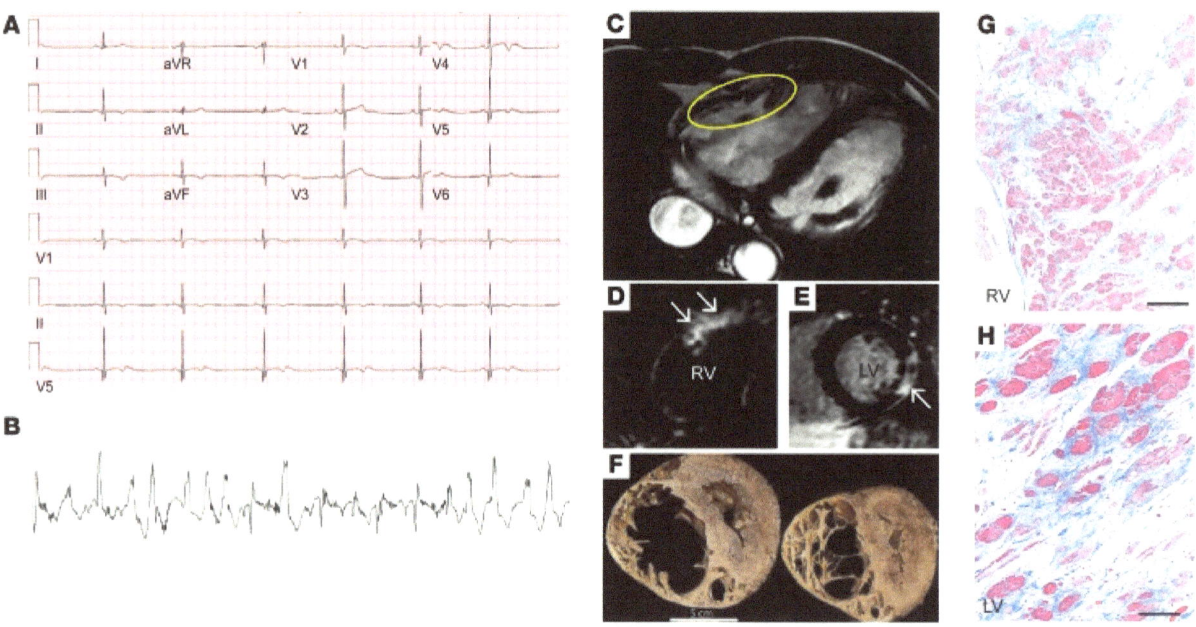

Fig. 33.47 Deceased proband harboring AnkB loss-of-function p.Glu1458Gly variant exhibits arrhythmogenic cardiomyopathy. (A) Surface 12-lead ECG. (B) Loop recording demonstrating nonsustained polymorphic VT. (C) Cardiac magnetic resonance short-axis image revealing moderate biventricular dilation; the yellow ring highlights focal "crinkling" of the subtricuspid region of the right ventricular free wall consistent with the "accordion sign." (D) Delayed enhancement imaging revealed scarring in the right ventricular (RV) free wall in a short-axis view (arrows) and (E) the left ventricular (LV) lateral wall (arrow) in a long-axis view. (F) Mid-transverse section of the autopsied heart revealing severe right ventricular dilation and wall thinning as well as concentric hypertrophy of the left ventricle. Histology of the (G) right ventricle showing severe fibrofatty infiltration of the free wall in association with extensive ventricular interstitial fibrosis and (H) left ventricle showing moderate hypertrophy with focal areas of fibrofatty muscular infiltration and widespread interstitial fibrosis. Scale bars: 160 μm (G) and 60 μm (H).

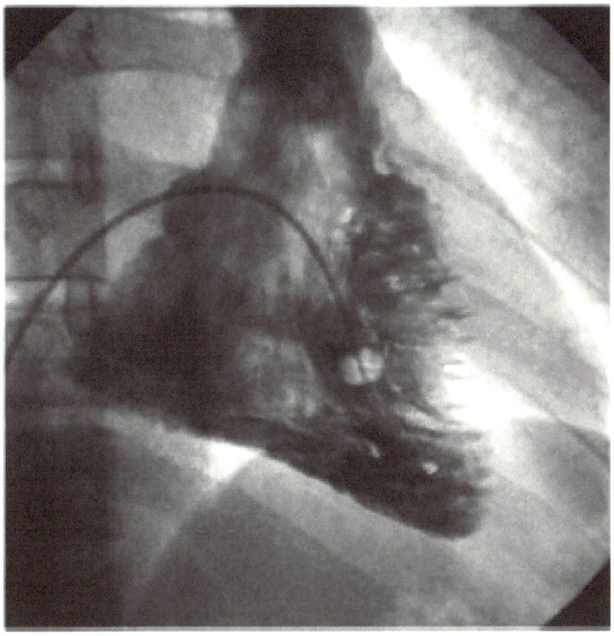

Fig. 33.48 Right ventriculogram showing akinetic/dyskinetic areas with diastolic septal bulge ("stack of coins") compatible with arrhythmogenic right ventricular dysplasia.

ventricular structure and assessing function in these patients and because the spectrum of the disease is broad and includes mild morphological forms with subtle manifestations. Magnetic resonance imaging, however, promises enhanced non-invasive diagnosis of this condition. The demonstration of right ventricular segmental or global dysfunction or substantial right ventricular cavity enlargement would support the diagnosis of right ventricular dysplasia; alternatively, thickening or enlargement of the left ventricle would be most consistent with athlete's heart.

Hypertrophic Cardiomyopathy: The greatest difficulty in distinguishing clinically between athlete's heart and structural heart disease most frequently arises with respect to HCM, since many of the other cardiac disorders that cause sudden death in a young athletic population can be identified independently of any changes in cardiac morphology typically associated with training. The basic definition of HCM used here is that of a patient (or athlete) with evidence of a hypertrophied and nondilated left ventricle in the absence of another cardiac or systemic disease that could itself cause hypertrophy of the magnitude present in that individual.

Wall Thickness: In the vast majority of competitive athletes, absolute left ventricular wall thickness is normal or only mildly increased (12 mm) In some athletes, however, the increase in left ventricular wall thickness may be more substantial, up to 16 mm, unavoidably raising the possibility of HCM. In patients with HCM, the increase in left ventricular

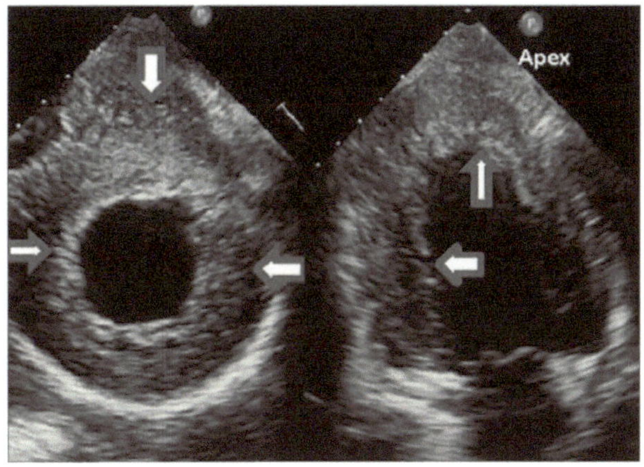

Fig. 33.49 Echocardiogram showing short axis (left) and two chamber view(right) in patient with HOCM affecting more than one segment including the apex (arrows).

wall thickness is usually marked; the average wall thickness reported in most echocardiographic studies of this disease is 20 mm, ranging to >50 mm. However, an important minority of patients with HCM show relatively mild left ventricular hypertrophy with wall thickness values in the range of 13 to 15 mm, and many of these patients are asymptomatic.Therefore, a diagnostic dilemma arises in those athletes who fall into this morphological "gray zone" between physiological hypertrophy and HCM. While this distinction cannot be resolved with certainty in some of these athletes, careful analysis of several echocardiographic and clinical features permits this diagnostic differentiation in most.

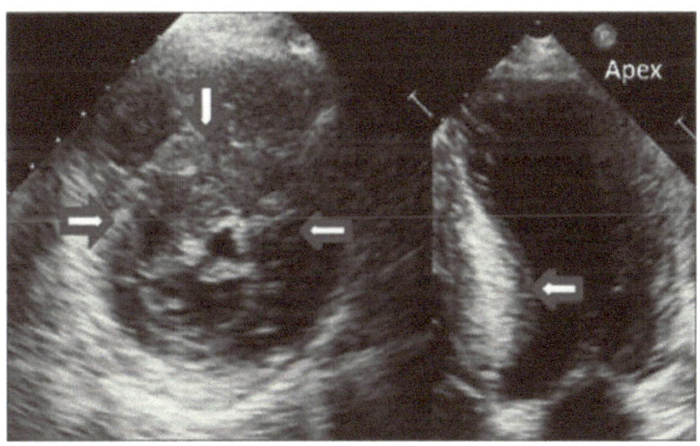

Fig. 33.50 Echocardiogram showing hypertrophy of more than one segment (arrows) in short axis and long axis but sparing the apex in patient with HOCM.

CARDIAC ARRHYTHMIA IN YOUNG ATHLETES (FIGS. 33.51–33.58)

Atrial Fibrillation

Treatment of atrial fibrillation in young athletes is similar to other young patient populations. There is little evidence that calcium channel blockers and α-blockers reduce episodes of atrial fibrillation, but rather make them less symptomatic when they occur. Antiarrhythmic drugs are typically quite effective in individuals without heart disease.

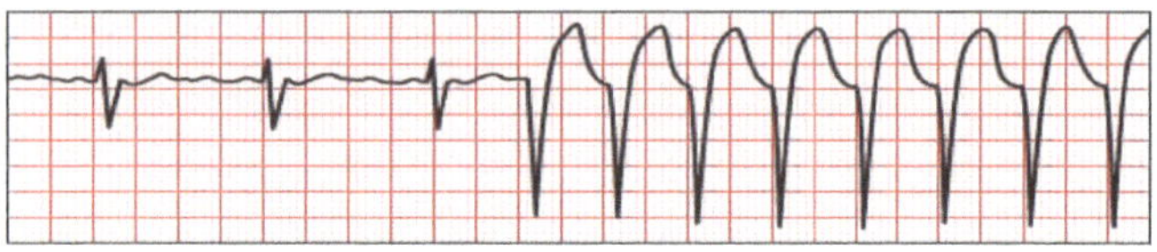

Fig. 33.51 ECG trace showing atrial fibrillation in a young athlete

Type 1C agents such as flecainide or propafenone are generally preferred as initial agents because of the safety profile and efficacy of these drugs. Rapid atrial flutter can be especially troubling with flecainide and for this reason a rate controlling agent such as a α-blocker or calcium channel blocker is generally recommended. The use of amiodarone is not advised because of the young age of the athletes and the long-term toxicity of amiodarone. Whether dronedarone will play a role in the management of atrial fibrillation in young athletes is not yet clear. Ablation of atrial fibrillation is a particularly attractive option for athletes as they generally are young, have normal hearts and face a lifetime of atrial fibrillation risk .Pulmonary vein isolation would be a reasonable first step in the ablation of atrial fibrillation in athletes with more aggressive ablation options reserved for those who fail pulmonary vein isolation.

Atrial flutter is unusual in the individual without heart disease; when present, a stress test and echocardiogram are necessary to rule out the presence of structural heart disease.

Radiofrequency ablation is preferable to antiarrhythmic agents in individuals with atrial flutter because of the high likelihood of cure and the low risk of the procedure. Anticoagulation in atrial fibrillation and atrial flutter is no different than in nonathletes.

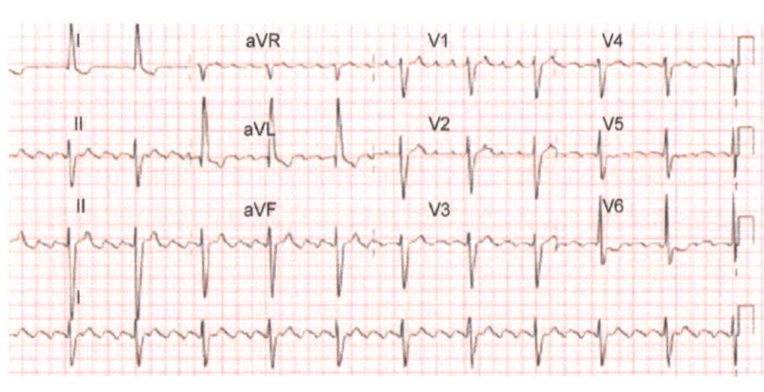

Fig. 33.52 ECG trace showing atrial flutter with 4:1 block. There are inverted flutter waves in II, III + aVF at a rate of 260 bpm. There are upright flutter waves in V_{1-2} (= anticlockwise circuit). There is 4:1 block, resulting in a ventricular rate of 65 bpm. The relatively slow ventricular response suggests treatment with an AV nodal blocking agent.

Wolf-ParkinsonWhite(WPW) Syndrome is not more common in the athlete, but athletes with WPW may be at higher risk for sudden death due to the high sympathetic drive seen with competition and with training.

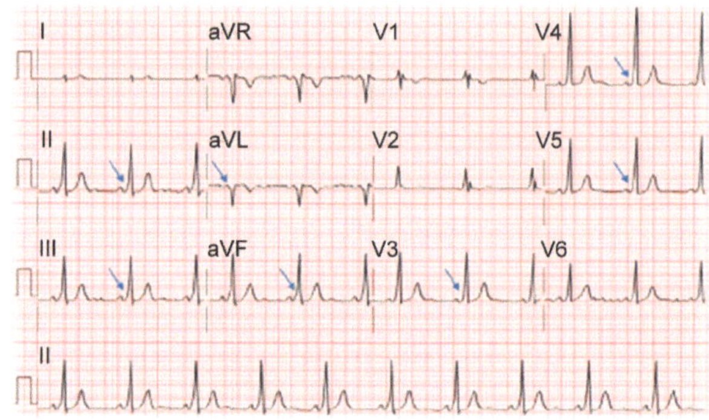

Fig. 33.53 ECG interpretation: PR interval <0.12 seconds, P waves of normal appearance.

QRS complex is wide, with a longer duration than 0.12 seconds; The presence of delta waves. Slow enrollment or thickening of the initial portion of the QRS complex (delta wave) is the most important criterion for diagnosis of Wolff-Parkinson-White syndrome. Delta wave length range between 0.02-0.07 seconds; Secondary changes of ST segment and T wave, which are showing a opposite direction from the QRS complex and delta wave.

For this reason most authorities recommended risk stratification of individuals with WPW .Risk stratification may be performed by rapid atrial pacing, by induction of atrial fibrillation in the electrophysiological laboratory and sometimes by stress testing. The 36th Bethesda guidelines recommend ablation for multiple bypass tracts or if the bypass tract can conduct rapidly enough to sustain a tachycardia of greater than 240 bpm. ESC Guidelines are more aggressive and recommend ablation for all asymptomatic WPW athletes age 12 years because of the relative ease of ablation and the life-long risk of SCD. In individuals who refuse ablation, competitive sports are allowed provided that short pre-excited cycle lengths of < 240 ms at rest and < 220 on isoproterenol or exercise during atrial fibrillation are not present. Both European and Bethesda Guidelines recommend radiofrequency ablation for the symptomatic athlete with WPW.

Supraventricular tachycardias such as AV nodal reentrant tachycardia, AV reciprocating tachycardia, and atrial tachycardia are not more common in athletes. Similar to non-athletes, when these arrhythmias occur initial treatment may be with beta-blockers and calcium channel blockers. However, in both the 36th Bethesda Guidelines and the

European Guidelines, definitive treatment such as ablation is generally preferred because of the young age and lifetime risk of these arrhythmias. Atrial premature contractions are common in many individuals and may be symptomatic or asymptomatic.

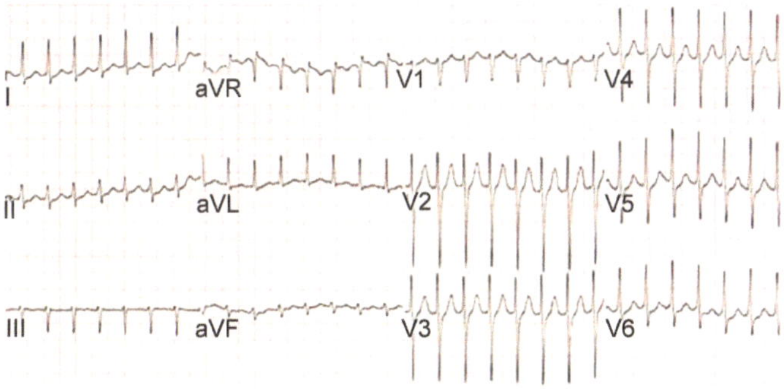

Fig. 33.54 ECG Showing Supraventricular tachycardia - AV nodal reentry. AV nodal reentry is a form of SVT that establishes its atrioventricular circuit entirely within the AV node. The heart rate is usually regular, between 150 to 250 bpm (below = 186 bpm). The QRS complex is narrow with a duration less than 0.2 seconds and a conduction ratio of 1:1. P waves are buried within the QRS compelx although they may be visible at the end of the complex as a distortion of the terminal forces. Due to the fact that atrial activation originates from the inferior aspect of the right atrium, P wave polarity is negative in leads II, III and aVF. This form of SVT is usually benign and is easily converted to sinus rhythm by vagal maneuvers.

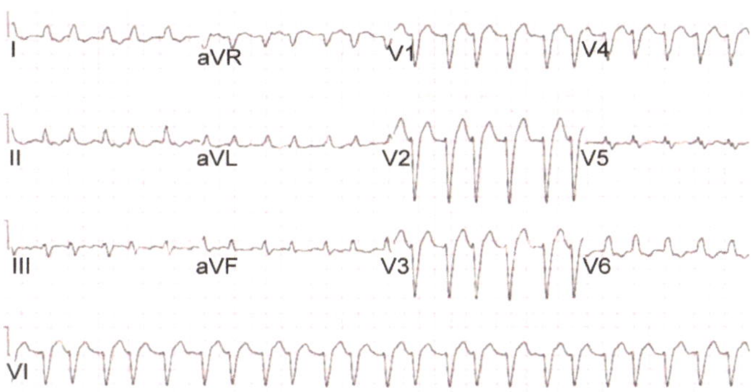

Fig. 33.55 ECG Findings: Supraventricular Tachycardia with Aberrancy

If symptomatic, atrial premature beats can be treated with â-blockers; however, reassurance is usually reasonable enough treatment.

Idiopathic Ventricular Tachycardia

The 2 most common cardiac regions for idiopathic ventricular tachycardias are the right ventricular outflow tract and the left posterior fascicle. Both of these ventricular tachycardias can be triggered by exercise and both these ventricular tachycardias are readily curable with ablation. They are also adenosine and verapamil sensitive. In individuals with these idiopathic ventricular tachycardias strong consideration should be given to ablation as the ablation is curative and of relatively low risk

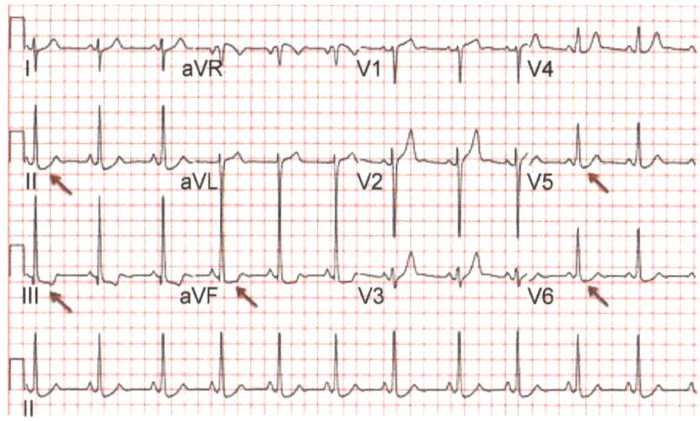

Fig. 33.56 Left-bundle branch block ventricular tachycardia with inferior axis (right ventricular outflow tract origin).

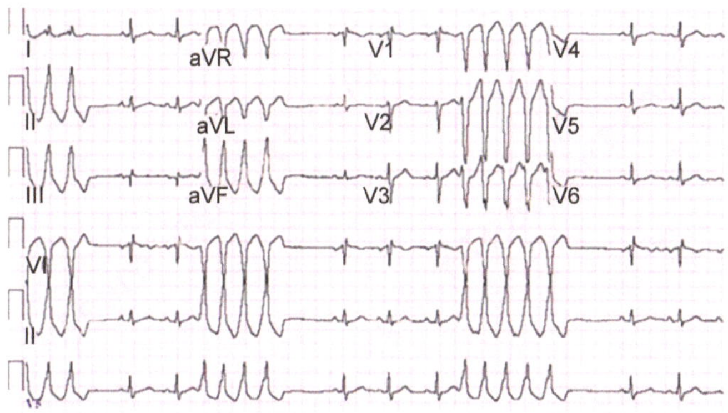

Fig. 33.57 ECGshowing Non-sustained Monomorphic Ventricular Tachycardia.

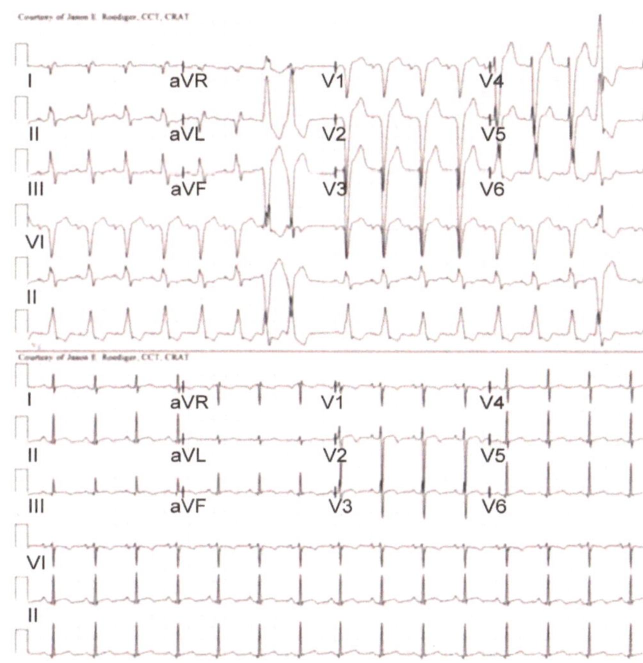

Fig. 33.58 12-lead ECGs from a 49-year-old black man with arrythmogenic cardiomyopathy. (TOP): Sinus tachycardia (rate about 101/min) with LBBB accompanied by RAD (here about 108°). Frequent multifocal PVCs (both singly and in pairs) and left atrial enlargement. (BOTTOM): Same patient about 5 months later status-post orthotopic heart transplant.

Deep vein thrombosis (DVT) or pulmonary embolism (PE) in athletes (Figs. 33.59–33.64)

The diagnosis of deep vein thrombosis (DVT) or pulmonary embolism (PE) in athletes, who exhibit classic symptoms (table 1), may be delayed or even missed because such medical problems are often not considered by healthcare providers or by the affected athlete. No studies have been done to determine whether athletes are at a higher, the same, or lower risk for developing blood clots than non-athletes. Blood clots are uncommon in young, healthy individuals – and most athletes are young and healthy. So, for that reason, DVT, PE, and arterial clots in athletes are not the norm.

To understand the problematic issues facing an athlete and the attending caregiver it is important to first understand the condition terminology. Our body is composed of an endless tunnel of arteries and veins through which blood

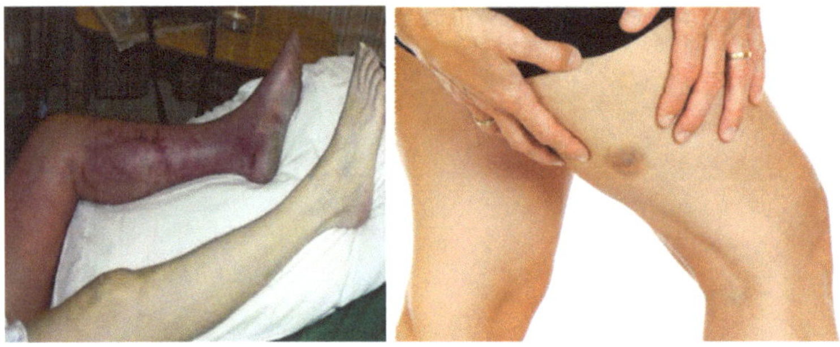

Fig. 33.59 Photographs of two athletes who developed venous thromboses after exhausitive competitive games.

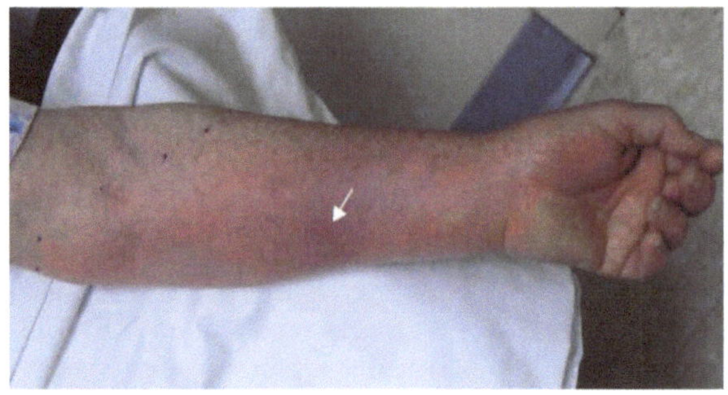

Fig. 33.60 Photographs of a athlete who developed venous thromboses after extensive exercise

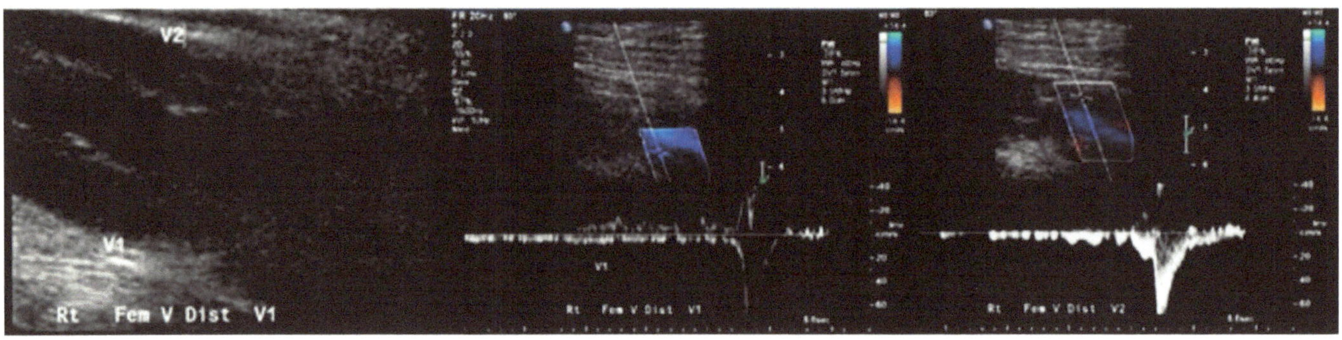

Fig. 33.61 The ultrasound image left) shows the distal femoral vein, which is duplicated. The wave form in both branches is also shown.

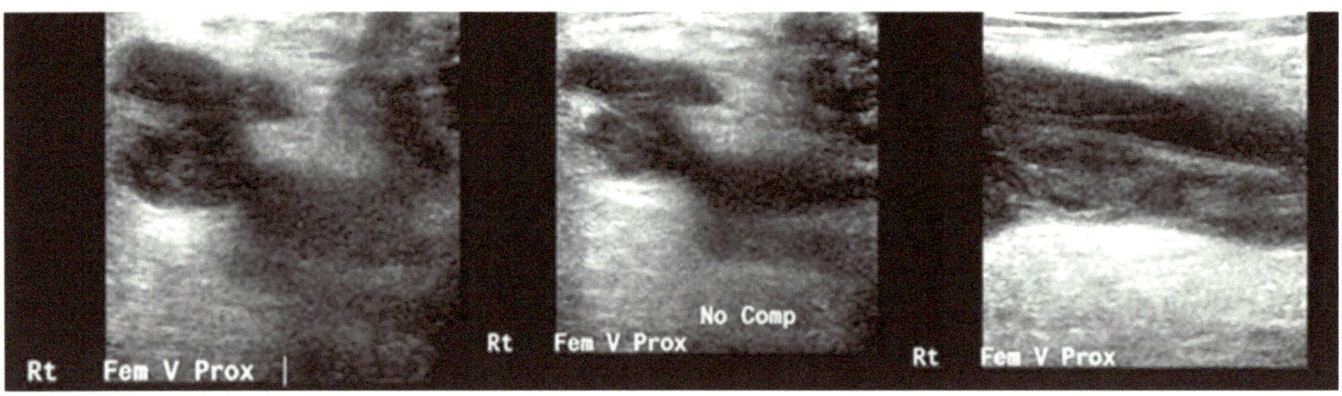

Fig. 33.62 These three views of the proximal femoral vein show the diameter of an occluding thrombus within the vessel. The middle image shows no compression of the vessel; the longitudinal image on the right shows the length of the thrombus. This clot extends into the profunda femoris and greater saphenous veins, as we shall see shortly. A clot this large can break away from the vessel wall becoming an embolus that may lodge in the pulmonary veins or go upward to occlude blood supply to the brain.

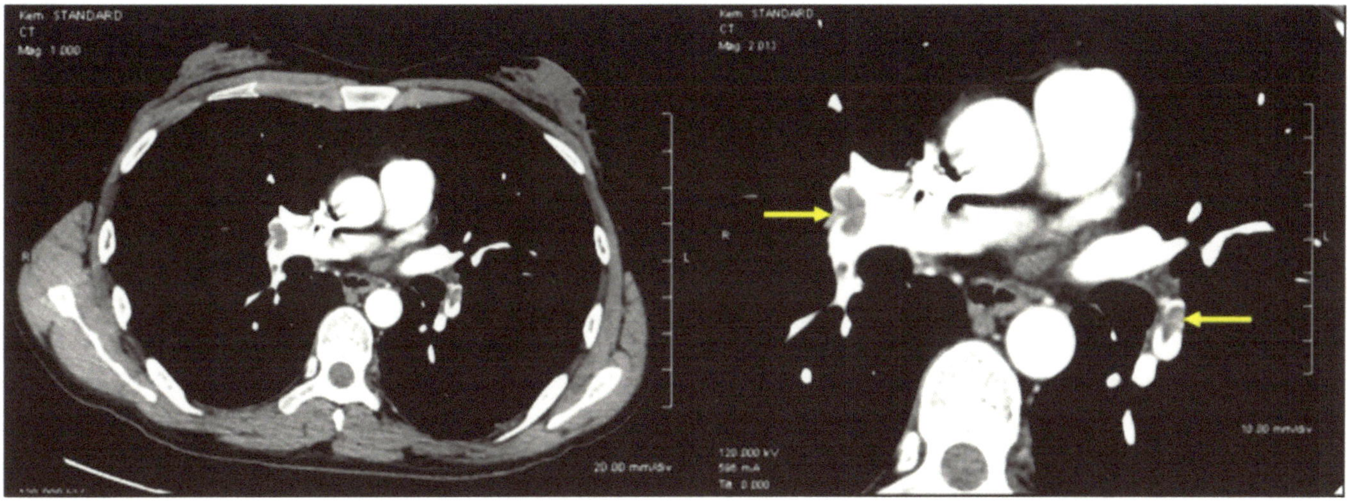

Fig. 33.63 These two axial CT images show profound pulmonary emboli. On the left the embolus almost completely blocks the right pulmonary artery (yellow arrow). Right image show an extensive saddle embolus forming in both pulmonary arteries and becoming extensive. Both of these types of pulmonary emboli are life threatening and require immediate medical attention.

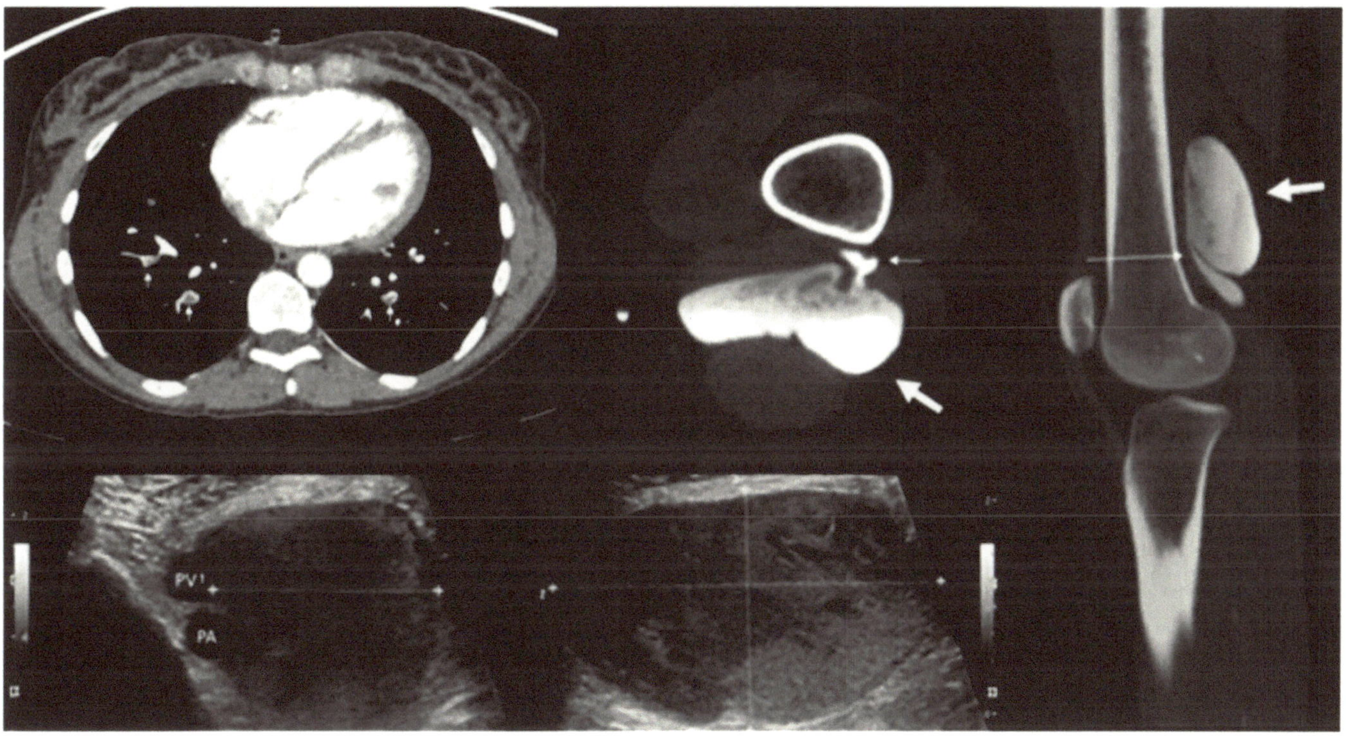

Fig.33.64 Popliteal vein aneurysm presenting as recurrent pulmonary embolism.

flows throughout the body. Arteries are the blood vessels through which the blood flows from the heart into the periphery: the brain, the internal organs, the legs, and the arms. A clot in an artery leads to stroke, heart attack, or limb threatening peripheral arterial clot causing a painful, cold, and pale extremity. Many people think of blood clots as a problem occurring in elderly people, but not in young and apparently healthy individuals. Symptoms may, therefore, be misinterpreted as something less serious. The leg symptoms from DVT are often interpreted as "muscle tear," a "Charlie horse," a "twisted ankle," or shin splints, while the chest symptoms from PE are attributed to a pulled muscle, costochondritis (inflammation of the joint between ribs and breast bone), bronchitis, or a "touch of pneumonia." Veins are the vessels through which blood is carried back to the heart. A clot in the deep veins of legs, arms, pelvis, abdomen, or around the brain is called a deep vein thrombosis (DVT). If a piece of clot breaks off from a leg or arm DVT it can travel into the lung causing a life threatening condition known as a pulmonary embolism (PE).

Athlete-Specific Risk Factors for Clots (Figs. 33.65–33.69)

Being apparently healthy and being an athlete does not prevent a person from developing blood clots. Several circumstances put the athlete, as well as the non-athlete, at increased risk for DVT and PE. Athletes, coaches and trainers should be particularly aware of these risk factors.

Blood clots can occur when:

- There is a disparity between the two systems that balance the clotting process in our blood; either
  - (A) Too much activity of the proteins and blood platelets that form clots (the procoagulant system), or
  - (B) Too little activity of the system that dissolves blood clots as they form (the fibrinolytic system)
- There is trauma to the blood vessel wall, as may occur after a bone fracture or in thoracic outlet obstruction
- Blood return from the extremities to the heart is impaired, such as when sitting with bent legs in cramped positions for a prolonged period of time;

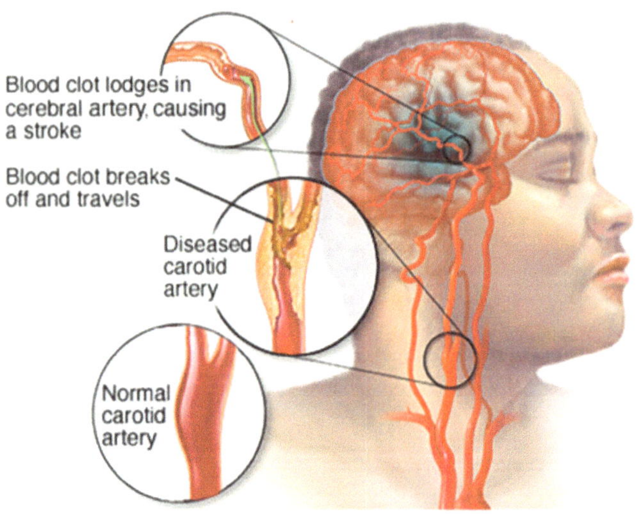

Fig 33.65 Illustration shows the pathogenesis of development of cerebral strok in athlete

- The blood is "thicker" than usual, as occurs when an athlete is dehydrated, using the drug erythropoietin (EPO), or has received excessive blood transfusions (blood doping).
- Unfortunately, there are few studies investigating the influence that physical training has on blood clot formation and dissolution. So, the exact net effect of training on this equilibrium is unknown. It is known, for example, that blood levels of the clotting protein "factor VIII" increase with exercise and that the elevation persists during recovery. Theoretically, this could lead to an increased risk of blood clots in athletes. However, data also indicate that the fibrinolytic system that dissolves blood clots is overactive in people who exercise. With this over activity present, the athlete would be protected from having a blood clot. Yet, the net effect of these changes in the athlete is not known.
- A detailed scientific discussion of the coagulation issues relevant to exercise and training can be found in a recently published review . However, the conclusions are sparse and vague, because of a lack of data and conflicting results from different studies.

Risk Factors for DVT and PE in Athletes

The most common clots occurring in athletes are DVT of the leg and PE. Factors that increase the risk for an athlete, as well as the non-athlete, are listed in table 2. A few unique risk factors predisposing the young and the athlete to DVT and PE are:

Thoracic Outlet Obstruction

In some individuals an extra (cervical) rib or excess muscle or tendon tissue compress the big vein in the upper chest (subclavian vein) that drains the blood from the arm. This compression typically gets worse when the arm is lifted up. This obstruction, often combined with repeated trauma to the vein (due to throwing activities or gymnastics maneuvers), may cause a DVT to form in this area, extending into the arm veins. This is termed "effort thrombosis" or "thoracic outlet obstruction/syndrome." If the DVT resolves, such as after clot buster treatment, resection of the extra rib or the excess tissue may be indicated to increase space in the thoracic outlet.

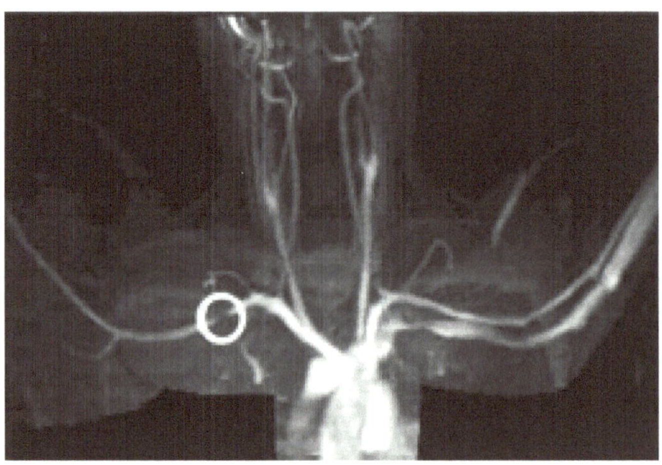

Fig.33.66 MRI scan of the thoracic outlet showing compression of the subclavian artery.

May-Thurner Syndrome

This is a common congenital anatomic variation that predisposes to DVT in the left leg, because the main left pelvic vein is compressed by the overlying main right pelvic

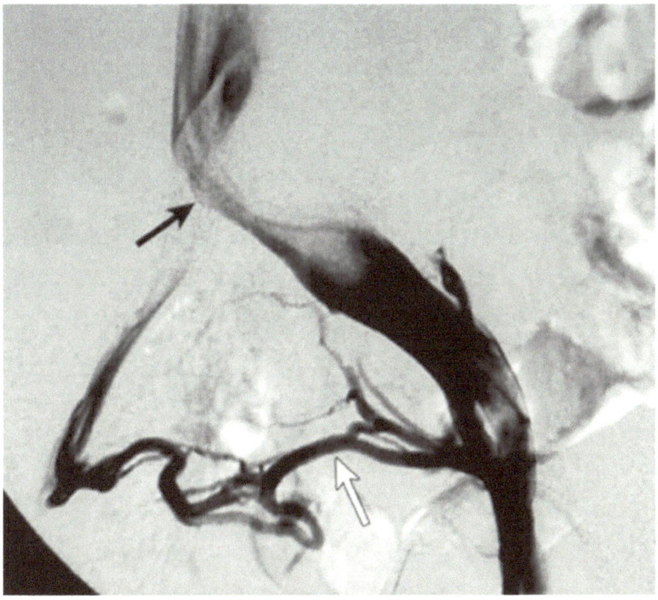

Fig. 33.67 Subtracted frontal venogram shows left iliac vein in May-Thurner syndrome. Note the compressed left common iliac vein (black arrow) and contralateral venous drainage via pelvic venous collaterals (white arrow).

artery. This increases the risk of clot formation at the site of this narrowing in the left pelvis with extension of clot down into the left leg. If the DVT resolves, such as after clot buster (thrombolytic) treatment, the narrowing can be opened up by a radiologist with a balloon angioplasty and then kept open by placing a stent.

Congenital Absence or Malformation of the Vena Cava

Congenital abnormalities of the anatomy of the big vein in the abdomen (vena cava) or pelvic veins can be a cause of DVT in young people. The abnormal anatomy probably leads to disturbed blood flow and an increased risk of clotting.

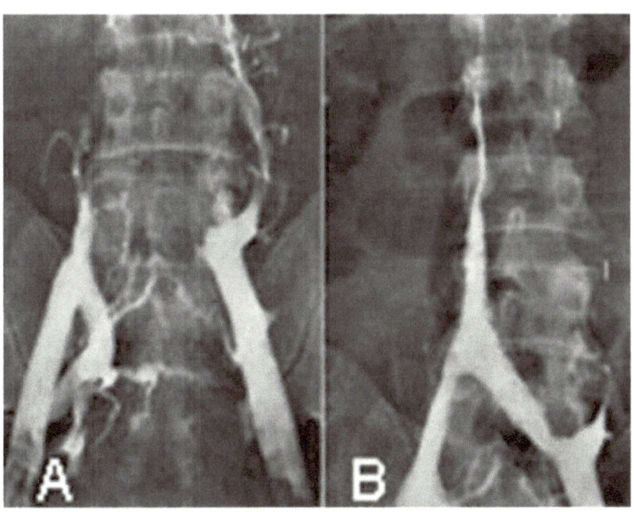

Fig. 33.68 (A) Occluded IVC and common iliac (B) After Urokinase infusion

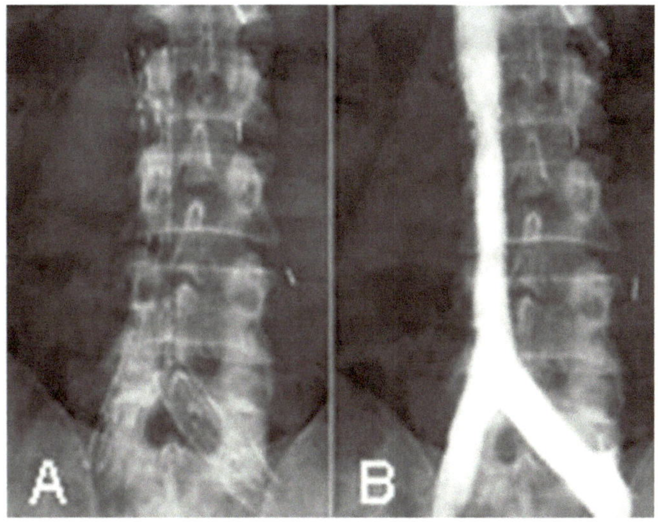

Fig.33.69 (A) After stent placement (B) Five month follow up venogram.

The patient was intravenously heparinized and prepared for thrombolysis. An ultrasound-guided puncture was performed in both popliteal veins with multiperforated 5F catheters. Both catheters progressed easily until the IVC. However, about 5 cm above the iliac vein confluence, the catheters stopped progressing at a site lateral to the IVC wall (Figure 1). Phlebography was performed, confirming a voluminous thrombosis with increased iliac arteries and extensive collateral circulation above those veins, with no contrast in the IVC. Due to the hypothesis of extrinsic IVC compression, thrombolysis was not performed.

Treatment decisions for people affected with blood clots must be individualized. This is particularly true for young, apparently healthy individuals, such as athletes. In thc case of unexplained DVT, testing for an inherited or acquired clotting disorder may be appropriate. When first diagnosed with the DVT, clot buster medication (fibrinolytic or thrombolytic therapy) should be considered to quickly dissolve the clot. However, clot buster treatment has not been systematically studied to determine whether it really decreases the risk for long-term damage to the veins of the leg and arm, i.e. the post-thrombotic syndrome.

Sudden Cardiac Arrest in Young Athletes

Each year between 10–12 million kids in the U.S. participate in sports. The tragedy of a sudden death in an otherwise "presumably healthy" child causes not only sadness, but concern as to how the death might have been prevented. Doctors are often asked, "is not there a test or something to prevent this? Depending on the studies I have read, the sudden cardiac death of a child or adolescent accounts for about 100 deaths a year in the U.S. The prevalence rate for sudden cardiac death is 1:100,000-200,000 and is higher among males than females. Statistics show that 90% of these sudden deaths occur immediately post training or competition with football and basketball having the highest incidence. In 2007 the American Heart Association came out with guidelines to evaluate athletes who may be at risk for sudden cardiac death. The most important screening mechanism has been found to be the "gold standard" in medicine, a thorough history and physical exam. The history that should be taken on any athlete who is being screened for sports participation should include a history of any unexplained or sudden death in a family member. Are there any family members with unexplained fainting episodes or seizures? Are there family members who had unexplained deaths (drowning or single car accidents)? Are there any family members with a known genetic disorder that predisposes to sudden cardiac death? The history should also ask about any fainting (syncope) in the athlete. After a good history is taken (which should be updated yearly), the child/adolescent needs a complete and thorough physical exam. This exam should include blood pressure measurements, and a careful cardiac exam looking for new murmurs. Symptoms such as palpitations during exercise, visual changes, fainting while exercising or immediately after exercise, and chest pain should all warrant further evaluation. Studies show that about half of pediatric patients who succumb to sudden cardiac death had experienced a warning sign. There are about 20 causes for SCD, with the most common causes being hypertrophic cardiomyopathy, anomalous coronary artery, and myocarditis. While some may advocate routine EKG screening and echocardiograms on athletes (this is done in Italy), many studies have been done which show that it would take the screening of 200,000 student athletes to prevent 1 death. At the same time you will certainly identify some children with clear risk factors for SCD, but for every positive finding there may be 10–20 athletes who have "borderline" or questionable findings that would require even more expensive follow up. These pediatric patients might also be told they cannot participate in sports during the evaluation time and some might be told that they cannot participate even if they were not found to have disease, but were excluded just due to liability concerns. There does not seem to be one right answer to this issue. If your child is going to begin competitive sports make sure to see your pediatrician for a complete physical exam including a good family history. Also advocate that your school have automatic external defibrillators viable at all times and personnel that know how to use them. That's your daily dose for today. We'll chat again tomorrow.

Risk of Sudden Death during Sports Performance (Figs. 33.70–33.81)

Little is known about the risk of sudden death associated with exercise in young competitive athletes, and whether the benefits of sports activity outweigh the hazards of exercise-related fatal events is a clinical dilemma. For the purpose of this consensus document, we consider young competitive athletic individuals who are aged 35 years or less and are engaged in a regular fashion in exercise training as well as participating in official athletic competitions. Competition is intended as an organized team or individual sport event, placing high premium on athletic excellence and achievement.

Characteristics of competitive athletes are their strong inclination to extend themselves physically to their limits and to improve performance. Recently, Corrado et al. assessed the incidence of sudden death in the athletic and non-athletic young population (12–35 years old) of the Veneto Region of Italy and showed that competitive sports activity enhances by 2.5-fold the risk of sudden death in adolescents and young adults. In this study, young competitive athletes who died suddenly were affected by silent cardiovascular diseases, predominantly consisting of cardiomyopathies, premature coronary artery disease, and congenital coronary anomalies.

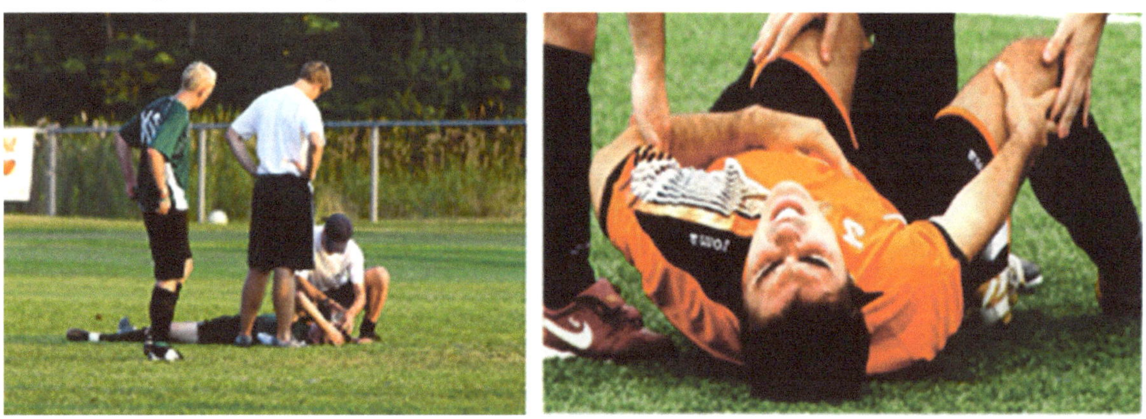

Fig. 33.70 Photographs showing unconscious athletes in the ground with resuscitative ground staff

Therefore, sports activity was not per se a cause of the increased mortality; rather, it acted as a trigger of cardiac arrest upon those underlying cardiovascular diseases predisposing to life-threatening ventricular arrhythmias. Thus, it seems ethically and clinically justifiable that every effort should be made to recognize in good time such diseases that the athlete is at risk, with the perspective that disqualification of affected individuals makes the prevention of athletic field death possible.

A variety of cardiovascular diseases have been identified as potential causes of sudden death in young competitive athletes (<35 years old). The vast majority of these deaths occur on the athletic field during severe exertion in the context of training or competition. Each of the responsible diseases is also known to cause sudden death in non-athletes.

1. Hypertrophic obstructive cardiomyopathy(HOCM)

Hypertrophic cardiomyopathy (HCM) is a primary disease of the myocardium (the muscle of the heart) in which a portion of the myocardium is hypertrophied (thickened) without any obvious cause, creating functional impairment of the cardiac muscle. It is a leading cause of sudden cardiac death in young athletes. The occurrence of hypertrophic cardiomyopathy is a significant cause of sudden unexpected cardiac death in any age group and as a cause of disabling cardiac symptoms. Younger people are likely to have a more severe form of hypertrophic cardiomyopathy.

2. Congenital coronary artery anomalies

Sudden and unexpected cardiac deaths in young subjects are rare, but tragic events in competitive athletes assume high public profile, and that unavoidably raise questions regarding the underlying pathological causes and clinical strategies to prevent these catastrophes . Various pathological investigations have reported that several structural cardiovascular abnormalities are responsible for sudden death in young athletes, but hypertrophic cardiomyopathy is the most common disease in U.S. autopsy-based series, and right ventricular cardiomyopathy predominates in young Italian athletes. Nevertheless, congenital coronary artery anomalies (CCAA) are frequently found (in about 20% of cases), and they represent the second most frequent disease responsible for athletic field deaths. Specifically, the wrong sinus coronary artery origin, that is, the left main artery arising from the right anterior sinus (ALMCA), and the right coronary artery originating from the left sinus (ARCA), with a proximal course between aorta and pulmonary trunk, are the most frequent occurrences of CCAA.

3. Myocarditis

Myocarditis is the reason for sudden cardiac death in 5-22% of athletes < 35 years of age. Actually, parvovirus B19 and human herpes virus 6 are the most important pathogens.

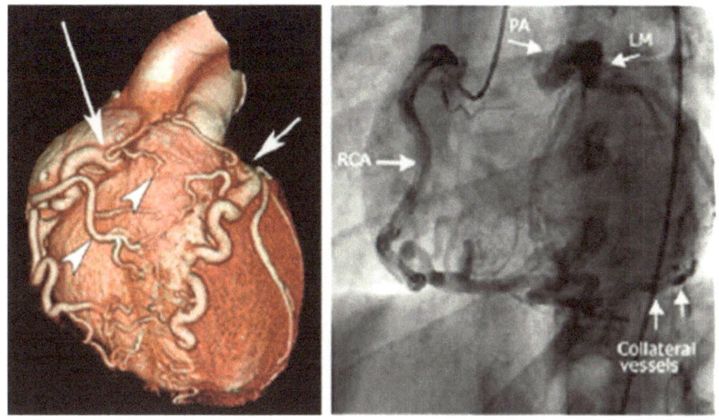

Fig 33.71 Cronary artery anomalies. (A) Three-dimensional volume-rendered multidetector CT angiogram shows dilated intercoronary collateral arteries (arrowheads), which connect the tortuous RCA (long arrow) to the LCA (short arrow). (B) Cine-Coronary angiography of the right coronary artery with collateral filling of the left coronary vascular territory, which connects directly to the pulmonary trunk.

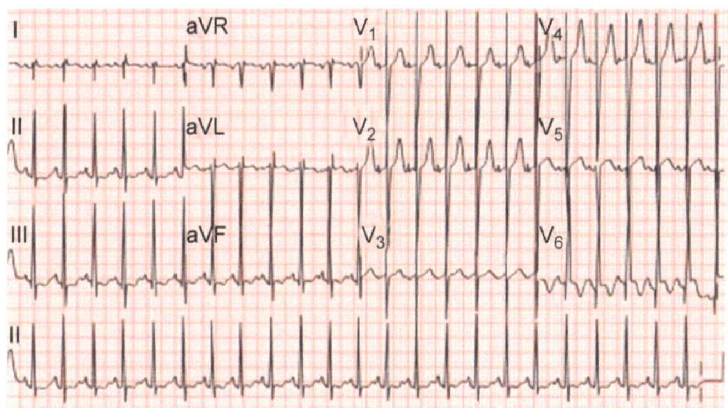

Fig.33.72 ECG presentation in patient with ALCAPA. Typical prominent Q waves are present in lead V6. Conversely, typical abrupt loss of R waves in midprecordial leads and prominent Q waves in leads I and aVL associated with ALCAPA are not present.

Clinical presentation of myocarditis is heterogeneous, with all courses between asymptomatic and fulminant reported. Especially in athletes it is important to take subtle discomforts seriously and initiate further evaluation. Electrocardiogram, laboratory parameters, serologic markers, and echocardiography are helpful in diagnosis of myocarditis, but are not specific. Magnetic resonance imaging (MRI) of the heart has become an important tool in the evaluation of patients with myocarditis and allows non-invasive appraisal of myocardial inflammation using late enhancement. However, MRI is not able to assess viral persistence. Therefore, endomyocardial biopsy (EMB) remains the gold standard in diagnosis of myocarditis. When considering EMB in these athletes one should not ignore spontaneous healing in 50% of patients with myocarditis. Contrariwise, specific therapy (*e.g.*, immunosuppression, interferon, immunoglobulins) for myocarditis is only feasible after getting results of EMB. When myocarditis is verified, athletes have to withdraw from sport for at least 6 months. Before restarting physical activity, a detailed examination is necessary and most of the patients will undergo another EMB. For prevention of myocarditis and sudden cardiac death it is recommended to stop elite sport for 4 weeks after an unspecific infection. Whether moderate sport can be started earlier is unclear.

4. Dilated cardiomyopathy

In an important minority of athletes, the increase in left ventricular diastolic cavity dimension that occurs with training overlaps with that characteristic of certain known pathological entities. For example, while left ventricular end-diastolic cavity dimension in athletes is usually in the range of 53 to 58 mm, in some individuals it may extend into what may be regarded as the pathological range of >58 mm and thereby resemble dilated cardiomyopathy. However, the absence of left ventricular systolic dysfunction is usually sufficient to distinguish this physiological ventricular enlargement induced by training from that due to dilated cardiomyopathy.

5. Marfan's syndrome

Marfan syndrome is an autosomal dominant genetic disease with variable penetrance, mostly caused by a mutation in the fibrillin-1 gene on chromosome 15. It has an increased risk for sudden death due to aortic dissection. It is characterized clinically by a diverse constellation of abnormalities variable in severity and involving primarily the ocular, skeletal, and cardiovascular organ systems.

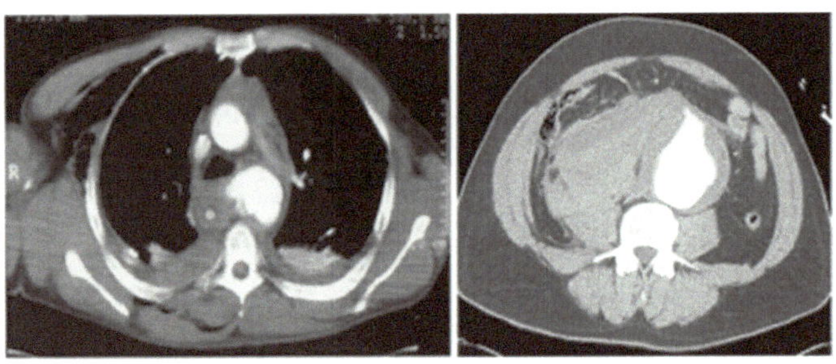

Fig.33.73 (A) Axial source image of CT angiography showing traumatic aortic dissection (B) Axial source image of CT angiog-raphy showing ruptured ascending aorta.

The disease has an estimated incidence of 1 in 5000-7000 and has been shown to be more common in taller athletes such as basketball and volleyball players because tallness is one of the phenotypic expressions of the syndrome. Diagnosis is made according to the Ghent nosology if major criteria are present in two organ systems and a third is involved, or when there is a family history of Marfan syndrome. Skeletal abnormalities include arm span to height ratio greater than 1.05, tall stature, arachnodactyly, hyperextensibility and ligamentous laxity, scoliosis, and chest wall deformity (pectus excavatum or carinatum), in addition to ectopia lentis (lens dislocation).

Cardiovascular manifestations that impact on prognosis consist of progressive dilatation of the aortic root or descending aorta which are predisposed to dissection and rupture; and mitral valve prolapse with associated mitral regurgitation or LV systolic dysfunction, which may occasionally be predisposed to ventricular tachyarrhythmias and sudden death.

Echocardiography can be used to measure and monitor the degree of aortic root dilation. The risk for aortic rupture is usually linked to marked enlargement of the aorta (transverse dimension greater than 50 mm). However, dissection can also occur with a normal (or near-normal) aortic root dimension. Weightlifting has been specifically associated with aortic dissection in athletes. The incidence of aortic dissection appears to decrease with earlier prophylactic surgical aortic root reconstruction and beta-blocker therapy.

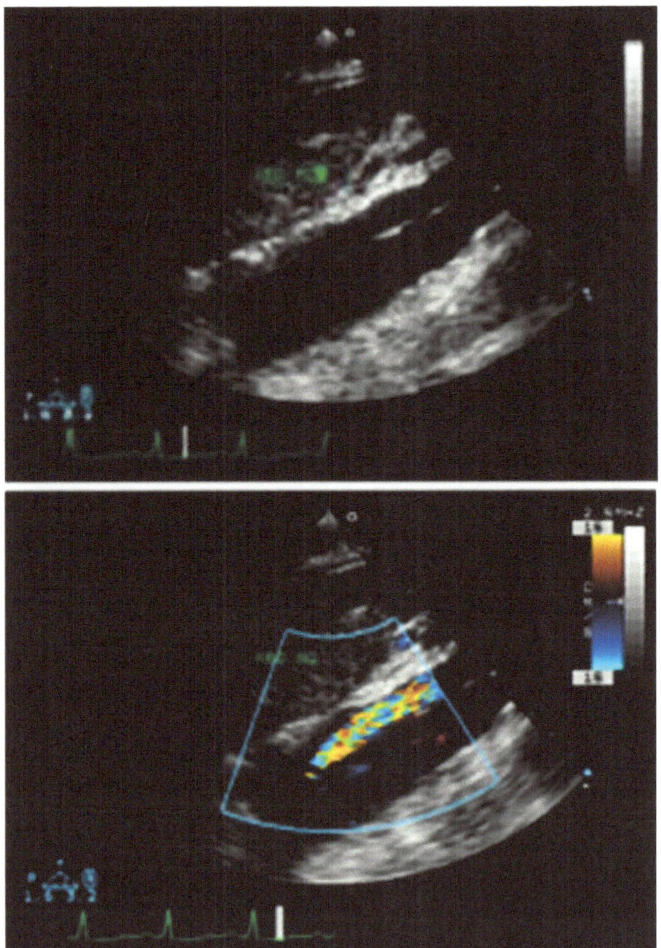

Fig.33.74 Marfan syndrome in athlete. An echocardiogram displaying the true lumen and false lumen of an aortic dissection. In the image to the left, the intimal flap can be seen separating the two lumens. In the image to the right, color flow during ventricular systole suggests that the upper lumen is the true lumen.

Athletes with Marfan syndrome can participate in low and moderate static/low dynamic competitive sports if they do not have any of the aortic root dilatation or moderate-to-severe mitral regurgitation or family history of dissection or sudden death in a Marfan relative. It is recommended, however, that these athletes have an echocardiographic measurement of aortic root dimension repeated every six months for close surveillance of aortic enlargement[

6. Right ventricular dysplasia (in one series)

Arrhythmogenic right ventricular dysplasia (ARVD) is a cardiomyopathy with several time-dependent clinical presentations. The clinical characteristics depend on the penetration grade of the disease. There are two different histological patterns consisting of a lipomatous and a fibrolipomatous form. The presence of arrhythmias in the ARVD syndrome constitutes an important risk factor for sudden cardiac death in athletes. In this article, we describe two professional endurance athletes who died suddenly. One of these athletes had asymptomatic ARVD, the other had symptomatic polymorphic ventricular tachycardias. Both athletes showed fatty penetration of the disease in both the right and left ventricle; one of them also showed fatty involvement at the atrial level and in the other there were signs of myocarditis consistent with ARVD. In the last few years magnetic resonance imaging has become an important diagnostic tool in patients with ARVD.

7. Cardiac sarcoidosis

Sarcoidosis is a multisystem granulomatous disorder of unknown etiology, characterized by "non-caseating granulomas" in different organs.

Clinical signs are variable and dependent on the organ involved. Although it is often asymptomatic in athletes, considering the high level of athletic performance and the related risks due to the potential heart involvement, a particular diagnostic flow-chart to consider some other diagnoses is required.

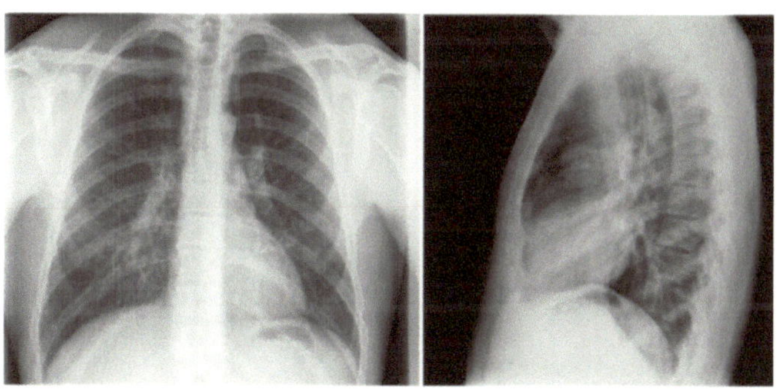

Fig. 33.75 The pictures of the chest by X-ray exam in two differ-ent visualizations show the pulmonary involvement as hilar lymphadenopathy in sarcoidosis in one of the competitive atheletes .

8. Aortic valve stenosis

In patients with aortic stenosis (AS), sudden death remains a particular concern. The following hypothesis have been proposed to explain the mechanism of sudden death in aortic stenosis:

1. An abnormal Betzold-Jarisch reflex (stimulation of left ventricular baroreceptors may lead to arterial hypotension, a fall in venous return and consequent bradycardia)
2. Ventricular tachyarrhythmias (inappropriate hypotension and a low cardiac output provoke coronary hypoperfusion, in patients who already have a predisposition through left ventricular hypertrophy)
3. Atrioventricular conduction disturbances (there is a contiguity between valvular-perivalvular calcification and the His-Purkinje system [there is also a high prevalence of conduction abnormalities in patients with AS])

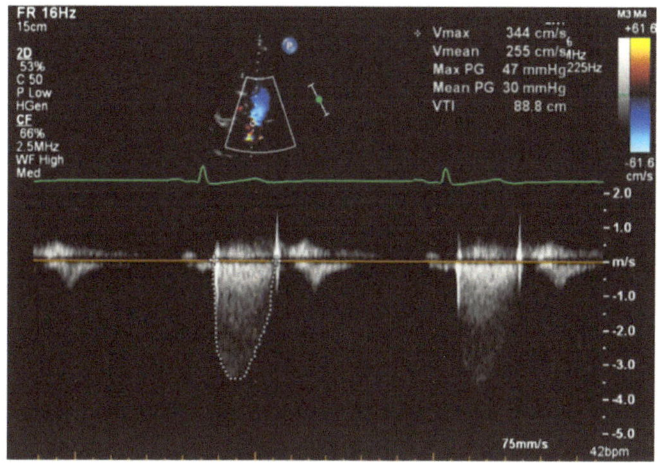

Fig.33.76 Echo- Doppler study showing increase in gradient in of the atheletes in aorticvalvular stenosis.

9. QT-interval prolongation syndromes

Numerous conditions are associated with SCD; the focus for this article is the Long QT Syndrome (LQTS) — a disorder of the heart's electrical system. The prolonged Q-T interval that can be detected via an electrocardiograph (ECG). This prolonged Q-T interval represents the slower than normal passing of the electrical signal through the ventricles of the heart. This congenital syndrome is often asymptomatic. In

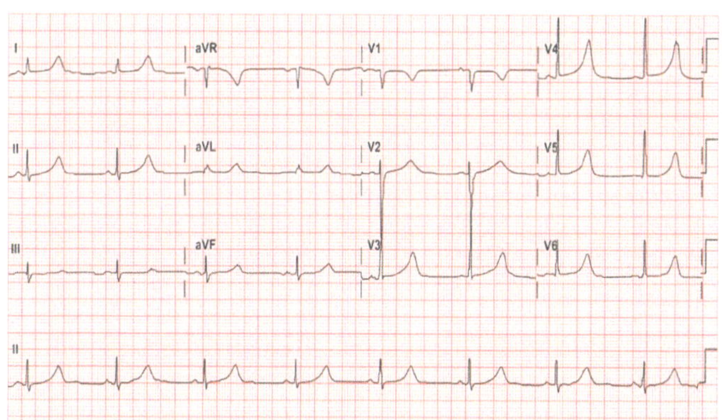

Fig. 33.77 ECG of an 18-year-old tennis player demonstrating a prolonged QT interval (> 500 msec) with T-wave notching (arrow).

some cases people with LQTS experience unexplained faints, seizures, or arrhythmias. Sudden death can be the first clinical manifestation. According to Pugh et al. (2011), genetic testing is available for people with prolonged QT on ECG and those with a family history of SCD. This test is particularly useful for patients who do not exhibit any of the symptoms that are typically associated with the condition. The diagnosis of LQTS should be considered for any athlete with a history of losing consciousness.

10. Acute aortic dissection

Acute aortic dissection can occur at the time of intense physical exertion in strength-trained athletes like weightlifters, bodybuilders, throwers, and wrestlers. Rapid rise in blood pressure and history of hypertension are the most common causes of aortic dissection in athletes. It is a very tragic event because of its high mortality rate of about 32% in young patients.

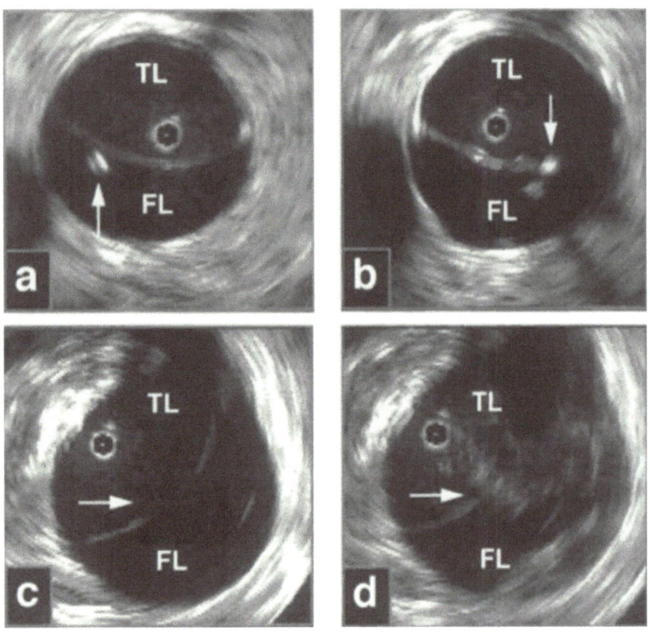

Fig.33.78 IVUS imaging during procedurein aortic dissection. (a) Tip of needle positioned against membrane before membrane was punctured (arrow). (b) Needle lying across membrane after puncture (arrow). (c) After fenestration, opening created in membrane is well visualized (arrow). (d) Satisfactory flow of contrast from one lumen into other (arrow). TL indicates true lumen; FL, false lumen.

11. Mitral valve prolapse

Mitral valve prolapse is probably the most common cardiac valve disorder, affecting approximately 5% of the population. Although it is genetically determined, its clinical manifestations do not usually become evident before adulthood. In the setting of a cardiology referral center, a mitral valve prolapse

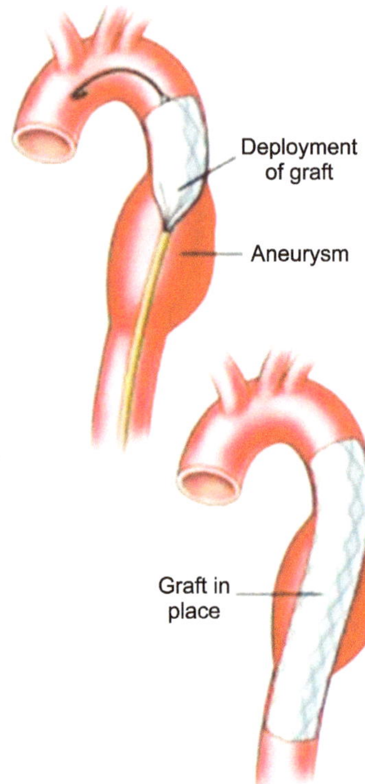

Fig. 33.79 Illustrations showing surgical repair in a athlete with Marfan. Syndrome.

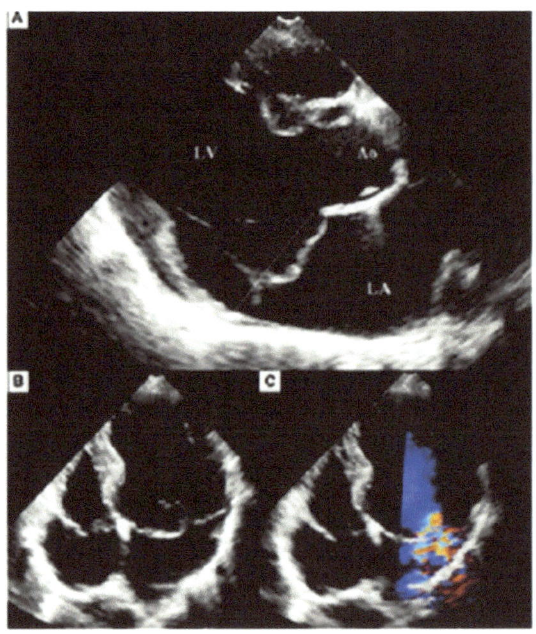

Fig.33.80 Mitral valve prolapse. (A) Echocardiographic paraster-nal long-axis view showing the mitral leaflets prolapsing more than 2 mm above the plane of the mitral annulus (dotted line) during systole in a child with Marfan syndrome. (B) Echocardiographic apical four-chamber view showing bileaflet prolapse in the same patient. (C) Colour Doppler view showing moderate mitral re-gurgitation. Ao: aorta; LA: left atrium; LV: left ventricle.

syndrome, consisting of non-specific symptoms, repolarization changes on the electrocardiogram and arrhythmias, has been identified.

The prognosis of mitral valve prolapse is generally favorable but infrequent complications do occur and include transient ischemic attacks, progression of mitral regurgitation with or without ruptured chordae tendineae, infective endocarditis and sudden death. The symptoms and the complications are not usually related to physical activity. A permissive attitude toward participation of patients with mitral valve prolapse in competitive athletics is probably warranted; however, it would appear reasonable to disqualify athletes with mitral valve prolapse in the following circumstances: history of syncope; disabling chest pain; complex ventricular arrhythmias, particularly if induced or worsened by exercise; significant mitral regurgitation; prolonged QT interval; Marfan's syndrome; and family history of sudden death.

12. Brugada Syndrome

Brugada Syndrome is a genetic disease resulting in a characteristic abnormal EKG pattern and increased risk of SCD. Arrhythmic events generally occur in early to mid adulthood (22-45 yrs of age), are more likely at night, and men are more likely to be affected. Current treatment relies upon the implantable cardioverter-defibrillator (ICD), which can detect and correct an abnormal and potentially lethal heart rhythm. There has been a great deal of progress in recent years identifying the genetic causes of Brugada Syndrome, with as many as 8 specific genes identified. Genetic screening is available for families with a history of Brugada Syndrome, and can help identify individuals who are at risk for SCD, and those who are not at risk.

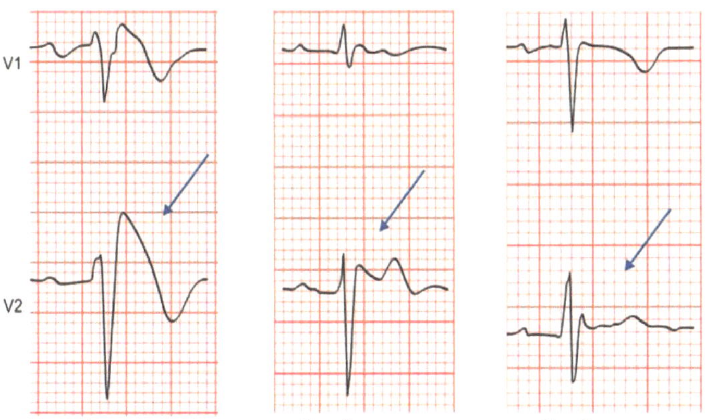

Fig.33.81 Three types of ST-segment elevation in Brugada syndrome, as shown in the precordial leads on ECG in the same patient at different times. Left panel shows a type 1 ECG pattern with pronounced elevation of the J point (arrow), a coved-type ST segment, and an inverted T wave in V1 and V2. The middle panel illustrates a type 2 pattern with a saddleback ST-segmentelevated by >1 mm. The right panel shows a type 3 pattern inwhich the ST segment is elevated and lt; 1 mm. According to aconsensus report (Antzelevitch, 2005), the type 1 ECG pattern is diagnostic of Brugada syndrome. Modified from Wilde, 2002.

MANAGEMENT OF CARDIOVASCULAR EMERGENCIES (FIG. 33.82)

Sudden cardiac arrest

Management of a cardiac emergency begins with prompt recognition, an accurate assessment and in uncertain cases the implementation of response protocols based on proper assumptions. SCA should be suspected in all cases of non-traumatic collapse, and in all cases in which an athlete is collapsed and unresponsive. There are a number of potential pitfalls when evaluating a collapsed athlete that may result in delayed recognition of SCA and resultant critical delays in resuscitation. Agonal breathing and occasional gasping often occur within the first minutes after SCA and can be misinterpreted as normal respirations. Accurate assessment of the presence or absence of a pulse in the emergency setting is also challenging and studies demonstrate that healthcare providers correctly diagnose pulselessness as little as 50% of the time. As a result, the 2010 American Heart Association and international guidelines for CPR recommend that healthcare providers spend no more than 10 s assessing for a definitive pulse, and that lay responders not check for a pulse at all. In addition, brief myoclonic or seizure-like activity occurs in approximately half of young athletes with SCA.20 Thus, SCA must be assumed in any athlete with seizure-like activity until cardiac arrest is effectively ruled out.

In cases of presumed or confirmed SCA, key steps in management must occur rapidly, and often simultaneously. These include:

(1) calling for help and activating the local emergency medical response system,
(2) beginning CPR with chest compressions.
(3) retrieving and applying a defibrillator (if available) for rhythm analysis and shock deployment (if indicated) as soon as possible. Most cases of SCA in the athletic setting are witnessed and involve more than one rescuer. Thus, one rescuer can perform CPR while another retrieves the AED if not already present.

Recent CPR guidelines changed the basic life support sequence from 'A-B-C' (Airway, Breathing and Chest compressions) to 'C-A-B' (Chest compressions, Airway and Breathing). In the A-B-C sequence, chest compressions are often delayed while the responder opens the airway to give mouth-to-mouth breaths or retrieves a barrier device or other ventilation equipment. By changing the sequence to C-A-B, chest compressions will be initiated sooner and may ensure that more victims receive chest compressions by rescuers unable or unwilling to provide ventilations. Hands-only (compression only) CPR is encouraged for the untrained lay rescuer and appears to achieve outcomes similar to those of conventional CPR (compressions with rescue breathing). Adequate chest compressions include a rate of 100/min with a depth of at least 2 inches, complete recoil of the chest in between compressions and minimisation of any pauses in compressions.

Chest compressions should be resumed immediately after shock delivery. Many victims will have pulseless electric activity or asystole after defibrillation. Thus, CPR is needed to provide perfusion to the myocardium during this critical period to decrease recurrent ventricular arrhythmias. Minimising the interval between stopping chest compressions and delivering a shock (ie, the preshock pause) also improves the chance of shock success and patient survival. Resuscitative measures should be continued until the victim becomes responsive or a non-cardiac cause of collapse is clearly identified.

Acute coronary syndromes

ACS should be suspected in any athlete presenting with chest pain. Knowledge of an athlete's medical history and risk factors for coronary artery disease is helpful to guide management. Some symptoms attributed to ACS, such as diaphoresis, dyspnoea, lightheadedness and nausea, may be more difficult to differentiate in the athletic setting. A focused assessment should include vital signs, heart and lung auscultation, and chest wall palpation as reproducible pain with palpation decreases the likelihood of ACS. When there is clinical suspicion for ACS, the athlete should be immediately removed from play, seated or laid supine and the local emergency medical system activated.

Treatment in haemodynamically stable patients includes aspirin 162–325 mg chewed and nitroglycerin 0.4 mg sublingual every 5 min up to three doses as needed for chest pain. If an AED is available, it should be retrieved as acute ischaemia increases the risk of ventricular arrhythmias and SCA. New guidelines do not recommend routine use of oral β-blockers and supplemental oxygen in the absence of hypoxia due to lack of evidence that shows a survival benefit. Patients with ACS or SCA are ideally transferred to hospital facilities capable of advanced cardiac care and immediate percutaneous coronary intervention with angiography or bypass surgery if indicated.

Prognosis

Although gross structural changes resemble those in some cardiac disorders, no adverse effects are apparent. In most cases, structural changes and bradycardia regress with detraining, although up to 20% of elite athletes have residual chamber enlargement, raising questions, in the absence of long-term data, about whether athlete's heart is truly benign.

ATHLETE-SPECIFIC CHALLENGES AND QUESTIONS

Most often, an active individual – be it an athlete or one who remains physically fit through routine training and exercise – is suddenly stymied by the affects of his/her clotting incident.

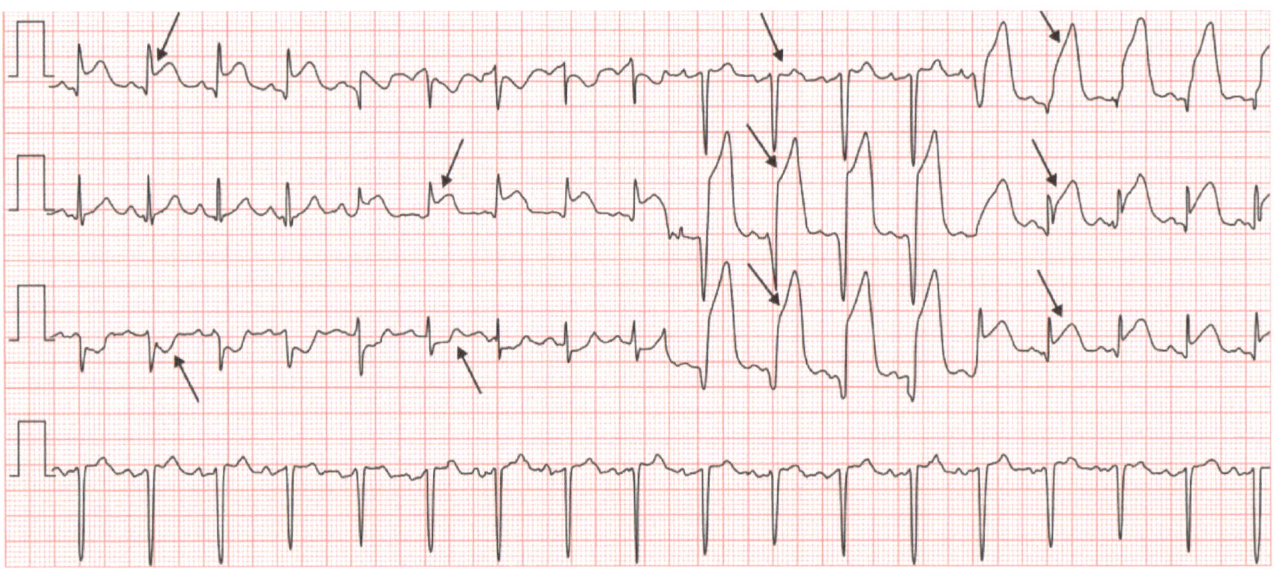

Fig. 33.82 ECG trace showing ST-segment elevation leads 1, AVL, V_1-V_6 and reciprocal changes in leads 11,11 and AVF in acute coronary syndrome (arrows).

Questions, lots of questions, are poised to the care-giver. Of paramount importance for the athlete are particularly the two following issues:

Can I continue my sport while on warfarin?

A solid medical assessment should be made whether the person who has had a blood clot can come off warfarin or should remain on it. Being on warfarin increases the risk for bleeding. Therefore, contact sports and sports with a risk for serious injury, such as football, hockey, basketball, soccer, gymnastics, alpine skiing, or boxing should not be pursued by a person on warfarin. However, athletes such as runners, bicyclists or triathletes may be able to continue their sport, but they should adapt their activities to avoid trauma that might put them at risk for bleeding (avoid situations leading to bicycle crashes, etc.). Individual blood thinning treatment plans can also be designed, such as (a) a decrease in warfarin dosage a few days prior to athletic events that would otherwise put the person at increased risk for bleeding, (b) switching the athlete who should be on long-term blood thinners to low molecular weight heparin shots during the athletic season and interrupting the shots for competitions that pose a risk for bleeding, (c) stopping blood thinners during the season and accepting a higher risk for blood clots during that time, but restarting warfarin during the off season. Finally, an athlete may decide to switch from a high risk bleeding competitive sport to one with a lower risk. Obviously, these are all very individual treatment decisions that should be thoroughly discussed between the patient's personal physician, the patient, and the team physician (if the patient is participating in a team sport).

How soon after a DVT or PE can I go back to training?

Patients with a DVT may have significant extremity swelling and pain which may improve only slowly over weeks and months. Some residual symptoms may persist long-term, this is termed "postthrombotic syndrome." It appears that being highly active one month after a DVT is not detrimental; it may, actually be beneficial and lead to less symptoms of post-thrombotic syndrome (reference 2). This can be used as an argument to encourage individuals to return to physical activity relatively soon after a DVT. Also, wearing individually fitted compression stockings decreases the long-term risk for post-thrombotic syndrome.

No official guidelines exist as to when and how quickly an athlete might return to exercising. Each patient will need an individualized exercise plan (an example is described in reference 3). It seems appropriate to refrain from any athletic activities for the first 10-14 days after an acute DVT or PE until the clot is more adherent to the blood vessel wall and the risk of having the clot break loose (causing a PE) has decreased. To lessen deconditioning during this period of relative inactivity, the athlete may do some strength training – arm and trunk exercises in the case of a leg DVT, leg and trunk exercises in the case of an arm DVT. The athlete may then increase activity between week 2 and 4 and return to pre-clot activity levels by week 4.

How to minimize the risk for clots?

Measures that the athlete and, for that matter, the non-athlete should take to minimize the risk for DVT or PE are listed in table 3. For the athlete the most important ones are probably to (a) avoid dehydration, and (b) take breaks when traveling long distances.

Psychosocial Implications

Athletes need to appreciate that significant deconditioning can occur after a DVT or PE. Depression can also set in after such a life-changing event. This is not surprising, given that athletes often view themselves as healthy and, from a health point of view, invincible, and now suddenly realize that they are vulnerable, sick, and sometimes even disabled. Patient support groups may be helpful in this situation, as may antidepressants.

Hypercoagulability in Athletes

Risk factors for thromboembolism are well known, and athletes are placed under conditions that can result in exposure to several of these risk factors, which include travel, trauma, immobilization, hemoconcentration, and polycythemia. Presence of a genetic hypercoagulable disorder adds additional risk. Overall management is no different than in nonathletes. Thrombolysis is strongly recommended for upper extremity deep venous thrombosis (DVT) coupled with surgical decompression of obstructive structures if indicated. Thrombolytic therapy does not appear to be necessary for treatment of lower extremity DVT. Prevention of DVT with travel can be achieved through general techniques such as leg exercises, hydration, and loose fitting clothes. Aspirin before travel shows some benefits of protection, but individuals at higher risk may need low molecular weight heparin. Athletes should be screened during preparticipation physicals for thromboembolic risk. Individuals on anticoagulation therapy should not participate in collision or contact sports. Return to play with gradual increase in intensity is recommended with careful monitoring for recurrent venous thromboembolism and management of post-thrombotic symptoms.

Key Recommendations in Athletes

Planning for cardiac emergencies in the athletic setting

- Establish an emergency action plan for each venue.
- Identify anticipated first responders (coaches, officials, administrators and the medical team) and provide training in Sudden cardiac arrest (SCA) recognition, cardiopulmonary resuscitation (CPR) and automated external defibrillators (AED) use.
- Develop an internal communication system and a means to activate the local emergency response system.
- Install AEDs in strategic locations and equip key medical staff with portable AEDs as needed to ensure early access to defibrillation (within 3 min of collapse)
- Register AEDs with the local emergency medical system.
- Identify the person responsible for AED maintenance.
- Determine routes for emergency vehicles to easily access each athletic venue in case of a cardiac emergency.
- Practice and review the emergency action plan at least annually with all potential first responders.
- Consider acquiring additional emergency equipment and medications depending on the population at risk and the experience of the medical providers.
- Coordinate onsite ambulances and other mobile responders for certain high-risk events.

Management of cardiac emergencies in the athletic setting

- Promptly recognise a cardiac emergency by maintaining a high level of suspicion.
- Assume SCA in any collapsed and unresponsive athlete.
- Avoid misdiagnosis as a result of agonal breathing and/or seizure-like activity.
- Elicit help from people nearby.
- Activate the local emergency response system.
- Begin chest compressions, retrieve an AED and apply it as soon as possible for defibrillation (if indicated).
- Continue CPR, AED use and resuscitative efforts until the victim becomes responsive or care is transferred to an emergency facility capable of advanced cardiac life support.
- In a conscious athlete suspected of having an acute coronary syndrome, provide aspirin and nitroglycerin, activate the emergency response system and monitor closely.

BIBLIOGRAPHY AND ACKNOWLEDGEMENT

Berg RA, Hemphill R, Abella BS, et al. Part 5: adult basic life support: 2010 American Heart Association Guidelines for Cardiopulmonary Resuscitation and Emergency Cardiovascular Care. *Circulation* 2010;122:S685–705.

Borjesson M, Dugmore D, Mellwig KP, et al. Time for action regarding cardiovascular emergency care at sports arenas: a lesson from the Arena study. *Eur Heart J*2010;31:1438–10.

Borjesson M, Serratosa L, Carre F, et al. Consensus document regarding cardiovascular safety at sports arenas: position stand from the European Association of Cardiovascular Prevention and Rehabilitation (EACPR), section of Sports Cardiology. *Eur Heart J* 2011;32:2119–24.

Corrado D, Basso C, Rizzoli G, et al. Does sports activity enhance the risk of sudden death in adolescents and young adults? *J Am Coll Cardiol* 2003;42:1959–63.

Crocco TJ, Sayre MR, Liu T, et al. Mathematical determination of external defibrillators needed at mass gatherings. *Prehosp Emerg Care* 2004;8:292–7.

Dahabreh IJ, Paulus JK. Association of episodic physical and sexual activity with triggering of acute cardiac events: systematic review and meta-analysis. *JAMA*2011;305:1225–33.

Drezner JA, Courson RW, Roberts WO, et al. Inter-association task force recommendations on emergency preparedness and management of sudden cardiac arrest in high school and college athletic programs: a consensus statement. *J Athl Train*2007;42:143–58.

Drezner JA. Preparing for sudden cardiac arrest—the essential role of automated external defibrillators in athletic medicine: a critical review. *Br J Sports Med*2009;43:702–7.

Drezner JA, Rao AL, Heistand J, et al. Effectiveness of emergency response planning for sudden cardiac arrest in United States high schools with automated external defibrillators. *Circulation* 2009;120:518–25.

Drezner JA, Rogers KJ. Sudden cardiac arrest in intercollegiate athletes: detailed analysis and outcomes of resuscitation in nine cases. *Heart Rhythm* 2006;3:755–9.

Eberle B, Dick WF, Schneider T, et al. Checking the carotid pulse check: diagnostic accuracy of first responders in patients with and without a pulse. *Resuscitation*1996;33:107–16.

Eckart RE, Scoville SL, Campbell CL, et al. Sudden death in young adults: a 25-year review of autopsies in military recruits. *Ann Intern Med* 2004;141:829–34.

Field JM, Hazinski MF, Sayre MR, et al. Part 1: executive summary: 2010 American Heart Association Guidelines for Cardiopulmonary Resuscitation and Emergency Cardiovascular Care. *Circulation* 2010;122:S640–56.

Harmon KG, Asif IM, Klossner D, et al. Incidence of sudden cardiac death in national collegiate athletic association athletes. *Circulation* 2011;123:1594–600.

Hazinski MF, Markenson D, Neish S, et al. Response to cardiac arrest and selected life-threatening medical emergencies: the medical emergency response plan for schools—a statement for healthcare providers, policymakers, school administrators, and community leaders. *Ann Emerg Med* 2004;43:83–99.

Hazinski MF, Nolan JP, Billi JE, et al. Part 1: executive summary: 2010 International Consensus on Cardiopulmonary Resuscitation and Emergency Cardiovascular Care Science With Treatment Recommendations. *Circulation* 2010;122:S250–75.

Henkel DM, Witt BJ, Gersh BJ, et al. Ventricular arrhythmias after acute myocardial infarction: a 20-year community study. *Am Heart J* 2006;151:806–12.

Katz E, Metzger JT, Marazzi A, et al. Increase of sudden cardiac deaths in Switzerland during the 2002 FIFA World Cup. *Int J Cardiol* 2006;107:132–3.

Kim JH, Malhotra R, Chiampas G, et al. Cardiac arrest during long-distance running races. *N Engl J Med* 2012;366:130–40.

Lapostolle F, Le Toumelin P, Agostinucci JM, et al. Basic cardiac life support providers checking the carotid pulse: performance, degree of conviction, and influencing factors.*Acad Emerg Med* 2004;11:878–80.

Larsen MP, Eisenberg MS, Cummins RO, et al. Predicting survival from out-of-hospital cardiac arrest: a graphic model. *Ann Emerg Med* 1993;22:1652–8.

Leusveld E, Kleijn S, Umans VA. Usefulness of emergency medical teams in sport stadiums. *Am J Cardiol* 2008;101:712–14.

Luiz T, Kumpch M, Metzger M, et al. Management of cardiac arrest in a German soccer stadium. Structural, process and outcome quality. *Anaesthesist* 2005;54:914–22.

Maron BJ, Doerer JJ, Haas TS, et al Sudden deaths in young competitive athletes: analysis of 1866 deaths in the United States, 1980–2006. *Circulation* 2009;119:1085–92.

Maron BJ, Estes NA. Commotio cordis. *N Engl J Med* 2010;362:917–27.

Maron BJ, Poliac LC, Roberts WO. Risk for sudden cardiac death associated with marathon running. *J Am Coll Cardiol* 1996;28:428–31.

Maron BJ Sudden death in young athletes. *N Engl J Med* 2003;349:1064–75.

Motyka TM, Winslow JE, Newton K, et al. Method for determining automatic external defibrillator need at mass gatherings. *Resuscitation* 2005;65:309–14.

Note:-It is a modified chapter with added newer text and figs . However many fis also have been transferred from chapter 44 of pediatric cardiology.

O'Connor RE, Brady W, Brooks SC, et al. Part 10: acute coronary syndromes: 2010 American Heart Association Guidelines for Cardiopulmonary Resuscitation and Emergency Cardiovascular Care. *Circulation* 2010;122:S787–817.

O'Doherty M, Tayler DI, Quinn E, et al. Five hundred patients with myocardial infarction monitored within one hour of symptoms. *Br Med J (Clin Res Ed)* 1983;286:1405–8.

Rea TD, Fahrenbruch C, Culley L, et al. CPR with chest compression alone or with rescue breathing. *N Engl J Med* 2010;363:423–33.

Ruppert M, Reith MW, Widmann JH, et al. Checking for breathing: evaluation of the diagnostic capability of emergency medical services personnel, physicians, medical students, and medical laypersons. *Ann Emerg Med* 1999;34:720–9.

Strike PC, Perkins-Porras L, Whitehead DL, et al. Triggering of acute coronary syndromes by physical exertion and anger: clinical and sociodemographic characteristics. *Heart* 2006;92:1035–40.

Swap CJ, Nagurney JT. Value and limitations of chest pain history in the evaluation of patients with suspected acute coronary syndromes. *JAMA* 2005;294:2623–9.

Thompson PD, Stern MP, Williams P, et al. Death during jogging or running. A study of 18 cases. *JAMA* 1979;242:1265–7.

Toresdahl BG, Drezner JD, Rao AL, et al. Outcomes of sudden cardiac arrest in US high schools: a prospective study from the national registry for AED use in sports. *Clin J Sport Med* 2011;20:137.

Tunstall Pedoe DS. Marathon cardiac deaths: the london experience. *Sports Med*2007;37:448–50.

Virmani R, Robinowitz M, McAllister HA. Non-traumatic death in joggers. A series of 30 patients at autopsy. *Am J Med* 1982;72:874–82.

Waller BF, Roberts WC. Sudden death while running in conditioned runners aged 40 years or over. *Am J Cardiol* 1980;45:1292–300.

Wassertheil J, Keane G, Fisher N, et al. Cardiac arrest outcomes at the Melbourne Cricket Ground and shrine of remembrance using a tiered response strategy-a forerunner to public access defibrillation. *Resuscitation* 2000;44:97–104.

Webner D, Duprey KM, Drezner JA, et al. Sudden cardiac arrest and death in United States marathons. *Med Sci Sports Exerc* 2012.

Wilbert-Lampen U, Leistner D, Greven S, et al. Cardiovascular events during World Cup soccer. *N Engl J Med* 2008;358:475–83.

Willich SN, Lewis M, Löwel H, et al. Physical exertion as a trigger of acute myocardial infarction. Triggers and mechanisms of Myocardial Infarction Study Group. *N Engl J Med*1993;329:1684–90.

34 Pre and Post-operative Care of Children with CHD

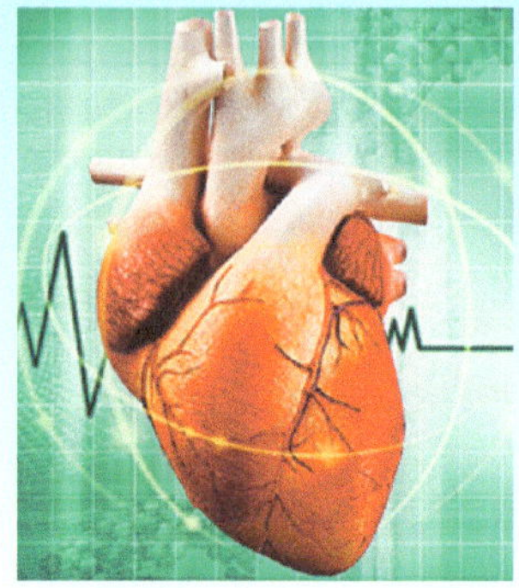

Stabilization during preoperative cardiac surgery especially in neonates has an important role to predict outcome for pediatric congenital heart surgery. An attempt has been made to elaborate general guidelines on how to diagnose and some anticipations for emergency treatments tailored by the type of congenital heart disease in neonates. Stabilization consists of medical treatment including emergent prostaglandin institution in some types of duct dependent lesion. The role of interventional catheterization such as patent ductus arteriosus (PDA) stent, balloon pulmonary valvotomy, etc. as modalities for stabilization before surgery was also elaborated. Some general and specific guidelines based on the type of surgeries for postoperative management were also discussed. This can be studied under two main headings

1.Initial treatment of critically ill neonates with cardiac defects
2.Postoperative cardiac intensive care therapy

1. Initial treatment of critically ill neonates with cardiac defects

The general features of various congenital heart defects, their clinical symptoms and treatment principles for the management of congenital heart defects that become symptomatic in neonates will be discussed. In this context, the special measures for the initial treatment of the most common defects are presented.

Incidence

Based on many epidemiological studies, the actual incidence of congenital heart defects is 8–11 per 1000 live births independent of ethical background, social welfare or medical standards. As a rule thumb nearly half of these children require any form of surgical or interventional intervention within the first year of life. With adequate management, more than 90% of these children can reach adulthood and lead a relatively normal life.

Symptoms

It is typical for the different congenital heart defects to present and become manifest at different times in early life. Of most importance are the very early phase when the patent ductus arteriosus closes for all ductal-dependent cardiac defects; the next important timeframe of clinical manifestation is the reduction in pulmonary vascular resistance (PVR) for defects with left-to-right shunt.

Typical leading symptoms for the presentation of congenital heart defects in neonates are as follows:

Heart failure or cardiogenic shock (usually in the first or second week of life if there is left heart obstruction; for shunt defects typically not until after the drop in pulmonary resistance at the age of 2–8 weeks)

Heart failure

The characteristic clinical signs of heart failure in neonates are as follows:

- Tachypnea, dyspnea, thoracic retractions
- Rarely but possible pulmonary edema mainly due t overflow
- Tachycardia
- Hepatomegaly
- Failure to thrive, difficulty in feeding, increased sweating, abnormal sleepiness
- Pallor, prolonged capillary refill time

It is evident that the clinical symptoms of neonatal heart failure are unspecific and may be similar to the clinical symptoms of sepsis. Therefore, many neonates with heart failure are treated for suspected sepsis. In particular, cardiac defects with left-sided obstruction (coarctation of the aorta, critical aortic stenosis, hypoplastic left heart syndrome), or typically become manifest as early as the first 1–2 weeks of life with the clinical symptoms of cardiogenic shock caused by early duct closure

Cyanosis

Cyanosis is a clinical sign that becomes evident when about 5% of the hemoglobin is deoxygenated. In neonates with polycythemia (Hb >20 g/dl), this may be present even without hypoxemia, in patients

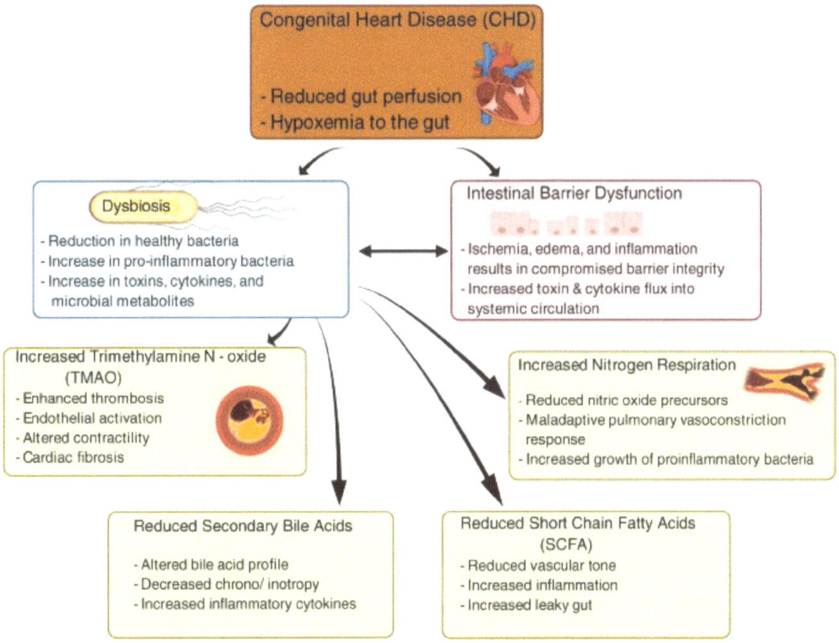

Fig. 34.1 Relationship of the microbiome and CHD. CHD results in reduced systemic perfusion and/or hypoxemia to the gut. This can lead to dysbiosis, an alteration in the normal gut flora, and reduced healthy bacteria and increased pro-inflammatory bacteria. These bacteria produce cytokine-like molecules, toxins, and metabolites. The byproducts induce intestinal barrier dysfunction, compromising the barrier integrity and a flux of toxins and cytokines into the systemic circulation. These metabolites lead to increased TMAO, which effects endothelial activation, increased thrombotic risk, altered cardiac contractility, and cardiac fibrosis. Dysbiosis also leads to reduced secondary bile acids, which decrease the inotropy in the heart, and increase circulating cytokines. There is also a reduction in short chain fatty acids, such as butyrate, which yield a reduction in vascular tone, increased gut inflammation leading to a "leaky gut". Increased nitrogen respiration leads to reductions in nitric oxide, maladaptive pulmonary vasoconstriction and promote further growth of pro-inflammatory bacteria. CHD, congenital heart disease; TMAO, trimethylamine N-oxide; SCFA, short chain fatty acids

Table 34.2 Classification of congenital heart defects which become symptomatic in the neonatal period

Group	Examples
Cardiac defects with ductal-dependent systemic circulation (left heart obstructions)	Critical aortic stenosis, hypoplastic left heart syndrome, interrupted aortic arch, critical coarctation of the aorta
Cardiac defect with ductal-dependent pulmonary circulation (right heart obstructions)	Critical pulmonary stenosis, pulmonary atresia with intact ventricular septum, pulmonary atresia with VSD, pronounced form of Tetralogy of Fallot, severe Ebstein's anomaly, tricuspid atresia with pulmonary atresia or high-grade pulmonary stenosis
Cardiac defects with parallel circulation	d-TGA—transposition of the great arteries
Cardiac defects with complete intracardiac mixing of blood	Total anomalous pulmonary venous connection, univentricular heart
Cardiac defects with a large left-to-right shunt symptomatic usually after 4–6 weeks	Large VSD, complete AVSD, large PDA, aortopulmonary window, Truncus arteriosus communis, univentricular hearts with unobstructed pulmonary blood flow

with anemia this may be overseen. To avoid this, pulse oximetry at all four limbs is the standard of care. Neonatal screening: Cyanosis in a newborn should be picked up by a neonatal screening program that measures saturation by pulse oximetry at all four extremities at the first day of life. It should be standard of care that all newborns should have this screening test. If the saturation is >95% and the control 12 h later is again >95%, a cyanotic heart defect can be ruled out. If the saturation is ≤95%, additional examinations (today—ECHO as the preferred method of choice) are needed. Hyperoxia test: The hyperoxia test is a more historical test and no longer useful in the times of ECHO. It was used to try and distinguish between cardiac and pulmonary cyanosis. In patients with pulmonary cyanosis, the oxygen saturation increases markedly after oxygen is given, while oxygen saturation is usually not significantly improved in those with cyanotic heart defects. This test lacks specificity and sensitivity to rule out or confirm cardiac defects. Both pre- and postductal oxygen saturation should be measured. Cardiac cyanosis can be the result of either reduced lung perfusion due to a right-to-left shunt, complete venous mixing in patients with total anomalous pulmonary venous return or intracardiac mixing of systemic and pulmonary venous blood. Methemoglobinemia is another rare cause for cyanosis. In addition, cyanosis can be caused by abnormality in the central nervous system (e.g., after cerebral hemorrhage or in cases with central apnea in premature neonates, etc.)

All newborns should have a neonatal screening for congenital heart defects immediately after birth and 12 h later. Today ECHO is the main diagnostic tool for secondary investigation and to rule out or confirm congenital heart defects. If the diagnosis can not be immediately confirmed by echocardiography, an attempt of treating the neonate with intravenous prostaglandin E1 is justified. The hyperoxia test is no longer standard of care. If there is no adequate increase in oxygen saturation in a cyanosed neonate, a congenital heart defect with ductal dependent lung perfusion must be assumed.

Heart murmur

As innocent murmurs are unlikely in this age group, a heart murmur in a neonate is always suggestive of a congenital heart defect. Usually, stenosis of the semilunar valves or AV valve insufficiency present immediately after birth due to a loud systolic murmur, the typical VSD murmur in a large VSD, for example, can often be not auscultated until after the pulmonary resistance has dropped and the pressure gradient between the left and right ventricles increases. In addition, in many critical heart defects, there might be no indicative heart murmur at all (e.g., d-TGA simplex, coarctation of the aorta).

Arrhythmias

Arrhythmias often present in neonates without structural heart defects (i.e., atrial flutter, congenital AV block) and therefore are rarely the first symptom of a congenital heart defect. An AV block may occur in association with an l-TGA or heterotaxy syndromes. Supraventricular tachycardia due to accessory conduction pathways occurs more frequently with an Ebstein anomaly. The most common arrhythmia in a newborn is atrial flutter that requires immediate electrical cardioversion after diagnosis with adenosine but usually presents without additional defects.

Hemodynamic situation

In a ductal-dependent defect survival depends on the persistence of a patent ductus arteriosus. In general, ductal-dependent systemic circulation must be distinguished from ductal-dependent pulmonary circulation. In patients with ductal-dependent systemic circulation, there is a high-grade obstruction of the structures of the left heart (mitral valve, aortic valve, arch and coarctation). To ensure sufficient systemic perfusion, the systemic circulation must be supplied with blood from the pulmonary circulation across the patent ductus arteriosus like in utero. In ductal-dependent pulmonary circulation, there is a high-grade right heart obstruction leading to cyanosis. Perfusion of the pulmonary circulation depends mainly on the blood supply from the aorta across the patent ductus arteriosus.In parallel circulations (d-TGA), survival depends on additional shunts (especially a sufficiently large atrial shunt) between the two circulations to enable mixing of the cyanosed and the arterialized blood. In cardiac defects with complete intracardiac mixing of blood, the resulting cyanosis is often only relatively mild; when excessive pulmonary blood flow due to the lack of pulmonary stenosis is often present simultaneously, this leads to pulmonary recirculation of the saturated blood. Heart failure usually develops as a result of the excessive pulmonary blood flow after 4–6 weeks. Based on this principle, congenital heart defects with a large left-to-right shunt do not become clinically symptomatic until the age of about 4–6 weeks; at that time, the PVR has dropped and the shunt between the systemic and pulmonary circulation increases dramatically. If left-sided heart obstruction is, however, also present (e.g., VSD with CoA), the symptoms may develop as early as the first week of life.

Diagnostic measures

Oxygen saturation

As a standard of care, oxygen saturation should always be measured in children both preductally (right hand) and postductally (lower limb). If there is a defect with ductal-dependent systemic circulation, the (postductal) oxygen saturation measured in the feet may be lower than the (preductal) saturation in the right hand. The brachiocephalic trunk branches off from the aortic arch well before the ductus arteriosus; therefore, it is safe to assume that the saturation measured in the right hand is equivalent to preductal saturation (except in the rare cases of a lusoric artery)

Blood gas analysis (BGA)

As metabolic acidosis is the typical finding in severe heart failure and cardiogenic shock, routine (arterial) BGA is recommended on multiple occasions. In addition, all BGA should measure lactate as surrogate of cardiac output and thereby tissue perfusion

Echocardiography (ECHO))

As mentioned before, today echocardiography is the diagnostic method of choice in all patients with a presumed cardiac defect or impaired circulatory situation. ECHO allows an accurate diagnosis of all significant cardiac defects that become symptomatic in the neonatal period. As modern standard of care, every neonatal unit must have ECHO and support of a pediatric cardiologist available on a 24/7 basis.

Hyperoxia test

In the time of ECHO, this test has only anecdotic relevance and lacks sensitivity and specificity. This test has been used to distinguish between cardiac or pulmonary central cyanosis. After breathing 100% oxygen for a few minutes, the cyanosis disappears or should be clearly reduced in pulmonary cyanosis and there is a relevant increase in arterial partial oxygen pressure. In cardiac cyanosis, the partial oxygen pressure should remain largely unchanged as the cardiac right-to-left shunt or inadequate pulmonary perfusion cannot be compensated by the administration of oxygen.

Pulse and blood pressure in all limbs

All neonates with suspected cardiac defect should have a pulse and blood pressure measurement at all 4 limbs. If a difference in blood pressure between the right arm (preductal) and the lower limbs (postductal) is then manifest or the peripheral pulses in the lower limbs cannot be palpated, this is a hint and leading findings of coarctation of the aorta or an interrupted aortic arch. This examination is helpful to assess systemic circulation.

In a large patent ductus arteriosus, there may be no difference in blood pressure between the upper and lower halves of the body even with relevant coarctation of the aorta or interrupted aortic arch. The saturations, however, vary substantially

Treatment

According to the different anatomic variations and physiologic situation, there is a substantial difference in the management of these children. The treatment principles for the various groups of congenital heart defects are presented below and based on the pathophysiology, the specific treatments of the individual heart defects in the neonatal period are described in this context.

Cardiac defects with ductal-dependent systemic circulation

In ductal-dependent systemic circulation, we should reestablish the prenatal circulation. Therefore, attempts must be made to provide as much blood as possible from the pulmonary circulation to supply the systemic circulation via the patent ductus arteriosus. As a result of this strategy, a saturation of 75–85% is adequate and saturations >85% that indicate excessive pulmonary blood flow should be avoided. The treatment principles of ductal-dependent systemic circulation are as follows:

- Provide patency of the ductus arteriosus with a continuous prostaglandin E1 infusion (initial dosage 20–50 ng/kg/min, to be reduced after ECHO assessment; caveat: Apnoea).
- Lower systemic vascular resistance:
  - o By reducing afterload: i.e., with sodium nitroprusside infusion
  - o If catecholamines are needed: Use preferably milrinone and/or dobutamine (vasodilatation effects); avoid vasoconstrictive effects of other catecholamines (dopamine, noradrenaline)
- Increase pulmonary resistance, increase pulmonary artery pressure:
  - o Avoid intubation, extubate early
  - o Avoid additional oxygen
  - o Aim for mild metabolic acidosis (pH 7.35)
  - o Aim for mild hypoventilation (pCO2 around 60 mmHg)
- In case of pulmonary edema caused by congestion and pulmonary overflow, give intravenous diuretics (1–2 mg/kg furosemide), ensure high PEEP (i.e., 10–15 cm H2O) and reduce prostaglandin E1 to a minimum (e.g., 10 ng/kg/min)

The administration of oxygen (SatO2 >85%) as a general measure and hyperventilation in children with ductal-dependent systemic circulation can lead to an acute decompensation of the hemodynamic situation.

Cardiac defects with ductal-dependent pulmonary circulation

The situation is reversed in ductal-dependent pulmonary circulation, but the prenatal situation should be achieved too. Again a saturation of 75–85% is adequate and saturations >85% should be avoided as they indicate inadequate pulmonary perfusion. The following measures can be useful to allow more blood to flow from the systemic circulation to the pulmonary circulation via the patent ductus arteriosus if needed:

- Secure patency of the ductus arteriosus via a prostaglandin E1 infusion (initial dosage 20–50 ng/kg/min).
- Lower pulmonary vascular resistance:

1Aim for mild metabolic alkalosis (use buffering) (pH 7.45–7.5)

2.Adjust ventilation for mild hyperventilation (pCO2 around 35 mmHg)

3.Increase FiO2

- Increase systemic vascular resistance and support systemic pressure by:
  - o Noradrenaline infusion
  - o Possibly also adrenaline infusion

Table 34.3 **Checklist for postoperative transfer**

Surgical aspects

- What were the intraoperative findings?compared to before
- What surgical technique was performed ?any problem
- what drainage was placed intraoperatively (eg ,pleural drainage,mediastinal drainage)?what is the assessment of post-operative result?
- Was an intraoperative TEE performed and what were the findings (residual gradient ,valve insufficiency ,residual shunt and myocardial function)?
- Did any intraoperative arrhythmia occure and how were they treated?
- Did any intraoperative bleeding occure and how were they treated?

Anesthesiological aspects

- Tube size and brand ,cuffed and uncuffed?
- Ventilation settings (Fio2 ,tidal volume ,rate,peak pressure and PEEP
- Central venous catheter :location of insetion ,size
- Arterial access:-location,size
- Was an LAor pulmonary artery catheter placed?
- Anesthetics and cardiac medication used (cathecolamines ,vasodilators,antiarrhythmics) and their dosages
- Heparinization and current coagulation levels
- Use of blood products (packed red cells ,platelet concenterates ,fresh frozen plasma)

Cardiopulmonary bypass

- Bypass time
- Aortic cross clamp time
- Cardiac arrest time
- Minimum temperature during bypass
- Was hemofilteration performed at the end of the bypass

o Use volume more generously
o Do not use dopamine

- Maintain rather high dosage of prostaglandin E1.

Prostaglandin

Prostaglandin E1 is given to maintain patency or reopen the ductus arteriosus in neonates with ductal-dependent defect. Due to its short half-life, it must be administered continuously intravenous. The initial dosage in a patient with a nearly closed duct is between 50 and 100 ng/kg/min. Based on the actual effect, this dosage can be reduced gradually to a minimum of 5–10 ng/kg/minThe most common side effects are as follows:

- Apnea (administer in readiness for intubation)
- Bradycadia
- Vasodilatation (pulmonary and systemic),hypotension
- Fever

(Cortical hyperostosis, periostitis only after long-term administration) Practical tip: When a prostaglandin infusion is required, always a second venous access should be inserted to ensure safe prostaglandin administration immediately via other access if the first one is dislocated. The second access can also be used for volume substitution in case of acute hypotension

Cardiac defects with parallel circulations

The only example of this cardiac defect is a transposition of the great arteries (d-TGA) together with its variations. The management of this situation is described in the specific treatment section

Cardiac defects with complete intracardiac mixing of blood

The different cardiac defects (i.e., univentricular hearts) in this group are also described in the following treatment section.

Cardiac defects with a large left-to-right shunt

When the pulmonary resistance drops after the first 4–6 weeks of life, the left-to-right shunt and thereby pulmonary blood flow will increase dramatically. Consequently, heart failure may develop caused by increased volume load, which must be treated medically (diuretics, ACE inhibitors, beta blockers, possibly digoxin or cathecholamines) until corrective surgery is performed. As additional oxygen will lower the pulmonary resistance and increase excessive pulmonary blood flow, no additional oxygen should be administered

Specific treatment of the most common symptomatic heart defects in the neonatal period

Left ventricle outflow tract obstruction lesion (i.e., critical aortic stenosis, coarctation of the aorta and interrupted aortic arch)

The initial management of these children has some common features:

- Shock therapy, including intubation and ventilation (high PEEP (>10 cm H2O) if there is pulmonary edema)
- Prostaglandin E1: initial dosage 50–100 ng/kg/min
- Oxygen: avoid excessive administration, use PEEP to improve oxygenation. (note: oxygen lowers pulmonary resistance and thus increases pulmonary blood flow)
- Use diuretics (furosemide), to manage pulmonary edema and lower preload
- Use catecholamines (dobutamine, adrenaline, NOT dopamine), preferably milrinone depending on blood pressure and myocardial function. (If there is a subvalvular stenosis, catecholamines should be administered with particular caution due to a possible increase in the obstruction.)
- Assess by ECHO and reduce afterload (e.g., sodium nitroprusside)
- Aim for moderate metabolic acidosis (target pH 7.35)
- Administer as little volume as possible; preferably only after cardiac function has recovered or is assessed to be stable in echocardiography

1. Critical aortic stenosis (AoS)

Hemodynamic situation

Due to the severe obstruction of the aortic valve, the left ventricular function usually is markedly impaired and cannot provide sufficient cardiac output for the systemic circulation which is supplied with blood from the pulmonary artery via the patent ductus arteriosus (i.e., prenatal situation). Left ventricular hypertrophy and possibly fibroelastosis have already developed in utero. This defect is often associated with other left heart obstructions (mitral stenosis,coarctation of the aorta, hypoplastic aortic arch—i.e., Shones complex). If a heart murmur is not already detected in the neonate, many patients with critical aortic stenosis present in severe cardiac shock. In addition, there is differential cyanosis.

In critical AoS with PDA-dependent systemic circulation (prostaglandin infusion), a left-to-right shunt at the atrial level is necessary to allow mixing of the oxygenated pulmonary venous blood via the right atrium, the right ventricle, the pulmonary artery and then the patent ductus arteriosus. A balloon atrial septostomy (Rashkind maneuver) may be necessary, if the shunt at the atrial level is not large enough,

Further procedure

If suspected ensure prompt transfer to a pediatric cardiac center for interventional catheterization and performance of balloon valvuloplasty (method of choice) or surgical commissurotomy (rarely required); possibly carry out an emergency Rashkind maneuver if there is a restrictive foramen ovale and inadequate left ventricular function after balloon valvuloplasty.

2. Coarctation of the aorta (CoA)

Hemodynamic situation

In patients with critical CoA, the lower half of the body is supplied with deoxygenated blood from the pulmonary artery via the PDA (differential cyanosis). When the ductus arteriosus closes, dramatic hypoperfusion of the body distal to the aortic isthmus occurs. The left ventricle has now suddenly contract against the pronounced obstruction and rapid decompensation occurs. Associations with other left heart obstructions (bicuspid aortic valve) or a VSD are common.

Further procedure

Again organize prompt transfer to a pediatric cardiac center for surgical correction, which is generally attempted after the hemodynamic situation has been stabilized. In some special conditions (e.g., for patients in poor general condition or with necrotizing enterocolitis—NEC), primary interventional catheterization with balloon dilatation or implantation of a coronary stent may be indicated for stabilization until surgery.

3. Interrupted aortic arch

Hemodynamic situation

There are different forms of an interrupted aortic arch and the perfusion of the lower half of the body depends however entirely on a patent ductus arteriosus (i.e., prostaglandin). A VSD is nearly always associated with this defect and other left heart obstructions occur occasionally. Again oxygen saturation should be measured preductally (right hand), as the preductal saturation reflects the situation of the perfusion and blood supply in the CNS and coronary arteries. The levels measured in the lower limbs correspond with pulmonary arterial saturation.

Further procedure

Prompt transfer to a pediatric cardiac center for surgical correction.

4. Hypoplastic left heart syndrome

Hemodynamic situation

In patients with a hypoplastic left heart syndrome (HLHS), both the pulmonary and systemic systems are supplied by the right ventricle. Although there are four forms of HLHS (i.e., MA and AoA, MS and AoA, MS and AoS, MA and AoS with VSD), retrograde coronary perfusion takes place in all across the ductus arteriosus with mixed blood from the pulmonary artery and retrogradely across the coarctation and ascending aorta. Within the first few hours of life, the drop in pulmonary resistance together with the manifestation of a coarctation causes the blood from the pulmonary artery to flow primarily into the pulmonary circulation. Therefore, the systemic circulation—together with the coronary arteries—is increasingly less perfused. Severe heart failure develops, which if untreated usually results in shock. As a result, there is severe metabolic acidosis but due to pulmonary recirculation, the oxygen saturation is only moderately reduced The higher the oxygen saturation is, the more the ratio of pulmonary to systemic perfusion changes are in favor of pulmonary over perfusion and systemic underperfusion. In addition, postnatal closure of the PDA enhances this fatal circulation with underperfusion of the systemic circulation and excessive pulmonary perfusion. It is important to note that oxygenated pulmonary venous blood from the left atrium can only reach the systemic circulation across a sufficiently large shunt to the right atrium (see above).

Initial treatment

- Shock treatment, including intubation and ventilation (but avoid ventilation if possible, as long as the pH is balanced); hyperventilation must be avoided
- Prostaglandin E1: initial dosage 50–100 ng/kg/min
- Avoid administering oxygen (additionally reduces pulmonary resistance and thus systemic perfusion), target saturation 70–85%
- Administer some furosemide (1–2 mg/kg) to lower preload or for pulmonary edema
- Catecholamine treatment is often required, but should be administered with restraint (can increase the myocardial oxygen consumption), give milrinoneor dobutamine if needed, do not use dopamine
- Possibly reduce afterload (e.g., sodium nitroprusside)
- For severe acidosis, large amounts of NaBic are often required to manage acidosis (doses up to 10 ml/kgbw of NaBic are common!)
- Aim for moderate metabolic acidosis (target pH 7.35, avoid over-buffering)
- As little volume as possible should be administered; preferably only after cardiac function has recovered or is assessed to be stable in echocardiography

Further procedure

If the atrial defect is restrictive (leading symptom: severe cyanosis, oxygen saturation <65%, seriously ill child), pulmonary congestion has developed and an emergency balloon atrial septostomy (Rashkind maneuver) may be needed. The patient should be transferred quickly to a pediatric cardiac center for surgery after stabilization (usually a Norwood procedure as the first step of three-stage Fontan palliation).

5. Right ventricle outflow tract obstruction lesion and pulmonary atresia with intact ventricular septum or ventricular septal defect, tetralogy of fallot, tricuspid atresia with pulmonary stenosis and Ebstein anomaly)

Initial treatment

- **Prostaglandin E1 infusion: initial dosage 50–100 ng/kg/min**

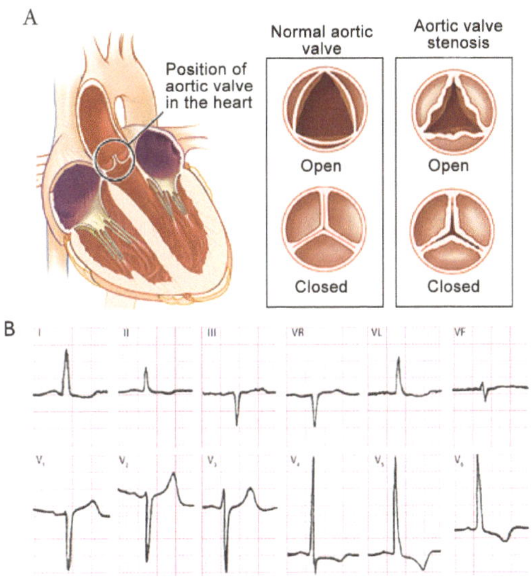

Fig. 34.2 (A) Showing anatomical features of normal and stenosed aortic valve (B) ECG trace shows left ventricular hy-pertrophy with strain pattern in severe valvular aortic stenosis.

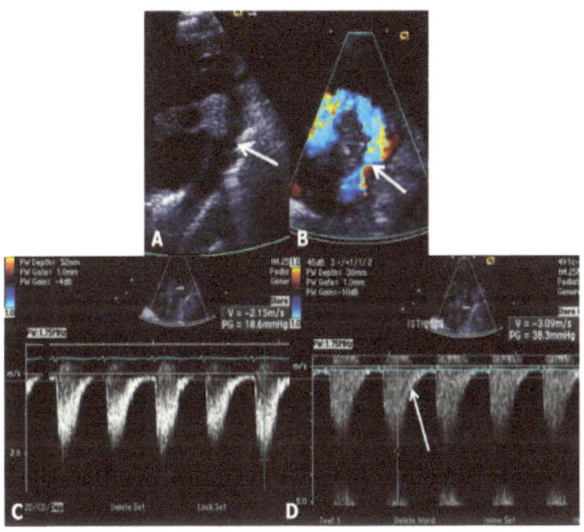

Fig. 34.3 Suprasternal notch views in a neonate with aortic coarctation; 2D (A) and color flow (B) images are shown. The arrows point to the site of coarctation. Doppler flow velocity increased from the aortic isthmus (C) to the DAo (D) along with diastolic extension (arrow in D).

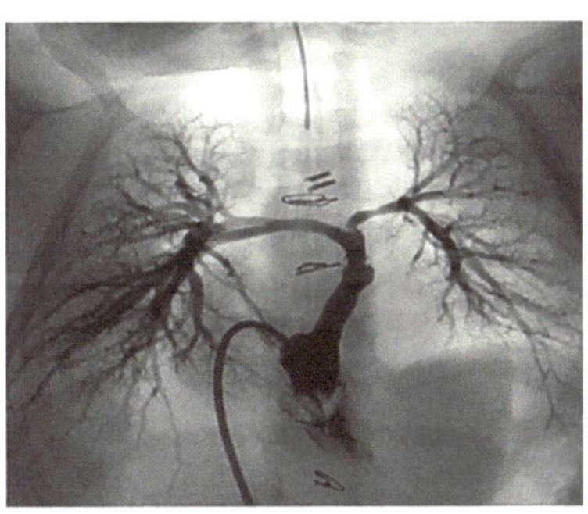

Fig. 34.4 Right ventriculography (antegrade approach) with Berman angiography balloon catheter (Arrow International Inc., Reading, PA) – cranially tilted frontal projection. Patient with hypoplastic right heart syn drome (weight 4 kg) after central shunt due to pulmonary artery hypoplasia.

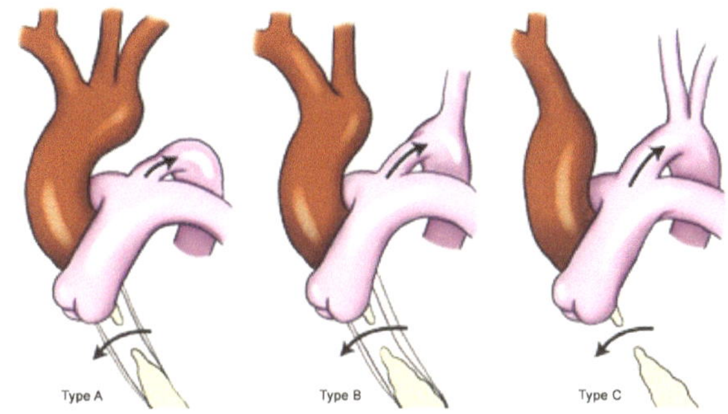

Fig.34.5 Diagram illustrating the different types of inter-rupted aortic arch. Type (A), Interruption of the arch distal to the left subclavian artery; Type (B), interruption of the arch between the left carotid artery and the left subclavian artery; Type (C), interruption of the arch between the innominate artery and the left carotid artery.

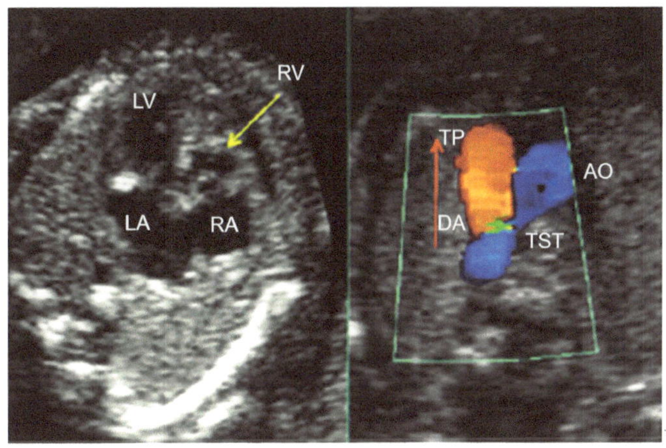

Fig. 34.6 Hypoplastic right ventricle (arrow) in a fetus with pulmonary atresia and intact ventricular septum (a). Color doppler of the 4-chamber view with asymmetric flow between the left heart and right heart. Pulmonary valve atresia can be diagnosed using color Doppler by visualizing the great vessels - aorta (Ao) and pulmonary trunk (TP) - in the upper thorax and demonstrating the retrograde flow from the descending aorta across the ductus arteriosus toward the pulmonary valve.

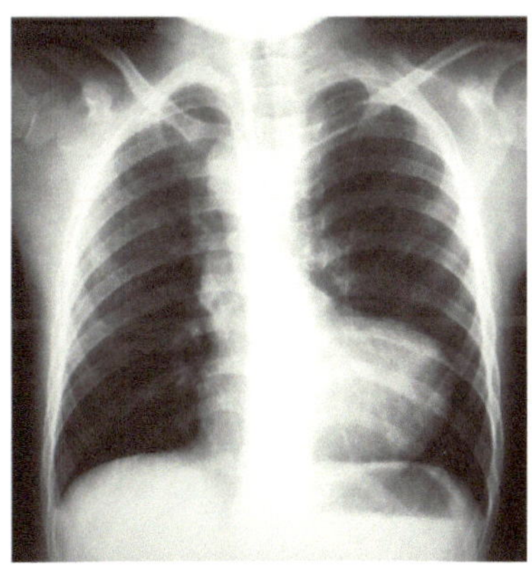

Fig.34.7 X-ray chest PA view shows counterclockwise eleva-tion of cardiac apex, marked RVH with abscence of pulmonary bay with peripheral pruning of pulmonary vasculature in a patient with Pulmonary atresia with intact IVS.

- **Initially more generous oxygen therapy (lowers pulmonary resistance)**
- **Initially more generous volume therapy (i.e., 20 ml/kg bw)**
- **Try to achieve mild metabolic alkalosis (use over-buffering) (pH 7.45–7.5)**
- **Possibly ventilation and mild hyperventilation (pCO2 around 35 mmHg)**
- **Possibly use an increase in systemic resistance (noradrenaline)**

6. Critical pulmonary stenosis

Hemodynamic situation

A critical pulmonary stenosis is a high-grade obstruction of the pulmonary valve with subsequent hypoxemia. As the right ventricle cannot drain into the pulmonary circulation, secondary hypoxia occurs due to a right-to-left shunt across the foramen ovale/ASD. The musculature of the RV is severely hypertrophic and the RV and tricuspid valve may sometimes be hypoplastic. To ensure oxygenation, the pulmonary circulation is supplied with blood from the aorta via the PDA.

Further procedure

After diagnosis and prostaglandin infusion organize transfer to a pediatric cardiac center for interventional catheter balloon valvuloplasty.

7. Pulmonary atresia with intact ventricular septum

Hemodynamic situation

In pulmonary atresia with intact ventricular septum, which can be judged as extreme form of pulmonary stenosis, the right ventricle cannot drain its blood normally to the PA. The majority of blood from the right ventricle either flows back into the right atrium due to tricuspid regurgitation. In addition in some cases, the right ventricle may be connected with the coronary arteries via myocardial sinusoids. In the latter case, the coronary arteries may have other problems and are stenotic so that coronary perfusion may depend on blood flow from the right ventricle (right ventricular dependent coronary circulation (RVDCC). Usually there is suprasystemic pressure in the right ventricle and the right ventricle is hypoplastictic various degrees. Again, the pulmonary circulation is supplied with blood from the aorta via the PDA to ensure oxygenation.

Further procedure

After stabilization, organize transfer to a pediatric cardiac center. In most cases, cardiac catheterization is needed to rule out myocardial sinusoids and coronary anomalies. In some cases, it is possible to open the right ventricular outflow tract by interventional catheterization or implant a stent into the PDA. Otherwise interim palliative surgery (opening the right ventricular outflow tract or aortopulmonary shunt) must be performed accordingly.

8. Tricuspid atresia

Hemodynamic situation

In tricuspid atresia, that may give an example for all univentricular heart defects, there is no continuity between the right atrium and ventricle, so the right atrium can drain into the left atrium only across a right-to-left shunt at atrial level. There are various forms of tricuspid atresia depending on the variations of obstructions of the right ventricular outflow tract or pulmonic valve. The RV is usually perfused from the LV across a VSD that is almost always present. The RV is hypoplastic to various extents. Oxygen saturation is identical in the aorta and pulmonary artery because of the complete mixing of blood.

Frequently stenosis and even atresia of the pulmonary artery occur and may have a negative effect on the blood flow to the pulmonary circulation. If there is atresia or a high grade stenosis of the pulmonary artery, perfusion of the lungs depends on a patent ductus arteriosus (see above). In addition, the great vessels can be in normal position or in transposition.

If there is no pulmonary stenosis and blood flow to the pulmonary circulation is unobstructed, the main symptom that may develop later on is heart failure (tachypnea, hepatomegaly, pallor, possible pulmonary edema), but this constellation is much less common.

Initial treatment

Initial treatment if there is no pulmonary stenosis (leading symptom: heart failure):

- Anticongestive treatment (diuretics, milrinone, rarely catecholamines)
- Restrictive volume therapy
- Restrictive oxygen therapy

Further procedure

Transfer to a pediatric cardiac center should be organized. If there is a restrictive atrial shunt (rare), an interventional catheter balloon atrial septostomy (Rashkind maneuver) may be needed. If there is inadequate pulmonary perfusion, a palliative aortopulmonary shunt is placed. The separation of circulations is performed later as multistep procedure (Fontan procedure).

9. Tetralogy of Fallot

Hemodynamic situation

In tetralogy of Fallot, there is a typical combination of a large VSD with overriding of the aorta, a subpulmonary and pulmonary stenosis, often combined with supravalvular stenosis of various degrees and a marked hypertrophy of the right ventricle. Cyanosis is determined by the extent of

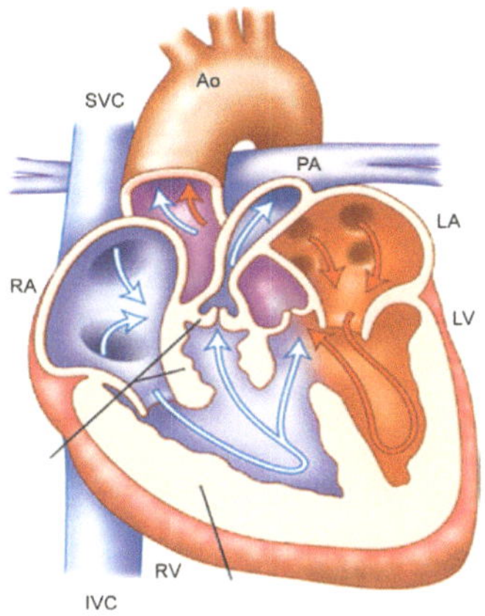

Fig. 34.8 Graphic representation of tetralogy of Fallot show-ing the classic features of this lesion: ventricular septal defect, pulmonary stenosis, overriding aorta (Ao), and right ventricular hypertrophy. The potential various levels of right ventricular outflow tract obstruction are noted (subvalvar, valvar, and supra-valvar). The right-to-left shunt across the ventricular septal defect (shown by the arrow) accounts for the presence of cyanosis in this defect. IVC inferior vena cava, LA left atrium, LV left ventricle, PA pulmonary artery, RA right atrium, RV right ventricle, SVC superior vena cava.

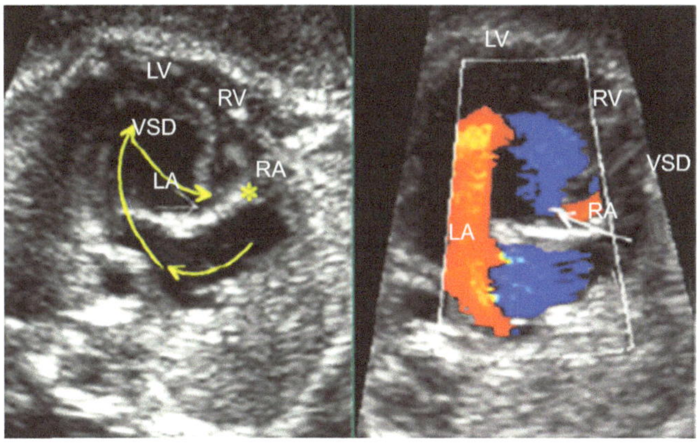

Fig.34.10 Tricuspid atresia (*) and ventricular septal defect (VSD). Arrows show the direction of flow; due to the atresia of the tricuspid valve, blood entering the right atrium cannot enter directly into the right ventricle and it flows to the left atrium, left ventricle and across the VSD to the hypoplastic right ventricle (right).

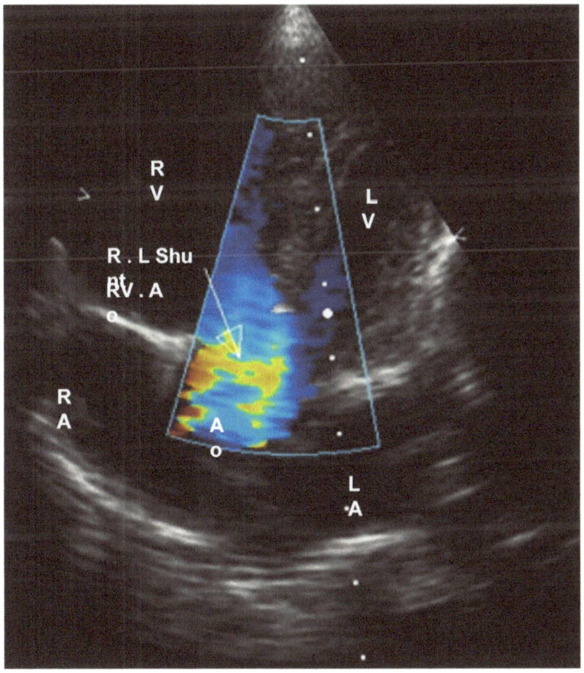

Fig. 34.9 Apical five chamber view in Tetralogy of Fallot in systole with right to left shunt.

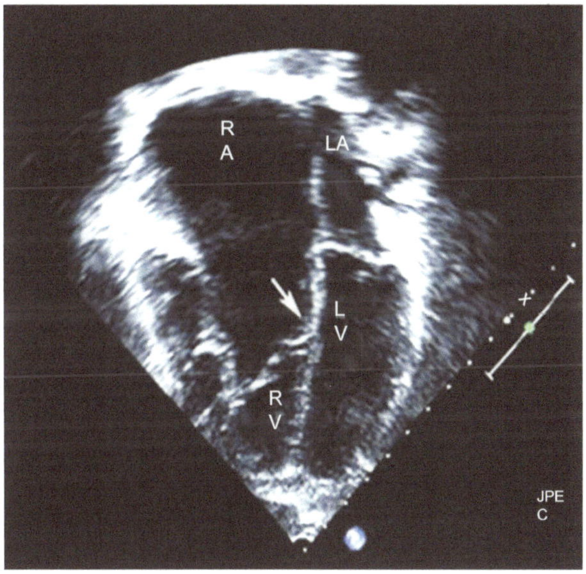

Fig.34.11 Ebstein anomaly of the tricuspid valve. Apical four-chamber echocardiogram in a patient with Ebstein anomaly demonstrates severe apical displacement of the septal leaflet of the tricuspid valve (arrow), with resulting "atrialization" of a large portion of the right ventricular sinus. The anterior leaflet of the tricuspid valve is large (often described as "sail-like") and has multiple attachments to the apex and anterior right ventricular wall (RV). LA, left atrium; LV, left ventricle, RA, right atrium.

the obstruction of the right ventricular outflow tract and thereby pulmonary blood flow. In most cases, this obstruction is only mild at birth, but becomes more significant during the first few weeks of life due to the increase in the infundibular stenosis. If there is pronounced stenosis of the right ventricular outflow tract (functional pulmonary atresia), the children may already develop symptoms with cyanosis or hypoxic spells even in the neonatal period. Hypercyanotic spells occur if there is a sudden increase in subpulmonary muscular obstruction of the RVOT (i.e., agitation) or an acute drop in peripheral vascular resistance (i.e., after feeding).

Treatment of a hypoxic-hypercyanotic spell

- Immediate sedation (e.g., ketamine IV 2–5 mg/kg, alternatively opiates, benzodiazepines)
- Oxygen therapy
- Increase in systemic resistance by
  1. pressing the child's flexed knee against the chest ("jack-knife position")
  2. if necessary infusion of vasoconstrictors (noradrenaline)
  3.. generous volume bolus (e.g., 20–50 ml/kg)
- Compensation of metabolic acidosis by buffering
- Possibly beta blockers (e.g., propranolol IV 0.01–0.1 mg/kg very slowly under monitor guidance)

Further procedure

Rapid transfer to a pediatric cardiac center is urgently needed.In most circumstances, interventional management can improve the hemodynamic situation (i.e., balloon dilatation of the pulmonary valve, stenting of the right ventricular outflow tract, stenting of a PDA). Only in few cases, early surgical correction is required today. In special situations (e.g., very small children), an aortopulmonary shunt is first placed as a palliative measure to ensure lung perfusion.

10. Pulmonary atresia with ventricular septal defect

Hemodynamic situation

From the hemodynamic aspect, this disease is an extreme form of Tetralogy of Fallot. Pulmonary perfusion is, however, dependent on a patent ductus arteriosus (prostaglandin infusion) or aortopulmonary collaterals.

Further procedure

After stabilization with prostaglandin infusion, a rapid transfer to a pediatric cardiac center should be organized. In cases with only membranous valvular atresia, an attempt can be made to open the valve by interventional catheterization (or with stent placement). In addition placing a stent in the PDA may help to achieve catch-up growth of the pulmonary vessels, which are almost always hypoplastic. If this intervention is not possible, an aortopulmonary shunt is placed as surgical palliation. After catch-up growth of the pulmonary vascular system, a continuity between the pulmonary vessels and the right ventricle is created surgically later (e.g., with a valved conduit

11. Ebstein's anomaly

Hemodynamic situation

In Ebstein's anomaly, there is apical displacement of the tricuspid valve into the right ventricle combined with moderate to severe tricuspid regurgitation and reduced flow from the small right ventricle to the pulmonary artery. The right atrium is markedly too massively dilated. A pronounced Ebstein's anomaly can already be symptomatic in the neonatal period. Cyanosis occurs due to a right-to-left shunt at the atrial level caused by minimal antegrade flow to the pulmonary artery. In addition, the gross dilatation of the heart may compress the lungs and impair pulmonary function.
The disease may often complicated by accessory pathways (Wolf-Parkinson-White syndrome).

Initial treatment

Besides initial treatment stated above, in Ebstein's anomaly:

- If there is heart failure, possibly catecholamines and diuretics
- If there is supraventricular tachycardia, it should be terminated with a vagal maneuver, adenosine, amiodarone, possibly cardioversion

Further procedure

The goal of surgical treatment is to reconstruct the tricuspid valve and close the ASD. If there is insufficient lung perfusion, it may be necessary to place an aortopulmonary shunt. If there is pronounced hypoplasia of the right ventricle, the univentricular Fontan pathway may be the only option. The overall prognosis is unfavorable for children who become symptomatic already in the neonatal period. These children require urgent transfer to a pediatric cardiac center.

12. d-transposition of the great arteries (d-TGA)

Hemodynamic situation

In d-TGA, there is parallel connection of the pulmonary and systemic circulations; the systemic venous blood is directed back into the aorta and the pulmonary venous blood is pumped back to the pulmonary artery. Survival is only possible if shunts between the two circulatory systems do exist. The most important is a patent foramen ovale or ASD as shunt at atrial level, so oxygenated blood can reach the systemic circulation via the right ventricle across this left-to-right shunt. A PDA has a favorable effect on

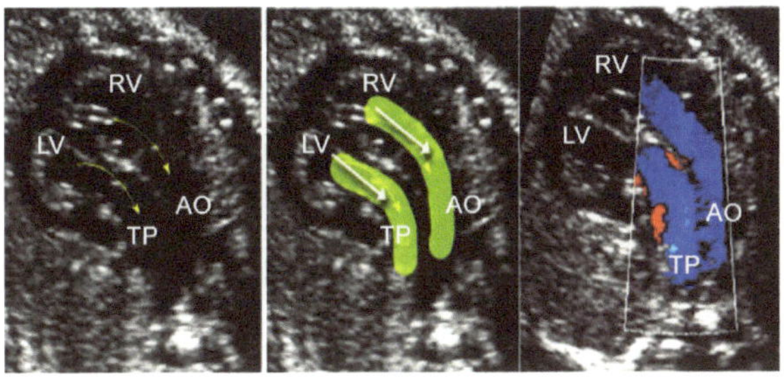

Fig.34.12 Fetal echocardiography shows transposition of the great arteries demonstrating the abnormal connection of the right ventricle (RV) with the aorta (AO) and the left ventricle (LV) with the pulmonary trunk (TP). Both great arteries show a parallel course.

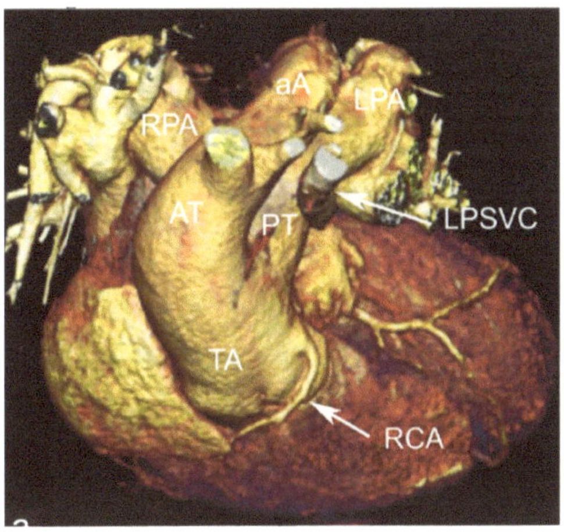

Fig.34.13 A yoing male patient with unrepaired truncus arteriosus (TA) admitted to adult congenital cardiology clinic for surgical operation. The three-dimensional volume-rendered cardiac computed tomography angiogram Oblique superior-inferior - maximum intensity projection view show an anatomical pattern consistent with TA Type IA with persistent left superior vena cava. The right coronary artery branches from the non-coronary sinus at the left side of the truncus.

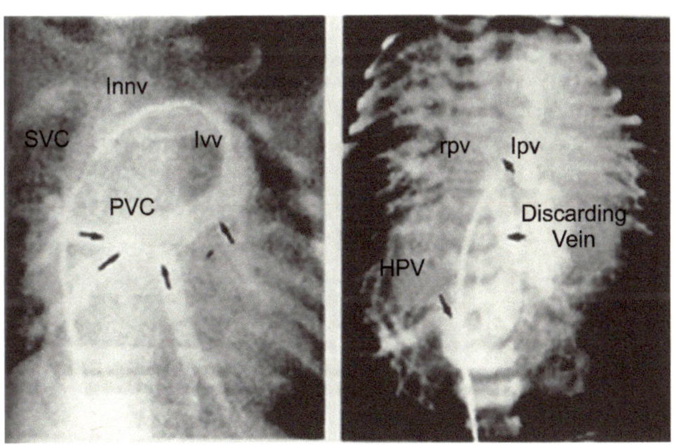

Fig. 34.14 Contrast angiography showing contrast material entering into pulmonary artery (PA)showing return of pulmonary venous blood (B)Left sided vertical vein with subsequent opacification of the right SVC (RSVC) in patient with total anomalous pulmonary venous connection.

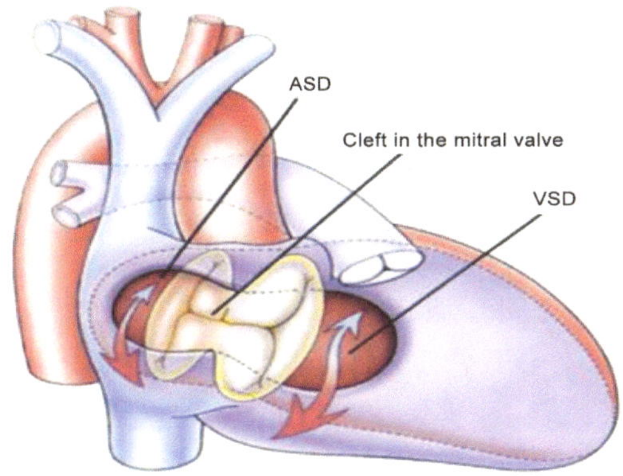

Fig. 34.15 Illustration showing disturbed anatomy and circula-tion in atrioventicular septal defect.

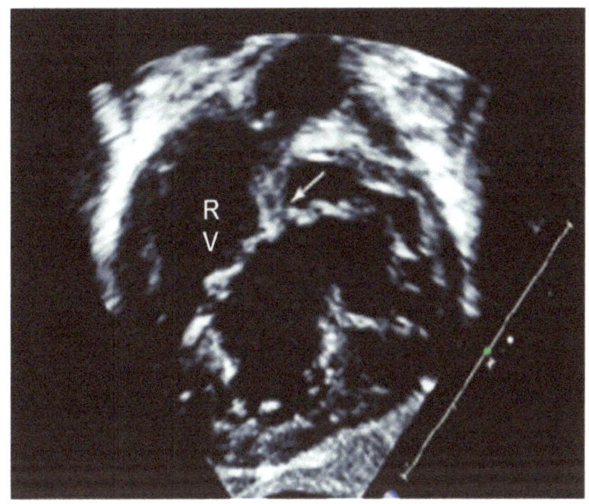

Fig.34.16 En-face echocardiogram view of complete common atrioventricular canal, Rastelli type (A) En-face imaging from sub-xiphoid view shows the multiple leaflets of the common atrioventricular valve; note the attachment of the superior bridging leaflet to the ventricular septum (arrow). RV, right ventricle.

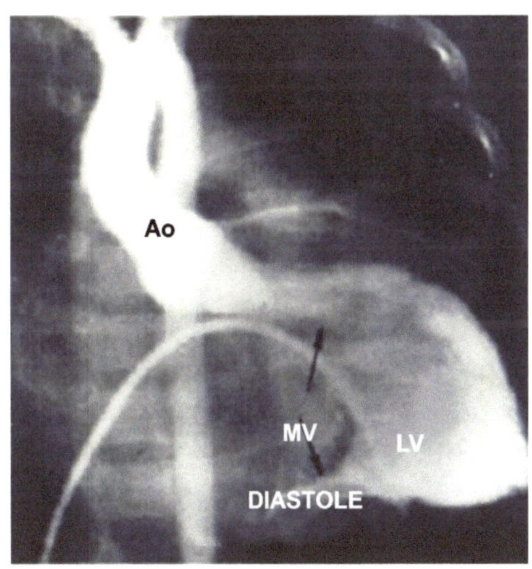

Fig. 34.17 Cine -angiocardiography showing goose neck defor-mity of LVOT in patient with septum primum defect.

oxygenation because PDA blood flow increases lung perfusion and as a result the volume load and pressure in the left atrium is increased, so the left-to-right shunt at atrial level increases and more oxygenated blood can reach the systemic circulation .

Oxygen application may act indirectly by reducing pulmonary resistance and thus increasing pulmonary perfusion and thereby left atrial volume load and pressure (caution: uncontrolled administration of oxygen can also lead to closure of the ductus arteriosus when used without prostaglandin). In addition to improve mixing between the two circulations, especially in "poor mixers," an attempt should be made to improve mixed venous saturation. If there is an associated large VSD, cyanosis is usually less pronounced.

Initial treatment

- Prostaglandin E1 infusion: initial dosage 50 ng/kg/min
- Generous volume therapy
- Aim for mild metabolic alkalosis (over-buffering) (pH 7.45–7.5, lowers pulmonary resistance)
- Oxygen therapy for severe cyanosis in neonates (caution: i nduces closure of the ductus arteriosus)
- If possible avoid intubation, ventilation and relaxation (lowers oxygen consumption and therefore increases mixed venous saturation. On the other hand, ventilation increases the intrathoracic pressure, which can impair mixing of the blood)
- Consider the improve cardiac output and thus mixed venous saturation by milrinone
- Generous treatment of anemia (improves oxygen supply)

Further procedure

If there is a restrictive shunt at the atrial level, a bedside interventional catheter balloon atrial septostomy (Rashkind maneuver) should be performed as soon as possible before transfer to a pediatric cardiac center. The surgical standard treatment is an arterial switch operation (Jatene procedure) within the first 2 weeks of life.

13. Truncus arteriosus communis

Hemodynamic situation

In a truncus arteriosus communis (TAC), only one vessel (common trunk) arises from the heart. The systemic and pulmonary circulation and the coronaries are here supplied from this trunk only. A VSD is almost always present. Since the blood follows the path of least resistance and tends to flow into the pulmonary circulation, there is usually excessive pulmonary blood flow after the drop in pulmonary resistance between the second and eighth weeks of life. In this situation, clinical signs of heart failure are already present in the first weeks of life. Due to the significant pulmonary recirculation, there is often only astonishingly mild cyanosis, although the trunk vessel contains only mixed blood.

Initial treatment

- Oxygen lowers pulmonary resistance and thus increases blood flow to the pulmonary circulation, leading to excessive pulmonary blood flow and increasing heart failure—therefore, use oxygen restrictively
- Treatment of heart failure: diuretics, possibly catecholamines (dobutamine) or phosphodiesterase inhibitor (milrinone), afterload reducer (ACE inhibitor, possibly sodium nitroprusside)
- If associated with an interrupted aortic arch: prostaglandin E1 infusion: initial dosage 50–100 ng/kg/min

Further procedure

Organize transfer to a pediatric cardiac center. The definitive correction with a Rastelli procedure is generally performed within the first weeks of life depending on the clinical signs of heart failure.

14. Total anomalous pulmonary venous connection (TAPVC)

Hemodynamic situation

Depending on the location of the anomalous connection of the pulmonary veins, we distinguish between supracardiac, cardiac, infracardiac and mixed forms. Please note that an infracardiac total anomalous pulmonary venous connection is regularly associated with an obstruction at the connection site.In a total anomalous pulmonary venous connection, all pulmonary veins drain into the systemic venous system and oxygenated blood is guided from there into the right atrium. The perfusion of the systemic circulation thus depends on a right-to-left shunt at the atrial level that is necessary for survival.

In a TAPVC without obstruction of the pulmonary vein, the hemodynamic situation is similar to that of a large ASD (volume overload of the right atrium, ventricle and pulmonary circulation)

Initial treatment

Total anomalous pulmonary venous connection with obstruction of the pulmonary vein:

- Oxygen therapy
- Intubation and ventilation with a high PEEP (>10 cm H2O) for pulmonary edema
- Lower PVR: hyperventilation, generous buffering (target pH 7.45–7.5), increase oxygen supply, possibly inhaled NO or prostacyclin IV
- Diuretics, possibly catecholamines for low cardiac output (caution: catecholamines can exacerbate pulmonary edema)

Further procedure

A TAPVC with obstruction of the pulmonary vein is an absolute cardiac surgery emergency that must be surgically corrected immediately. Dilatation with or without stent implantation can treat the stenosis of the pulmonary vein in individual cases, so that the surgical repair can be performed after the child is stabilized. If there is a restrictive atrial shunt or if surgical correction is not possible immediately, an interventional catheter balloon atrial septostomy (Rashkind maneuver) may be considered.

15. Complete atrioventricular septal defect

Hemodynamic situation

In a complete atrioventricular septal defect (AVSD, AV canal), both segments of the ventricular and atrial septum in the region of the AV valves are absent and the development of the AV valves is also impaired. This malformation results in a large left-to-right shunt that increases when the pulmonary resistance drops within the first weeks of life. Children with a complete AVSD usually develop heart failure when the pulmonary resistance drops after 2–8 weeks of life. The situation can be complicated by (mainly systemic) AV valve insufficiency

Note trisomy 21 is frequently associated with AVSD. All neonates with trisomy 21 must therefore have an ECHO examination at an early age.

Initial treatment

- Avoid oxygen (excessive pulmonary blood flow is increased)
- Pharmacological treatment of heart failure: diuretics, ACE inhibitors, beta blockers, rarely catecholamines (possibly digoxin?)

Further procedure

The corrective surgery is generally performed at the age of 4–6 months and it may be necessary earlier if conservative heart failure treatment is unsuccessful.

11. Postoperative cardiac intensive care therapy

The following remarks apply primarily to those patients that are transferred immediately after surgery from the surgical operating room and their early postoperative period in the pediatric cardiac intensive care unit (PCICU).

Basics

One of the main requirements for providing good quality of care in a PCICU is to understand that the job of the intensive care physician starts far before the operated child is admitted to the PCICU. Detailed information on the case of the child is required in advance before the day of admission. The PCICU intensivist must be aware of and understand the hemodynamics of the cardiac defect (i.e., check the ECHO, cath data, etc.), possible complicating or concomitant diseases, the actual planned surgical repair or procedure and the usually possible perioperative and postoperative complications.

Every intensive care physician should be familiar with the major steps of cardiac surgery in general and the specific steps and details of the case to be admitted. These steps include the whole process of surgery from opening the thorax and the mediastinum, thereafter arterial and venous cannulation for the cardiopulmonary bypass, initiation of cardiopulmonary bypass, cardioplegic arrest and finally, the restoration of cardiac function at the end of the operation including decannulation and closure of the thorax. To obtain this crucial understanding, every intensivist should visit the cardiac theatre on a regular basis and observe about 50 surgeries per year. In complex cases, the intensivist should work together in the time after decannulation or weaning of the bypass with the anesthetist before admission of the patient to the PCICU.

Preparation of the bed place

The majority of patients will be admitted on a planned and forseable basis. Before the patient is transferred to the PCICU, a careful and standardized preparation of the bed/ place must be completed to avoid unnecessary misunderstanding and streamline the admission process. This preparation may vary from unit to unit but generally includes the following:

- Preparation of the ventilation equipment, adjustment of the settings to the estimated patient-specific parameters, checking of the ventilation bag and mask, oxygen delivery, suction equipment and catheters. In addition, it must be determined by contacting the operating theatre or by assessment of the preoperative information whether iNO (nitric oxide) ventilation is required and possible with the ventilation equipment
- Medication plan: The prepared medication plan should be tailored to the patients' age and weight and include the medication and calculated dosages for the presumed standardized postoperative treatment (i.e., sedation, pain therapy, antibiotics, catecholamines, vasodilators, diuretics, fluid therapy and infusions). The perfusors and flushing solutions should be purged and primed before the patient is transferred to the PCICU
- Monitoring: The bedside monitor is checked beforehand and the patient-specific alarms according to reference values for age and disease are set
- Administrative tasks: Unit specific paperwork is prepared and an X-ray order for the first postoperative X-ray and laboratory order for the first laboratory tests should be prepared

A. Postoperative transfer of the patient to the ICU

In order to understand the physiology of the patient, a detailed handover from the different disciplines treating the patient during surgery is necessary. The checklist in Table 2 contains some common and useful questions that the ntensive care physician should discuss with the surgeons, anesthesiologists and cardiac technicians/perfusionists at transfer. The information is crucial and may have direct impact on the subsequent PCICU management.

Table 34.1. Checklist for postoperative transfer.

Surgical aspects
- What were the intraoperative findings? Compared to before?
- What surgical technique was performed? Any problems?
- What drainages were placed intraoperatively (e.g., pleural drainage, mediastinal drainage)?
- What is the assessment of postoperative result?
- Was an intraoperative transesophageal echocardiography performed and what were the findings (residual gradient, valve insufficiency, residual shunt, myocardial function)?
- Did any intraoperative arrhythmias occur? How were they treated?
- Did any intraoperative bleeding problems occur? How were they treated?

Anesthesiology aspects
- Tube size and brand, cuffed and uncuffed?
- Ventilation settings (FiO_2, tidal volume, rate, peak pressure and PEEP)
- Central venous catheter: location of insertion, size
- Arterial access: location, size
- Was an LA or pulmonary artery catheter placed?
- Anesthetics and cardiac medication used (cathecolamines, vasodilators, anti arrhythmics) and their dosages
- Heparinization and current coagulation levels
- Use of blood products (pack red cells, platelet concentrates, fresh frozen plasma)

Cardiopulmonary bypass
- Bypass time
- Aortic cross clamp time
- Cardiac arrest time
- Minimum temperature during bypass
- Was hemofiltration performed at the end of the bypass?

B.Initial examination after transfer to the ICU

Immediately after the patient is admitted to the ICU, the most important clinical parameters must be assessed by the admitting physician and the nurses involved to confirm that the patient is in a stable and safe situation:

- Respiration: Is the chest moving? How are thorax/chest movements? Symmetrical lung expansion? Adequate expansion? How is the Oxygen saturation? FiO_2?

- Circulation: Palpation of peripheral pulses (femoral, brachial), visual check of pressure parameters on the monitor (arterial blood pressure, CVP, if inserted pulmonary artery pressure or LA pressure) and check of capillary filling time (normal<2–3 s)

- Diuresis: Is the urine bag filled? How much? Is the bladder filled despite urine catheter? Does the urine look clear or hemolytic? Does the patient appear edematous (puffy) or rather dehydrated?

- Bleeding: Are the drains connected to suction? How much is in the bag and how quick is it filling? Are the secretions dark red (venous blood), bright red (arterial blood), yellowish or clear (serous), warm (fresh) or cold (older)?
- Neurology: is the patient sedated/anesthetized, what is the status of the pupils, are there spontaneous movements and is the patient breathing against the ventilator?

- Body temperature
- Assessment of catheters, lines and cables inserted

During this gross examination to assess the patient's stability, the patient is connected to the bedside monitor system and other equipment. The arterial and central venous accesses are connected with the pressure transducers, set to zero and activated again. The patient is also connected to the ventilator and the drainages set to suction (in general, the suction pressure is set at around 15 cm H_2O). In addition, the external pacemaker is checked for proper function.

In parallel, the first blood samples are taken and include an arterial and central venous blood gas analysis, an ACT and a survey of different pathology markers to asses organ function. The first blood gas analysis including electrolyte status provides information on the ventilation situation, the hemodynamic status (lactate, central venous saturation) and electrolyte metabolism (especially potassium). A standard limb ECG is then recorded, a chest X-ray arranged and finally, an initial exploratory echocardiography (ECHO) performed as a standard in every patient.

C. Further postoperative management

Fluid intake

As capillary leak is a normal reaction to bypass and the subsequent inflammatory process induces edema of all organs, the amount of free water intake should be limited postoperatively. Therefore, fluid intake is ideally reduced to 30–50% of the normal maintenance on the first postoperative day and then increased day by day to 75 and finally 100% on the following days.Patients, however, who underwent cardiac surgery without cardiopulmonary bypass (e.g., resection of an aortic coarctation, PDA ligature) do not require any restriction of postoperative fluid intake.As soon as the children are able to drink, oral fluid intake should not be restricted any more.

Ventilation

The majority of patients are ventilated after cardiac surgery when they arrive in the PCICU. Pulmonary function is affected by a large variety of preoperative, intraoperative and postoperative factors. Important examples to be considered are listed below:

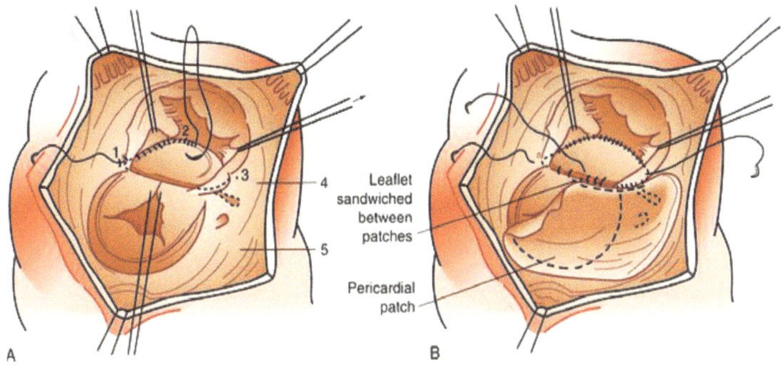

Fig. 34.18 Repair of Complete AtrioventricularDefect Using Two-Patch Technique.

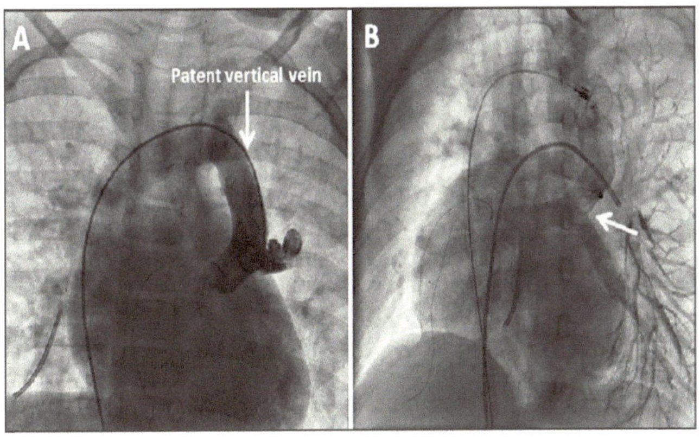

Fig.34.19 (A) Cine angiogram of a patient showing injection in the vertical vein using pigtail catheter, (B) closure of patent vertical vein using Amplatzer vascular plug II causing impingement of pulmonary vein by the distal disc.

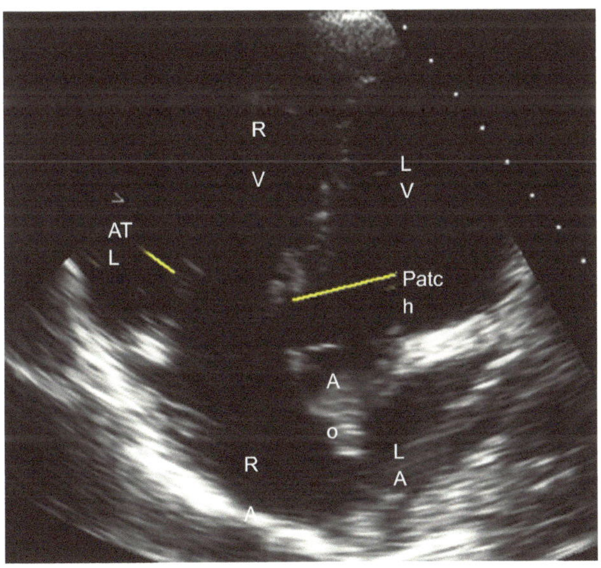

Fig. 34.20 Apical five chamber (5C) view after TOF repair, showing the patch in the subaortic region where the VSD (ventricular septal defect) was closed. ATL: anterior tricuspid leaflet.

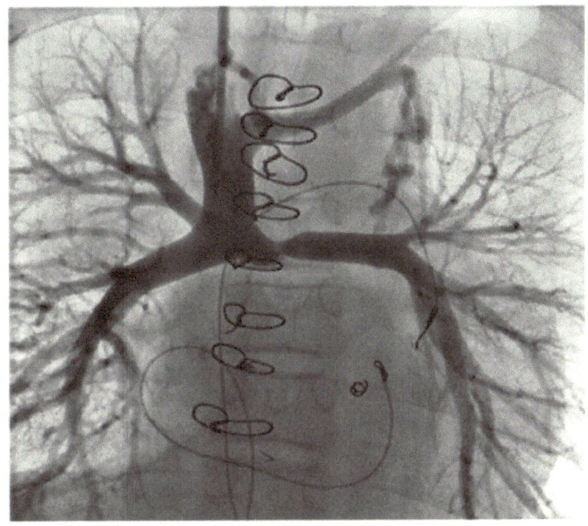

Fig. 34.21 An angiogram with radiocontrast dye injected us-ing a pigtail catheter showing the patient's Blalock-Taussig shunt connecting the innominate artery to the right pulmonary artery. Blalock-Taussig shunt, also known as Blalock-Thomas-Taussig shunt, is a palliative procedure designed to increase pulmonary arterial blood flow in patients with right ventricular outflow tract obstruction (e.g. tetralogy of Fallot).

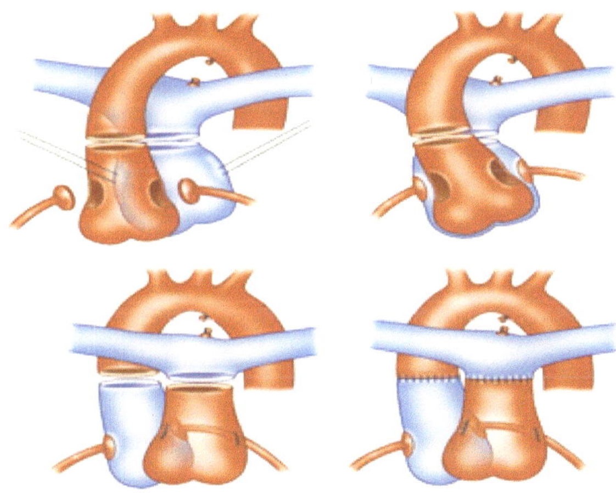

Fig.34.22 Graphic representation of the arterial switch operation in d-transposition of the great arteries. Upper left panel, the ductus arteriosus/ligamentum is divided, and the great arteries are transected above the level of their native semilunar valves and roots. Coronary artery buttons are then removed from the typically anterior and rightward aorta. Upper right panel, the coronary arteries are translocated to the posterior "neoaortic" root (native pulmonary root). Left lower panel, the Lecompte maneuver is performed allowing for the main pulmonary artery to be mobilized in front of the neoaorta. Right lower panel, the aortic anastomosis is completed and after repairing the defects in the native aorta ("neopulmonary artery") where the coronary buttons were removed, the pulmonary arterial anastomosis is completed.

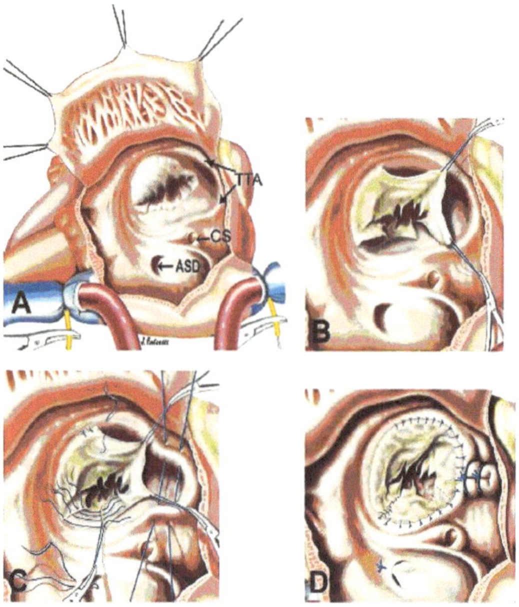

Fig.34.23 Operative steps for Ebstein anomaly repair. (A) Opened right atrium showing displacement of the tricuspid valve. TTA, true tricuspid annulus; ASD, atrial septal defect; CS, coronary sinus. (B) Detached part of the anterior and posterior leaflet as a single piece. (C) Clockwise rotation of the posterior leaflet edge to be sutured to the anterior leaflet septal edge and plication of the true tricuspid annulus to bring the valve to a uniform level. (D) Completion of valve attachment to the true tricuspid annulus and closure of the atrial septal defect. Used with permission from Elsevier Thorac Cadiovasc Surg. 2007 Jan;133(1):215-23).

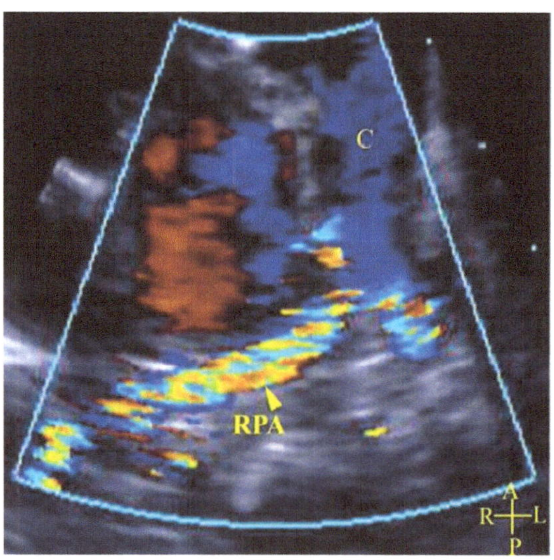

Fig. 34.24 Parasternal short-axis view. Severe right pulmonary artery stenosis (RPA) (yellow arrow head) following truncus arteriosus repair demonstrated by color Doppler. C, conduit; RPA, right pulmonary artery.

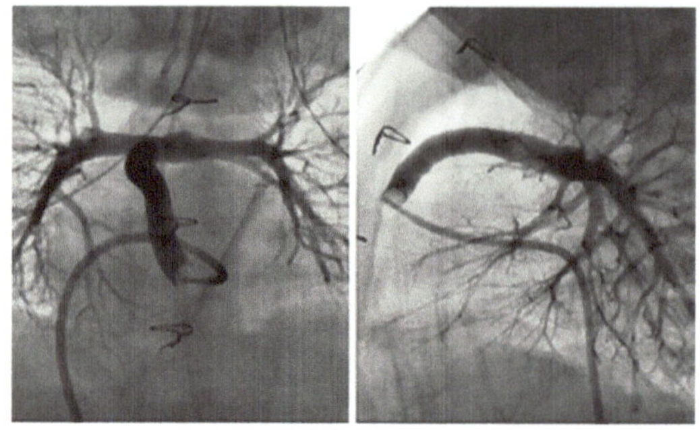

Fig.34.25 Postero-anterior (left) and lateral angiograms (right) performed in a subject with a ring-reinforced Gore-Tex right ventricle to pulmonary artery Sano shunt. Here there is relative uniformity of the conduit caliber along its length with no narrowing.

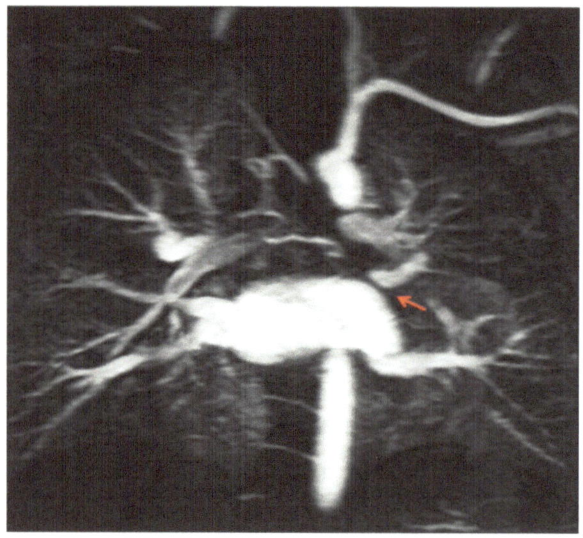

Fig. 34.26 Follow-up CT scan performed after repair of total anomalous pulmonary venous connection (TAPVC). The right upper pulmonary vein (RUPV) appears severely stenosed (red arrow).

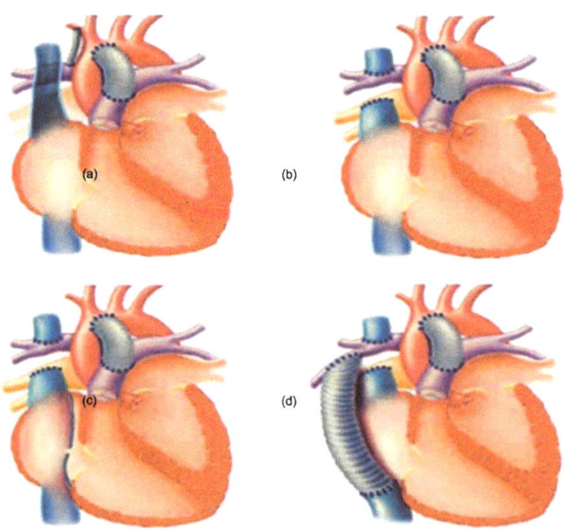

Fig.34.27 Stages in the repair of functional single ventricles (a) Norwood; (b) bidirectional Glenn; (c) lateral tunnel; (d) ext-racardiac conduit.

Table 34.4 Typical postoperative problems and the most common causes

Problem	Common causes
Blood pressure too high	Pain, fear, catecholamines, excessive. fluid volume, result of the abrupt drug discontinuation (beta blockers, ACE inhibitors); typical postoperative problem after correction of an aortic coarctation. Rare. causes: cerebral seizures, hypoglycemia (counter regulation)
Blood pressure too low	Hypovolemia, low cardiac output: limited myocardial function, pericardia.I effusion, arrhythmia (junctional ectopic tachycardia, AV block), exces:;ive drainage lo$$, hemorrhage, excessive. diuresis; vasodilators, anaphylaxis, sepsis, shock, pneumothorax
Central venous pressure. (CVP) too low	Fluid deficit (excessive. drainage losses, hemorrhage, exces:;ive diuresis, volume intake too low)
Central venous pressure. (CVP) too high	Tense/stiff patient (reaction to wake up, insufficient sedation in ventilation patients); impaired right ventricle function. In patients with univentricular heart, a high CVP suggests poor systemic ventricular or a relevant AV va)ve regurgitation. Other causes are. a pericardia) tamponade or pneumothorax
Arterial saturation too low	Atelectasis, hypoventiJation, technical problems with the ventilation device, disconnected/obstructed tube, pneumothora.x, pleural effusion, pneumonia, pulmonary edema, pulmonary hemorrhage, secretion, right to Jeft shunt
Arterial saturation too high	In patients with univentricular hearts, saturation over 85% suggest an imbalance between pulmonary and systemic perfusion: excessive blood flow to the lungs and diminished supply to the systemic circulation
Bradycardia	Sinus bradycardia, AV block
Tachycardia	Narrow QRS complexes: sinus tachycardia, supraventricular tachycardia, JET Wide QRS complexes: ventricular tachycardia
Increase in Jactate	Poor systemic perfusion, seizures, gut ischemia

Table 34.5: *Presents normal hemodynamics and oxygen consumption in children*

Age (weight/BSA)	*Cardiac output (ml/min)*	*Heart rate*	*Stroke volume (ml)*	*Oxygen consumption (ml/min*	*ml/min/m–*
Newborn (3.2 kg/0.2 m–)	700–800	145	5	36–54	180–270
6 months (8 kg/0/42 m–)	1000–1600	120	10	70–100	167–238
1 year (10 kg/0/5 m–)	1300–1500	115	13	85–110	170–220
2 years (13 kg/0.59 m–)	1500–2000	115	18	91–123	154–211
4 years (17 kg/0.71 m–)	2300–2375	105	27	110–150	155–211
5 years (19 kg/0.77 m–)	2500–3000	95	31	115–170	149–221
8 years (28 kg/0.96 m–)	3400–3600	83	42	150–208	156–200
10 years (35 kg/1.1 m–)	3800–4000	75	50	190–250	122–227
15 years (50 kg/1.4 m–)	5000–6000	70	85	300–400	120–200

- **Preoperative factors:**
  1. Preexisting excessive pulmonary blood flow (wet lung congestion)
  2. Preexisting pulmonary hypertension (left-to-right shunt)
  3. External compression of the airways, for example, due to vascular rings or prominent pulmonary arteries
- **Intraoperative factors:**
  1. Atelectasis due to surgical manipulation in the thorax or lack of ventilation during the bypass
  2. Edema development due to the effect of cardiopulmonary bypass and SIRS
  3. Trauma of the lung
- **Postoperative factors:**
  1. Swollen mucosa (SIRS)
  2. Atelectasis
  3. Lung edema as a result of a postoperative increased lung perfusion. Typical examples are after a shunt procedure or operative opening of circulation in the lungs in pulmonary atresia or severe stenosis ("reperfusion edema")
  4. Impaired respiratory mechanics due to postoperative diaphragmatic paresis
  5. Pain-related reduction in respiratory capacity (surgery drains)
  6. Respiratory depression caused by drugs
  7. Pneumothorax, pleural effusions
  8. Bleeding through MAPCAS

Settings of the ventilator

Volume-controlled ventilation is the ventilation of choice in every cardiac patient after cardiac surgery. In many ventilators, a setting with a pressure control combination (i.e., PRVC-mode) can be chosen. Hereby markedly, lower rates are usually used (e.g., 20/min for neonates) in the sedated patient. The tidal volume is usually set to 10–15 ml/kg. A relatively long inspiration time is usually selected initially. The PEEP is around 5–10 mmHg and an FiO2 value is selected at which oxygen saturation of over 95% can be achieved. When the patients waking up, the volume controlled mode is combine with a SIMV mode. In spontaneous breathing patients, the following values can be used as references for the age-specific respiratory rate:

- Neonates: 40/min
- Infants: 25–30/min
- Toddlers: 25/min
- School-age children: 20/min
- Adolescents: 15/min

Again, in the controlled situation, the rate settings used are much slower. The following situations are important variants from these initial settings of the ventilator:

- Univentricular heart: In univentricular hearts, the balance between systemic and pulmonary circulation is very important to avoid pulmonary overcirculation at the cost of inadequate systemic perfusion. At an oxygen saturation of around 75–85%, a nice balance between systemic and pulmonary perfusion is achieved (Qp/Qs = 1:1). Therefore, the target oxygen saturation in these patients is approximately 80%. Uncritical oxygen administration must be avoided.

- Fontan circulation: In these patients, the transpulmonary blood flow is depending completely on the intrathoracic pressure and pulmonary vascular resistance. Theoretically, a high PEEP increases the intrathoracic pressure and thus reduces passive blood across the pulmonary vascular system. A lower PEEP level (<5 mmHg) is therefore often recommended for Fontan patients. On the other hand, a higher PEEP also increases the residual functional capacity and reduces atelectases, so better lung perfusion can be achieved via the Euler–Liljestrand reflex. It has been advocated earlier to ventilate Fontan patients without PEEP—this management strategy is inappropriate and no longer recommended.

- Pulmonary hypertension: Pulmonary vascular resistance is reduced by a low pCO2, a high pH and a high FiO2. To use this principle, patients with known or presumed pulmonary hypertension (i.e., large VSD, older age, truncus, etc.) should be ventilated using mild hyperventilation (Target pCO2: 30–35 mmHg) and with higher than normal FiO2 to achieve an oxygen saturation of around 100% and a paO2 of more than 150 mmHg

Infection prophylaxis

Cardiopulmonary bypass reduces the capacity of the immune system to act against bacterial infections and so postoperative antibiotic prophylaxis is always given for children after cardiac surgery. The antibiotics used and the duration of antibiotic treatment are, however, subject of some controversy. First or second generation cephalosporins are frequently used, for example, cefazolin 30 mg/kg/dose every 8 hourly. For an uncomplicated postoperative course, many centers carry out antibiotic prophylaxis for 2–3 days (6–9 doses, until the drains are out) although hardly any evidence-based data for this procedure are available. For patients with an open sternum or peritoneal dialysis or ECMO, no additional management is required but prolonged treatment is often used in many centers. Antibiotic prophylaxis is then continued for 24 h post-chest closure or ECMO/PD removal.

Sedation

In most centers, a combination of an opiate (morphine, fentanyl) and a benzodiazepine (midazolam) is administered intravenously continuously in the initial postoperative period. Propofol is often used in older children who are sedated for only a short period. No time (2–3 days) or dose (3–8 mg/kg/h) limitation applies in these cases. Lactate levels should be checked on a routine basis.

Analgesia

Surgery itself and the drains in the body after surgery is painful procedure. To reduce postoperative pain, a fixed and standardized combination of non-steroidal analgesics

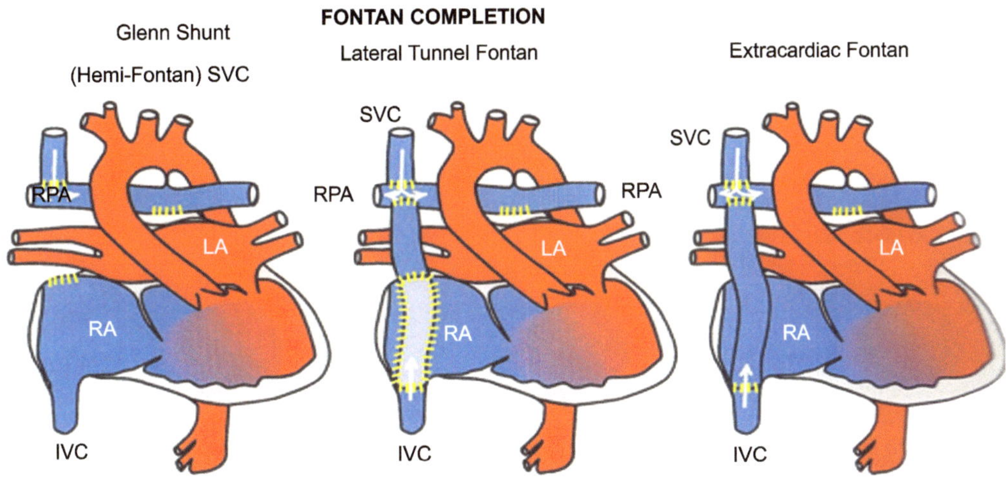

Fig. 34.28 Illustration showing Fonton completion procedure with different approaches such as Glenn shunt(Hemi-Fonton ,Lateral Tunnel Fonton and Extracardiac Fonton.

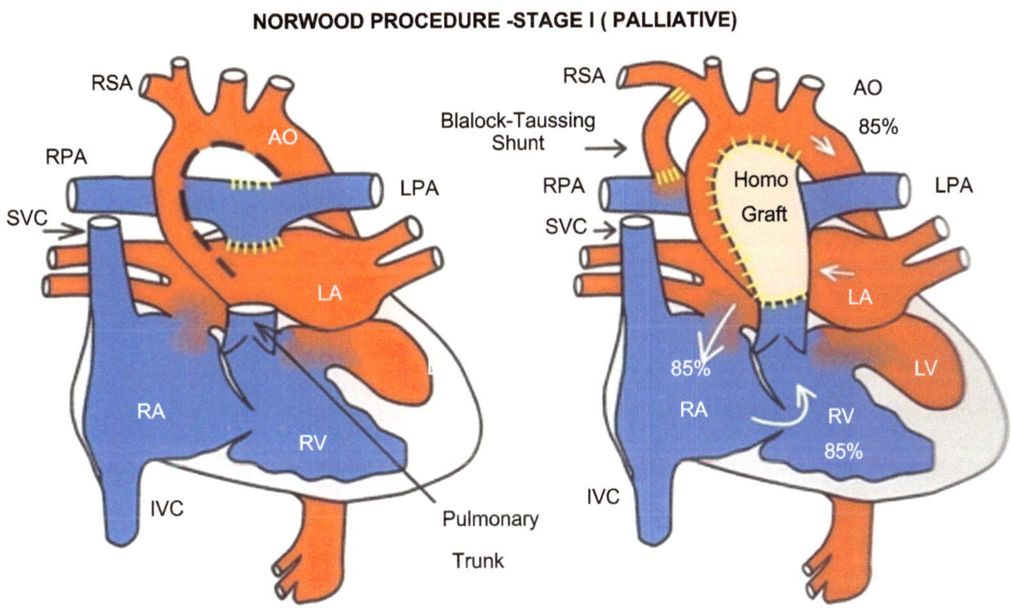

Fig. 34.29 Illustration showing various palliative steps in NORWOOD Procedure –stage I.

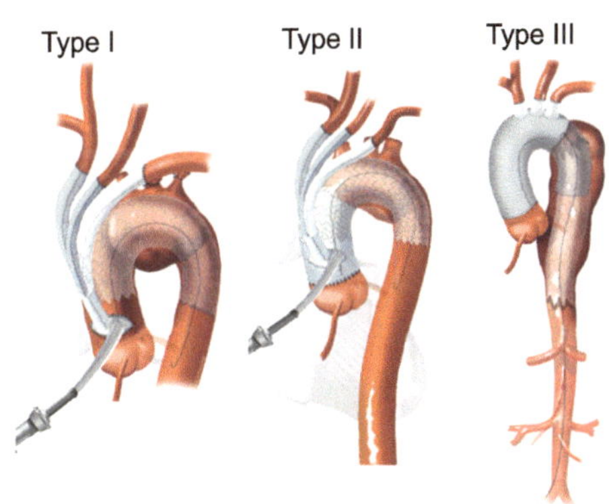

Fig. 34.30 Hybrid aortic arch repair Types I, II and III

(i.e.,paracetamol, ibuprofen) and opiates (morphine, fentanyl) is usually used for analgesia for the first 2–3 days. Patient-controlled analgesia with a PCA pump is also applicable for older children (who can already play a video game).

Kidney function

Kidney function nearly always deteriorates in patients who have undergone cardiac surgery. The use of cardiopulmonary bypass leads to renal impairment and intraoperative fluid loading and inflammatory reactions that result in fluid retention. A negative fluid balance is therefore targeted postoperatively

Urine excretion reflects a combination of cardiac function and cardiac output in combination with kidney function. In general, a urine excretion of at least 2 ml/kg/h after cardiac surgery is a minimum to ensure adequate fluid balance. Patients most often have a combination of pre-renal kidney failure (low cardiac output, capillary leak, volume deficit) in combination with the direct effects of SIRS on the kidney itself. In addition, a low systemic blood pressure and, in case of ascites, a high intra-abdominal pressure leads to a low perfusion pressure in the kidneys (aggressive drainage of ascites). Other less common examples of renal kidney failure are renal vein thrombosis or iatrogenic kidney damage (aminoglycosides, cyclosporin A). Post-renal kidney failure can be caused by obstructions in the region of the efferent urinary tract (e.g., obstruction of the urinary catheter or the urethra) or simply by increased intra abdominal pressure caused by capillary leak and ascites

Suitable diuretics in the postoperative phase are primarily loop diuretics (Furosemide, ethacrynic acid). They are administered as a bolus or as a continuous infusion if the response is inadequate. The combination with theophylline sometimes enhances the effect. If excretion is insufficient or the fluid balance is clearly positive, peritoneal fluid drainage, or peritoneal dialysis should be initiated early

Low cardiac output syndrome (LCOS)

There is a variety of factors that can result in myocardial dysfunction and subsequent low cardiac output postoperatively. Typically, they include an inflammatory reaction to cardiopulmonary bypass, myocardial ischemia and inadequate myocardial function as a result of the intraoperative clamping of the aorta, intraoperative hypothermia, a reperfusion edema, or if a surgical procedure was performed using a ventriculotomy—direct myocardial damage, coronary ischemia, inadequate cardioplegia, mechanical alteration, or an infection.

Symptoms

Typical clinical signs of low cardiac output are as follows:

- Tachycardia
- Oliguria
- Delayed capillary filling time (>3–4 s)
- Hypotension
- Decreased pulse pressure
- Reduced mixed venous saturation (Note: a difference between arterial and mixed venous saturation not <20–25% suggests sufficient cardiac output and adequate oxygen supply)
- Metabolic acidosis (BE less than −5)
- High lactate level (>3 mmol/l)

Treatment

The treatment of low cardiac output has to focus on the underlying causes which should be eliminated if possible. The following measures depending on the hemodynamic situation are commonly used as follows:

- Volume substitution (in case of hypovolemia)
- Inotropic support (catecholamines (i.e., adrenaline, dobutamine), phosphodiesterase inhibitors, intravenous calcium)
- Afterload reduction (sodium nitroprusside, phosphodiesterase inhibitors)
- Consider hormonal therapy for hypotensive resistance to epinephrine and vasopressors: cortisol for suspected adrenal insufficiency, IV or oral triidothyronine (T3) for euthyroid sick syndrome (low T3 levels with LCOS symptoms)
- Chronotropic support (pacemaker therapy, positive chronotropic drugs)
- Treatment of arrhythmias (amiodarone)
- Ventilation strategy
- Reduction in oxygen consumption (sedation, cooling)
- Mechanical circulatory support (ECMO, LVAD)

Pulmonary hypertensive crisis

Based on the underlying anatomy and pathophysiology, many patients may have a significant elevation of pulmonary pressures or pulmonary vascular resistance before surgery. Typical heart defects for this are those with high flow and pressure driven left-to-right shunt defects (large VSD, AVSD, Truncus, etc.) and those with unrestricted flow over a long period (i.e., >6 or 12 months of age). Postoperatively, there may be a rapid and critical increase in pulmonary arterial pressure or pulmonary vascular resistance in certain situations (i.e., agitation, external stimulation such as suctioning, pain, etc.). The result of a rapid increase in PVR is a standstill of the trans-pulmonary blood flow with secondary congestion in the right atrium (high CVP) and ventricle and drop in pressure in the left atrium and ventricle (low CO and BP). Ultimately, cardiac output collapses and the coronaries are not perfused. The following patients are at a particularly high risk for this type of crisis:

- Patients with already increased pulmonary vascular resistance preoperatively (primary pulmonary hypertension)
- Neonates within the first week of life
- Patients with pulmonary venous hypertension (e.g., within the context of a total anomalous pulmonary venous connection or mitral stenosis)
- Older children with a still uncorrected high flow and pressure shunt defects that led to an increase in pulmonary vascular resistance (e.g., complete AV canal, large VSD, truncus)

The following factors may increase pulmonary vascular resistance:

- Hypoxia
- Acidosis (pH <7.3, BE less than −5)
- High partial pressure of carbon dioxide (paCO2 >50)
- Polycythemia
- Atelectasis
- Agitation

The following factors may reduce pulmonary vascular resistance:

- Oxygen administration
- Alkalosis
- Hyperventilation
- NO inhalation (nitric oxide)
- Recruitment of atelectatic lung segments

Prophylaxis of a pulmonary hypertensive crisis is crucial, the acute management as well as the prophylaxis of a pulmonary hypertensive crisis includes the following measures:

- Sufficient analgesia and sedation or relaxation for 1–2 days
- Oxygenation (paO2 >150)
- Optimizing the ventilation (adequate PEEP)
- Slightly alkalotic pH level (target pH 7.4–7.5) and mild hyperventilation (paCo2 30–35)
- Pharmacological vasodilators (NO, iloprost, prostacyclin)
- Avoidance of unnecessary manipulations such as too frequent suctioning

Postoperative features of heart defects with a univentricular heart

The large group of heart defects with a univentricular physiology may pose great challenges to postoperative intensive care in the PCICU. These patients include those with a hypoplastic left heart syndrome, tricuspid atresia, or a double inlet left ventricle. The most important principles in the postoperative treatment of these patients are presented below. As an example, the three-stage surgical procedure for patient with a hypoplastic left heart syndrome is explained. In general, palliation in a Fontan procedure is made with the goal of achieving complete separation of the pulmonary and systemic circulation to eliminate cyanosis. The lungs are perfused passively from the vena cavae without any pumping chamber in between. The single ventricle supplies only the systemic circulation and thereby has a reduced volume load.

The three stages are as follows:

- Norwood procedure or Damus-Kaye-Stansel procedure with a shunt
- Upper cavopulmonary anastomosis (Glenn procedure, "hemi Fontan")
- Total cavopulmonary anastomosis (Fontan procedure)

Norwood procedure

The Norwood procedure is the first step for patients with a hypoplastic left heart syndrome toward separation of the circulatory systems by a Fontan procedure. There are several modifications of this surgical procedure (classical Norwood, Norwood-Sano-procedure). The principal goal is to form a neo-aorta from the pulmonary artery and the hypoplastic aorta that can supply the systemic circulation with blood without a pressure gradient (i.e., unobstructed systemic blood flow). To achieve this, the pulmonary artery and the hypoplastic aorta are anastomosed distal to the valves. Additional patch material is usually required for the reconstruction of the aortic arch and excision of the coarctation. In this manner, a strong vessel for systemic perfusion is created. The pulmonary artery is transected shortly before the pulmonary artery bifurcation and in most cases, pulmonary perfusion is ensured via an aortopulmonary shunt or Sano shunt (placement of a conduit through right ventricular to pulmonary artery).

To achieve the unobstructed inflow to the heart and outflow from the pulmonary veins, an atrial septectomy is also performed. There is a balance between the pulmonary and systemic circulatory systems when arterial saturation is between 75 and 85% (Qp/Qs = 1). Typical problems after a Norwood procedure are low cardiac output, capillary leak caused by SIRS and hypoxemia.

Low cardiac output

As a typical result of the long bypass time required or even prolonged circulatory arrest, a systemic inflammatory response syndrome (SIRS) of various degrees occurs in these neonates. As a consequence, myocardial function is usually markedly impaired so that a certain and often higher amount of catecholamine support is always needed postoperatively. Other possible causes of inadequate systemic perfusion are increased pulmonary perfusion at the expense of systemic perfusion (Qp/Qs >1; leading symptoms: arterial saturation>85%, tachycardia, hypotension, oliguria, metabolic acidosis). To manage this situation, an attempt is made by reducing the afterload of the systemic circulation and increasing pulmonary resistance. AV valve insufficiency or arrhythmias can also cause or deteriorate low cardiac output.

Hypoxemia

Hypoxemia (i.e., saturation <70%) can be the result of an imbalance between pulmonary and systemic

Table 34.6 Specific early postoperative problem and complications (modified from Schwartz and Millar 2009 in Roger's Handbook of Pediatric Intensive care).

Cardiac defect/operation	Specific early postoperative problems and complications
ASD closure	Sinus node dysfunction, left heart failure/pulmonary edema in older children and adults
VSD closure	Pulmonary hypertensive crisis, complete AV block, JET, residual shunt
AV canal correction incompetence	Pulmonary hypertensive crisis, complete AV block, JET, AV valve stenosis or
PDA ligation	Injury to the recurrent laryngeal nerve (vocal cord paralysis) or the thoracic duct (chylothorax), accidental ligation or injury to surrounding vessels (especially left p pulmonary artery, aorta
Truncus arterious correction	Pulmonary hypertensive crisis, truncus valve stenosis or incompetence, right ventricular dysfunction
Aortopulmonary window (correction)	Pulmonary hypertensive crisis, coronary ischemia
Anomalous pulmonary venous connection (correction)	Pulmonary hypertensive crisis, atrial arrhythmia, residual stenosis of the pulmonary veins or pulmonary vein anastomosis with the left ventricle, high left ventricular filling pressure due to the relatively small left atrium and ventricle
Fallot correction	Right ventricular diastolic dysfunction (poor compliance of the hypertrophic ventricle), JET, complete AV block, residual pulmonary stenosis, residual VSD, pulmonary insufficiency after a transannular patch
Pulmonary atresia with intact ventricular septum	Right ventricular dysfunction, myocardial ischemia due to right ventricle dependent coronary circulation, circular shunting due to creation of an aortopulmonary shunt and opening of right ventricular outflow tract
Aortic stenosis correction	Residual stenosis, disruption of left ventricular diastolic function, aortic insufficiency, AV block
Ross procedure	Coronary ischemia
Konno procedure	Coronary ischemia, obstruction of the right ventricular outflow tract, arrhythmias (e.g., AV block), mitral regurgitation
Subaortic stenosis (resection)	Residual stenosis, mitral valve injury, (ventricular) arrhythmia, AV block
Coarctation of the aorta (resection)	Residual obstruction, paraplegia, post-coarctectomy syndrome, unmasking an aortic valve stenosis, injury to the recurrent laryngeal nerve, chylothorax
Interrupted aortic arch (correction)	Residual obstruction, compression of the left main bronchus by the aorta, injury to the recurrent laryngeal nerve, chylothorax
Mitral stenosis correction	Pulmonary hypertensive crisis, residual stenosis, mitral regurgitation, left ventricular dysfunction
Creation of an aortopulmonary shunt	Imbalance between systemic and pulmonary perfusion, shunt leak, shunt thrombosis, pulmonary edema, coronary ischemia
Pulmonary artery banding	Cyanosis, insufficient banding (excessive pulmonary blood flow), Qp-Qs mismatch
Norwood procedure	Low cardiac output, imbalance between systemic and pulmonary perfusion, residual obstruction of the aortic arch, AV valve insufficiency, SIRS
Superior cavopulmonary anastomosis (Glenn, Hemifontan)	Cyanosis, hypertension, edema/congestion of the upper half of the body, Chylothorax
Fontan completion	Ascites, pleural effusions, edema, cyanosis, low cardiac output, arrhythmias
TGA (switch operation)	Coronary ischemia, left ventricular dysfunction, neo aortic insufficiency, peripheral pulmonary stenosis
TGA (Mustard/Senning atrial baffle procedure)	Pulmonary or systemic venous obstruction, atrial arrhythmias
Bland-White-Garland syndrome (correction)	Myocardial dysfunction, mitral regurgitation

circulations to the detriment of the pulmonary circulation—for example, in an obstruction of the aortopulmonary shunt or increased pulmonary resistance. Other causes are typical pulmonary problems such as atelectasis, a pleural effusion, edema, or pneumonia. Peripheral cyanosis occurs with low cardiac output or increased oxygen consumption (leading symptom: reduced systemic venous saturation).

Superior cavopulmonary anastomosis

The aim of a superior cavopulmonary anastomosis is to allow passive blood flow from the upper half of the body into the pulmonary circulation. The superior vena cava is anastomosed in an end-to side manor with the pulmonary artery and thereby the systemic venous blood from the upper half of the body then flows passively to the lungs without an intermediate pumping chamber and is oxygenated there. The systemic venous blood from the lower half of the body does not reach the lungs, but is mixed with the pulmonary venous blood in the heart and pumped into the systemic circulation. The systemic circulation thus contains mixed blood. The saturation of these children is usually about 80–85%.

The aim of a superior cavopulmonary anastomosis is to allow passive blood flow from the upper half of the body into the pulmonary circulation. The superior vena cava is anastomosed in an end-to side manor with the pulmonary artery and thereby the systemic venous blood from the upper half of the body then flows passively to the lungs without an intermediate pumping chamber and is oxygenated there. The systemic venous blood from the lower half of the body does not reach the lungs, but is mixed with the pulmonary venous blood in the heart and pumped into the systemic circulation. The systemic circulation thus contains mixed blood. The saturation of these children is usually about 80–85%. Typical postoperative problems are increased pressure in the superior vena cava, hypertension and hypoxemia.

Elevated pressure in the superior vena cava

In a superior cavopulmonary anastomosis, elevated pressure in the superior vena cava suggests an obstruction in the area of the cavopulmonary anastomosis or pulmonary circulation or elevated pulmonary vascular resistance.The difference in pressure between the superior vena cava and atrium (transpulmonary gradient) should be <10 mmHg. A high pressure in the superior vena cava can restrict cerebral outflow and lead to marked edema in the upper half of the body (superior vena cava syndrome).After this operation, patients should be positioned with the upper body elevated (about 45°, half sitting position). Elevated intrathoracic pressure from mechanical ventilation additionally hinders passive blood flow from the superior vena cava into the pulmonary circulation and patients should therefore be quickly extubated.

Hypertension

Temporary hypertension during the first few postoperative days is not unusual in these patients. The elevation of intracranial pressure that is necessary to maintain adequate cerebral perfusion pressure may be one reason. Aggressive lowering of the blood pressure should therefore be avoided but normal arterial pressures should be obtained.

Hypoxemia

Saturation levels below 75% following a superior cavopulmonary anastomosis can be caused by many reasons all resulting in a reduction in pulmonary perfusion. This may be due to an obstruction in the area of the anastomosis or pulmonary vessels. Another possible explanation is that blood from the upper half of the body is conducted past the alveoli, for example, if there are venovenous collaterals (connections between the systemic and pulmonary veins), the azygos vein was not ligated by the surgeon, a left sided superior vena cava has reopened or arteriovenous collaterals (connections between the pulmonary arteries and veins) have gained importance.

In the early postoperative phase, arterial saturation can often be improved by attempting mild hypoventilation. Slightly elevated pCO_2 (>50 mmHg) causes vasodilatation of the cerebral vessels, so more blood flows to the brain. Since this allows relatively more blood to reach the upper half of the body, more blood is conducted through the SVC and into the lungs and becomes oxygenated. In addition, the blood can also be slightly alkalized by administering sodium bicarbonate (target pH >7.4).

Total cavopulmonary anastomosis (Fontan procedure)

In a Fontan procedure (total cavopulmonary anastomosis), the pulmonary and systemic circulation are finally completely separated by anastomosing the inferior vena cava also with the pulmonary circulation. A tunnel is created that connects the inferior vena cava with the pulmonary artery. This tunnel may pass either through the atrium (intracardiac Fontan) or alternatively outside the heart (extracardiac tunnel). It should be standard to leave a small shunt between the Fontan tunnel and the atrium (i.e., Fontan fenestration) that functions as an overflow (right-to-left shunt) if the resistance in the pulmonary circulation is too high and not all of the systemic venous blood can enter the pulmonary circulation. This may have the disadvantage of mild hypoxemia but the positive effects (improved systemic circulation, decompression of the venous side, less ascites, edema, etc.) clearly overweigh the disadvantage of lower saturations.

When the Fontan circulation is completed, all of the systemic venous blood (exception: coronary sinus) flows passively into the pulmonary circulation without passing through a pumping ventricle. The oxygenated blood is then pumped into the systemic circulation by the univentricular heart. Typical postoperative problems are low cardiac output, hypoxemia, effusions, arrhythmias and thrombosis.

Low cardiac output

In Fontan patients, low cardiac output can often occur due to low preload (hypovolemia), increased pulmonary resistance, or an obstruction in the area of the systemic venous outflow

Table 34.7: *Medications for pediatric resuscitation* and arrhythmias

Medication	*Dose*	*Remarks*
Adenosine	0.1 mg/kg (maximum 6 mg) Repeat: 0.2 mg/kg (maximum 12 mg)	Monitor ECG Rapid IV/IO bolus
Amiodarone	5 mg/kg IV/IO; repeat up to 15 mg/kg Maximum: 300 mg	Monitor ECG and blood pressure Adjust administration rate to urgency (give more slowly when perfusing rhythm present) Use caution when administering with other drugs that prolong QT (consider expert consultation)
Atropine	0.02 mg/kg IV/IO 0.03 mg/kg ET* Repeat once if needed Minimum dose: 0.1 mg Maximum single dose Child 0.5 mg Adolescent 1 mg	Higher doses may be used with organophosphate poisoning
Calcium chloride (10%)	20 mg/kg IV/IO (0.2 mL/kg)	Slowly
Epinephrine	0.01 mg/kg (0.1 mL/kg 1:10 000) IV/IO 0.1 mg/kg (0.1/kg 1:1000) ET* Maximum dose: 1 mg IV/IO; 10 mg ET	Adult dose: 5–10 mL
Glucose	0.5–1 g/kg IV/IO	D10W: 5–10 mL/kg D25W: 2–4 mL/kg D50W: 1–2 mL/kg
Lidocaine	Bolus: 1 mg/kg IV/IO Maximum dose: 100 mg Infusion: 20–50 1/4 g/kg per minute ET*: 2–3 mg	
Magnesium sulfate	25–50 mg/kg IV/IO over 10–20 min faster in torsades Maximum dose: 2 g	
Naloxone	< 5 y or 20 kg: 0.1 mg/kg IV/IO/ET* 5 y or > 20 kg: 2 mg IV/IO/ET*	Use lower doses to reverse respiratory depression associated with therapeutic opioid use (1–15 1/4 g/kg)
Procainamide	15 mg/kg IV/IO over 30–60 min Adult dose: 20 mg/min IV infusion upto total maximum dose 17 mg/kg	Monitor ECG and blood pressure Use caution when administering with other drugs that prolong QT (consider expert consultation)
Sodium bicarbonate	1 mEq/kg per dose IV/IO slowly	After adequate ventilation

†IV indicates intravenous; IO intraosseous; and ET, via endotracheal tube

Flush with 5 mL of normal saline and follow with 5 ventilations

(tunnel stenosis, anastomosis stenosis). Therefore, higher volume requirements are often necessary in these patients. In addition, poor ventricular function or AV valve insufficiency and arrhythmias can also cause low cardiac output.

Arrhythmias

As the completion of the Fontan procedure require surgical manipulation at the atrium and the area of the sinus node, atrial arrhythmias may occur and sinus node dysfunction is typical. A pacemaker (atrial stimulation) sometimes becomes necessary.

Hypoxemia

Cyanosis can be the result of a relevant right-to-left shunt across a tunnel fenestration. In addition, the usual pulmonary problems (i.e., pleural effusion, atelectasis, pneumonia) can also lead to hypoxemia. Reduced pulmonary perfusion, caused by arteriovenous or venovenous collaterals can also cause hypoxemia in Fontan patients.

Pleural effusions and ascites are common immediately after surgery. They can be the result of elevated venous pressure and volume load required and may lead to considerable postoperative complications

Thrombosis

Based on the low flow in the Fontan circuit, these patients are at an increased risk of developing venous thrombosis. This risk is increased especially if there is low cardiac output. Most centers therefore recommend lifelong anticoagulation for Fontan patients. There is, however, no uniform opinion with respect to the duration or the form of anticoagulation (vitamin K antagonists or platelet aggregation inhibitors). While many different anticoagulation regimens are used in small children (no anticoagulation, aspirin, warfarin), there is a general consensus that anti-coagulation is obligatory in patients after puberty.

Table 34.8 : *Medications for pediatric resuscitation* and arrhythmias

Medication	*Dose*	*Remarks*
Adenosine	0.1 mg/kg (maximum 6 mg) Repeat: 0.2 mg/kg (maximum 12 mg)	Monitor ECG Rapid IV/IO bolus
Amiodarone	5 mg/kg IV/IO; repeat up to 15 mg/kg Maximum: 300 mg	Monitor ECG and blood pressure Adjust administration rate to urgency (give more slowly when perfusing rhythm present) Use caution when administering with other drugs that prolong QT (consider expert consultation)
Atropine	0.02 mg/kg IV/IO 0.03 mg/kg ET* Repeat once if needed Minimum dose: 0.1 mg Maximum single dose Child 0.5 mg Adolescent 1 mg	Higher doses may be used with organophosphate poisoning
Calcium chloride (10%)	20 mg/kg IV/IO (0.2 mL/kg)	Slowly
Epinephrine	0.01 mg/kg (0.1 mL/kg 1:10 000) IV/IO 0.1 mg/kg (0.1/kg 1:1000) ET* Maximum dose: 1 mg IV/IO; 10 mg ET	Adult dose: 5–10 mL
Glucose	0.5–1 g/kg IV/IO	D10W: 5–10 mL/kg D25W: 2–4 mL/kg D50W: 1–2 mL/kg
Lidocaine	Bolus: 1 mg/kg IV/IO Maximum dose: 100 mg Infusion: 20–50 1/4 g/kg per minute ET*: 2–3 mg	
Magnesium sulfate	25–50 mg/kg IV/IO over 10–20 min faster in torsades Maximum dose: 2 g	
Naloxone	< 5 y or 20 kg: 0.1 mg/kg IV/IO/ET* 5 y or > 20 kg: 2 mg IV/IO/ET*	Use lower doses to reverse respiratory depression associated with therapeutic opioid use (1–15 1/4 g/kg)
Procainamide	15 mg/kg IV/IO over 30–60 min Adult dose: 20 mg/min IV infusion upto total maximum dose 17 mg/kg	Monitor ECG and blood pressure Use caution when administering with other drugs that prolong QT (consider expert consultation)
Sodium bicarbonate	1 mEq/kg per dose IV/IO slowly	After adequate ventilation

†IV indicates intravenous; IO intraosseous; and ET, via endotracheal tube
Flush with 5 mL of normal saline and follow with 5 ventilations

Table 34.9 *Medications to maintain cardiac output and for postresuscitation stabilization*

Medication	*Dose range*	*Comment*
Inamrinone	0.75–1 mg/kg IV/IO over 5 minutes; may repeat × 2 then: 2–20 µg/kg per minute	Inodilator
Dobutamine	2–20 mg/kg per minute IV/IO	Inotrope; vasodilator
Dopamine	2–20 mg/kg per minute IV/IO	Inotrope; chronotrope; renal and splanchnic vasodilator in low doses; pressor in high doses
Epinephrine	0.1–1 mg/kg per minute IV/IO	Inotrope; chronotrope; vasodilator in low doses; pressor in higher doses
Milrinone	50–75 µg/kg IV/IO over 10–60 min then 0.5–0.75 µg/kg per minute	Indilator
Norepinephrine	0.1–2 µg/kg per minute	Inotrope; vasopressor
Sodium nitroprusside	1–8 µg/kg per minute	Vasodilator; prepare only in D5W

IV indicates intravenous; and IO intraosseous
Alternative formula for calculating an infusion:
Infusion rate (mL/h) - [weight (kg) × dose (µg/kg/min) × 60 (min/h)]/concentration µg/mL

BIBLIOGRAPHY AND ACKNOWLEDGEMENT

- Kansy A, Tobota Z, Maruszewski P, Maruszewski B. Analysis of 14,843 neonatal congenital heart surgical procedures in the European Association for Cardiothoracic Surgery Congenital Database. Ann Thorac Surg. 2010; 89:1255-9.
- Allen HD, et al. Moss and Adams' heart disease in infants, children and adolescents including the fetus and young adult. Philadelphia: Lippincoẽ Williams & Wilkins; 2008.
- Bakshi KD, Vaidyanathan B, Sundaram KR, Roth SJ, Shivaprakasha K, Rao SG, et al. Determinants of early outcome after neonatal cardiac surgery in a developing country. J Thorac Cardiovasc Surg. 2007;134:765-71.
- Bove T, Francois K, De Groote K, Suys B, De Wolf D, Verhaaren H, et al. Outcome analysis of major cardiac operations in low weight neonates. Ann Thorac Surg. 2004; 78 :181-7.
- Brown KL, Ridout DA, Hoskote A, Verhulst L, Ricci M, Bull C. Delayed diagnosis of congenital heart disease worsens preoperative condition and outcome of surgery in neonates. Heart. 2006;92:1298-302.
- Chang AC, et al. Pediatric cardiac intensive care. Philadelphia: Lippincoẽ Williams & Wilkins; 1998.
- Choudhary SK, Bhan A, Sharma R, Mathur A, Airan B, Saxena A, et al. Repair of total anomalous pulmonary venous connection in infancy: experience from a developing country. Ann Thorac Surg. 1999;68:155-9.
- Cloherty JP, Eichenwald EC, Stark AR. Manual of neonatal care. Philadelphia: Lippincoẽ Williams & Wilkins; 2008.
- Culbert EL, Ashburn DA, Cullen-Dean G, Joseph JA, Williams WG, Blackstone EH, et al. Quality of life of children after repair of transposition of the great arteries. Circulation. 2003;108:857-62.
- Derrick G, Cullen S. Transposition of the great arteries. Curr Treat Options Cardiovasc Med 2000;2:499–506.
  Driscoll DJ. Fundamentals of pediatric cardiology. Philadelphia: Lippincoẽ Williams & Wilkins; 2006.
- Jacobs JP, Mavroudis C, Jacobs ML, Lacour-Gayet FG, hypoplastic left heart syndrome. Pediatrics 2007;119:109–117.
- Tchervenkov CI, William Gaynor J, et al. Lessons learned from the data analysis of the second harvest (1998-2001) of the Society of Thoracic Surgeons (STS) Congenital Heart Surgery Database. Eur J Cardiothorac Surg. 2004;26:18-37.
- Newburger JW, Spray TL, Moller JH, Iezzoni LI. Consensus-based method for risk adjustment for surgery for congenital heart disease. J Thorac Cardiovasc Surg. 2002;123:110-8.
- Kumar RK, Tynan MJ. Catheter interventions for congenital heart disease in third world countries. Pediatr Cardiol. 2005;26:241-9. Kumar RK. Delivering pediatric cardiac care with limited resources. Ann Pediatr Cardiol. 2014;7:163-6.
- Masse L, Antonacci M. Low cardiac output syndrome: Identification and management. Crit Care Nurs Clin North Am. 2005;17:375-83.
- Padley JR, Cole AD, Pye VE, Chard RB, Nicholson IA, Jacobe S, et al. Five-year analysis of operative mortality and neonatal outcomes in congenital heart disease. Heart Lung Circ. 2011;20 :460-7.
- Park MK. Pediatric cardiology for practitioners. Philadelphia: Mosby Elsevier; 2008.Pre and Postoperative Management of Pediatric Patients with Congenital Heart Diseases
- Reddy VM, McElhinney DB, Sagrado T, Parry AJ, Teitel DF, Hanley FL. Results of 102 cases of complete repair of congenital heart defects in patients weighing 700 to 2500 grams. J Thorac Cardiovasc Surg. 1999;117:324-31.
- Saxena A, Sharma M, Kothari SS, Juneja R, Reddy SC, Sharma R, et al. Prostaglandin E1 in infants with congenital heart disease: Indian experience. Indian Pediatr. 1998;35:1063-9.
- Shukla VV, Nimbalkar SM, Ganjiwale JD, John D. Direct cost of critical illness associated healthcare expenditures among children admitted in pediatric intensive care unit in rural India. Indian J Pediatr. 2016;83:1065-70

35 Prevention of Cardio-vascular Ailments with Yogic Asanas In Children

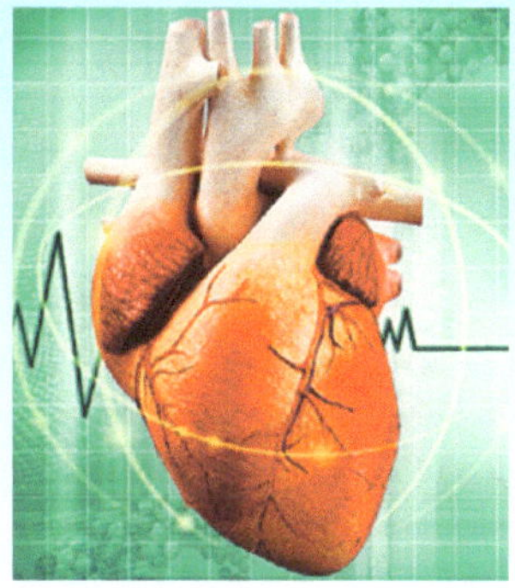

The American Academy of Pediatrics (AAP) recommends yoga as a safe and potentially effective therapy. It can help children and adolescents cope with emotional, mental, and physical conditions while improving behavioral health Yoga was born thousands of years ago in India. The word "yoga" means "to yoke" or unite the mind, body, and spirit Yoga typically focuses on three areas - physical postures (asanas), breathing techniques (pranayama), and meditation (dhyana). There are many different types of yoga, among which Hatha yoga, Iyengar Yoga, Bikram Yoga, and Vinyasa yoga are more popular

What Science Says About Yoga for Kids ?

Studies have been done to see the effect that yoga has on children. The practice has been proven to increase focus and decrease anxiety when it comes to schoolwork and studying. It has also been found to promote mindfulness for kids who do yoga regularly. These studies have also shown that practicing yoga is associated with decreased violence in schools by providing a way for kids to release pent-up energy, stress, and anger.Yoga is a powerful tool for children and teenagers to have as they face the stresses of school, social drama, and peer pressure, among other challenges.

Yoga involves practicing balance and giving heavy sensory input. This is why it is a great tool for kids who have sensory processing disorders. The sensory benefits of yoga, in particular, make it useful for children on the autism spectrum.There are many advantages to beginning a yoga practice at an early age. It provides a strong foundation for a child to have as they grow up.

- Yoga is known for improving flexibility and balance. But did you know that yoga can also boost cardiovascular health?

- Yoga is an ancient practice that involves holding and moving through a series of postures or poses. It focuses on flexibility and strength-building and can also include meditation and breathing exercises to help calm the mind.

- The poses and stretches performed in yoga can also reduce chronic pain. Many of the postures are weight-bearing postures, which help strengthen bones and muscles. Yoga for cardiovascular health includes simple poses to promote flexibility, stress relief, and relaxation.

- Yoga also improves heart health by increasing circulation and blood flow. In addition, practicing yoga can help lower blood pressure, cholesterol, and blood glucose levels, as well as the heart rate — which can all add up to a lower risk of hypertension, stroke, and heart disease.

Children of the Age Group of 3-10 Years

Children less than 10 years of age can do upto 10 seconds staying in the final stage of any asana / Yoga practice. The total time for the kid's Yoga session should be not more than 20 minutes. Children are advised not to perform asana for long duration and breathe holding practices (Kumbhaka). Yoga for children involves gentle Yoga stretches and movements, often mimicking animals, and incorporated with games. Imaginative stories about Yoga practices are the best methods of teaching Yoga to kids. Always demonstrate the posture, rather than explaining it. Use the same method when trying to correct their poses, during practical sessions.

- Avoid extreme forward and backward bending asanas.
- Avoid head stand and hand standing asanas.
- Avoid over stretching or pushing too hard while practicing Yoga.
- Yogic practice should be done in an empty or light stomach.
- Children should practice Yoga under the supervision of an expert/ trained Yoga teacher with proper guidance and never alone.
- If child complains of any discomfort while or after practicing Yoga, he / she should be given full attention and medical help, if needed

• Never compare the children with each other. Encourage them in each and every session for discipline to sit properly.
• It's always appreciated to teach Yoga with affection and deal all their reactions tenderly.
• Basic principles of Yoga like Yama and Niyama should be emphasized while teaching Yoga practices to get better results.

Adolescents upto the Age of 18 Years

- There should not be any competitive attitude while practicing Yoga.
- Girls should avoid Yoga practices during menstruation or they can do relaxing practices.
- The practice sequence of asanas should be initial to advance in order, followed by Pranayama, Bandhas, Mudras, Relaxation and Meditation
- Asanas should not be practiced in haste or by applying any sort of undue force under any circumstances.
- Attain the final position step by step and maintain the same with closed eyes for an inward awareness within the whole body.
- Maintenance of the final posture in asana is always beneficial as per one's capacity.
- Yogic practice should be done on an empty stomach or light stomach.
- It is the period of changing from childhood to adulthood, which needs practice of the posture done with more time and awareness.
- Adolescent ages usually have a negative body image due to bodily / hormonal changes and teaching with all such considerations and encouraging them, is needed.
- Physical movements from one posture to another provide strength, endurance, flexibility to joints a nd muscles of the growing adolescents and facilitate positive health.
- Explain what they are doing by telling teens about each practice and how the practice will be beneficial for them. Create conducive atmosphere for them so that they can share their experiences without any hesitation

Easy Yoga Poses and Their Health Benefits

Children, in particular, can greatly benefit from a regular yoga practice for many reasons. These benefits include but are not limited to:

1. Sensory input
2. Balance
3. Release of excess energy
4. Helping with anxiety/depression
5. Better sleep
6. Focus
7. Relaxation
8. Stress reduction
9. Better alignment of the body/posture
10. Increased strength

Due to the many ways children can benefit from a regular yoga practice, some schools have begun to integrate yoga into their curriculum, programs, and philosophies. However, this change has only been made in a fraction of schools worldwide, and a lot of kids do not receive the opportunity to do and learn about yoga.Yoga can be done outside of school as well, and children can also practice at home with family. Doing yoga with parents is a great bonding experience for everyone involved and also gives kids some often needed one-on-one time.For kids, yoga is very different from what it is for adults. While many are used to a quiet, calming, hour-long class, children cannot sit still for very long. Yoga can be done through storytelling, singing songs, dancing, playing games, and even while watching yoga on TV.There are many amazing yoga poses for children to do, and each kid is different. Therefore, some poses may benefit one child more than the others depending on the individual need.

Here is a list of 10 easy great yoga poses for kids to do:

1. Easy sitting pose (Sukhasana)
2. Child's pose (Balasana)
3. Half-lotus pose (Ardha Padmasana)
4. Cobra pose (Bhujangasana)
5. Wide-angle seated forward bend (Upavistha Konasana)
6. Seated forward fold (Paschimottanasana)
7. Butterfly pose (Baddha Konasana)
8. Tree pose (Vrksasana)
9. Warrior I (Virabhadrasana I)
10. Corpse pose (Savasana)

Others (see below)

35.1. Easy sitting pose (Sukhasana)

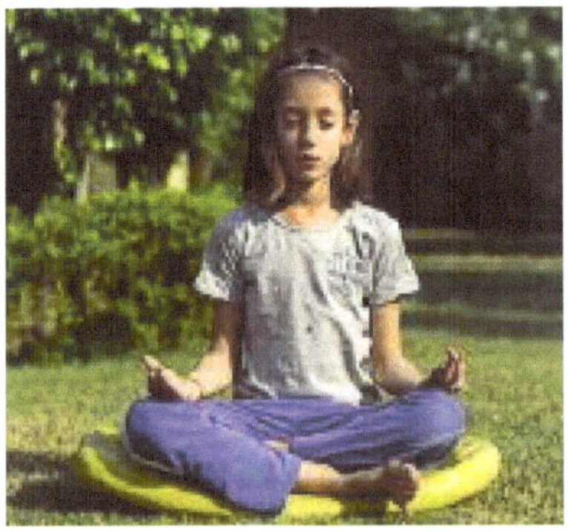

The easy sitting pose is one of the easier poses to do, hence the name. It involves sitting up straight with the legs crossed; many kids know this as the "crisscross applesauce.

How to do this pose:

1. Sit on the ground with the back nice and tall.
2. Cross the legs, bringing the knees toward the ground.
3. The hands can be on the knees facing up, or they can be together at heart center.
4. This pose can be held for multiple breaths or when meditating.

Benefits :

- Promoting relaxation
- Increasing focus
- Correcting posture
- Strengthening the muscles in the back
- Increasing flexibility in the hips and legs
- Decreasing stress

This pose can be practiced while taking deep, calming breaths or while focusing on a specific thought or image.

35.2 Child's pose (Balasana)

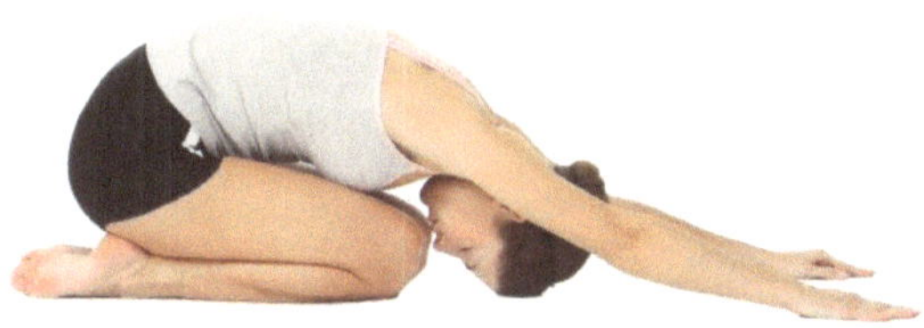

The child's pose is another simple pose to do, and it involves sitting back on the heels and folding forward, bringing the arms out in front of the body, and resting the forehead on the ground. By curling up like this, one can feel held

How to do this pose:

- Start on the hands and knees.
- Press the hips back toward the heels.
- The arms can be stretched out in front of the body or curled down by the sides.

Benefits

- Promoting relaxation
- Reducing stress
- Grounding oneself
- Calming oneself
- Increasing flexibility and strength in the ankles, legs, and hips
- Releasing tension from the body (specifically the upper body)

This pose mimics what it feels like to be in the womb. Therefore, for a child, this pose is incredibly comforting and grounding. This pose is also helpful in settling down a child when they are overwhelmed, upset, or hyper, but it can also be used just for relaxing in general.

35.3 Half-lotus pose (Ardha padmasana)

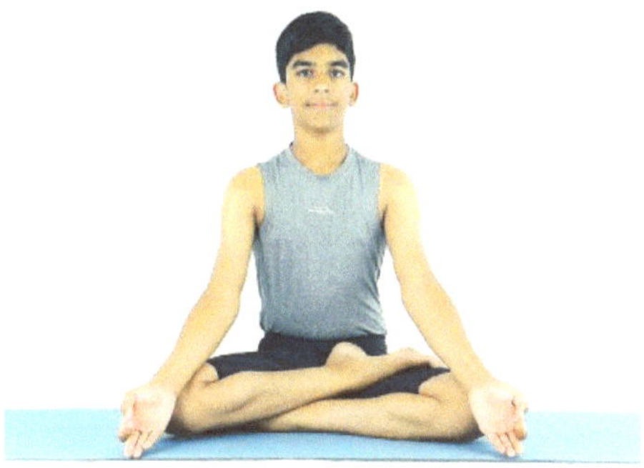

How to do this pose:

- Sit down on the ground.
- Fold the legs in front of the body.
- Bring one leg on top of the other, flexing the feet.
- Do the same on the other side.
- Benefits of this pose include but are not limited to:
- Promoting relaxation
- Grounding oneself
- Increasing creativity
- Strengthening awareness
- Increasing flexibility in the hips and legs
- Correcting posture
- Releasing tension from the body (specifically the upper body)

Benefits :

Half Lotus stretches the muscles around the pelvis, legs, and ankles. It helps you maintain flexibility in your gluteal muscles and the deep rotator muscles of your hips. It can help stretch the piriformis, which is useful if you have symptoms of sciatica. Your piriformis can tighten from being inactive (sitting too much) or due to running and other vigorous activity. Half Lotus helps promote good posture. It is a calming pose for your mind and is restorative.

35.4 Cobra pose (Bhujangasana)

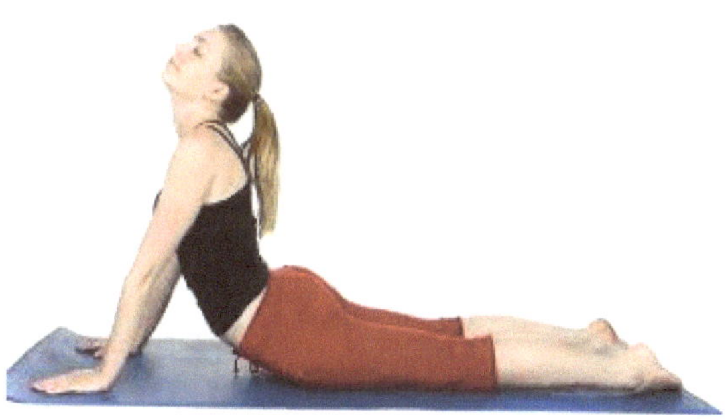

The cobra pose is a very fun pose that includes laying on the belly, bringing the hands flat to the ground beneath the shoulders, and straightening the arms just enough to lift the chest up. When doing this pose, one should make sure to only press up as far as one can go using the muscles in the back. This prevents overextending and keeps the body safe.

How to do this pose:

- Start on the belly.
- Bring the hands flat to the ground under the shoulders.
- Using the back muscles and the core, lift up.
- Hold the pose for a few breaths.

Benefits of this pose include but are not limited to:

- Increasing positivity
- Decreasing stress
- Strengthening the muscles in the chest, arms, and back, and abdomen
- Increasing creativity
- Strengthening awareness
- Correcting posture
- Reducing fatigue
- Promoting proper circulation

A fun way to do this pose is for one to lie on the ground with the hands flat, take a deep breath in, and then press up into the cobra pose while hissing like a snake. This is a very fun way for kids to practice this exercise, and it usually ends with lots of giggles.

35.5 Wide-angle seated forward bend (Upavistha konasana)

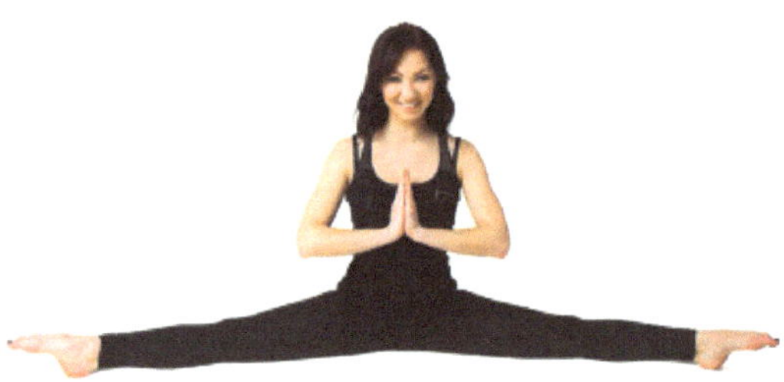

How to do this pose:

- Sit on the ground with the legs out to the sides and the feet flexed (to protect the hamstrings).
- Bring the arms up.
- Fold over the legs as far as comfortable.
- Hold for a few breaths

Benefits of this pose include but are not limited to:

- Strengthening muscles in the core and spine
- Increasing flexibility in the legs and hips
- Correcting posture
- Improving digestion
- Decreasing frequency of belly aches
- Promoting relaxation

Another fun way to perform this wide-angle seated forward bend is as a team. To do this stretch, two people can face each other, bringing the feet out to the side and touching them together. Both people can then join hands and carefully take turns pulling each other deeper into the pose. As one person leans forwards, the other leans back.

35.6 Seated forward fold (Paschimottanasana)

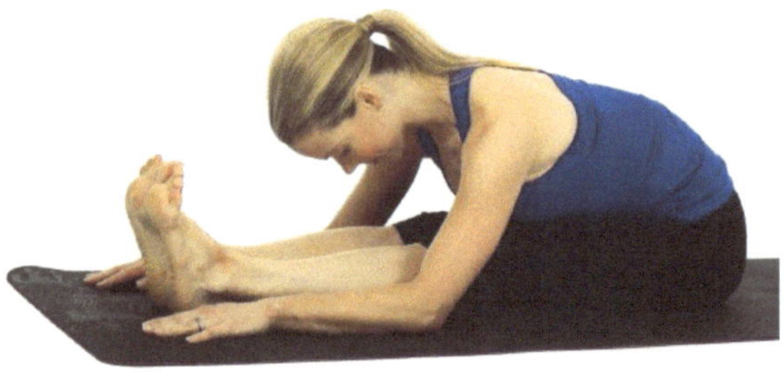

How to do this pose:

- Bring the legs out in front of the body, flexing the feet.
- Bring the arms up.
- Fold forward as far as comfortable.
- If the feet cannot be reached, reach for the legs.
- Hold for a few breaths.

Benefits of this pose

- Promoting relaxation
- Decreasing stress
- Improving digestion
- Decreasing frequency of belly aches
- Decreasing anxiety
- Relieving headaches
- Reducing fatigue

The seated forward fold is similar to the wide-angle seated forward bend. The difference, however, is that instead of having the legs out to the sides, the legs are out in front of the body, creating a much different stretch

35.7 Butterfly pose (Baddha konasana)

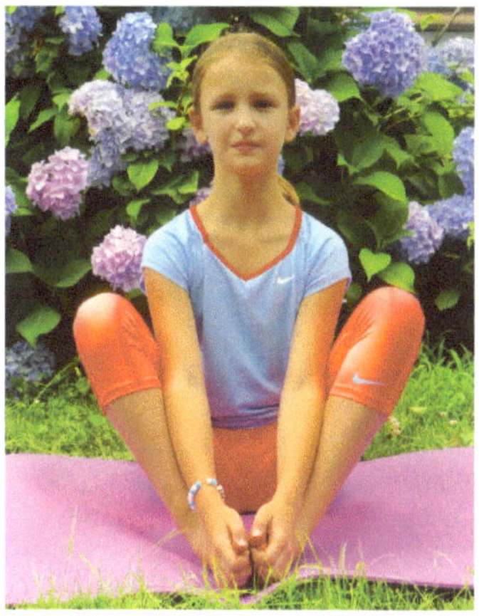

How to do this pose:

- Sit on the ground with the feet together and the knees out to the sides.
- This pose can be held while flapping the legs like butterflies or while breathing deeply.
- Hold for a few breaths.

Benefits

- Promoting creativity
- Strengthening the muscles in the legs and abdomen
- Improving digestion
- Decreasing anxiety
- Calming oneself
- Relieving headaches
- Reducing fatigue
- Grounding oneself

The butterfly pose is very popular with kids. It allows for super fun bonding experiences, especially between parents and their kids. By sitting with the feet flat together and the knees out to the side, the child can flap their knees up and down like wings and tell a story or imagine flying.

35.8 Tree pose (Vrksasana)

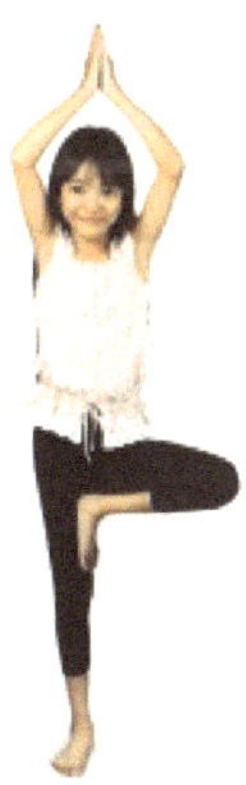

The tree pose is often a favorite among children. While challenging, the pose has many variations, making it accessible for people of all ages and abilities

How to do this pose:

- Shift the weight into one foot and bring the other foot to the ankle, shin, or thigh.
- Bring the arms up or the hands together at the chest.
- Focus on an unmoving spot or object.
- Hold for a few breaths.
- Do the same to the other side.

Benefits

- Promoting creativity
- Strengthening the muscles in the legs, hips, glutes, and core
- Promoting balance
- Providing sensory input
- Correcting posture

Kids love to turn this pose into a competition to see who can hold it the longest. A fun way of practicing the tree pose is to imagine roots coming down from the feet in the ground and to lift the arms to create "branches."

35.9 Warrior pose I (Virabhadrasana I)

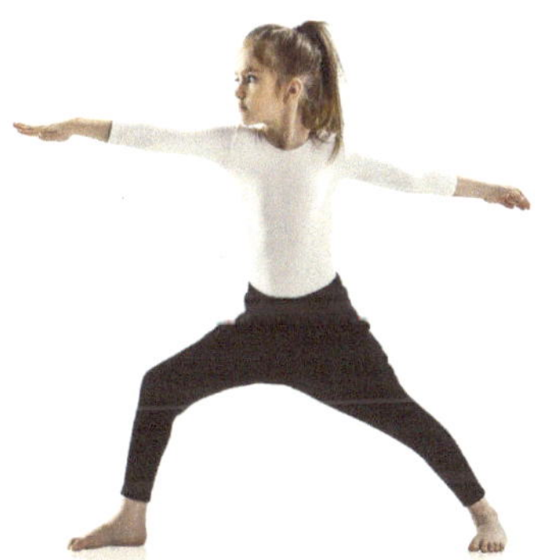

How to do this pose:

- Step into a high lunge, bending the front leg at a 90° angle.
- Bring the back foot flat to the ground at a 45° angle.
- Bring the arms up to the sky, keeping the hips squared.
- Hold for a few breaths.

Benefits

- Strengthening the muscles in the legs, hips, chest, arms, and back
- Promoting balance
- Providing sensory input
- Correcting posture

- Increasing circulation
- Increasing focus
- Decreasing stress
- Reducing anxiety
- Promoting calmness and meditation

While all of the warrior poses are fun to practice, warrior I in particular emphasizes balance, strength, and focus. Therefore, it is a great pose to do with kids.

35.10 Corpse pose (Savasana)

The corpse pose is a very simple pose to do and just involves lying flat on the ground with the arms by the sides and the legs straight out in front of the body. This is usually when one meditates during a yoga practice

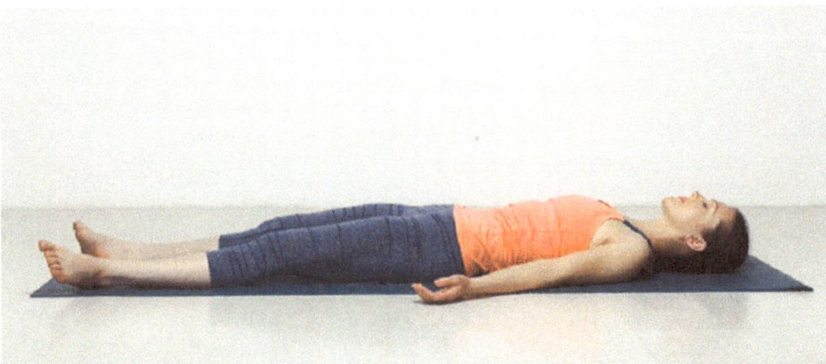

How to do this pose:

- Lie on the ground with the arms by the sides and the legs out in front of the body
- Hold this pose during meditation or deep breathing exercises

Benefits

- Promoting creativity
- Decreasing anxiety
- Promoting relaxation
- Calming oneself
- Grounding oneself
- Increasing focus

There are lots of online meditations for kids, but they can also create their own by thinking of a fun or happy place and focusing on everything that is seen there.

35.11. Bridge Pose (Setu Bandha Sarvangasana)

This rejuvenating backbend gives a good stretch to the spine and thighs.

How to do this pose:

- Lie on the back.
- Bend the knees a little and keep the feet flat on the floor, hip-width apart.
- The knees and ankles must be in a straight line.

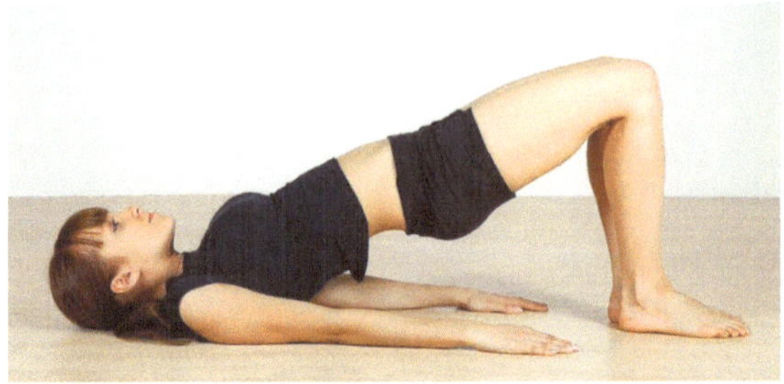

- Place the arms in a resting position beside the body, with the palms downwards.
- Take a deep breath and lift the lower, middle, and upper back off the floor.
- Balance the body in a way that the arms, shoulders, and feet support the body weight.
- Keep the buttocks tight.
- Have the fingers interlaced, and hands pushed to the ground to help lift the torso higher.
- Let your child hold this posture for as long as they are comfortable and breathe slowly while they are in thepose.
- Exhale and release.

Benefits of this pose

Stretches and opens the shoulders, thighs, hips, and chest portion; strengthens the back and hamstrings; increases the flexibility of the spine

Caution

: If your kid faces difficulty in making the pelvis lift from the floor, slide a sturdy bolster under their sacrum to rest their pelvis. In case of any neck or shoulder pain, take assistance from a professional to hone the steps.

35.12 Bow Pose (Dhanurasana)

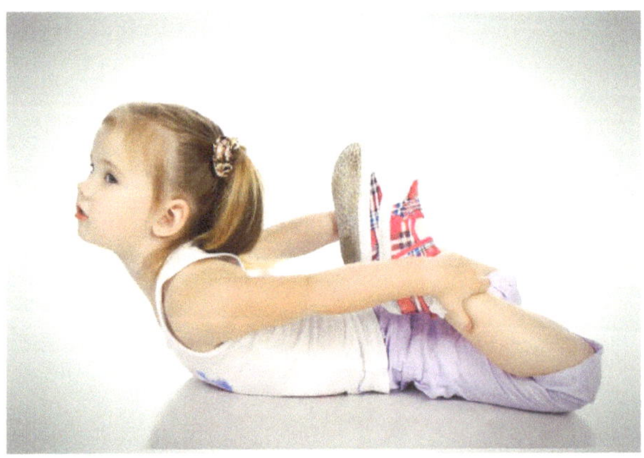

This rejuvenating backbend gives a good stretch to the spine and thighs.

How to do this pose:

- Lie on the back.
- Bend the knees a little and keep the feet flat on the floor, hip-width apart.
- The knees and ankles must be in a straight line.
- Place the arms in a resting position beside the body, with the palms downwards.
- Take a deep breath and lift the lower, middle, and upper back off the floor.
- Balance the body in a way that the arms, shoulders, and f eet support the body weight.
- Keep the buttocks tight.
- Have the fingers interlaced, and hands pushed to the ground to help lift the torso higher.
- Let your child hold this posture for as long as they are comfortable and breathe slowly while they are in the pose.
- Exhale and release.

Benefits of this pose

Stretches and opens the shoulders, thighs, hips, and chest portion; strengthens the back and hamstrings; increases the flexibility of the spine

Caution

If your kid faces difficulty in making the pelvis lift from the floor, slide a sturdy bolster under their sacrum to rest their pelvis. In case of any neck or shoulder pain, take assistance from a professional to hone the steps

35.13 Boat Pose (Naukasana)

This balancing yoga pose might help kids to de-stress and revitalize.

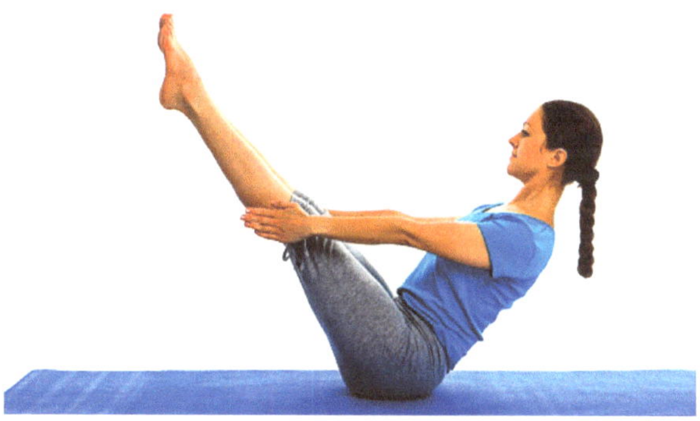

How to do this pose:

- Lie down flat with feet aligned together and arms on the sides.
- Keep the arms and fingers outstretched in the direction of the toes.
- Inhale and while exhaling, lift the chest and feet off the ground, to form a 'V' shape.
- This will build tension and stretch in the core.
- The weight of the body will solely rest on the hips.
- The eyes, hands, and toes should align straight.
- Hold the breath and retain the posture for a few seconds.
- Exhale slowly while bringing the body down to the neutral position. And relax.

Benefits of this pose

Strengthens the core, arm muscles, shoulders, and thighs; it is great for the liver and kidneys; helps reduce constipation and alleviates digestive problems.

Caution

: If your kid suffers from any chronic disease or spinal cord problems, avoid the pose.

35.14 Lion Pose (Simhasana)

Might help your child de-stress with this animal asana; have them roar and enjoy.

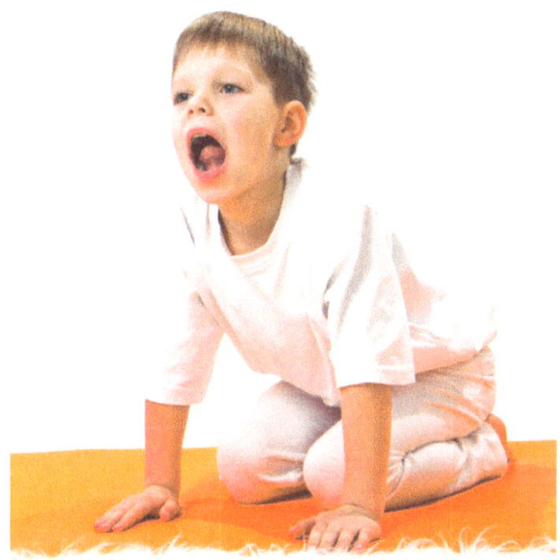

How to do this pose:

- Sit with the hips on the heels.
- Rest the palms on the knees.
- Start inhaling from the nose, and while you're on it, stick your tongue out.
- Keep the eyes wide open, exhale through the mouth, and make a sound of a roaring lion (Haaa).
- Many yoga schools suggest that you either concentrate looking at the tip of the nose or in the middle of the eyebrows.

Benefits of this pose

A great yoga stretch for the lungs, throat, and the respiratory tract; regulates the functioning of the tonsils and the immune system; reduces stress, anger, and anxiety; suitable for a hyperactive child.

Caution

Do not repeat this for more than five times.

A daily routine of yoga activity will make your child more disciplined and focused on their activity and gives them the strength to face stress. Start with one or two yoga poses to practice initially, and then you can have them try more as they get used to the practice.

35.15 Mountain Pose (Tadasana

This is a foundational pose for all the standing asanas and could be a calm-down yoga pose for children.

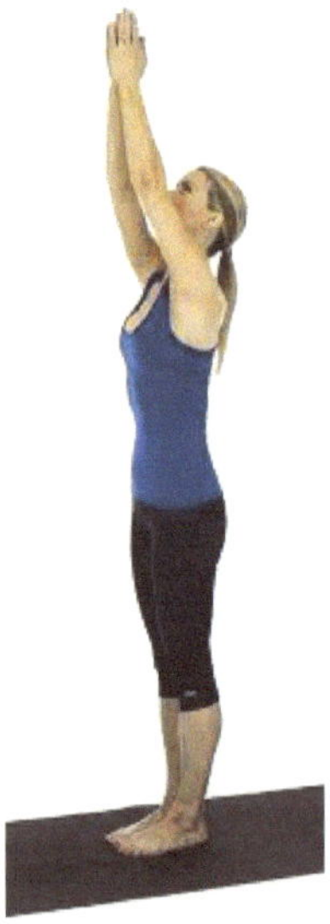

How to do this pose:

- Stand straight and tall.
- Spread the legs a few inches apart and spread the toes.
- Keep the arms alongside the body.
- The shoulders must be relaxed and not stiff.
- Raise the arms above your head.
- Hold the posture and breathe slowly.
- Retain as long as comfortable.

Benefits of this pose

Improves posture, strengthens the thighs, legs, and ankles; firms the abdomen and hips; improves sleep

Caution

: No cautions to follow up.

35.16 Nadi Sodhana Pranayama For Kids and Youngs

'Prana' is the Sanskrit name for 'energy'. 'Paranayama' refers to yogic breathing.Yogic breathing is when you are breathing in through the nose and out through the nose.When you are doing any other exercise you are normally encouraged to breathe in through the nose and out through the mouth. Yogis breathe in through the nose and out through the nose when practicing asanas.For example, when you are sitting in padmasana you should try to breathe in this way taking very long in breaths and out breaths through the nose.There are many different types of pranayama or breathingtechniques SodhanaPranayama **Nadi Sodhana Pranayama** is known as alternate nostril breathing:A 'nadi' is a tubular organ of the body like an artery providing a passage for the flow of prana or energy. Sodhana means to purify or cleanse so the object of Nadi Sodhana Pranayama is to purify the nerves

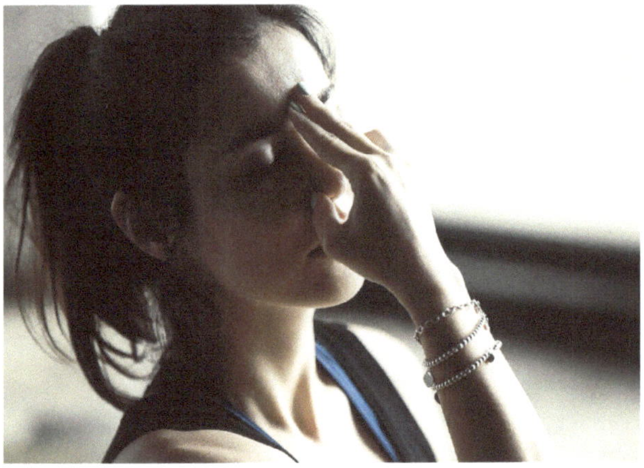

How to do this pose:

Sit in a comfortable position like padmasana
Stretch the left arm. Rest the back of the left wrist on the left knee.
Perform Jnana Mudra with the left hand.
Bend the right arm at the elbow. Bend the index and middle fingers towards the palm, keeping them passive.
Bring the ring and little fingers towards the thumb.
Place the right thumb on the right side of the nose just below the nasal bone, the ring and little fingers on the left side of the nose just before the nasal bone.
Press the ring and little finger to block the left side of the nose completely, empty the nose completely with the right nostril.
Inhale slowly, steadily and deeply through the right nostril fill the lungs to the brim. During this inhalation the left nostril is completely blocked by the ring and little fingers.
After full inhalation, block the right nostril completely with the pressure of the thumb and release the pressure of the ring and little fingers on the left nostril. Exhale slowly, steadily and deeply through the left nostril.
Empty the lungs completely.
Inhale through the left nostril slowly, steadily and deeply filling the lungs to the brim.
After full inhalation through the left nostril, block it and exhale through the right nostril adjusting the pressure of the right thumb on the right nostril.

Benefits of Nadi Sodhana Pranayama

The benefit of nadi shodhana pranayama is that the blood in our bodies receives a larger supply of oxygen that normal breathing. You feel refreshed, your mind becomes still and your nerves are clamed and purified. This pranayama is especially beneficial for those suffering from high / low blood pressure. Once you have mastered this pranayama technique, the next step is to lengthen each inhalation and exhalation and retain the breath between changing nostrils.

35.17 Frog Pose (Mandukasana) for Kids

The word Mandukasana has been derived from the Sanskrit word. It consists of two words manduk and asana. The meaning of 'manduk' is Frog and 'asana' is showing a yoga posture. In the final stage, the asana seems to like a frog, hence the name. It is one of the important sitting yoga poses to give appropriate massage to the abdominal organs. It is helpful to make your stomach flat by burning the extra fats from the belly.

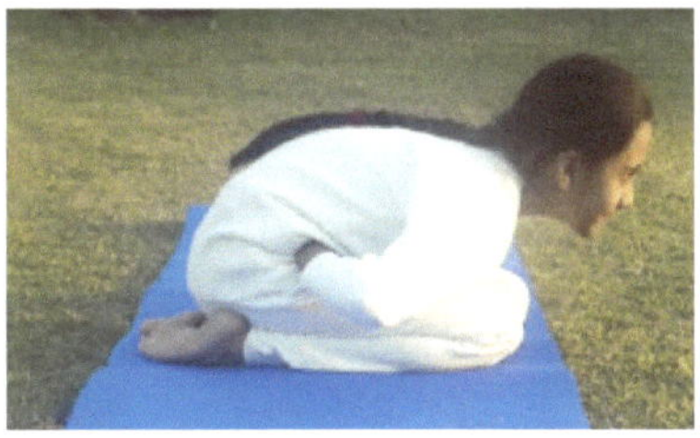

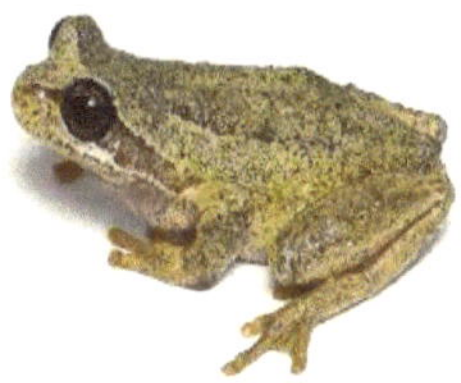

How to do this pose:

The simple steps to do Mandukasna are given below. By following this technique, one can perform Mandukasna even oneself.

- Sit in Vajrasana.
- Now, make fists where thumbs should be inside.
- Put the fists at the naval region.
- Inhale deeply.
- Exhale bend forward and put maximum pressure on the naval area.
- While bending forward, your chest should touch your thigh and look ahead with open eyes just like a frog.
- Maintain the pose as long as you can do.
- Inhale-exhale slowing while maintaining the pose.
- Come to Vajrasana with a deep inhale.
- Perform it 3 to 5 times.

Benefits of this pose

- It massages the entire abdominal organs. Thus, good for the smooth functioning of these organs.
- It controls weight. Thus effective for those who are longing for weight loss and making the stomach flat.
- It is beneficial in the case of constipation and indigestion.
- It is helpful to release unwanted gases from the stomach thus making you feel relaxed and calm.
- It helps to control diabetes by stimulating the pancreas.
- Dislocated naval can be corrected by performing this asana.
- It should be practiced by those who have asthmatic conditions.
- It strengthens the back if practice technically right.

Generalized precautions before starting pranayama.

Below are few generalized precautions before starting pranayma.

- If you have any chronic medical condition, seek advice from your doctor.
- Always breathe through the nose unless specifically asked to do so.
- There should not be any strain during pranayama practice. Lungs are delicate organ; ensure that your breathing is not beyond limits.
- Do not make loud sounds during breathing. Keep the breath rhythmic and steady.
- Pranayama should not be practiced immediately after meals. You can do pranayama at least three hours after meals.
- Beginners should not hold breath. When you become comfortable with basics of pranayama, learn to hold breath under the guidance of an expert teacher.
- If you feel tired or discomfort, stop doing pranayama, lie down in shavasana while carrying out normal breathing. Consult your yoga teacher.
- Do not practice pranayama if you are too tired, relax for 10-15 minutes in shavasana before doing pranayama.
- If you do yoga asanas and pranayama, practice yoga asanas before pranayama. After practicing asanas, relax in shavasana
  before doing pranayama. Do not do any strenuous exercise after pranayama.
- Pranayama should not be practiced in a hurry.
- Do pranayama outdoors or in a well ventilated room.
- Pranayama should not be practiced when the lungs are congested.

BIBLIOGRAPHY AND ACKNOWLEDGEMENT

- Folleto JC, Pereira KR, Valentini NC. The effects of yoga practice in school physical education on children's motor abilities and social behavior. International journal of yoga. https://www.ncbi.nlm.nih.gov/pmc/articles/PMC4959326/. Published 2016.
- Kaley-Isley LC, Peterson J, Fischer C, Peterson E. Yoga as a complementary therapy for children and adolescents: a guide for clinicians. Psychiatry (Edgmont (Pa. : Township)). https://www.ncbi.nlm.nih.gov/pmc/articles/PMC2945853/. Published August 2010.
- Woodyard C. Exploring the therapeutic effects of yoga and its ability to increase quality of life. International journal of yoga. https://www.ncbi.nlm.nih.gov/pmc/articles/PMC3193654/. Published July 2011.
- Stephens I. Medical Yoga Therapy. Children (Basel, Switzerland). https://www.ncbi.nlm.nih.gov/pmc/articles/PMC5332914/. Published February 10, 2017.
- Kanchibhotla D, Kulkarni S, Singh S. Effectiveness of a Comprehensive Yoga Program on Convicted Extremist Offenders. International journal of yoga. https://www.ncbi.nlm.nih.gov/pmc/articles/PMC6937884/. Published 2020.

36

Artificial Intelligence in Pediatric Cardiology. A Review

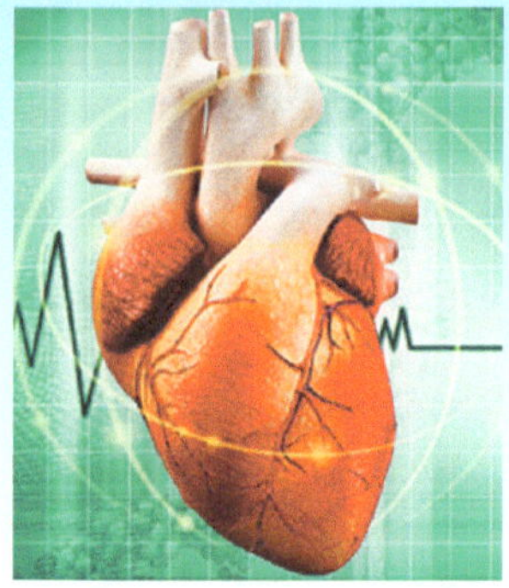

The discipline of pediatric cardiology has evolved as a specialty over the past 60 years, deriving its roots from attempts to treat congenital heart diseases .Congenital heart diseases (CHD), in the wake of the burden of mortality and morbidity they bring in, have always been an issue of concern. A total of 3.12 million babies in the United States were born with congenital heart disease, and around 13.3 million individuals are living with congenital heart anomalies . CHD has a multifactorial etiology that consists of environmental stressors and genetic factors and accounts for 80% of all forms of CHD . Pediatric heart diseases remain a global burden on health services and are associated with lifelong comorbidities that carry into adulthood, ultimately decreasing the quality of life for children . The last decade has seen the increasing prevalence of hypertension and other 'adult' heart diseases among the pediatric population, especially adolescents, which has counterpoised the falling burden of rheumatic heart disease in the same age group. Advancements in pediatric cardiology care and surgical technology have helped with significant reductions in mortality . However, while high-income countries saw the mortality rates of CHD reduce by half, the needs for surgical care and advanced imaging for pediatric patients are unmet in middle- and lower-income countries .The absence of a timely diagnosis for suspected pediatric heart diseases significantly delays timely treatment and often presents a diagnostic dilemma. The clinically suspected diagnosis of CHD is confirmed by echocardiography, which can even be conducted during pre- and postnatal screening . The diagnosis thus requires adequate clinical suspicion, health infrastructure, and a skilled workforce .The growth of artificial intelligence (AI) in the context of medicine has contributed immensely to the streamlining of clinical processes and decision making in health care since 1960 . The concept of machine learning (ML) is integral to the evolution of AI. ML is defined as the ability of machines to learn tasks from a large amount of previous data and be able to predict the same for future instances . As a result, AI has multiple key applications in the diagnosis, surveillance, prevention, and intervention of congenital heart diseases and has created major advancements in pediatric cardiology as a specialty . Due to its widespread ability to improve the diagnostic value of cardiac magnetic resonance imaging (MRI), echocardiograms (ECHO), computer tomography (CT) scans, and electrocardiographs (ECG), AI can augment the diagnostic accuracy of pediatric heart diseases .

While AI has already found its applications in a multitude of specialties, the notion of its use in almost any medical specialty is conceivable. CHD is an interesting area where AI can be applied owing to the burden of CHDs in pediatric and adult populations. AI-based algorithms have expanded their application in various domains of pediatric cardiology including but not limited to screening, clinical examination, diagnosis, image processing, prognosis, risk stratification, and precision medicine . Surprisingly, the full extent of AI applications in all stages of care for patients with congenital heart diseases has not yet been discussed. Evolving literature has pinpointed the efficiency of machine-learning algorithms in the interpretation of heart murmurs, a common sign of congenital heart diseases .The recent utilization of deep-learning computer networks has demonstrated the ability to perform MRI segmentation, allowing clinicians to detect valvular defects simultaneously in all four of the heart's chambers .Based on our knowledge, there is only one systematic analysis of a case series of atrial septal defect repair with robotic assistance and AI; the full extent of AI applications in all stages of care for patients with CHD has not yet been discussed. The objective of this systematic review is to compile all existing literature on AI applications in the specialty of pediatric cardiology with a focus on CHD. The review will attempt to appraise the evolving literature and compile clinically relevant data that can serve as a source of health information for clinicians.

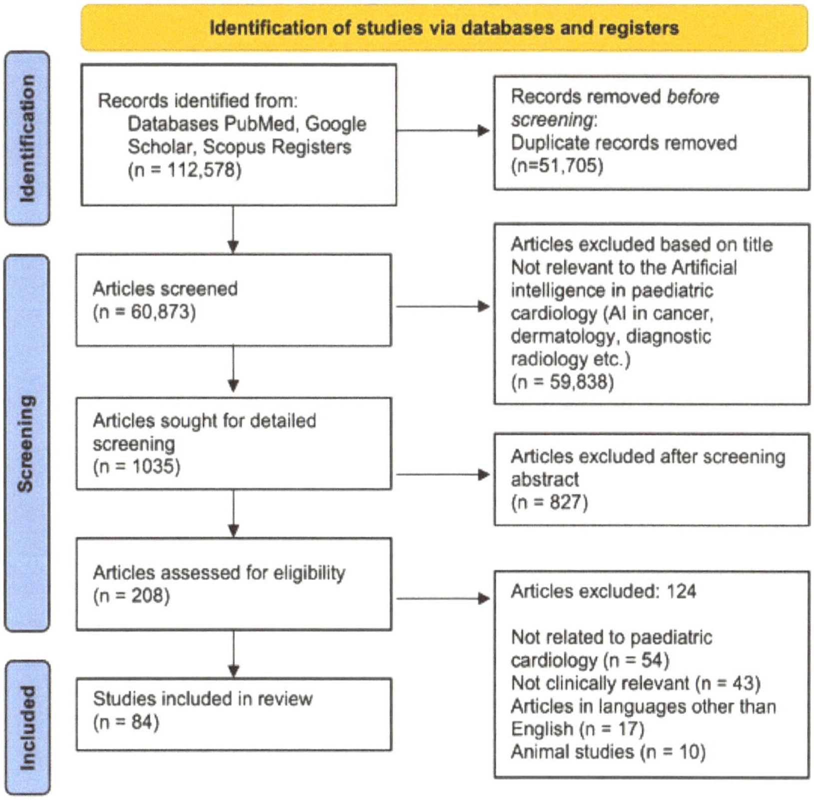

Fig. 36.1 Flow diagram showing selection process of studies included

AI and Murmurs

AI has the potential to improve the validity of auscultatory findings for diagnosing CHD .The limitations of objective performance data have restricted wide acceptability so far . The auscultatory findings of CHD are integral to the clinical diagnosis and have the benefit of being a low-cost tool, but are subject to clinical expertise, which becomes a limitation in resource-limited countries and creates a need for support to the clinician that is objective and reportable by even peripheral health workers. The lack of trained cardiologists at the peripheral level leads to an unavoidable miss of a timely clinical diagnosis of CHD, contributing to delayed intervention and thus a poor prognosis .The emergence of AI-based digital stethoscopes and cloud reporting for telemedicine has helped with the timely diagnosis and early intervention of CHD in reported samples . The AI-based technologies also seem affordable, helping the current interest. The use of an intelligent diagnostic system based on AI algorithms such as wavelet analysis and artificial neural networks has shown a specificity of 70.5% and a sensitivity of 64.7% . The developments in AI for detecting cardiac murmurs have shown promise in terms of sensitivity but still require clinical validation before wide clinical recommendation

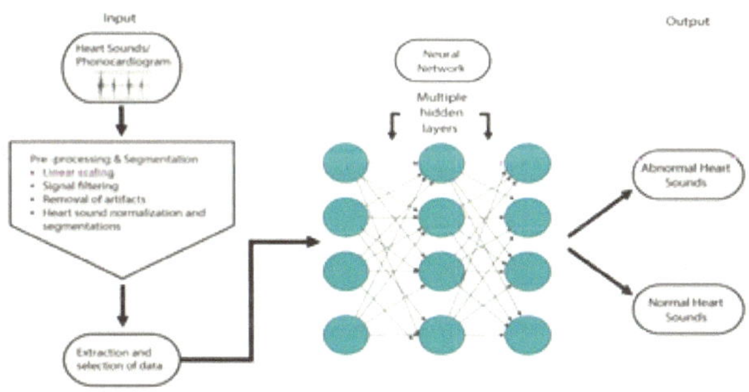

Fig.36.2 A model of application of neural networks in pediatric cardiology.

Image Processing with AI

Chest x-ray

CHDs present with some classical chest x-ray signs that can help with suspicion of the disease, including boot-shaped heart (Tetralogy of Fallot), egg-on-string (Transposition of Great Arteries), snowman sign (Total Anomalous Pulmonary Venous Return), scimitar sign (Partial Anomalous Pulmonary Venous Return), gooseneck sign (Endocardial cushion defects), a figure of three (Coarctation of Aorta) and box-shaped heart (Ebstein anomaly) .Chest radiography being easy, cost-effective, and readily available allows a direct or collaborative diagnostic approach to CHD. The evolution of deep learning models and machine learning models and the establishment of defined pediatric datasets have allowed the entry of AI for use in the pediatric population . AI can be immensely beneficial in various steps of imaging such as ordering tests, reporting communication, enhancing the quality of images, and aiding radiologists in interpreting images

MRI

Cardiac MRI has evolved as a precise method for structural and functional evaluations of the heart . The technology has evolved over the years from traditional techniques such as cardiac gating and the suspension of breathing to newer advanced techniques of high-field-strength magnets, high-performance gradient hardware and ultrafast pulse sequences. In the discipline of magnetic resonance imaging, the advancement of AI has allowed for shorter scan times, resulting in higher patient satisfaction; it also reduces errors by minimizing motion artefacts caused by patient movement. The segmentation of cardiac chambers helps visualize them better and aids in diagnosis. Currently, we do this manually, and a shift to AI will help with a faster diagnosis and reduce variation between different analysts .

Echocardiography

New AI-based technologies have revolutionized modern medicine in obtaining fetal echocardiograms with improved precision and accuracy. Combining it with machine learning has been quintessential in making predictions of future variables associated with disease progression using retrospective patient data. It has helped in eliminating limitations associated with a lack of expertise in fetal echocardiology, fetal movements, and fetal heart size . Machine learning-based systems have been useful in differentiating pathological versus physiological hypertrophic remodeling of the heart . Deep learning models have demonstrated superiority in terms of sensitivity and specificity up to 76% and 88%, respectively, in diagnosing atrial septal defect (ASD) compared with pediatric cardiologists who demonstrated sensitivity and specificity of 53% ± 0.04 and 67% ± 0.10 respectively .Automation, AI, and machine learning are game-changing as complementary tools to physicians and in areas with limited expert medical personnel or cardiologists.Fetal intelligent navigation echocardiography (FINE) has presented as a novel method for fetal echocardiographyusing "intelligent navigation" technology to obtain nine standard views—four-chamber, aortic arch, three vessels, and trachea—and display abnormalities with great sensitivity helping to detect CHD . New AI-based technologies have revolutionized modern medicine in obtaining fetal echocardiograms with improved precision and accuracy. Combining it with machine learning has been quintessential in making predictions of future variables associated with disease progression using retrospective patient data. It has helped in eliminating limitations associated with a lack of expertise in fetal echocardiology, fetal movements, and fetal heart size . Machine learning-based systems have been useful in differentiating pathological versus physiological hypertrophic remodeling of the heart . Deep learning models have demonstrated superiority in terms of sensitivity and specificity up to 76% and 88%, respectively, in diagnosing atrial septal defect (ASD) compared with pediatric cardiologists who demonstrated sensitivity and specificity of 53% ± 0.04 and 67% ± 0.10 respectively .Automation, AI, and machine learning are game-changing as complementary tools to physicians and in areas with limited expert medical personnel or cardiologists.Fetalintelligentnavigation echocardiography (FINE) has presented as a novel method for fetal echocardiography using "intelligent navigation" technology to obtain nine standard views—four-chamber, aortic arch, three vessels, and trachea—and display abnormalities with great sensitivity helping to detect CHD .

ECG

The use of deep learning (DL), an application of AI, in the field of adult cardiology has been well studied . Its application in pediatric cardiology has become especially relevant due to its potential for allowing early diagnosis, and thus better prognosis, in congenital heart diseases (CHDs). DL models such as convolutional neural network (CNN) and recurrent neural network (RNN) are used in conjunction with electrocardiograms, which remain the staple diagnostic tool for CHDs, to provide enhanced diagnostic information that is otherwise only deduced with input from specialists . Convolutional neural networks can perform image processing and classification, providing an advantage of extracting additional ECG information that would otherwise either be undetected . While the efficiency and utility of using AI models with ECGs for CHDs is evident, the enhancement of the interpretability and training of deep learning models is still needed for widespread implementation .

Prognosis and Risk Stratification

AI-based algorithms have proven to be of great help for pediatric cardiology in the clinical examination, diagnosis, procedural planning, and management of cardiac interventions AI models have also aided with the extraction of patient data for risk stratification and ambulatory health monitoring from wearables. Machine learning (ML)-based models such as optimal classification trees (OCTs) have accurately predicted mortality, postoperative mechanical ventilatory support time (MVST), and hospital length of stay (LOS) even with nonlinear data in patients with a history of congenital heart surgery . Similarly, ML algorithm-based models, extreme gradient boosting (XGBoost), and RCRnet have accurately predicted preoperative mortality odds in patients with CHDs and statistically significant prognostic indicators along with risk stratification markers in patients with Tetralogy of Fallot and left-to-right shunt CHDs, respectively . Importantly, the far-reaching utility of AI-based models in risk stratification and prognostic predictions is the trainability of models to work with various data cohorts .

Planning and Management of Cardiac Interventions

The current approach to planning and the execution of interventions in CHD relies primarily on generic treatment protocols derived from biological data and set guidelines. As such, there is a lack of tailor-made interventions based on each patient, which would drastically improve outcomes and post-intervention prognosis . Artificial intelligence (AI), with its applications in the form of machine learning (ML) and deep learning (DL) among many, has emerged as a tool aiding the creation of personalized intervention plans as well as an accurate data extractor to ascertain potential post-operative sequelae . The supervised machine learning models such as k-nearest neighbor classifier (KNN) and support vector machine classifier (SVM) have also aided in the intra-operative assessment of cardiac fluid kinematics, which are significant determinants of successful congenital heart surgeries . The subsequent post-operative management of CHDs is imperative for maintaining the structural fluid dynamics and thus the prognosis. This could be done seamlessly with the help of recurrent neural networks based on ML models and deep learning models, allowing for an integrated system that can enhance survival outcomes in pediatric patients .

AI in Cardiac Surgeries

AI can revolutionize pediatric surgery in all stages of surgery: preoperative, intraoperative and post-operative. Preoperative risk assessment and decision-making can be made easier by the tremendous processing and analyzing capacity of AI-enabled algorithms. Surgical decision support systems using ANN can predict post-op outcomes and can prevent morbidity and mortality arising from poor risk assessment pre-operatively.

Tech-enhanced (Hitech) operation theaters can enable intraoperative interventions and decision support and bring about a paradigm shift in telesurgery; it is especially useful in cardiac surgeries, where manual segmentation of retrieved images (CT/MRI) can take an unreasonable amount of time. Humans embarked on this path successfully when Xiaowei Xu et al. utilized AI to perform a cardiac surgery remotely in a patient having complications of long-standing ASD through the backbone of 5G technology. This was possible since AI replaced manual segmentation and provided accurate results in just two minutes compared to the traditional manual segmentation which takes 2–3 h even by experts . In this situation, the authors helped a patient who could not be transported to another hospital due to her frail condition; we can extend the same advantage to a remote inaccessible location especially in rural areas and developing countries . Postoperative AI can help in various aspects such as ambulatory patient monitoring post-discharge with AI wearables and automated risk stratification of patients to enable stricter follow-ups. Mahayni AA et al. described an ECG based AI algorithm that predicts ventricular dysfunction post-surgery, predicts long-term mortality in cardiac surgeries. Such algorithms can be developed and implemented for pediatric surgical procedures and drastically improve surgical outcomes.

AI in other Pediatric Heart Diseases

Kawasaki disease (KD) is an acquired pediatric vasculitis that can lead to coronary artery aneurysms and acute coronary syndrome . Very little is known about the pathogenesis of Kawasaki disease but a recent study using AI-guided signatures reveals a shared pathology with Multisystem inflammatory syndrome in children (MIS-C), COVID-19 associated vasculitis in children. Both these syndromes share systemic inflammatory storm with similar cytokines such as IL15/IL15RA. Such AI-based investigative approaches will further elucidate its complex pathogenesis and help decipher novel diagnostic and therapeutic targets

The appropriate and timely management of Kawasaki disease can significantly reduce the coronary complications associated with Kawasaki disease which contribute greatly to mortality in adulthood . AI-based approaches can prove to be extremely crucial in predicting the risk of developing a coronary aneurysm. It is widely known that Kawasaki patients with intravenous immunoglobulin resistance are at a higher risk of developing coronary artery aneurysms, but most scoring models present for predicting the resistance are impractical. Wang T et al. describe a machine learning-based model on patient data that can predict intravenous immunoglobulin resistance in Kawasaki disease patients successfully. The scope for several such prediction models is possible with the advent of AI and can support clinical decisions to improve patient outcomes . Distensibility changes in a coronary artery can be used to predict acute coronary disease in these patients. Benovoy M et al. calculated these changes in KD using an automated deep learning approach and correlated it with the severity of OCT (Optical coherence tomography) findings of KD-related CA damage . Despite, the limited studies using AI-based approaches, AI has the potential to revolutionize risk stratification and prognosis estimation of Kawasaki disease as well as paving way for newer drug targets by elucidating the pathogenesis.

RHD—The screening of RHD requires the clinician's expertise, and hence the grass-root level is limited by a lack of skilled human resources. Automatic diagnosis of echo-detected RHD is feasible and can form the core of the screening programs of the future covering the workload of experts . Recent data has also shown promise for a convolutional neural network-based deep learning algorithm to identify heart sounds as 'rheumatic' with an overall accuracy of 96.1% having 94.0% sensitivity and 98.1% specificity . Therefore, AI can form the backbone of future global screening programs for RHD.

AI Algorithms in Pediatric Cardiology

In many areas of pediatric cardiology, AI-based algorithms can be beneficial, including: (1) clinical examination and diagnosis, (2) image processing, (3) fetal cardiology, (4) prognosis and risk stratification, (5) precision cardiology, and (6) planning and management of cardiac interventions. Machine learning algorithms are a very promising tool for diagnosing and assessing critical and non-critical CHD; however, extensive research is still required to develop interpretable, robust, and generalizable models for clinical application, especially in light of the extreme heterogeneity of complex CHD. Various such AI algorithm models have gained interest over the past decade, and the present time has seen many motivating developments.

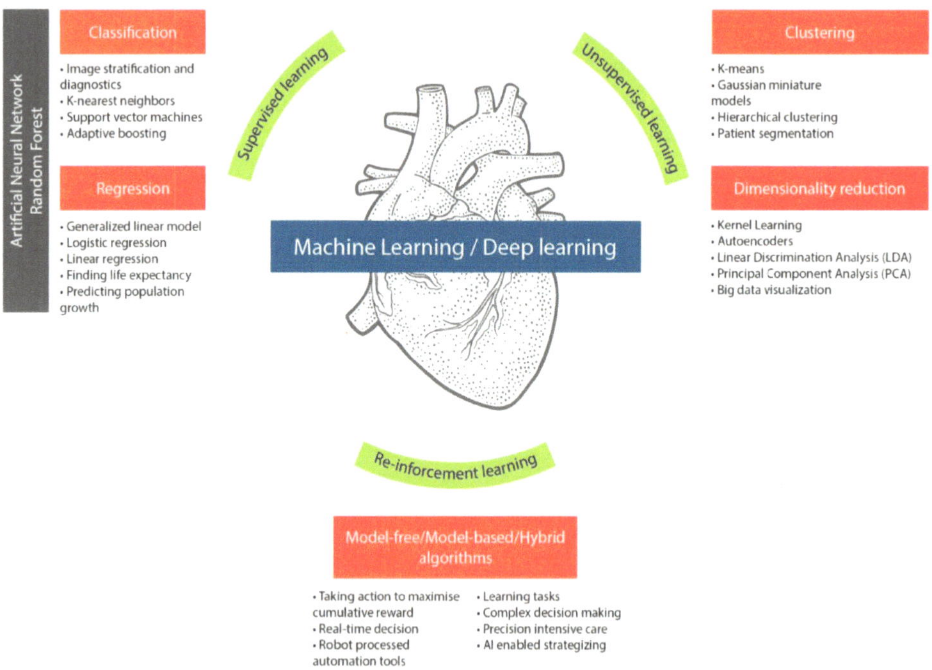

Fig. 36.3 AI-based algorithms and pediatric cardiology.

AI is rapidly growing, and its significance in clinical practice cannot be negated. It plays a crucial part in augmenting and standardizing care by adding to a physician's skills and expertise. The role of AI in pediatric cardiology has greatly evolved over the past two decades . It picks up subtle or unrecognizable features, preventing missed diagnoses and leading to a better prognosis. Physicians can combine their clinical expertise with AI to enhance their outputs in the domains of prevention, predictive intervention, and health maintenance. AI can make use of continuous data received from wearable devices to offer insight into patients' behaviors and health trends. These features of AI empower the professional to provide the best care to the patient earlier in the course of the disease, helping to improve prognosis and leading to better outcomes.

AI seems to be the tool of rich and economically advanced countries, but it can be the magic wand for risk stratification troubles in lower- and middle-income countries (LMICs). AI has the potential to reduce global health inequalities . It can help serve LMICs by bridging gaps in equity, availability, affordability, and accessibility . For instance, the major addition of AI is a reduction in the costs of dimensions requiring expensive equipment and specialized expertise, including tools of screening and planning that are unavailable in most hospitals, especially in LMICs. AI-based innovations can help overcome resource-constrained environments.The advent of AI has allowed smart tools to assist peripheral health workers in helping with a rough screening at the doorstep and in peripheral areas having poor doctor–patient ratios .

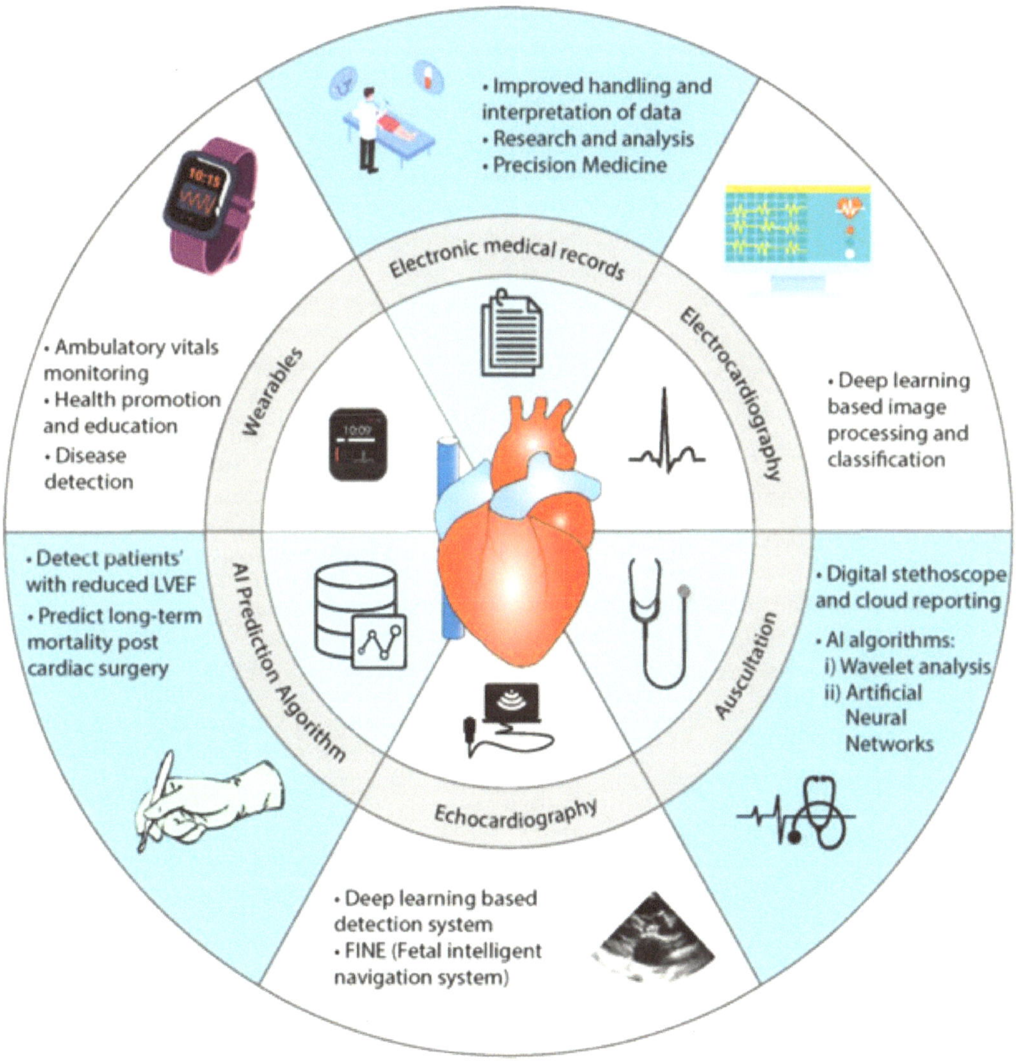

Fig. 36.4 Diagnostic and prognostic applications of AI in Pediatric Cardiology

The availability of skilled cardiologists to diagnose CHD in remote locations will require a giant leap in these countries. AI-based medical equipment can aid peripheral health care providers in helping with screening and referral. It can also help in terms of teleconsultation and remote radiology . Furthermore, with the availability of AI-based chatbots or virtual avatars and characters, we can offer greater help to populations suffering from stigmatizing pathologies (such as HIV/AIDS and psychiatric pathologies). This therefore can aid in improving access to health care and follow-up services. One of the biggest challenges to health care is language, with improving translation tools, AI can help cover this area well too .

AI: An Efficient Physician Assistant

The full-blown implementation of AI still is resisted by physicians and health care staff fearing inaccuracies, the exclusion of social variables, and possible unemployment. The mechanization of health care, loss of empathy, and human touch to this extent often invite skepticism from the traditional medical community. Despite the fear-mongering and skepticism of loss of human touch and jobs, we opine AI can be an efficient aid to physicians rather than a replacement . It can streamline insurance reviews, provide real-time data analysis, and assist in research. It can reduce the burden on physicians and burnout rates in the medical community. Thus, application in appropriate areas can contribute to the overall enhancement of health care delivery and experience .

Challenges to AI in Pediatric Cardiology

The incorporation of AI into pediatric cardiology has several challenges. The data available for pediatric cardiology is still very limited which is necessary to train AI algorithms to identify, assess and reduce inherent biases and overfitting. Furthermore, the heterogeneity in cardiac anatomy and the rarity of individual disease entities make data accessibility and AI incorporation into pediatric cardiology difficult. We can cater to this limitation by pooling data from all the different hospitals to get a large data set . Imaging in the pediatric population has another challenge owing to their smaller size and frequent movements during imaging, which lead to higher motion artifacts. This poses a technical challenge, for instance, requiring higher spatial resolution in the MRI . The doctor and patient may hesitate to use AI to replace the current protocols. The incorporation of AI will require health care providers to learn interpret data and accurately understand the many model parameters or model architectures. This challenge is being tackled in different ways. For example, some works have incorporated more intuitive interfaces in the models aiding easier interpretation .Additionally, AI is evolving and several ethical concerns are arising. These concerns include informed consent to data access, data security and privacy, algorithm fairness and biases, and transparency . Currently, there are no well-defined laws or regulations in place to address the legal and ethical issues that may arise with AI use in health care settings. However, as AI continues to grow and be used, laws and regulations can certainly be explored to ensure algorithmic transparency and protect data privacy.

Conclusions

AI can be touted as the next revolution in medicine. From making physicians' lives easier to enabling research with ease, it has variegated applications in the working environment as well as in the management of patients. Pediatric cardiology is a specialty requiring a great skill set in cognition and interpretation which makes it an ideal candidate for AI incorporation. AI has been successfully integrated into clinical examination, image interpretation, diagnoses, prognosis, risk stratification, precision medicine, and treatment in pediatric cardiology. The advent of AI has facilitated medicine to be more accurate and precise, but it is still a work in progress with challenges and limitations. Despite the roadblocks, we optimistically opine that AI with its current pace will streamline approaches in pediatric cardiology.

Bibliography and Acknowledgement

- Ahmad M.S., Mir J., Ullah M.O., Shahid M.L.U.R., Syed M.A. An Efficient Heart Murmur Recognition and Cardiovascular Disorders Classification System. Australas. Phys. Eng. Sci. Med. 2019;42:733–743.doi: 10.1007/s13246-019-00778-x. [PubMed] [CrossRef] [Google Scholar]
- Ali F., Hasan B., Ahmad H., Hoodbhoy Z., Bhuriwala Z., Hanif M., Ansari S.U., Chowdhury D. Detection of Subclinical Rheumatic Heart Disease in Children Using a Deep Learning Algorithm on Digital Stethoscope: A Study Protocol. BMJ Open. 2021;11:e044070. doi: 10.1136/bmjopen-2020-044070. [PMC free article] [PubMed] [CrossRef] [Google Scholar]
- Andrisevic N., Ejaz K., Rios-Gutierrez F., Alba-Flores R., Nordehn G., Burns S. Detection of Heart Murmurs Using Wavelet Analysis and Artificial Neural Networks. J. Biomech. Eng. 2005;127:899–904. doi: 10.1115/1.2049327. [PubMed] [CrossRef] [Google Scholar]
- Arafati A., Hu P., Finn J.P., Rickers C., Cheng A.L., Jafarkhani H., Kheradvar A. Artificial Intelligence in Pediatric and Adult Congenital Cardiac MRI: An Unmet Clinical Need. Cardiovasc. Diagn. Ther. 2019;9:S310–S325. doi: 10.21037/cdt.2019.06.09. [PMC free article] [PubMed] [CrossRef] [Google Scholar]
- Arnaout R., Curran L., Chinn E., Zhao Y., Moon-Grady A. Deep-Learning Models Improve on Community-Level Diagnosis for Common Congenital Heart Disease Lesions. arXiv. 2018 doi: 10.48550/arxiv.1809.06993.1809.06993 [CrossRef] [Google Scholar]

- Aufiero S., Bleijendaal H., Robyns T., Vandenberk B., Krijger C., Bezzina C., Zwinderman A.H., Wilde A.A.M., Pinto Y.M. A Deep Learning Approach Identifies New ECG Features in Congenital Long QT Syndrome. BMC Med. 2022;20:162. doi: 10.1186/s12916-022-02350-z. [PMC free article] [PubMed] [CrossRef] [Google Scholar]
- Basu K., Sinha R., Ong A., Basu T. Artificial Intelligence: How Is It Changing Medical Sciences and Its Future? Indian J. Dermatol. 2020;65:365. doi: 10.4103/ijd.IJD_421_20. [PMC free article] [PubMed] [CrossRef] [Google Scholar]
- Bayers S., Shulman S.T., Paller A.S. Kawasaki Disease. J. Am. Acad. Dermatol. 2013;69:513.e1–513.e8. doi: 10.1016/j.jaad.2013.06.040. [PubMed] [CrossRef] [Google Scholar]
- Begic E., Gurbeta Pokvic L., Begic Z., Begic N., Dedic M., Mrsic D., Jamakovic M., Vila N., Badnjevic A. From Heart Murmur to Echocardiography—Congenital Heart Defects Diagnostics Using Machine-Learning Algorithms. Psychiatr. Danub. 2021;33:236–246. [PubMed] [Google Scholar]
- Benke K., Benke G. Artificial Intelligence and Big Data in Public Health. Int. J. Environ. Res. Public Health. 2018;15:2796. doi: 10.3390/ijerph15122796. [PMC free article] [PubMed] [CrossRef] [Google Scholar]
- Benovoy M., Dionne A., McCrindle B.W., Manlhiot C., Ibrahim R., Dahdah N. Deep Learning-Based Approach to Automatically Assess Coronary Distensibility Following Kawasaki Disease. Pediatr. Cardiol. 2022;43:807–815. doi: 10.1007/s00246-021-02790-z. [PubMed] [CrossRef] [Google Scholar]
- Bertsimas D., Zhuo D., Dunn J., Levine J., Zuccarelli E., Smyrnakis N., Tobota Z., Maruszewski B., Fragata J., Sarris G.E. Adverse Outcomes Prediction for Congenital Heart Surgery: A Machine Learning Approach. World J. Pediatr. Congenit. Heart Surg. 2021;12:453–460. doi: 10.1177/21501351211007106. [PubMed] [CrossRef] [Google Scholar]
- Blue G.M., Kirk E.P., Sholler G.F., Harvey R.P., Winlaw D.S. Congenital Heart Disease: Current Knowledge about Causes and Inheritance. Med. J. Aust. 2012;197:155–159. doi: 10.5694/mja12.10811. [PubMed] [CrossRef] [Google Scholar]
- Bodenhofer U., Haslinger-Eisterer B., Minichmayer A., Hermanutz G., Meier J. Machine Learning-Based Risk Profile Classification of Patients Undergoing Elective Heart Valve Surgery. Eur. J. Cardiothorac. Surg. 2021;60:1378–1385. doi: 10.1093/ejcts/ezab219. [PubMed] [CrossRef] [Google Scholar]
- Bozkurt B., Germanakis I., Stylianou Y. A Study of Time-Frequency Features for CNN-Based Automatic Heart Sound Classification for Pathology Detection. Comput. Biol. Med. 2018;100:132–143. doi: 10.1016/j.compbiomed.2018.06.026. [PubMed] [CrossRef] [Google Scholar]
- Chang A. Artificial Intelligence in Pediatric Cardiology and Cardiac Surgery: Irrational Hype or Paradigm Shift? Ann. Pediatr. Cardiol. 2019;12:191. doi: 10.4103/apc.APC_55_19. [PMC free article] [PubMed] [CrossRef] [Google Scholar]
- Chang J.C., Binuesa F., Caneo L.F., Turquetto A.L.R., Arita E.C.T.C., Barbosa A.C., Fernandes A.M.D.S., Trindade E.M., Jatene F.B., Dossou P.-E., et al. Improving Preoperative Risk-of-Death Prediction in Surgery Congenital Heart Defects Using Artificial Intelligence Model: A Pilot Study. PLoS ONE. 2020;15:e0238199. doi: 10.1371/journal.pone.0238199. [PMC free article] [PubMed] [CrossRef] [Google Scholar]
- Chen C., Qin C., Qiu H., Tarroni G., Duan J., Bai W., Rueckert D. Deep Learning for Cardiac Image Segmentation: A Review. Front. Cardiovasc. Med. 2020;7:25. doi: 10.3389/fcvm.2020.00025. [PMC free article] [PubMed] [CrossRef] [Google Scholar]
- Chou F.-S., Ghimire L.V. Identification of Prognostic Factors for Pediatric Myocarditis with a Random Forests Algorithm-Assisted Approach. Pediatr. Res. 2021;90:427–430. doi: 10.1038/s41390-020-01268-7. [PubMed] [CrossRef] [Google Scholar]
- Davies R., Babu-Narayan S.V. Deep Learning in Congenital Heart Disease Imaging: Hope but Not Haste. Heart. 2020;106:960–961. doi: 10.1136/heartjnl-2019-316496. [PubMed] [CrossRef] [Google Scholar]
- Decourt C., Duong L. Semi-Supervised Generative Adversarial Networks for the Segmentation of the Left Ventricle in Pediatric MRI. Comput. Biol. Med. 2020;123:103884. doi: 10.1016/j.compbiomed.2020.103884. [PubMed] [CrossRef] [Google Scholar]
- DeGroff C.G., Bhatikar S., Hertzberg J., Shandas R., Valdes-Cruz L., Mahajan R.L. Artificial Neural Network–Based Method of Screening Heart Murmurs in Children. Circulation. 2001;103:2711–2716. doi: 10.1161/01.CIR.103.22.2711. [PubMed] [CrossRef] [Google Scholar]
- Dias R.D., Shah J.A., Zenati M.A. Artificial Intelligence in Cardiothoracic Surgery. Minerva Cardioangiol. 2020;68:532–538. doi: 10.23736/S0026-4725.20.05235-4. [PMC free article] [PubMed] [CrossRef] [Google Scholar]
- Diller G.-P., Babu-Narayan S., Li W., Radojevic J., Kempny A., Uebing A., Dimopoulos K., Baumgartner H., Gatzoulis M.A., Orwat S. Utility of Machine Learning Algorithms in Assessing Patients with a Systemic Right Ventricle. Eur. Heart J. Cardiovasc. Imaging. 2019;20:925–931. doi: 10.1093/ehjci/jey211. [PMC free article] [PubMed] [CrossRef] [Google Scholar]
- Diller G.-P., Kempny A., Babu-Narayan S.V., Henrichs M., Brida M., Uebing A., Lammers A.E., Baumgartner H., Li W., Wort S.J., et al. Machine Learning Algorithms Estimating Prognosis and Guiding Therapy in Adult Congenital Heart Disease: Data from a Single Tertiary Centre Including 10,019 Patients. Eur. Heart J. 2019;40:1069–1077. doi: 10.1093/eurheartj/ehy915. [PMC free article] [PubMed] [CrossRef] [Google Scholar]
- Diller G.-P., Lammers A.E., Babu-Narayan S., Li W., Radke R.M., Baumgartner H., Gatzoulis M.A., Orwat S. Denoising and Artefact Removal for Transthoracic Echocardiographic Imaging in Congenital Heart Disease: Utility of Diagnosis Specific Deep Learning Algorithms. Int. J. Cardiovasc. Imaging. 2019;35:2189–2196. doi: 10.1007/s10554-019-01671-0. [PubMed] [CrossRef] [Google Scholar]
- Diller G.P., Orwat S., Vahle J., Bauer U.M.M., Urban A., Sarikouch S., Berger F., Beerbaum P., Baumgartner H. Prediction of Prognosis in Patients with Tetralogy of Fallot Based on Deep Learning Imaging Analysis. Heart. 2020;106:1007–1014. doi: 10.1136/heartjnl-2019-315962. [PubMed] [CrossRef] [Google Scholar]
- Ding Y., Gudapati V., Lin R., Fei Y., Packard R.R.S., Song S., Chang C.-C., Baek K.I., Wang Z., Roustaei M., et al. Saak Transform-Based Machine Learning for Light-Sheet Imaging of Cardiac Trabeculation. IEEE Trans. Biomed. Eng. 2021;68:225–235. doi: 10.1109/TBME.2020.2991754. [PMC free article] [PubMed] [CrossRef] [Google Scholar]
- Dozen A., Komatsu M., Sakai A., Komatsu R., Shozu K., Machino H., Yasutomi S., Arakaki T., Asada K., Kaneko S., et al. Image Segmentation of the Ventricular Septum in Fetal Cardiac Ultrasound Videos Based on Deep Learning Using Time-Series Information. Biomolecules. 2020;10:1526. doi: 10.3390/biom10111526. [PMC free article] [PubMed] [CrossRef] [Google Scholar]

37 Transformative Technology Of 3D Printing In Congenital Heart Disease

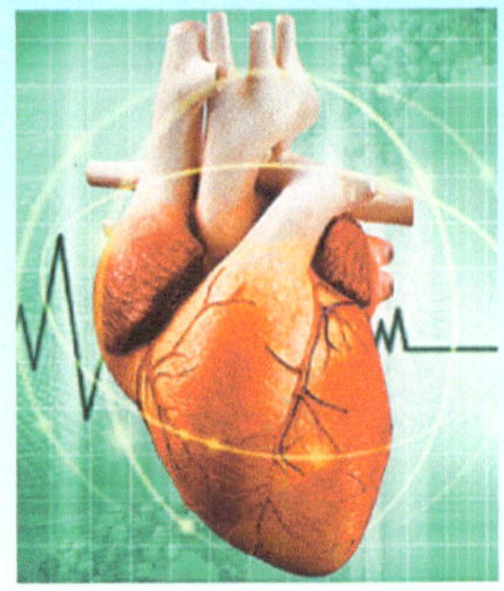

Survival in congenital heart disease has steadily improved since 1938, when Dr. Robert Gross successfully ligated for the first time a patent ductus arteriosus in a 7-year-old child. To continue the gains made over the past 80 years, transformative changes with broad impact are needed in management of congenital heart disease. Three-dimensional printing is an emerging technology that is fundamentally affecting patient care, research, trainee education, and interactions among medical teams, patients, and caregivers. This paper first reviews key clinical cases where the technology has affected patient care. It then discusses 3-dimensional printing in trainee education. Thereafter, the role of this technology in communication with multidisciplinary teams, patients, and caregivers is described. Three-dimensional (3D) printing is an additive manufacturing technique with increasing use in health care. As a fabrication technique 3D printing was recently listed by the McKinsey Global Institute as a "disruptive technology that will transform life, business and the global economy,"

1. Scope of Congenital Heart Disease and the Need for Transformative Care

The prevalence of CHD is approximately 9 in 1,000 live births. Survival rates vary by disease complexity, with long-term survival (>20 years) at approximately 95% for simple CHD, 90% for moderate complexity, and 80% for severe, complex CHD . Overall survival rates have steadily increased for even the most complex CHD , although survival alone is not a sufficient outcome measure in the current era.Other important metrics include the following: long-term morbidity; reintervention rates; length of hospitalization; neurodevelopmental outcomes; cost to the health care system; and patient or caregiver satisfaction. Obtaining the best outcomes requires an impact at multiple levels, including patients and caregivers, individual clinicians, the medical team and the health care system. 3D printing is a disruptive technology that is affecting each of these key areas in CHD.

The earliest papers on cardiovascular 3D printing were published in the early 2000s. Binder et al. showed feasibility from echocardiographic data in 2000, and Pentacost et al. produced 3D models replicating cardiac embryology from photomicrographic data in 2001. Soon thereafter, datasets from computed tomography (CT) or magnetic resonance imaging (MRI) were used to produce 3D cardiac models of increasing complexity , with a steady rise in publications in the past decade shows the applications of 3D printing in medicine, broadly categorized as surgical planning, education, and manufacturing of custom parts. Given that a 3D model is a replica of a patient's anatomy, models may be used for precise pre-surgical planning and simulation . Patient-specific pre-surgical planning may potentially reduce time spent in the operating room (OR) and result in fewer complications. In turn, this may lead to shorter post-operative stays, decreased reintervention rates, and lower health care costs. Given the relatively recent use of 3D printing in CHD, there are currently no data supporting these presumed outcomes. Most of the evidence in published reports is qualitative, through case reports and series. Emerging reports from other surgical subspecialties appear promising. Recent data from craniofacial reports suggest that 3D printing can improve outcomes, including saving time in the OR and thus translating to direct cost savings .

3D Printing Technology and Options for Cardiovascular Printing

Several recent publications have described the process of medical 3D ., summarized as these key steps:-

- Acquisition of a high-resolution 3D imaging dataset
- Segmentation of the anatomy using specialized post-processing software
- Computer-aided design to refine the design, add cut-planes, or include elements required for model stability
- Creation of a 3D file in a format recognized by the 3D printer, usually in the Surface Tessellation Language or stereolithography (STL) file format
- Printing of the physical model

3D printing technologies may be categorized as photopolymeric (the use of light to harden a deposited photopolymer), thermoplastic (extruding melted thermoplastics in layers to build up a model), or powder fusion (a process that fuses ceramic or metal powder by using an adhesive or laser beam to create a 3D object).. Printer resolution for higher-end medical-grade printers is in the order of micrometers, well within the resolution needed to print cardiac structures. Principally, there are 2 main types of cardiac models: "blood-pool" and "hollow" models. Blood pool models are solid 3D representations of the blood pool within the cardiac chambers and vessels . They are created by segmenting the blood pool signal, usually from contrast-enhanced CT or MRI, after which the 3D object is printed. Noncardiovascular structures such as airways or soft tissue may also be included for printing. These models provide excellent visualization of the great vessels, extracardiac vasculature, and surrounding structures such as airways or the esophagus. The drawback of these types of models is their limited views of intracardiac anatomy.

Hollow models are created by applying a mesh representing myocardium and vessel walls around the blood pool signal and then digitally removing the blood pool signal to show the intracardiac cavities. The end result is a hollow model showing the intracardiac anatomy in detail. These models are usually sectioned along a pre-determined cut-plane with 2 or more sections showing the intracardiac anatomy.

A subtype of the hollow models consists of intact hollow models. These models also show the intracardiac anatomy but are printed intact (i.e., without a cut-plane), thereby resulting in the most accurate representation of the heart as it sits in the chest. When printed in a flexible material, these models allow cardiothoracic surgeons to use standard surgical approaches and see the anatomy from a "surgeon's perspective," as they would for the actual case. Thus, these models are ideal for surgical simulation, especially when they are printed in materials that can be cut, can hold suture, and can allow engraftment of foreign materials (e.g., patch, cannula).

Applications of 3D Printing in CHD

Several publications have described the use of 3D printing in CHD, spanning the spectrum from atrial or ventricular septal defects (ASDs, VSDs) to the most complex cardiac lesions . Published reports have been summarized in a recent textbook on cardiac 3D printing .

A selection of cases is now reviewed to show the main applications of 3D printing in CHD. These cases were selected from a cohort of pediatric and adult patients with CHD at our institution who underwent 3D printing. Most of these cases were printed for surgical planning and simulation; others with unique or rare anatomy were printed for trainee education. The majority of cases had complex CHD, with a median complexity score of 3 (simple = 1, moderate = 2, great = 3) . Most of the cases printed for surgical planning were high-risk surgical candidates, and the median Society of Thoracic Surgeons-European Association for Cardio-Thoracic Surgery mortality category (1 to 5) was 4.

Planning complex intracardiac repair

Three of 1,000 patients born with CHD require catheter-based or surgical intervention early in life . Outcomes are significantly affected by the complexity of the underlying anatomy and perioperative factors, including cardiopulmonary bypass time, ischemic time, or circulatory arrest time .3D models allow the visualization and understanding of complex spatial relationships and enable precise pre-surgical planning.

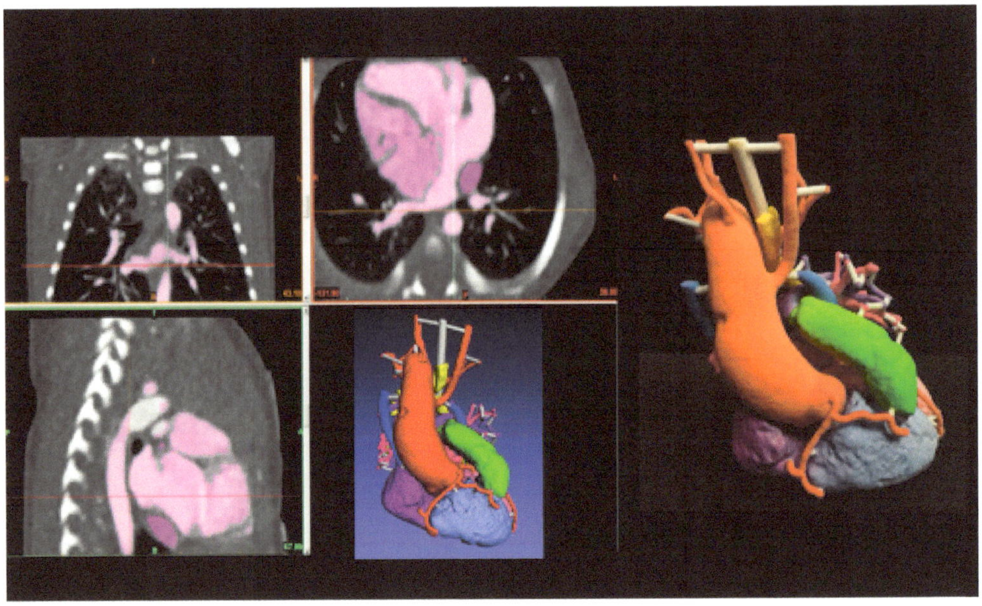

Fig.37.1 Blood Pool Cardiac 3D Model images on the left show the segmented blood pool signal. The model is shown on the right.

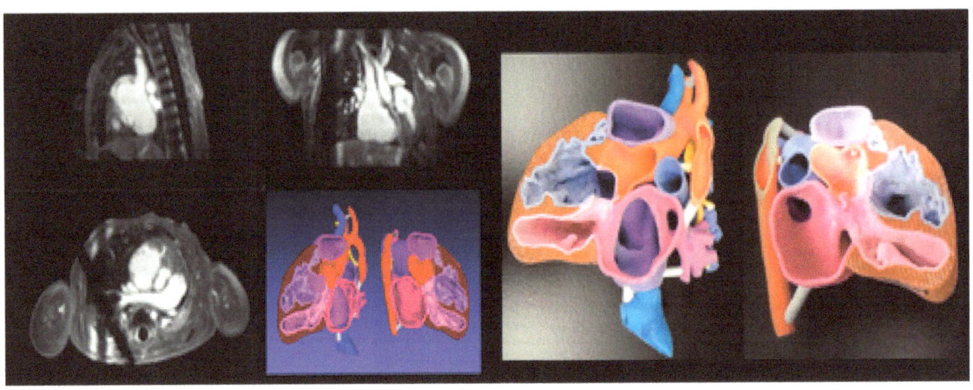

Fig.37.2 Hollow Cardiac 3D Model Showing Intracardiac Anatomy

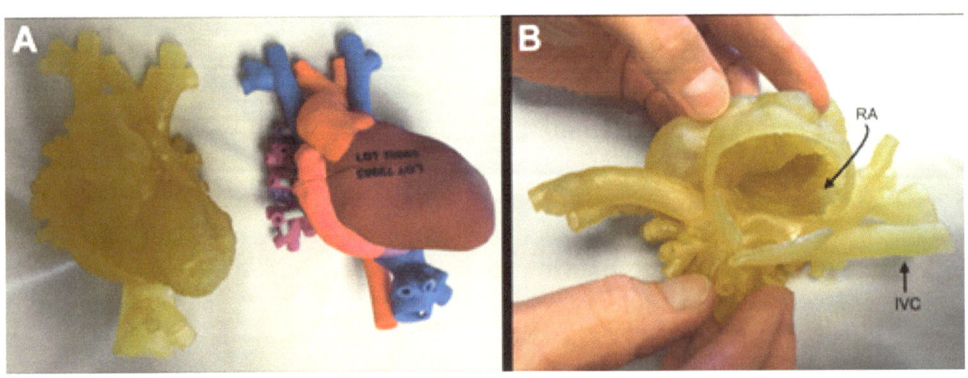

Fig.37.3 Models for Surgical Planning (A) Flexible hollow model printed intact with corresponding rigid multicolor model. (B) The "surgeon's view" through a right atriotomy. IVC = inferior vena cava; RA = right atrium.

A common application in CHD is planning repair of a double-outlet right ventricle (DORV) requiring a complex intracardiac baffle. This is typically a high-risk operation, Society of Thoracic Surgeons-European Association for Cardio-Thoracic Surgery category Several other groups have reported the use of 3D printing to plan complex intracardiac repairs in patients with multiple VSDs or DORV

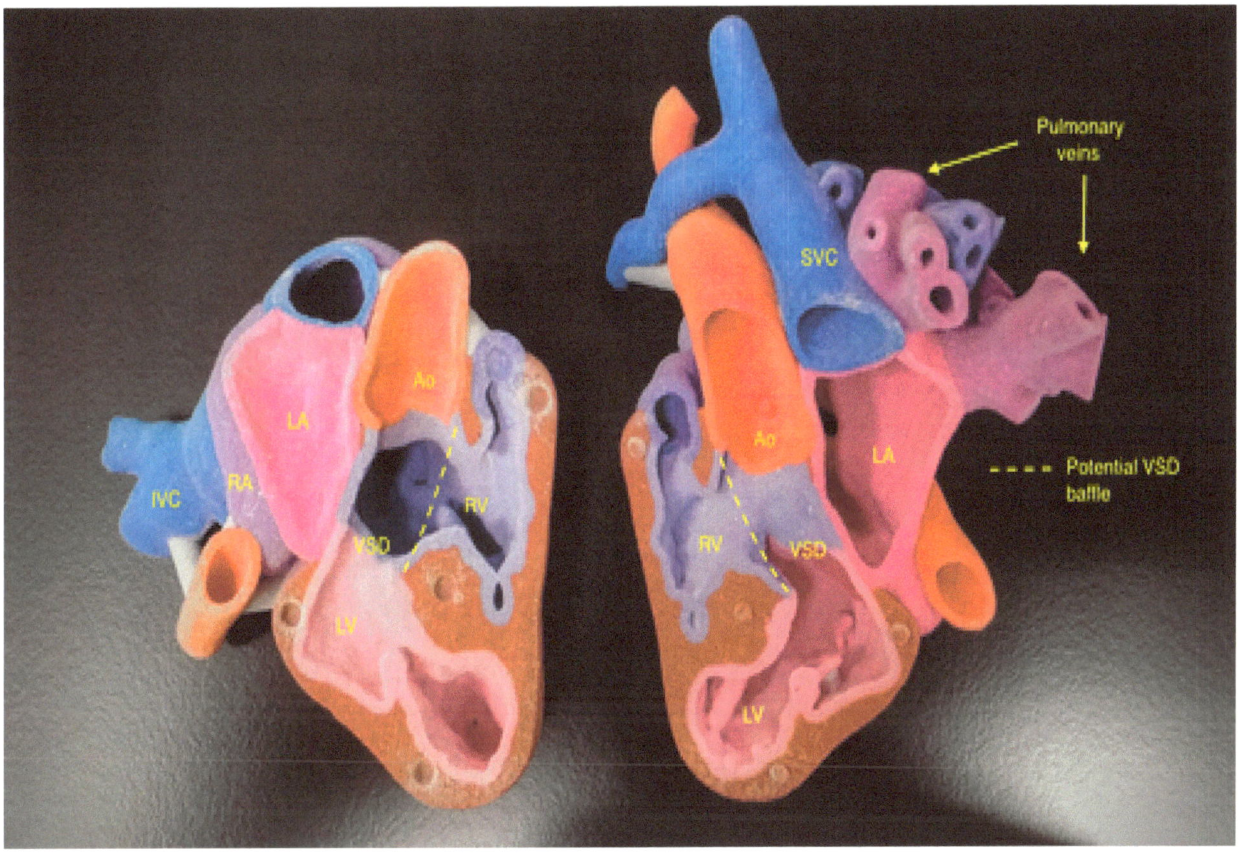

Fig.37.4 3D Model of Double Outlet RV Showing Relationships Among Ventricles, VSD, and Outflows The dashed line indicates the potential ventricular septal defect (VSD) baffle pathway to achieve a 2-ventricle repair. Ao = aorta; LA = left atrium; LV = left ventricle; RV = right ventricle; SVC = superior vena cava;

Surgical simulation

The ultimate in pre-surgical planning using 3D models is one in which a "simulated surgery" is performed, as illustrated by the next case. The patient was a 3 1/2-year-old male child with heterotaxy, asplenia syndrome with complex single ventricle anatomy, and abnormal systemic and pulmonary venous connections . He had previously undergone bilateral bidirectional superior cavopulmonary connections (bilateral Glenn procedure) as part of single ventricle palliation. 3D printing was performed to plan his next surgery, a total cavopulmonary connection (aka Fontan). Two 3D models were printed; 1 multicolor with an axial cut-plane and a second flexible intact-heart model (no cut-plane) for surgical simulation. The internal anatomy of both models was identical. By using the models, detailed pre-surgical planning was performed. Specifically, the models were used to plan placement of the Fontan conduit (intracardiac or extracardiac) and to evaluate its relationship with systemic veins and impact on pulmonary veins. The model was also used to simulate "plan A," "plan B," or "bailout" scenarios, each with a unique surgical plan. This level of detailed surgical simulation is not feasible with current standard of care (e.g., 3D volumetric rendering), and it shows the added value of 3D printed models.

Extracardiac and vascular surgery

3D printing can be a valuable tool to plan extracardiac and vascular surgery in patients with CHD. 3D models are helpful for planning high-risk unifocalization surgery,. The 3D models show spatial relationships among the aorta, aortopulmonary collaterals (APCs), pulmonary veins, and airways that enabled detailed pre-surgical planning. Precise visualization of the complex relationships between APCs and surrounding structures enables easier identification and surgical manipulation during the case, thereby reducing operative time and potentially improving the surgical outcome.This patient underwent a right modified Blalock-Taussig-Thomas shunt to the right-sided APCs . followed by a left modified Blalock-Taussig-Thomas shunt and, ultimately, successful unifocalization. 3D printing for pulmonary atresia and MAPCAs offers significant benefits over current standard of care, also described in prior publications .

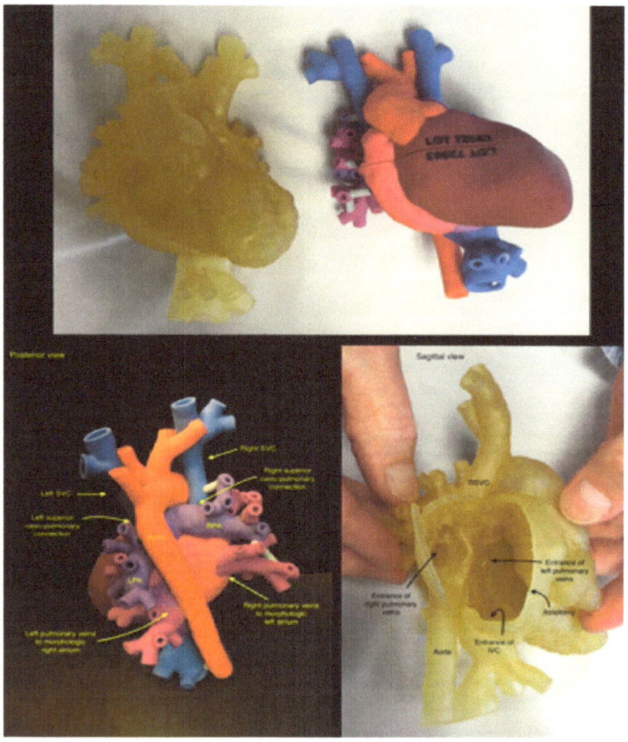

Fig.37.5 Simulated Surgery for Complex Total Cavopulmonary Connection Planning Using Flexible, Intact-Heart Model LPA = left pulmonary artery; RPA = right pulmonary artery; RSVC = right superior vena cava;

Ventricular assist device and heart transplant

An endpoint of many patients with CHD is heart failure requiring a ventricular assist device or heart transplant. 3D printing can aid in ventricular assist

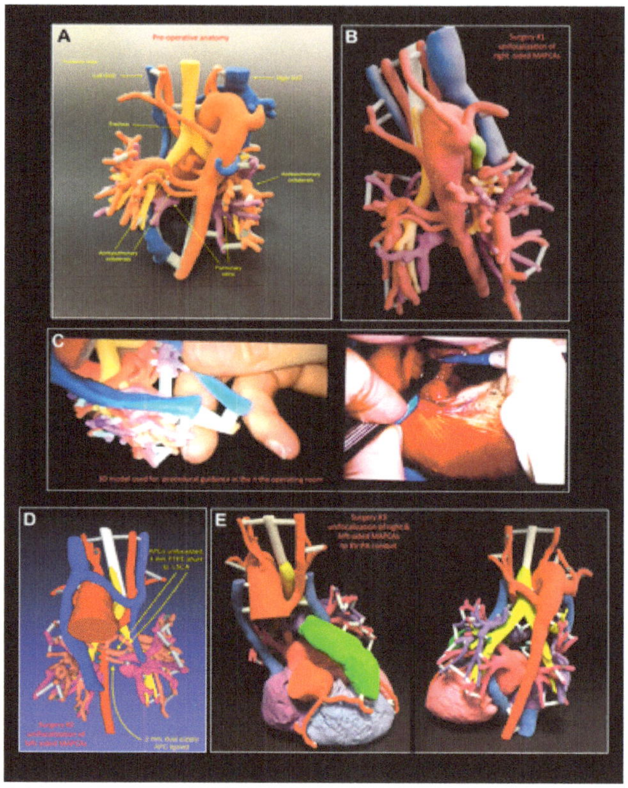

Fig.37.6 Staged Repair of Tetralogy of Fallot, Pulmonary Atresia, and MAPCAs

(A) Pre-operative anatomy. (B) Unifocalization of right-sided major aortopulmonary collateral arteries (MAPCAs) and small right pulmonary artery (PA)–to–right modified Blalock-Taussig-Thomas shunt. (C) Use of 3D model in the operating room for procedural guidance. (D) Unifocalization of left-sided major aortopulmonary collateral arteries–to–left modified Blalock-Taussig-Thomas shunt. (E) Right ventricular (RV)–to–pulmonary artery conduit placement (green) to unifocalized major aortopulmonary collateral arteries and takedown of bilateral modified Blalock-Taussig-Thomas shunts. APC = aortopulmonary collateral; LSCA = left subclavian artery; PTFE = polytetrafluoroethylene; SVC = superior vena cava.

device placement and optimizing function in complex CHD, as recently described by Farooqi et al and Saeed et al. . 3D printing can also assist with transplant planning for recipients with complex CHD More recently, a Melody valve was placed in a left ventricular–to–left superior vena cava conduit for conduit stenosis. 3D printing was performed to plan key components of the transplant, including thoracic entry,cannulation options, conduct of bypass, and graft-donor connections. 3D printing for transplant planning has been previously described for patients with complex pre-transplant anatomy .

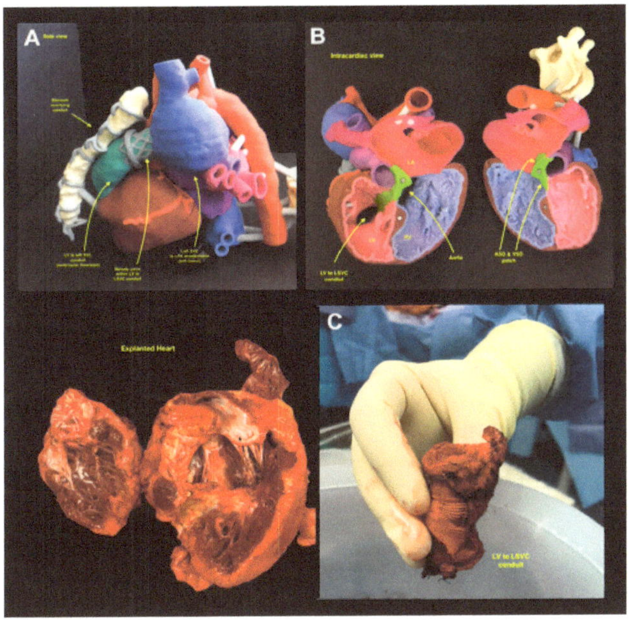

Fig.38.7 **Heterotaxy, Unbalanced Atrioventricular Canal, Ventricular Inversion, Modified Fontan**

(A) 3D model showing a left ventricle (LV)–to–left superior vena cava (LSVC) conduit and left-sided Glenn procedure that complicates transplantation of a normal donor heart.
(B) Intracardiac anatomy. (C) Intraoperative findings: explanted heart and a left ventricle–to–left superior vena cava conduit, showing accuracy of the 3D model. ASD = atrial septal defect;

Airway abnormalities

In CHD cases, the airways may be involved in the pathophysiology or need to be accounted for in surgical planning, as demonstrated earlier in the case with tetralogy of Fallot with pulmonary atresia and MAPCAs. In some CHD lesions, airways may be directly affected by the cardiovascular disease. Examples include vascular rings (Figure 10A), where aberrant vessels cause airway compression, or compression from dilated pulmonary arteries in tetralogy of Fallot with absent pulmonary valve.Airway compression or tracheobronchomalacia can significantly add to morbidity of patients with CHD from prolonged ventilator dependence. 3D printing recently led to a momentous breakthrough in the management of these patients with the use of 3D printed bioresorbable airway splints. In this series 3D printed splints were implanted without complications and resulted in patency of the airway. If successful in larger cohorts, this application of 3D printing will dramatically change the management and outcomes for these challenging patients. Other applications of 3D printing in otolaryngology and airway abnormalities were recently reviewed by VanKoevering et al.

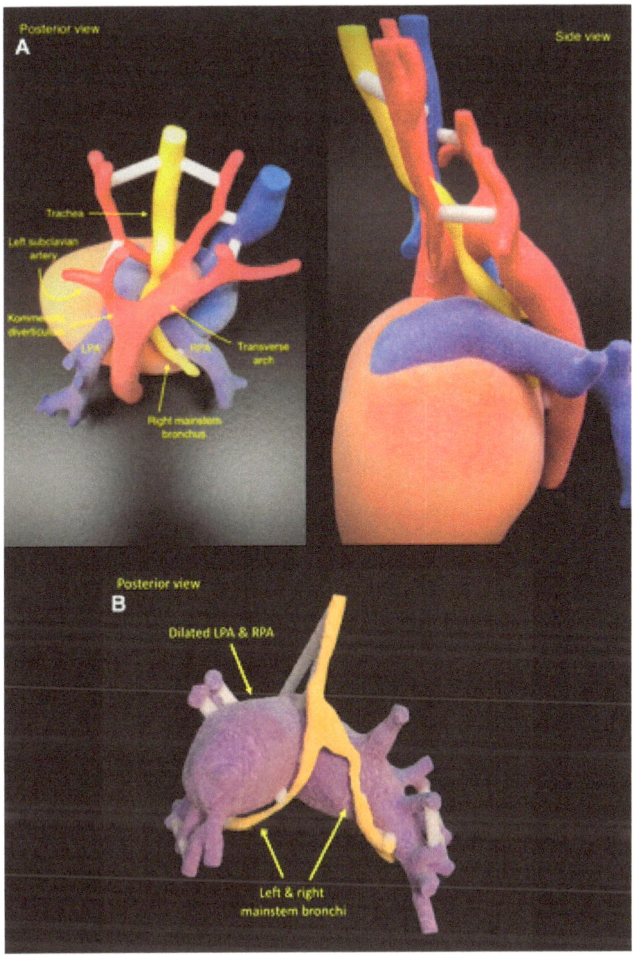

Fig.37.8 **Airway Abnormalities in Congenital Heart Disease**

(A) Vascular ring with posterior compression of trachea by a circumflex transverse arch coursing behind the aorta. (B) Severe branch pulmonary artery dilation in tetralogy of Fallot with absent pulmonary valve with compression and malacia of bilateral mainstem bronchi Airway compression or tracheobronchomalacia can significantly add to morbidity of patients with CHD from prolonged ventilator dependence.

3D printing recently led to a momentous breakthrough in the management of these patients with the use of 3D printed bioresorbable airway splints.In this series 3D printed splints were implanted without complications and resulted in patency of the airway. If successful in larger cohorts, this application of 3D printing will dramatically

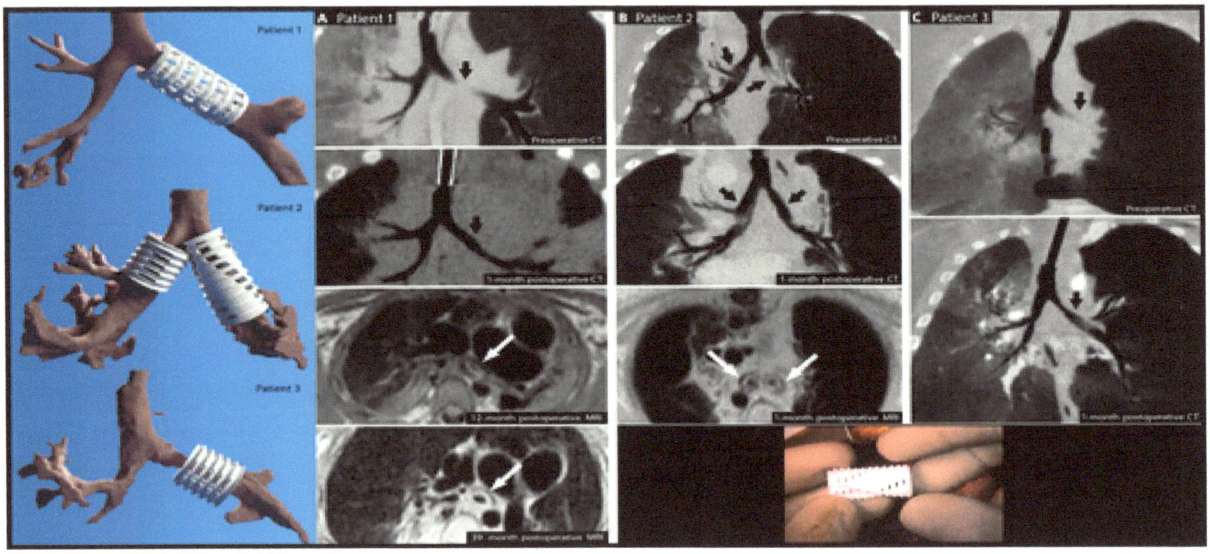

Fig.37.9 Bioresorbable Airway Splint Manufactured From Polycaprolactone With a Bellowed Design to Promote Expansion and Growth Over Time

change the management and outcomes for these challenging patients. Other applications of 3D printing in otolaryngology and airway abnormalities were recently reviewed by VanKoevering et al.

Catheter-based interventions

3D printing has been used for catheter-based interventions in CHD, although to a lesser degree compared with cardiothoracic surgery. Some noteworthy applications include the following: percutaneous pulmonary valve implantation, reported as early as 2007 ; coarctation procedures ; and stenting for aortic arch hypoplasia. Other reported applications include transcatheter ASD closure, double-lobed left atrial appendage closure , caval valve implantation , and stenting of Mustard baffle obstruction 3D printing is of particular interest in noncongenital structural heart disease, including transcatheter mitral and aortic valve interventions.. Potential benefits in interventional cardiology include visualization of complex anatomy that leads to decreased radiation and contrast from fluoroscopy and angiography and improved procedural outcome. Other benefits may include device development and testing in models that replicate abnormal anatomy . Finally, a key benefit may be feasibility testing for complex or borderline cases, as in the case of this 15-year-old male patient from our institution with repaired tetralogy of Fallot who met the criteria for pulmonary valve replacement.MRI measurements indicated that his right ventricular outflow tract dimensions were borderline large for transcatheter pulmonary valve replacement; thus, a 3D model was made in flexible material to trial pre-stenting as a precursor to transcatheter pulmonary valve replacement. The 3D model showed feasibility of the catheter-based strategy, and the procedure was carried out, with subsequent successful implantation of a transcatheter pulmonary valve, thereby avoiding surgery.

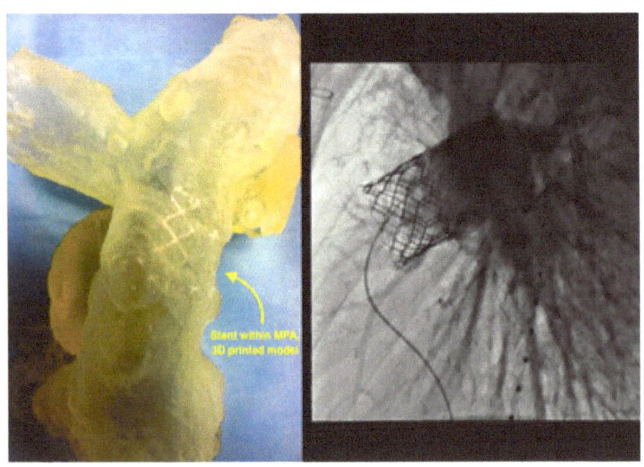

Fig.37.10 3D Printed Model in a Case of TOF With Borderline Large PA Measurements Image on the left shows a stent within main pulmonary artery (MPA). Image on the right is an angiogram taken after successful transcatheter implantation of pulmonary valve. PA = pulmonary artery; TOF = tetralogy of Fallot.

Impediments to greater use of 3D models incatheter-based procedures include tissue characteristics of the models that do not respond to balloons and stents in the same way as native tissue. Moreover, current models do not reflect the physiological environment encountered during catheterization, with nonpulsatility a major limitation of static models. Both these limitations may be overcome with future iterations of 3D models,

Adults with congenital heart disease

Approximately 85% of children with CHD now survive into adulthood , and adults with CHD (ACHD) now outnumber children . There are an estimated 5 million adult survivors in the United States alone . Over the past few decades the proportion of all deaths in patients with CHD has shifted from infants to the ACHD population . Similar to their pediatric counterparts, risk factors that worsen ACHD outcomes include complex anatomy, prior surgeries, and length of time spent on cardiopulmonary bypass . Although the challenges involving complex ACHD are considerable, 3D printing may help in their management by applications described

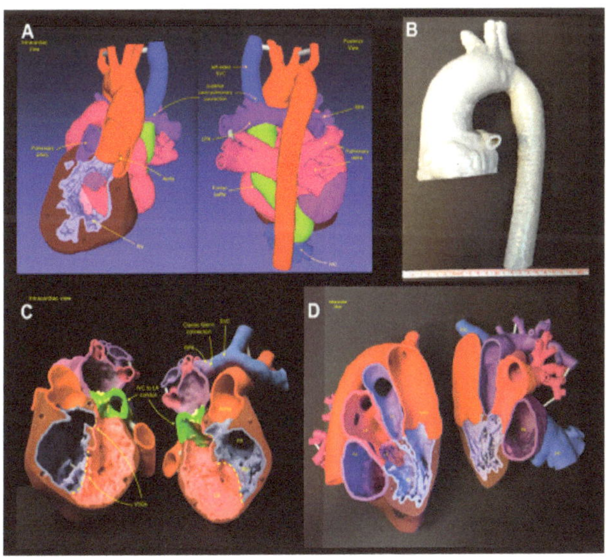

Fig 37.11 **3D Models of Adults With Congenital Heart Disease**

(A) A 31-year-old patient with dextrocardia, a double-outlet right ventricle (DORV), and a Fontan procedure.
(B) A 19-year-old patient with a bicuspid aortic valve (not shown) and a severely dilated aortic root and ascending aorta.
(C) A 40-year-old patient with a double-outlet right ventricle, 2 VSDs, and classic Glenn and modified Mustard procedures (conduit from inferior vena cava [IVC] to left atrium [LA], in green).
(D) A 45-year-old patient with a left dominant unbalanced atrioventricular canal, a double-outlet right ventricle, and right ventricular outflow tract obstruction.

Accuracy and Quality Assurance in Cardiac 3D Printing

Accuracy in medical 3D printing is of paramount importance, although published reports on this topic are limited. Accuracy is defined by comparison with a gold standard, and in the case of 3D printed models, 1 metric of accuracy is comparison with operative findings. At our institution, the quality assurance process is driven by feedback from our surgical colleagues and findings in the OR. Between February 2015 and May 2017, the average accuracy score for 21 3D printed models at our institution was 4 of a possible 5 points when the surgeon compared model anatomy with findings in the OR. A similar quality assurance process was described by Hermsen et al. for surgical models of hypertrophic obstructive cardiomyopathy. We have found that direct and ongoing communication among the imaging, modeling, and surgical teams is essential for maintaining high levels of accuracy. In addition, model accuracy may be diminished if there is a significant delay between acquisition of source images and time of surgery. In infants and young children somatic growth and evolution of the pathophysiology can produce relatively large changes to the anatomy as time passes; thus, the pre-operative imaging and 3D modeling should be performed close to the time of anticipated surgery.Besides direct comparison with OR findings, other metrics of accuracy include comparison with source images and user feedback. Olivieri et al. reported that 3D printed models from echocardiographic data were comparable in measurements of VSDs when compared with source images. Yoo et al. reported data from 50 surgeons after undergoing a Hands-on Surgical Training course using 3D models.The majority of cardiothoracic surgeons reported that the 3D models were of "excellent" or "good" quality for surgical simulation . Finally, accuracy of 3D models may be judged in terms of their ability to recreate native physiology, not just anatomy. The innovative work of Vukicevic et al. has shown the ability to recreate "hemodynamics" of abnormal aortic valves in 3D models, with Doppler characteristics nearly identical to those of the patient's own diseased valve

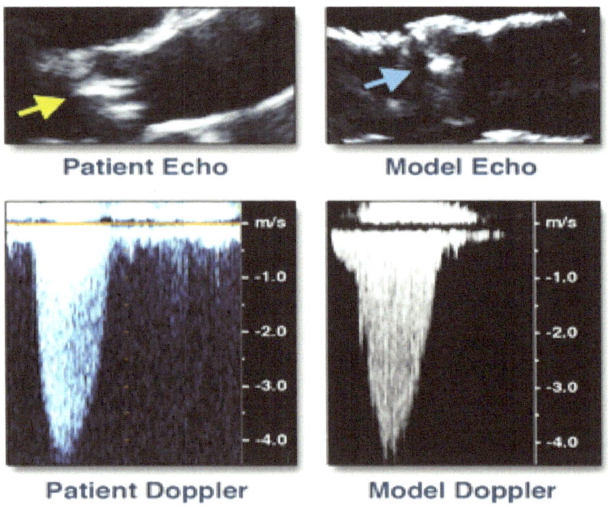

Fig.37.12 Patient and Model Doppler Comparisons Doppler profile of a patient's echocardiogram on the left, compared with the Doppler image from the 3D printed model on the right. Arrows point towards the aortic valve from the patient's echocardiogram (left) and model (right).

3D Printing for Trainee Education and Surgical Simulation

Another arena where 3D printing can bring about transformative change is in the education and training of the next generation of physicians. This is an established practice in neurosurgery and otolaryngology , with more recent application in cardiology . Although medical training has long followed the practice of "see 1, do 1, teach 1," use of 3D models in education represents a paradigm shift from an apprenticeship model to a simulator-based learning method that complements traditional mentored training .3D models in CHD can reduce the learning curve for cardiac trainees in 3 key areas:

- Understanding complex 3D anatomy
- High-fidelity simulation experiences
- Exposure to rare cases

As a tool for surgical simulation, 3D printing has been applied toward septal myectomy for hypertrophic obstructive cardiomyopathy , vascular procedures, and complex congenital procedures, as described by Yoo et al.

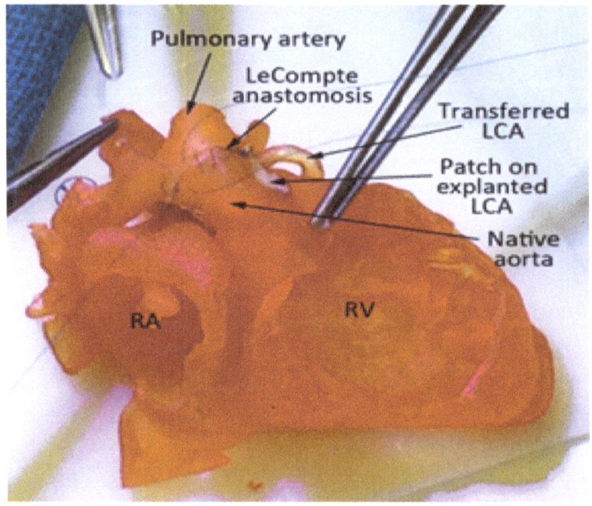

Fig.37.13 Simulated Arterial Switch Operation From a Hands-on Surgical Training Course for Cardiothoracic Surgeons Reproduced with permission from Yoo et al. LCA = left coronary artery.

In addition to allowing practice on highly accurate simulators, the 3D models expose trainees to pathological features they may rarely encounter. This shifts the practice of surgery from an "opportunity-based" to a "curriculum-based" experience. For experienced practitioners, models may be used for lifelong learning, for maintenance of certification, or for practice before challenging cases. Thus, a repository of 3D printed cardiovascular models with the spectrum of CHD would be an ideal educational resource The 3D print Heart Library at the National Institutes of Health is a good example of this concept. Electronic 3D models may supplement traditional learning methods. Finally, virtual reality displays may be used as complementary platforms to interact with electronic 3D models, with several robust options currently available

3D Printing to Facilitate Communication Within the Medical Teamandfor Counseling Patients and Families

Cardiac surgery and perioperative care are conducted in a multidisciplinary setting requiring highly skilled and specialized teams. Communication among specialists is essential for avoiding errors and optimizing patient outcomes . 3D models provide clarity, and they are cornerstones around which multiple subspecialists can gather to discuss the pathological condition, surgical plan, anticipated outcomes, and perioperative care. In so doing, they may reduce medical errors, a postulate that deserves further investigation.

In addition to facilitating communication among medical team members, 3D models enable better communication between the medical team and patients or their caregivers . The models can help the patient or caregiver better understand the disease process, risks, benefits, and alternatives. Anecdotally, our institutional practice is to counsel patients and families by using 3D models if a model has been printed for a case. Eleven caregivers who completed a questionnaire for cardiac models between 2014 and 2017 reported that the models were "very helpful" (score 5 of 5) to improve understanding of the anatomy. Similarly, Biglino et al. reported that 3D models could help improve the family's experience with medical care when models were used for counseling. More data are needed on the potentially powerful impact of 3D printing in patient and family education and shared decision making.

Advanced Applications and Future Directions

3D printing is rapidly evolving in medicine, with technical improvements in printers and software fueling new and exciting applications in patient care, innovation, and research. In cardiovascular medicine, a major limitation is high-resolution printing of structures currently not well resolved by CT or MRI, such as atrioventricular valves or the atrial septum. 3D printing from 3D echocardiography could potentially overcome these limitations, with some promising early results.3D printing from angiographic imaging could expand options, currently largely unexplored . The next evolution in 3D printing would be "multimodality" printing, with a model created by combining key elements of the anatomy from different imaging modalities. True co-registration of a highly accurate dataset is a technical challenge, and there are some early feasibility data. In addition to advances in 3D dataset acquisition and post-processing, the next major step forward in 3D printing will likely be driven by improvements in printer technology and print materials. "Tissue mimicking" materials currently under development would enable the creation of more life-like models that replicate the patient's unique anatomy and physiology. Currently there are highly accurate noninvasive methods to assess cardiac function and blood flow , including methods to assess 3D information over the cardiac cycle, thereby providing "4D" function and flow. These multivariate datasets could be integrated into 3D models to build holistic models to advance our understanding of cardiac disease. As 3D models achieve more realistic states, they may be used to study pathophysiology, predict long-term outcomes, and choose optimal treatment plans or surgical repairs. Recent studies have analyzed blood flow in deformable models , including flow characteristics in patients with hypoplastic left heart syndrome following Norwood arch reconstruction. Finally, bioprinting offers the potential to make the leap from printing "life-like" to living tissue itself. This revolutionary technology is in its infancy; however, several techniques now exist that can deposit bioinks in precise locations to build up complex tissue constructs . Bioprinting has been applied to print anatomically shaped cartilage structures , skin , implants for bone growth , and even a 3D printed "bionic ear" Within cardiology, researchers have reported techniques to print vasculature, myocardium, and valves . These applications and bioprinting techniques were recently reviewed by Duan . Although current and future applications of 3D printing are exciting and potentially game-changing, broad adoption is currently hampered by the costs of modeling and printing. The cost of a 3D printing center to a medical program is considerable, and at minimum it includes the cost of segmentation software, a medical-grade 3D printer, material costs, and personnel with 3D printing expertise. Some of the costs may be lowered by printing off-site through commercial vendors, although with inherent trade-offs in long-term costs and turn-around time. These are evolving issues, and the ultimate viability of medical 3D printing will in large part depend on the impact it has on improving patient care.

2. 3D Printing Applications For Percutaneous Structural Interventions In Congenital Heart Disease

The past several decades have seen remarkable advancements in percutaneous interventions for treatment of congenital heart disease (CHD). These advancements have been significantly aided by improvements in noninvasive diagnostic imaging. The use of three-dimensional (3D) printed models for planning and simulation of catheter-based procedures has been demonstrated for numerous cardiac defects and has been shown to reduce complications, procedure times, and limit radiation exposure. This paper reviews the process by which patient-specific 3D cardiac models are produced, as well as numerous applications of these models for use in percutaneous interventions in CHD.

Image postprocessing

Prior to creating a 3D model, a volumetric imaging dataset is acquired. CT and MRI are the most commonly used modalities for creating 3D reconstructions, although echocardiography and rotational angiography have also been used. Preference of one modality over another depends largely on the experience of the center, the structure of interest, and age of patient. CT has been shown to be the easiest modality for model creation as it allows for particularly detailed segmentation of great vessels and intracardiac anatomy due to high spatial resolution

Alternatively, MRI or contrast-enhanced magnetic resonance angiography offers whole heart 3D datasets while avoiding radiation exposure, which is preferred in younger patients. More recently, there have been several reports on the use of 3D echocardiography in creating 3D reconstructions. Novel echocardiographic transducers as well as advancements in software and hardware have enhanced echocardiographic images, making them more suited for 3D modeling The use of echocardiography is beneficial as it is more widely available and avoids both radiation exposure and the necessity of radiocontrast administration. This modality, however, has an inferior tissue-to-blood pool contrast, which makes image segmentation significantly more challenging. Echocardiography is also the preferred means by which to visualize cardiac valves and the atrial septum, which are poorly delineated in both CT and MRI. Hybrid imaging techniques have also been developed, which combine cross-sectional datasets with ultrasound in order to create complete heart models with embedded valve leaflets for more comprehensive visualization of intracardiac anatomy.

Following the acquisition of the imaging dataset, a 3D rendering is created through a process known as segmentation[8]. The files are first uploaded as a DICOM (Digital Imaging and Communications in Medicine) dataset into 3D visualization software, such as Mimics (Materialise, Belgium), or open-source software, such as 3D Slicer (Slicer Wiki). Pixel-intensity-based thresholding is then employed to highlight the blood pool within the desired region. Subsequently, regions of interest are isolated through manual or semi-automatic techniques. The process of segmentation is the most time-consuming step of creating a 3D reconstruction. Accuracy of the model is largely determined by blood pool-to-tissue contrast, spatial resolution of the imaging technique, motion artifact of the image, and the technician's understanding of anatomic relationships]. The 3D rendering is then imported as a stereolithography (stl) file into a 3D visualization software, such as 3-Matic (Materialise, Belgium), or open source programs, such as Blender or Owlet, for postprocessing to establish a print-compatible model.This process involves converting the object into a meshed surface file, hollowing the model, smoothing surfaces, and trimming vessels or chamber walls in order to visualize the area of interest[5]. The 3D rendered object is converted into a computer-aided design format that can be converted into a physical object using a 3D printer. Once complete, the 3D rendering undergoes rapid prototyping on a 3D printer. Capabilities of 3D printers vary based on build volume, layer resolution, materials, and colors available. The print technology utilized should be chosen based on the specific goal of the heart model. In making this decision, the material needed, level of detail, and turnaround time are all taken into consideration. Options for 3D printing include fused deposition modeling (FDM), Colorjet, Polyjet printing, and selective laser sintering. In FDM, a thermoplastic filament is extruded in a specified pattern that immediately hardens. This process typically has a shorter turnaround time and comes at a significantly lower cost. Colorjet printing is an additive manufacturing technology in which a core material is spread in thin layers and solidified by extrusion of a color binder. This technology allows for recreation of highly complex geometries in relatively short production times[. Polyjet printing, in contrast, allows for higher resolution printing of multiple materials in different colors, but it is much more costly and thus less often employed for routine modeling. This technique enables the use of flexible, translucent materials, which are optimal for rehearsing surgical procedures as they can be cut, retracted, and sutured in order to effectively simulate procedures. Additionally, selective laser sintering utilizes a high-power laser to fuse metal or ceramic powder, resulting in a highly accurate model. This method, however, is often cost prohibitive in comparison to other techniques. For each technique, the print material is sequentially layered, and the final model is encased in support material, which can be removed manually or by soaking in a solution.

Clinical applications

The use of 3D printed models has been described widely for numerous percutaneous interventions for the treatment of CHD. One of the most well described interventions in which 3D models play a role is transcatheter valve implantation. These procedures represent the fastest growing area of innovation in the field of pediatric interventional cardiology, with numerous devices developed in the last decade. Transcatheter valve replacements are beneficial because they enable proceduralists to correct valve regurgitation or stenosis without the need for repeat surgical interventions over the course of the patient's life. Among these procedures, pulmonary valve replacement in repaired cases of Tetralogy of Fallot and aortic valve replacement for aortic stenosis or regurgitation are the most widely described. Poterucha et al. described a case of repaired tetralogy of Fallot in which the native right ventricular outflow tract (RVOT) was deemed to be unfavorable for percutaneous intervention. A 3D model of the RVOT was then developed using 3D rotational angiography, which helped the interventionalist identify a landing zone for implantation of a Melody Valve (Medtronic, Fridley, Minnesota). A study by Shievano and colleagues showed that the use of 3D printed models allowed for more accurate selection of candidates for successful percutaneous pulmonary valve implantation (PPVI) than 3D MRI reconstructions alone. Qian et al. demonstrated the use of 3D printed models of the left ventricular outflow tract (LVOT) and aortic root of patients with aortic stenosis. The models approximated the precise anatomy and flexibility of the LVOT, which had substantial tissue calcifications, and were used to test valve implantation prior to the procedure. This permitted the proceduralists to assess the feasibility of the intervention and predict paravalvular leak after transcatheter aortic valve replacement. To test paravalvular leak, the models underwent analysis of strain distribution using a maximum bulge index, which aided in prediction of the degree of leakage following percutaneous valve implantation. This technique ultimately assisted in identifying ideal candidates for percutaneous rather than surgical intervention Along the same lines, Ripley et al. studied the use of 3D models to replicate patient-specific aortic root anatomy prior to transcatheter aortic valve replacement and they found that the models provide insight into how the patient anatomy will interact with implanted medical devices. This enables interventionalists to predict potential challenges in device placement and complications during or following the procedure

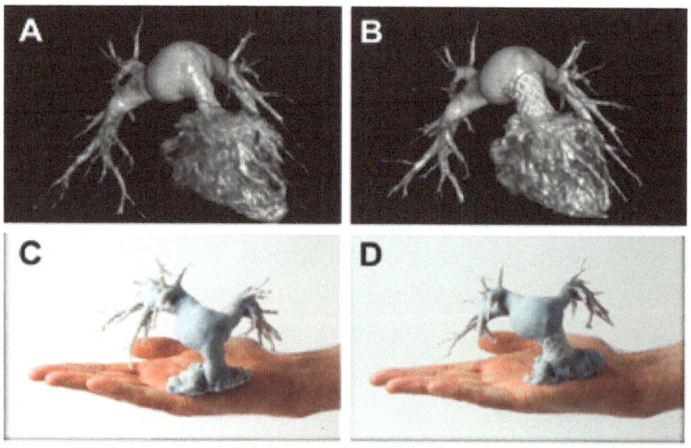

Fig.37.14 3D DynaCT reconstruction and 3D printed models: pre-Melody valve implantation in the RVOT (A, C); and post-Melody valve implantation in the RVOT (B, D). Reprinted with permission from Poterucha et al.. 3D: three-dimensional; RVOT: right ventricular outflow tract

An increasing number of devices have become available for atrioventricular valve repair using a percutaneous approach. Little et al. reported a case in which a 3D printed model was used to aid in procedural planning for a patient undergoing mitral valve repair with Mitraclip (Abbott, Abbott Park, Illinois). This group printed a multi-material 3D model in order to produce more realistic, deformable valve leaflets and recreate subvalvular calcium deposits within the adjacent myocardium. The model was then used to aid in the selection and sizing of the specific clip It enabled more accurate determination of a landing point for the device that avoided adjacent calcified tissue, and provided direct visualization of the effect of the implant on surrounding valve morphology and function Scanlan and colleagues performed a study in which patient-specific pediatric atrioventricular valves were modeled from 3D echocardiography[. The valves were printed and molded using custom software. The molded silicone valves were shown to be significantly more realistic for cutting and suturing, thus enhancing pre-procedural simulation. The technique is presently too time and labor intensive for widespread implementation

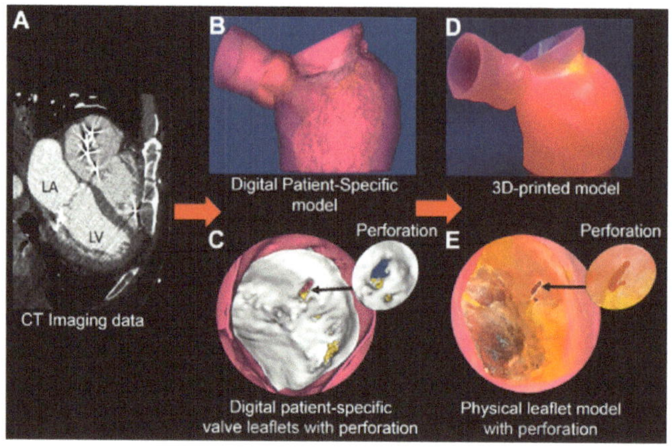

Fig.37.15 CT images (A) are used to create a digital model (B) and to assign tissue properties (C); the multi-material patient-specific 3D model (D, E) is then printed to replicate the mitral valve leaflet geometry, regional calcium deposition, and pathology. Reprinted with permission from Little et al. CT: computed tomography; 3D: three-dimensional

3D printed models are commonly used as guides for percutaneous closure of complicated atrial and ventricular septal defects. Velasco Forte et al. described a case in which a flexible, translucent 3D model was developed from a cardiac MRI in order to simulate the correction of a sinus venosus atrial septal defect (ASD). The model in this case allowed the interventionalists to accurately assess the anatomy and precise spatial relationships among the superior vena cava (SVC), left atrium (LA), and an anomalous pulmonary vein (PV). The model was also used to determine the length of the stent required to close the defect and assess the positioning of the stent necessary to redirect blood flow from the anomalous PV to the LA without obstructing flow from other vessels. Ultimately, a custom stent was successfully implanted into the SVC to close the sinus venosus ASD and commit the anomalous PV drainage correctly to the LA.

Another technically challenging percutaneous intervention that has the potential to be enhanced by patient-specific 3D printed models is endovascular stenting of the aorta in cases of aortic hypoplasia or coarctation. Placement of a stent within the aorta can result in many complications including stent migration, stroke, and occlusion of head and neck vessels by the stent itself. Valverde et al. presented a case in which a 3D model of a hypoplastic transverse aortic arch was created that closely mimicked the distensibility of the native vasculature and its response to stent delivery. In the case described, the endovascular stenting procedure was simulated on the printed model under fluoroscopic guidance prior to the percutaneous intervention. This simulation provided the proceduralists the opportunity to devise an optimal interventional approach, as well as determine the appropriate stent size, length, and position within the aorta3D printed models have recently been described for use in patients undergoing left atrial appendage (LAA) closure. Occlusion of the LAA in patients with atrial fibrillation significantly reduces thromboembolic risk in those who have contraindications to systemic anticoagulation. Given the variable dimensions and morphology of the LAA, accurately sizing and positioning an occluder device in the orifice of the LAA can be challenging. Additionally, implanting a sub-optimally sized device to occlude the orifice can result in complications such as peri-device leakage, thrombus formation, device migration, and cardiac injury.Fan et al. conducted a study assessingthe utility of 3D printed models created from 3D trans-esophageal echocardiography to aid in the selection of an appropriately sized device . They found that device sizing based on 3D-printed models was associated with higher implantation success, shorter procedural times, and fewer complications. Iriart et al. described their technique of printing the entire left atrium and atrial septum in addition to the LAA in order to determine the optimal orientation for transseptal puncture during device placement. They also found that the models are invaluable in training physicians and fellows and augmenting communication with patients.

Percutaneous closure of patent ductus arteriosus (PDA) is another intervention that has the potential to benefit from the use of 3D printed models. Particularly in adult cases, the PDA can be long, tortuous, and calcified, which makes catheter-based device placement challenging. Matsubara and colleagues presented a case in which patient-specific 3D printed models were created to detail the precise anatomy of the proximal aorta, aortic arch, PDA, and pulmonary artery.These models allowed for selection of a particular device and exact size. They also allowed the interventionalists to simulate and practice device deployment within the models themselves, thereby decreasing fluoroscopic and procedural times.

3D models can be instrumental in decision making to determine feasibility of transcatheter intervention.

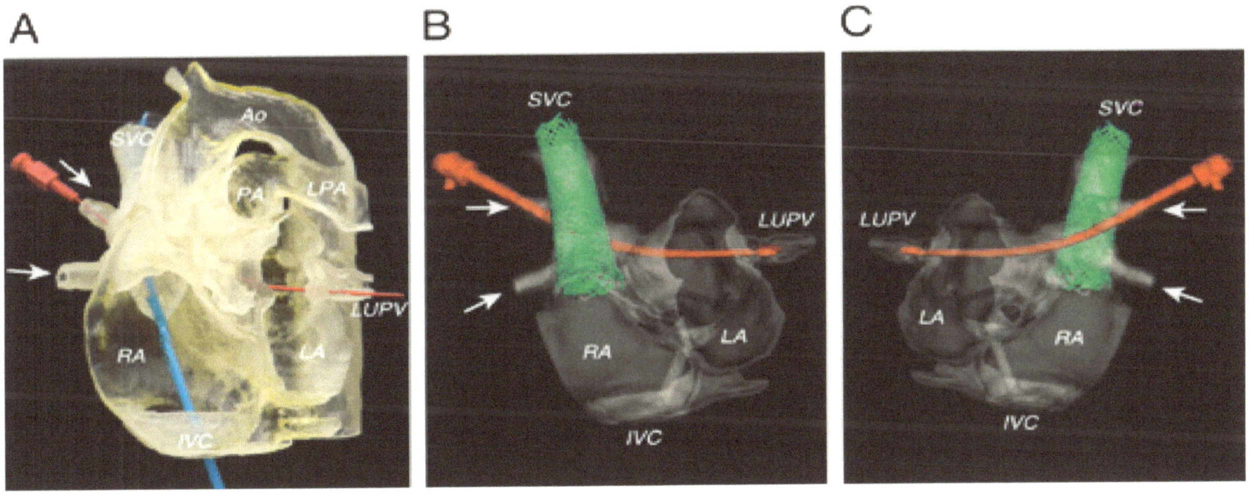

Fig.37.16 The flexible, translucent model (A) was examined to assess the relationship of the anomalous PVs (arrows) to the SVC and LA. A balloon-mounted stent catheter was placed in the SVC to RA junction (blue catheter), while a dilator (red) was passed from the anomalous right upper PV to the left upper PV. This model allowed for calculation of the length of the stent required to close the defect and redirect the flow of the partial anomalous pulmonary venous drainage toward the LA. CT of the model was performed using 3D rotational X-ray acquisition, shown from anteroposterior (B) and postero-anterior views (C) (dilator in red; stent in green). Reprinted with permission from Velasco Forte et al.[18]. PV: pulmonary vein; SVC: superior vena cava; LA: left atrium; RA: right atrium; CT: computed tomography; 3D: three-dimensional

A recent case at our center involved a 78-year-old patient with a sinus venosus atrial septal defect with partial anomalous pulmonary venous return of the right upper pulmonary vein (RUPV) to the superior vena cava. A 3D model was created from a cardiac CT to demonstrate the relationship between the anomalous pulmonary venous return, atrial communication, and left atrium for potential use of a covered stent toreroute the RUPV flow. Although the cross-sectional imaging was helpful in delineating the pulmonary venous anatomy, the 3D model provided a much clearer picture of the spatial relationship among the RUPV, superior vena cava, and the left atrium. It was determined that use of a covered stent would result in occlusion of the RUPV in the position needed to ensure stent stability and avoid embolization.Thep atient will undergo surgical intervention for this congenital heart defect.Finally, We described a case in which a large fistula, arising from the left coronary artery to the right atrium, was modeled in order to devise an approach for interventional closure.The 3D printed model enabled the interventionalists to consider several different approaches to transcatheter closure of the fistula .

Practicing the device closure on the 3D model demonstrated the feasibility of using a venous approach to access the fistula and provided insight on the optimal device to use for the procedure, with the goal of ultimately limiting procedure time and thereby reducing radiation exposure

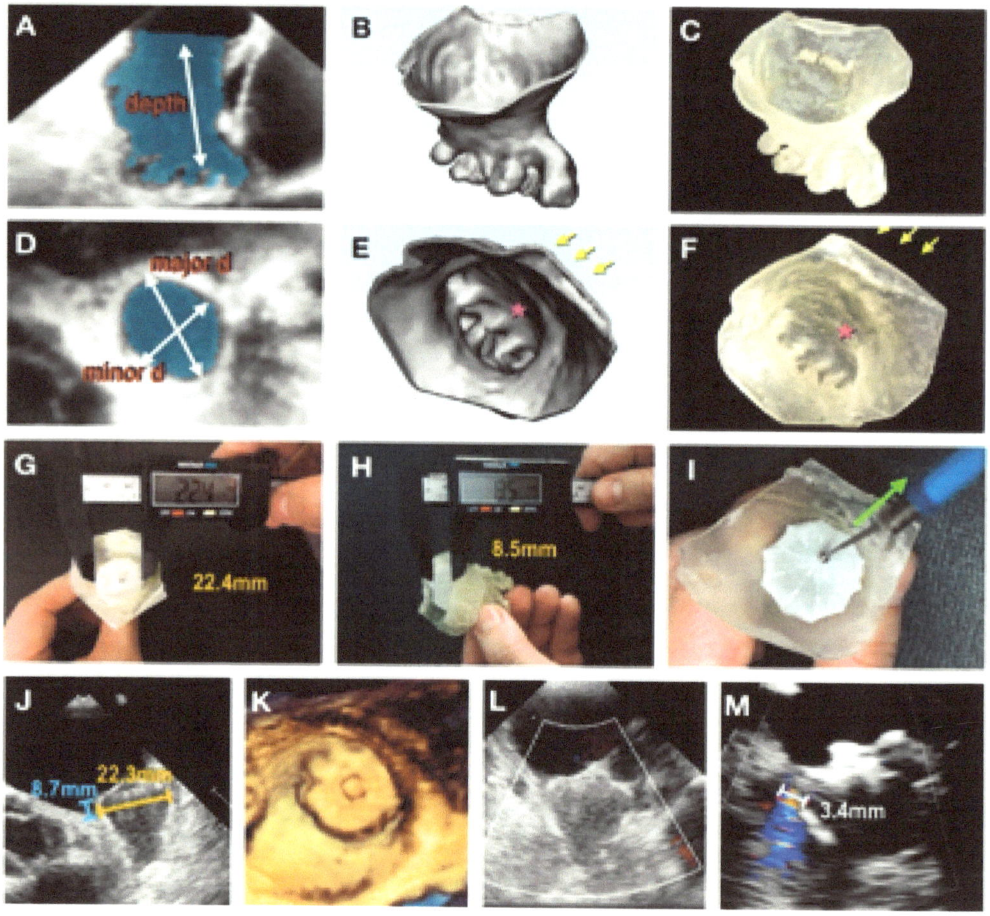

Fig.37.17 Echocardiography-based 3D printing of patient-specific models. Segmentation of LAA (shaded area) from 3D TEE data (A, D) is turned into a digital object (B, E), and printed using tissue-mimicking material (C, F). The major and minor ostial diameters and depth of the LAA are measured. Arrows denote pulmonary vein ridge; stars denote appendicular trabeculations. Closure devices are then sized and placed within the 3D model (G-I), and device compression and (H) protrusion are measured using a digital caliper. Device stability is assessed using the tug-test (I). Device placement visualized on TEE (J-L), and color Doppler assessment showing no peri-device leak (M). Reprinted with permission from Fan et al. LAA: left atrial appendage; TEE: trans-esophageal echocardiogram; CT: computed tomography; 3D: three-dimensional

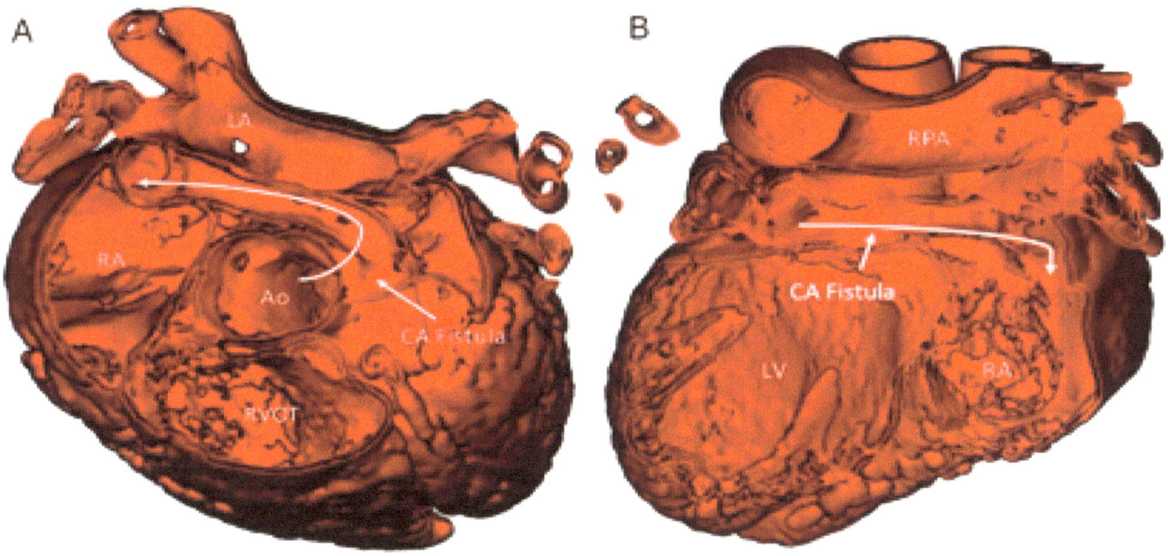

Fig. 37.18 The course of the coronary fistula (CAF) is viewed from a short axis view of the heart. From the leftward aspect of the aortic root, it courses posterior to the aorta (Ao) and rightward to drain into the right atrium (RA) (A); coronal view of the heart, as viewed from the posterior aspect, reveals the course of the CA fistula, almost parallel to the right pulmonary artery (RPA) from left to right to drain into the right atrium (B). CA: coronary artery; LA: left atrium; RVOT: right ventricular outflow tract

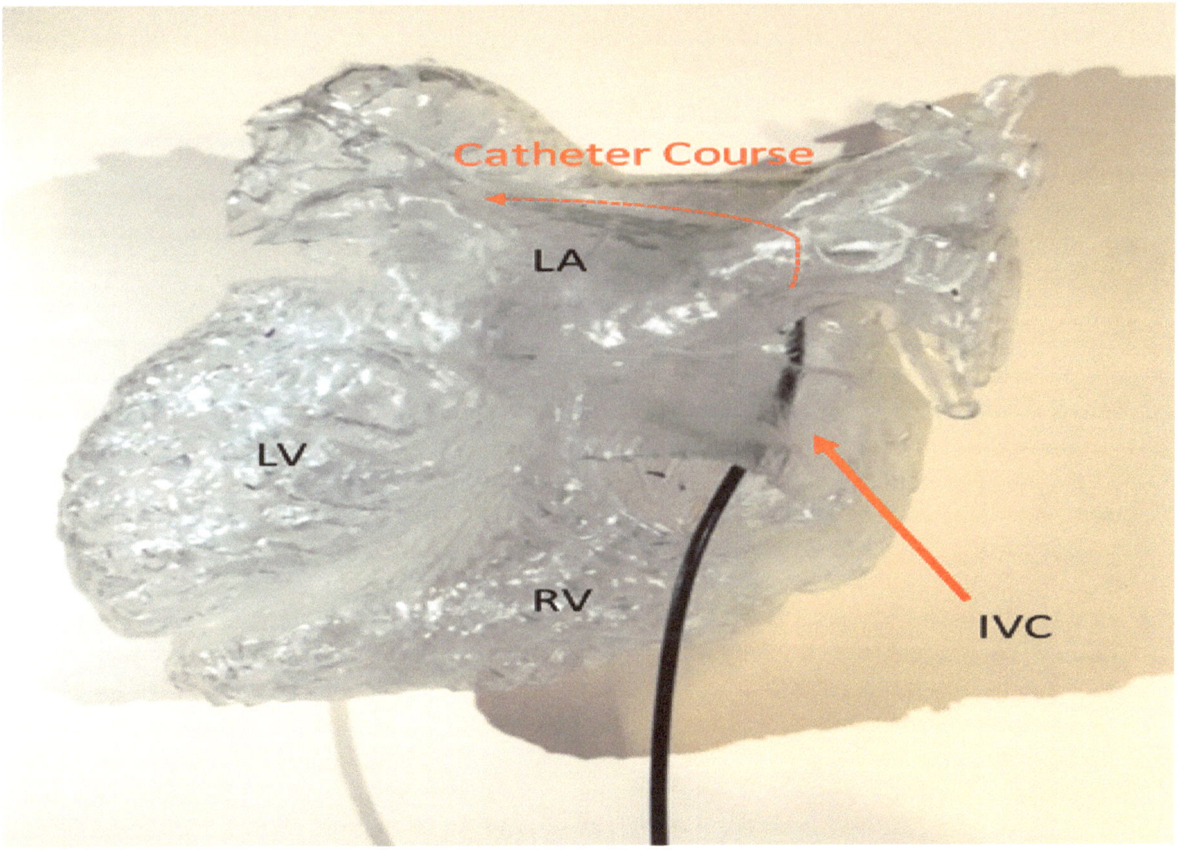

Fig.37.19 3D printed model of the CA printed in a clear resin (Formlabs, Somerville, MA) allows planning of the transcatheter approach to closure of the fistula as viewed from the posterior aspect. A catheter courses from the inferior vena cava through the fistula (red dotted line). 3D: three-dimensional; CA: coronary artery; LA: left atrium; LV: left ventricular; RV: right ventricular; IVC: inferior vena cava

Limitations

There are numerous limitations to creating and using 3D printed models that have prevented widespread adoption in most programs. A major consideration is that the creation of 3D models is a time-intensive process requiring familiarity with segmentation and computer automated design software, as well as an in-depth understanding of cardiac morphology. There is no standardized approach to creating these models, which can ultimately result in a wide variation in the quality of models produced. This was evidenced by Burkhardt et al. in an article evaluating the inter-operator variability in modeling the RVOT based on the threshold chosen for the initial segmentation. Another limitation is that rigid, or even flexible, 3D printed models only provide a snapshot of the cardiac structure at a specific point in the highly dynamic cardiac cycle, thus limiting our understanding of how these structures will change over the course of one heartbeat. Finally, creation of these models, while helpful in procedural planning, is not reimbursed by most insurance companies, and the prohibitively high cost of the software and 3D printing equipment significantly limits their utility on a routine basis. More studies are required to further assess the cost-effectiveness and diagnostic accuracy of these models prior to widespread implementation in the field of pediatric cardiology.

Future directions

Recently, there has been movement toward developing materials that more closely mimic the feel and behavior of myocardium, valve leaflets, and vessel walls. Novel materials combined with the use of multiple imaging modalities could also aid in enhanced identification of valve tissue, chordae tendineae, and other structures that are less well defined with current methods. Developing models that accurately mimic both healthy and pathologic tissue would be invaluable in implementing these models routinely. This advancement would not only allow for more accurate procedural planning but also be invaluable in training surgeons and interventionalists..Further advances in imaging techniques and software to ease the burden of segmentation would allow for more widespread implementation of this technology to a broader range of conditions.

Finally, 3D printing has the potential to aid in the design and construction of patient-specific catheter-based devices for numerous percutaneous interventions, which would further help to decrease procedural complications and improve long-term outcomes.

Conclusion

3D printed models have become increasingly invaluable tools in the field of pediatric cardiology. These models improve diagnostic ability, guide perioperative planning, and have thereby ushered in a vast array of new surgical and interventional approaches and techniques. Interventional cardiology has particularly benefitted from the advancement of 3D modeling, as the models can be used to devise and adjust procedural approaches and practice percutaneous procedures, which has the potential to drastically reduce complications, decrease procedure times, and significantly limit radiation exposure. Ultimately, the use of 3D models has significantly improved our ability to practice personalized medicine and has helped to enhance the care of patients with cardiac defects through percutaneous procedures.

3. 3D Printing in Congenital Heart Dseases

Congenital heart diseases causing significant hemodynamic and functional consequences require surgical repair. Understanding of the precise surgical anatomy is often challenging and can be inadequate or wrong. Modern high resolution imaging techniques and 3D printing technology allow 3D printing of the replicas of the patient's heart for precise understanding of the complex anatomy, hands-on simulation of surgical and interventional procedures, and morphology teaching of the medical professionals and patients. CT or MR images obtained with ECG-gating and breath-holding or respiration navigation are best suited for 3D printing. 3D echocardiograms are not ideal but can be used for printing limited areas of interest such as cardiac valves and ventricular septum.Although the print materials still require optimization forrepresentation of cardiovascular tissues and valves, the surgeons find the models suitable for practicing closure of the septal defects, application of the baffles within the ,

Table 37.1 Imaging techniques applicable for 3D Tprinting of heart models

Imaging Modality	Imaging Techniques
Computed tomography (CT)	• ECG-gated breath-held contrast-enhanced angiography • Non-ECG-gated contrast-enhanced angiography
Magnetic resonance (MR)	• Non-contrast 3D SSFP (steady state free precession) imaging • Non-ECG-gated 3D FLASH (fast low angle shot) angiography using gadolinium -based extracellular contrast agent • ECG-gated respiration-navigated 3D IR (inversion recovery) FLASH angiography using gadolinium-based blood pool contrast agent (Gadofoveset: ABLAVAR®, Lantheus Medical Imaging, Inc. MA, USA) • ECG-gated respiration-navigated 4D MUSIC (multiphase steady-state imaging with contrast enhancement) using ultra-small supermagnetic iron oxide (USPIO: Ferumoxyol, AMAG Pharmaceuticals, Lexington, MA, USA)
Ultrasound	• 3D grey-scale echocardiography • 3D color or power Doppler echocardiography
X-ray angiography	• Rotational CT angiography

ventricles reconstructing the aortic arch, and arterial switch procedure. Hands-on surgical training (HOST) on models may soon become a mandatory component of congenital heart disease surgery program. 3D printing will expand its utilization with further improvement of the use of echocardiographic data and image fusion algorithm across multiple imaging modalities and development of new printing materials. Bioprinting of implants such as stents, patches and artificial valves and tissue engineering of a part of or whole heart using the patient's own cells will open the door to a new era of personalized medicine

Applicable medical imaging techniques

Any medical images acquired in 3D demonstrating the blood pool distinct from the myocardium and vessel wall can be used for 3D printing . Ideally, electrocardiographic (ECG) gating and breath-holding or respiration navigation is required to avoid artifact from cardiac and respiratory motion. However, the images obtained without ECG-gatingand/or free breath ingare still applicable for 3D printing if it is not aimed to show small structures such as coronary arteries. The volume data with isotropic resolution is preferred.ECG-gated CT angiograms provide a spatial resolution of 0.3–0.7 mm and are the most commonly used images among currently applicable imaging modalities in 3D printing of cardiovascular structures. In CT angiography, it is important to time the scanning when all cardiac chambers are homogeneously enhanced. It is also important to inject a generous amount of saline chaser to minimize the artifact from undiluted contrast medium remaining in the superior or inferior vena cava and its tributaries. Although MR angiograms may provide <1 mm spatial resolution, high resolution imaging is at the expense of significant compromise in signal-to-noise ratio. If there is no significant stenotic lesion or valvular regurgitation that cause artifact from turbulent flow, non-contrast 3D SSFP (steady state free precession) imaging provides the images of sufficient quality. However, contrast-enhanced angiography is required in most cases with congenital heart disease. In conventional MR angiography using an extracellular contrast agent

ECG-gating is hardly applicable and a degree of artifact from cardiac motion is unavoidable. ECG-gated and respiration-navigated 3D FLASH (fast low angle shot) angiography using blood-pool contrast agent (Gadofoveset: ABLAVAR®, Lantheus Medical Imaging, Inc. MA, USA) provides excellent images with homogeneous distribution of contrast medium and no significant artifact from turbulent flow Most recently, ultrasmall superparamagnetic iron oxide (USPIO: Ferumoxyol, AMAG Pharmaceuticals, Lexington, MA, USA) that is used for treatment of iron deficiency anemia has been tried for angiography in children with excellent results and can certainly be applied for 3D printing. Ultrasound is not an ideal imaging modality for 3D printing because of the limited access windows for imaging and abundant artifacts from bones and air. However, certain parts of the heart such as atrial and ventricular septa can be imaged appropriately for 3D printing . Although the results are not satisfactory, cardiac valve leaflets can also be imaged and printed with ultrasound data. Lastly, rotational CT angiograms obtained from modern x-ray angiographic equipment can be used for 3D printing

Post-processing of image data

The postprocessing procedure includes:

1) segmentation, 2) conversion of the DICOM (Digital Imaging and Communication in Medicine) file to the STL (Stereolithography or Standard Tessellation Language) or other file fomat for 3D printing, and 3) computer aided design (CAD)

The blood pool is segmented using thresholding algorithm with manual adjustment . The better the image quality, the easier the segmentation process. When the boundary between the blood pool and the myocardium or vessel wall is not readily recognizable by automated thresholding, extensive manual work using drawing, erasing and regional thresholding tools and interpolation of the data between the slices are required. The manual work requires in depth understating of normal and pathological anatomy as well as its appearance on cross-sectional imaging. Once segmentation is completed, the 3D volume data is converted to a file format for 3D printing

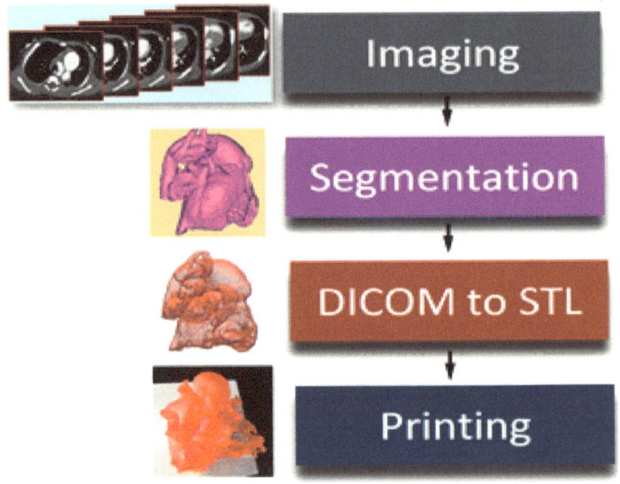

Fig.37.20 Diagram showing the steps in data processing for 3D printing. DICOM, digital imaging and communication in medicine; STL, stereolithography, standard tessellation language or standard triangle language

The file format conversion process includes a user-defined number of iterations for smoothing of the surface of the object. The lower number of iteration provides the models that are close to what are in the original image data, while the surface of the model may appear rough. The higher number of iteration provides a smoother surface of the model, while the detail of the surface anatomy is compromised to a certain extent. The operator needs to define the optimum number of iteration and smoothing factor according to the purposes of 3D printing. As the current imaging technologies do not provide good images of the cardiac valves, it is advisable to demarcate the annuli of the cardiac valves on the model. By marking a few points on the attachment of the valves to the wall using CAD program, an interpolated line of valve insertion is created and assigned a thickness . The graphically designed annuli of the cardiac valves are then added to the model. For the assessment of congenital heart diseases, two types of heart models are valuable: cast models of blood pool and wall models for endocardial surface representation. Cast models provide an excellent overview of the anatomy. Wall models provide detailed information regarding the endocardial surface anatomy. It is ideal to have the entire wall of the heart and vessels represented in the 3D print models

To achieve this goal, both inner and outer boundaries of the cardiac cavities and vessels (endocardial and epicardial surfaces for the heart) should be delineated. Although achievable, it is a time consuming process to delineate the outer boundary of the wall as the signal intensities of the myocardium and vessels are not distinctively different from those of the adjacent mediastinal tissues. Furthermore, a complete wall model requires a large amount of expensive print material, while it is stiff and heavy. As the surgeons operate mostly on the inside of the heart, it is generally sufficient if the endocardial surface anatomy is accurately shown on the models.

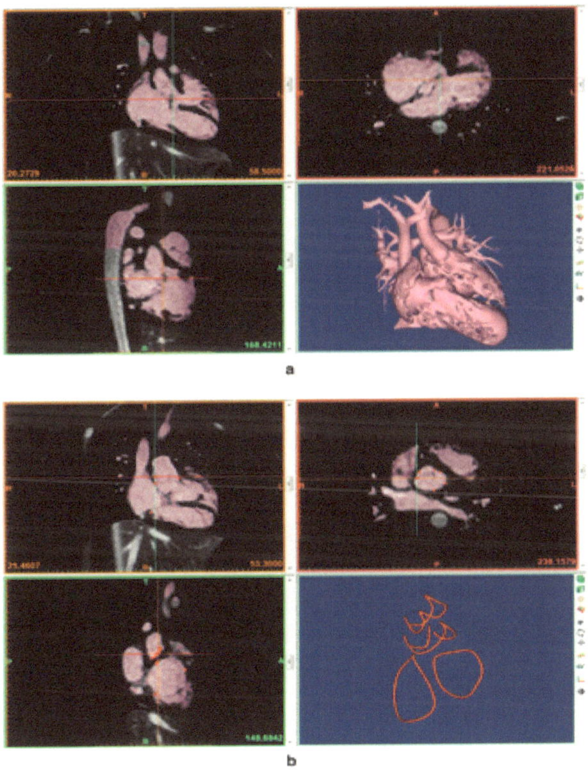

Fig.37.21 Segmentation process in a commercially available software program (Mimics®, Materialise, Leuven, Belgium) using magnetic resonance angiograms from a patient with congenitally corrected transposition of the great arteries with a ventricular septal defect. a Segmentation using thresholding and manual edition with a volume rendered image on the right lower panel. b Linear representation of the cardiac valvar attachments. A few points of attachment sites of each cardiac valve were marked and connected using a tool called "spline"

The endocardial surface anatomy can be represented by graphically adding a shell on the surface of the cavity cast that is clearly and distinctly definable. The result is a negative of the cast model with a wall of an arbitrary thickness . In order to visualize the inner surfaces of the heart and vessels, a few windows are made on the shell. For surgical practice, the entry window for surgical procedure is opened and the model is mounted on the plate to provide a stable position and to restrict movement of the model during the procedure . However, such shelling process is not applicable for representation of the lumens of small and tightly packed vessels such as peripheral pulmonary arteries and veins.

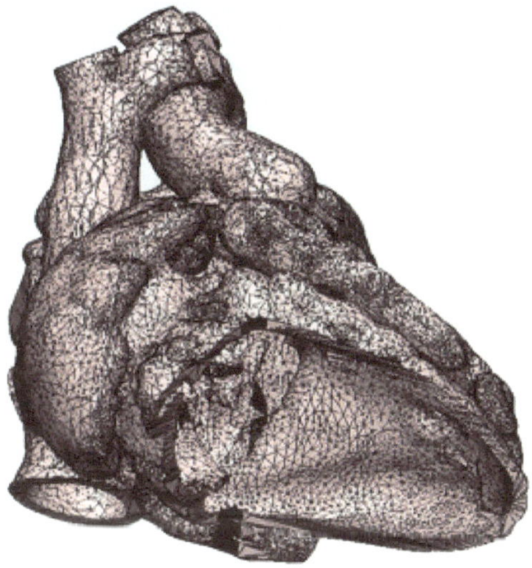

Fig.37.22 Surface geometry in STL (Stereolithography or Standard Tessellation Language) . The surface of the object is divided into a number of triangles without any gap and overlap

3D printing process

The STL files are loaded to the software program of the 3D printer and the materials are assigned to the files for printing. Most commercially available 3D printers are designed for building rigid plastic models, while a few printers are capable of building models with soft rubber-like materials. Ideally, the printing material should have the physical properties such as consistency, elasticity, tensile strength,tear resistance and memory capacity are similar to those of human soft tissue.

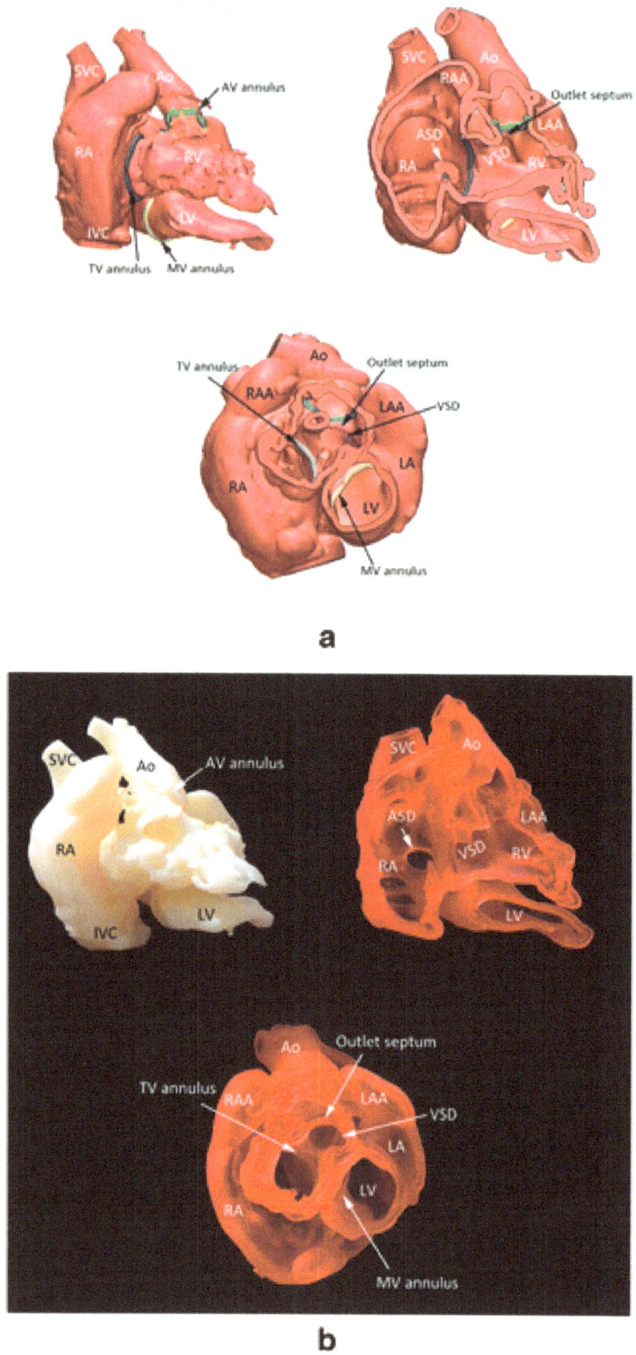

Fig.37.23 Screen-display of the STL files (a) and photographs of the corresponding models (b) in a case with so-called twisted or criss-cross heart with transposition of the great arteries and a ventricular septal defect (VSD). Cast model (top left), wall model after removal of the anterior free wall of the right atrium and right and left ventricles (top right), and wall model with the apical two thirds of the ventricles removed (bottom) are shown. The cardiac valve annuli are marked by the spline curves that were graphically designed as shown in Fig. 2B. Ao, aorta; ASD, atrial septal defect; AV, aortic valve; IVC, inferior vena cava; LA, left atrium; LAA, left atrial appendage; LV, left ventricle; MV, mitral valve; SVC, superior vena cava; TV, tricuspid valve

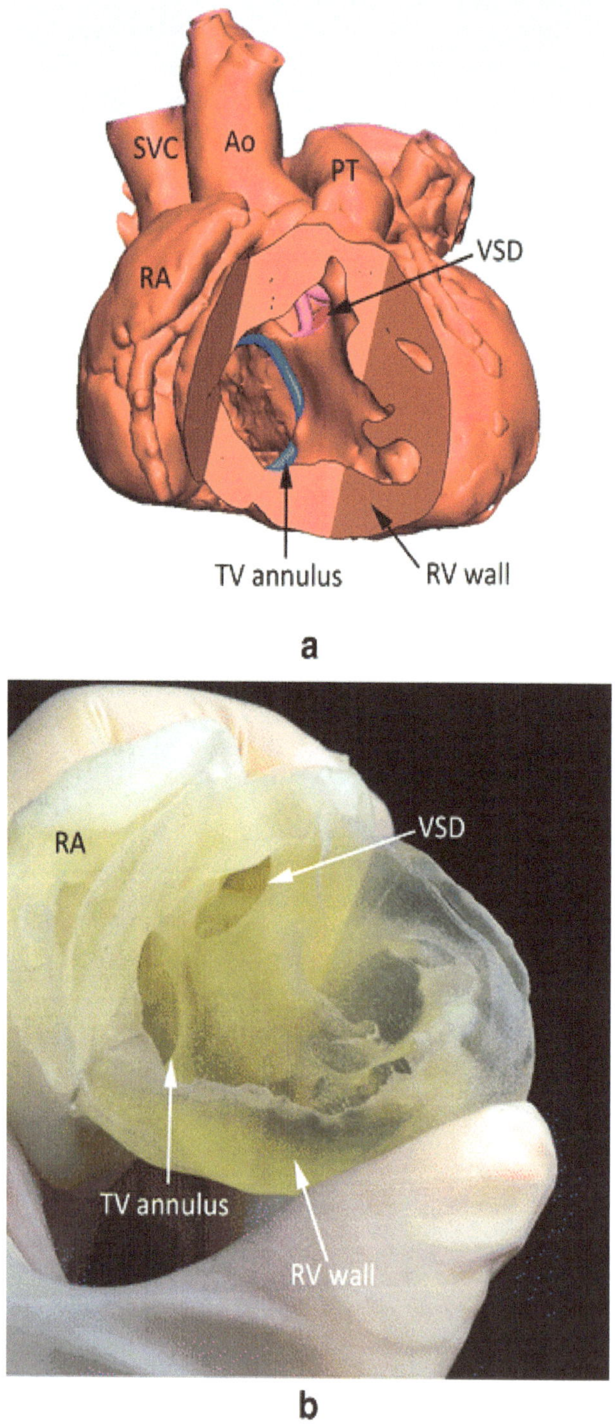

Fig.37.24 Screen-display (a) and photograph (b) of the 3D print model of the heart with tetralogy of Fallot. The full thickness of the myocardium was carefully segmented with both endocardial and epicardial boundaries delineated by thresholding and manual editing. Although it is considered ideal, the postprocessing was time consuming and the model is stiff to be used for surgical simulation. Ao, aorta; PT, pulmonary trunk; SVC, superior vena cava; TV, tricuspid valve; RA, right atrium; RV, right ventricle; VSD, ventricular septal defect

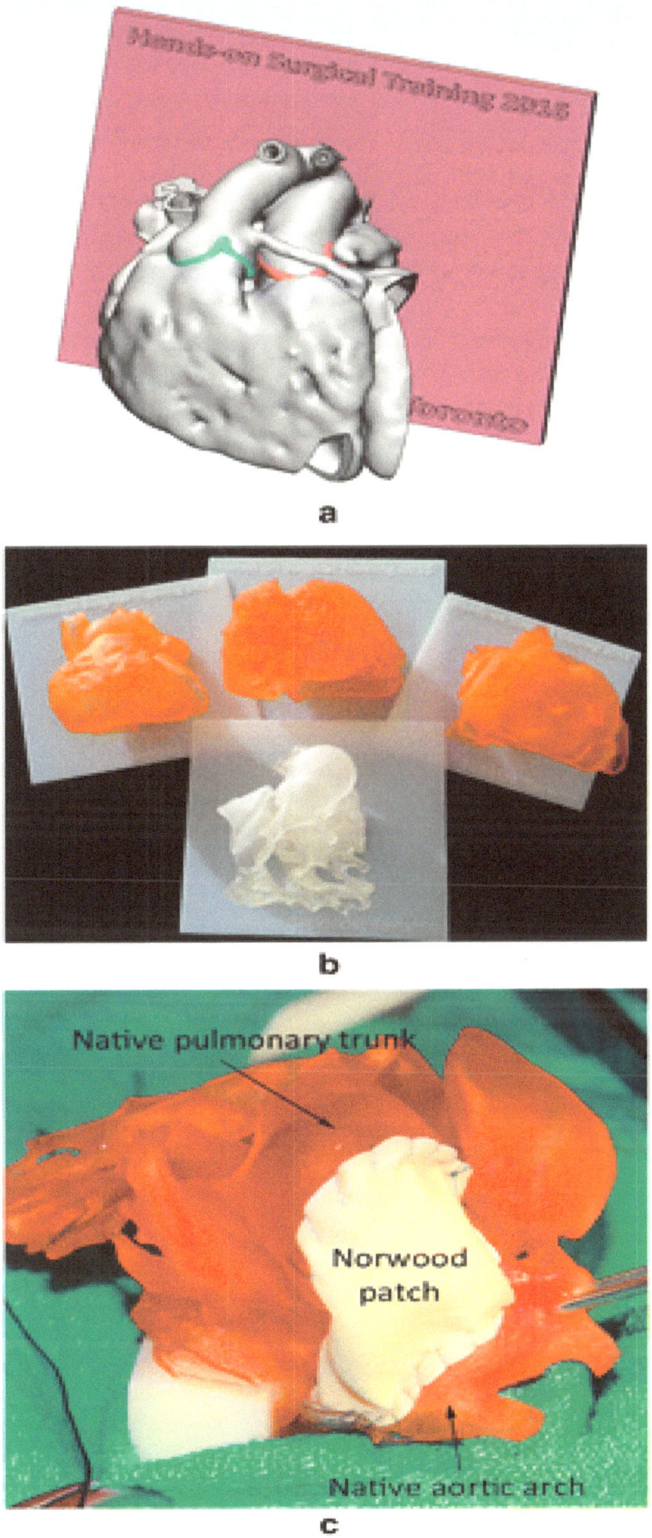

Fig.37.25 Models for surgical practice or training. a Screen-display of the STL file shows the heart mounted on a graphically designed platform. b Four example models for surgical training. c A 3D print model with hypoplastic left heart syndrome on which a surgeon underwent a Norwood procedure

Among the existing 3D printers, the printers using polyjet technology and photopolymer resin materials (Objet Connex Series printer and TangoPlus FullCure resin, Stratasys Ltd, Minnesota, USA, and Projet 5500X printer and Visijet CE NT-Elastomeric Natural resin, 3DSystems, Rockhill, USA) provide the physical properties of the printed models closest to those of human soft tissue, allowing simulated surgical and interventional procedures. If the purpose of 3D printing is for demonstration of the anatomy of the heart, any commercially available printer with an acceptable print resolution can be used

With current 3D printing technology, 3D printing typically takes 3–10 hours to build a single piece of the heart model depending on its size. After the model is completely built, it is harvested and the supporting material and/or the unused print materials are washed out with a waterjet, blown away with an airjet or melted down with chemicals and water. Depending on the materials used and the complexity of the geometry, this cleaning process takes a few minutes to an hour. Powder-based models require curing with chemicals and heat. Although some printers build the models with multiple colors, others provide limited color options. When the printed model is white or faintly colored, one may want to dye the model with a slightly dark color for improved perceptual representation of the complex surface anatomy.

Current applications

Planning and simulation for surgical and interventional procedures.

Preoperative assessment with 3D print models reduces the degree of uncertainty as regards to the patient's specific anatomy. In selected cases, 3D printing can contribute to an improved outcome as precise preoperative understanding of the complex anatomy may obviate or shorten lengthy exploration, and therefore operation and cardiopulmonary bypass time can be reduced . Surgical procedure on a patient with congenital heart disease is usually performed through a midline sternotomy or lateral thoracotomy and a small incision in the wall of an atrium, an arterial trunk or, rarely, a ventricle. As the patient's thorax and heart sizes are small in children the actual surgical scene is difficult to inspect especially from the assistant's position during the surgery. If the sterilized models showing the important surgical anatomy of the patient's heart.were given to the surgical team, the primary operator's procedure would be facilitated with precise and streamlined assistance from the assistants. In addition, 3D print models made of flexible material can be used for practice surgery before the real operation.

For preoperative assessment of congenital heart diseases, we typically make three models for each case: a cast model of blood pool for the overview, a wall model with the atrial and ventricular free wall partly removed for the atrial and ventricular septal anatomy, and a wall model with the apical halves to two thirds of the ventricles removed for the anatomy of the bases of the ventricles . As discussed, a model mounted on a plate can be provided for preoperative surgical practice The most common indication was double outlet right ventricle where the feasibility of intraventricular baffling procedure should be accurately assessed before undergoing biventricular repair . In this regard, 3D print models certainly provide the surgeons with clear and undisputable information. Although it is rare, so-called twisted or criss-cross heart is an important indication for 3D printing . In these cases, the spatial relationship of the cardiac chambers and great arteries and overall intracardiac anatomy are difficult to understand and explain.

With the 3D print models in the observer's hands, complex anatomy can be understood instantaneously and requires no explanation using ambiguous terminology introduced in the description of this particular pathology

For the surgical simulation, the print materials are still far from ideal and the representation of the cardiac valves is limited. The print material does not represent tissue properties of myocardium and enocardial and epicardial linings, limiting assessment of the tissue response to the surgical procedure or deployment of medical devices. In our limited experience, however, the surgeons find the models suitable for practicing surgical simulation procedures such as closure of the septal defects, application of the baffles within the ventricles, reconstructing the aortic arch, and arterial switch procedure (Fig. 6). 3D print models are also used for interventional procedures to test whether the size and shape of the device would fit the patient's specific anatomy and to practice the intended procedure

Contemporary morphology teaching with 3D print models

Traditionally, pathological specimens removed from the patients during autopsy or heart transplantation are used for cardiac morphology teaching. Although the specimens are valuable

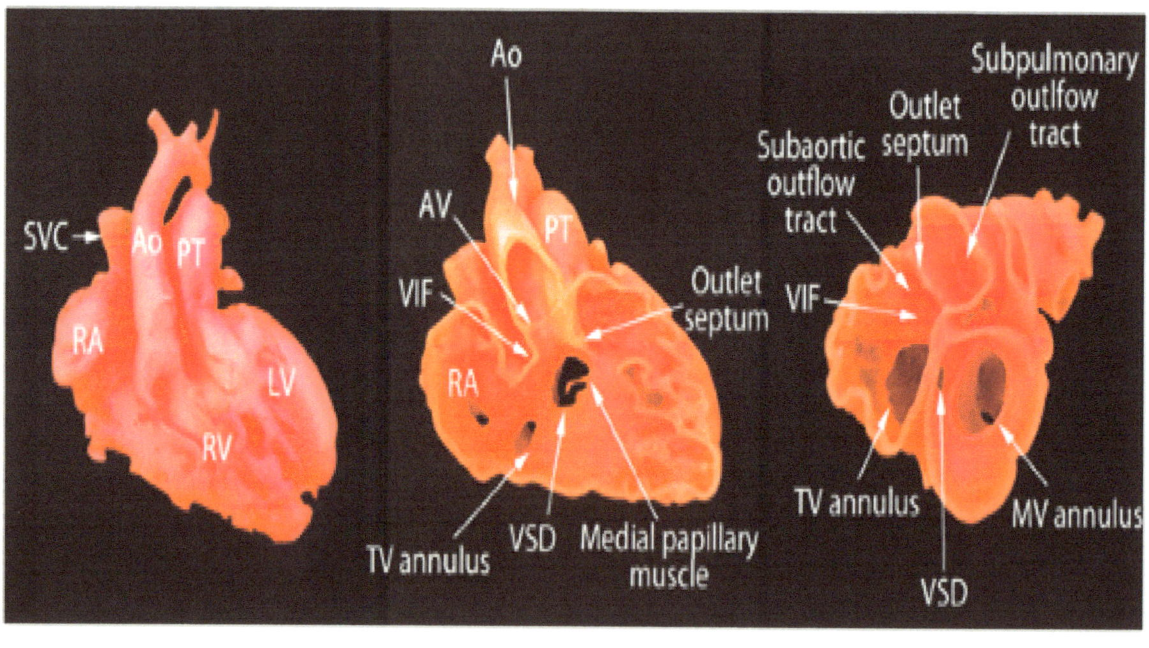

Fig.37.26 Photographs of the 3D print models of a case with double outlet right ventricle. Although echocardiograms showed that the ventricular septal defect (VSD) is remote from both arterial valves, 3D models show that the VSD is able to be routed to the aortic valve allowing biventricular repair. Ao, aorta; AV, aortic valve; LA, left atrium; LV, left ventricle; MV, mitral valve; SVC, superior vena cava; TV, tricuspid valve; VIF, ventriculoinfundibular fold

educational resources, they are scarce and do not represent the whole spectrum of pathology. With improvement of the surgical and medical management of congenital heart diseases and changing concept on human right issues regarding retention of the removed human organs in the pathology laboratory, fewer specimens will be available. On the other hand, the existing specimens are exposed to wear and tear. 3D print models are great educational resources . By using the living patients' imaging data, almost entire varieties of congenital heart diseases can be covered with 3D print models. The pathological features can be demonstrated in any desired planes or views. Any number of models can be reproduced and shared, and access to the models is not limited. With current technology, however, the valve tissues and myocardial pathology are hardly reproducible. Despite such a limitation, contemporary morphology teaching sessions using 3D printed educational model sets have increasingly been introduced in international and national meetings in the last few years

3D print models are helpful in education of the patients and their parents. The patient's cardiovascular pathology and the intended or previously performed surgical or interventional procedures are easy to understand when they are explained using 3D print models.

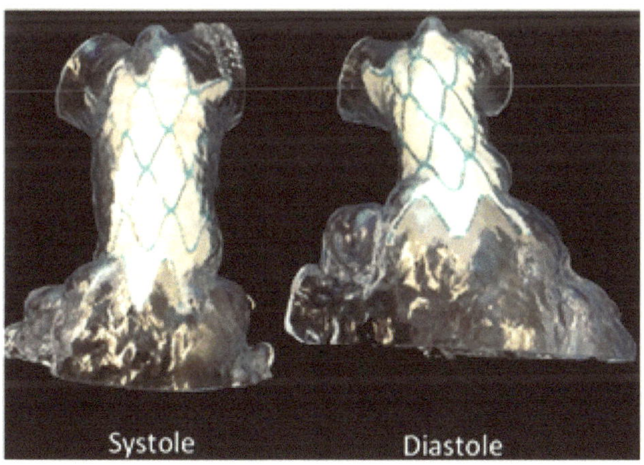

Fig.37.27 Photographs of the 3D print models of right ventricular outflow tract obtained in systole and diastole from a patient with severe pulmonary regurgitation after repair of tetralogy of Fallot. The fitness of the stent in the outflow tract was tested for both systole and diastole before the procedure

Hands-on surgical training (HOST)

Learning surgical techniques in congenital heart disease is challenging. As discussed, the size of the heart in children is usually small and the access routes for the procedure are limited for observation. In addition, the rarity of certain congenital heart diseases further limits the opportunity to learn and to improve the surgical skills. 3D printed models are great resources for surgical training . The supervisors can take unlimited time in showing their procedures. The trainees can take enough time in learning and practicing surgical procedures and repeat the procedures until they feel confident. To the experienced surgeons, 3D print models can be used for development of the new procedures or to improve their surgical skills for rare diseases.

In a personal communication, one of our senior surgeons commented that it usually takes a few years for the surgeons to learn how to do the Norwood operation in hypoplastic left heart syndrome and that he should have been able to learn the procedure overnight if 3D print models of a few cases with different pathologic variations would have been available for practice. We organized or supported three HOST courses in the last 12 months. All three courses were successful with high audience satisfaction [Yoo SJ, Spray T, Austine E, van Arsdell GS, et al. Hands-on surgical training (HOST) on congenital heart surgery using 3D print models. In preparation].

We strongly advise the surgeons and trainees to practice their surgical skills on 3D print models first before performing the specific operation on the patients.

Current limitations

The limitations of 3D printing occur in all stages, during imaging, postprocessing and printing. Precise representation of any moving anatomical structures requires high spatial and temporal resolutions. With currently available imaging technologies, it is difficult to image the fine moving structures such as valve leaflets and chordae tendinae with the image quality sufficient enough for 3D printing.

These fine structures are important as the abnormalities in these structures are usually associated with significant hemodynamic functional consequences and require delicate surgical repair. As discussed, 3D printing has significant limitations in using the data from ultrasound which is the primary and cheapest imaging technology in cardiac imaging. Segmentation of the required structures in postprocessing software programs primarily relies on thresholding of signal intensities. When the adjacent structures do not have distinctly different signal intensities allowing automatic boundary detection, extensive time-consuming manual editing is required and the accuracy is significantly compromised

It is ideal to print the heart using flexible materials with the physical properties similar to that of the human myocardium and valve tissues, especially when practice procedures were to be performed on the models. There are only a few flexible print materials, each of them being able to be used on a specific type of printer only. The surgeons find the models made of flexible material are more difficult to be sewn and easily torn or cut through as compared to real human myocardium or vessels

The most important limiting factor in applications of 3D printing in patient care and teaching medical professionals is its high cost rather than its utility. The available software programs, printers and printing materials are expensive. Postprocessing is labor-intensive and often requires the hands of experienced imagers. Although 3D printing is also called rapid prototyping, it is fundamentally a time consuming process to build any object by adding numerous layers. The expenses per case can be unbearably high for small programs

Although most 3D printers are provided with the company's own specification regarding print resolution, reports on its reproducibility and accuracy in human applications are scarce and prospective studies in larger cohorts are required. Nonetheless, it is of no doubt that 3D models are very helpful in understanding the complex morphology and spatial relationship among the structures. However, the models should be carefully reviewed in conjunction with the standard imaging findings as certain degrees of distortion and abbreviation of the information are inevitable during postprocessing and printing.

As have been the cases for any other procedures in their early developing phases when the objective data are lacking or scarce, it will take time for the insurance and its governing organizations to recognize 3D printing as a standard medical procedure and provide reimbursement for the service. In this respect, prospective clinical trials on use of 3D printing in congenital heart disease surgery and surgical training are crucially important to prove the cost-benefit of this newly developing technology.

Future direction

Of little doubt, 3D printing will be widely used in the medicine of congenital heart diseases. Hands-on surgical training will gradually become an essential component in the surgical training programs. For rare and complex surgical procedures, hands-on training on the 3D print models will be the prerequisite requirement for performing the procedure on the patients. Currently available print materials are not satisfactory for surgical practice. High quality silicone appears closest to the myocardial tissue and best suited for surgery. Currently, silicon models can be made using injection molding technology where silicone is infused into the 3D printed mold . Shiraishi et al used urethane to produce models with rubber-like consistency using molding technique . Although 3D printers using silicon as the printing material are not available, a few commercial companies have recently announced the plans for release of silicone-based printer in the near future

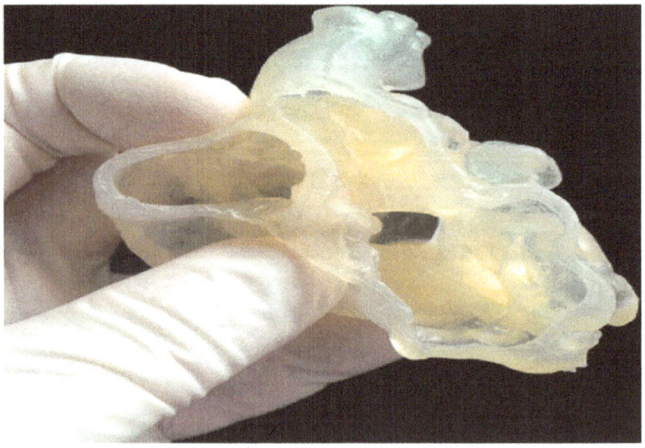

Fig 37.28 Photograph of a model made of silicone using injection molding technique

As discussed, each imaging modality has its own strengths and weaknesses. Both contrast-enhanced CT and MR are excellent in visualization of the blood pool, while ultrasound is far superior to CT and MR in the demonstration of the anatomy and function of the cardiac valves and chordae tendinae. Image fusion is to improve the image content by combining useful information from multiple imaging modalities . The process requires precise image registration process for spatial coordination between the images from different imaging modalities and mathematical algorithm for combining data from different sources. Image fusion technology will certainly enhance the image quality by compensating the weaknesses of each imaging modality and reduce the extent of artifact. 3D printing can be used for personalized implants such as stents, surgical patches and artificial valves . 3D printing has also been experimentally used for tissue engineering such as cardiac valves. Using 3D printing, a scaffold is printed and the cardiac progenitor cells are laid down with matrix for growth . While a clinically viable product has not yet been fabricated, tissue printing eventually will allow fabrication of the implants made of the patient's own stem cells and possibly obviate drug testing on animals by testing on bioprinted human tissues or organs

Conclusions

3D printing has found its niche applications in the medicine of congenital heart diseases. 3D print models allow instantaneous understanding of any complex anatomy and simulation or hands-on training of surgical and interventional procedures. It has made a small revolution in teaching and surgical practice. We expect that Hands-on surgical training (HOST) will soon become a mandatory component of the congenital heart disease surgery programs. 3D printing will expand its utilization with further improvement of imaging and printing technologies and development of new printing materials. Bioprinting and tissue engineering will open the door to the new era of personalized medicine.

Bibliography And Acknowledgement

- Anwar S., Singh G.K., Petrucci O., Eghtesady P., Woodard P.K. and Billadello J.J. : Adult congenital heart disease. In: Rapid Prototyping in Cardiac Disease . Edited by Farooqi K.M. . Cham, Switzerland: Springer International Publishing 2017: 99.
- Anwar S., Singh G.K., Varughese J.et al. : "3D printing in complex congenital heart disease: across a spectrum of age, pathology, and imaging techniques". J Am Coll Cardiol Img 2017; 10:953.
- Armillotta A, Bonhoeffer P, Dubini G, Ferragina S, Migliavacca F, Sala G, et al. Use of rapid prototyping models in the planning of percutaneous pulmonary valved stent implantation. Proc Inst Mech EngH.2007;221(4):407–16.
- Armillotta A, Bonhoeffer P, Dubini G, et al. Use of rapid prototyping models in the planning of percutaneous pulmonary valved stent implantation. Proc Inst Mech Eng H 2007;221:407-16.
- Barach P., Johnson J.K., Ahmad A.et al. : "A prospective observational study of human factors, adverse events, and patient outcomes in surgery for pediatric cardiac disease". J Thorac CardiovascSurg2008;136:1422.
- Bernhard J.-C., Isotani S., Matsugasumi T.et al. : "Personalized 3D printed model of kidney and tumor anatomy: a useful tool for patient education". World J Urol 2016; 34: 337.
- Bhatla P., Tretter J.T., Ludomirsky A.et al. : "Utility and scope of rapid prototyping in patients with complex muscular ventricular septal defects or double-outlet right ventricle: does it alter management decisions?". Pediatr Cardiol 2017; 38: 103.
- Biglino G, Capelli C, Wray J, Schievano S, Leaver LK, Khambadkone S, et al. 3D-manufactured patient-specific models of congenital heart defects for communication in clinical practice: feasibility and acceptability. BMJ Open. 2015;5(4):e007165.
- Biglino G., Capelli C., Taylor A.M. and Schievano S. : 3D printing cardiovascular anatomy: a single-centre experience. In: New Trends in 3D Printing . Edited by Shishkovsky I.V. . London, UnitedKingdom:InTechOpen2016: 1.
- Biglino G., Capelli C., Wray J.et al. : "3D-manufactured patient-specific models of congenital heart defects for communication in clinical practice: feasibility and acceptability". BMJ Open 2015; 5. e007165–5.
- Binder T.M., Moertl D., Mundigler G.et al. : "Stereolithographic biomodeling to create tangible hard copies of cardiac structures from echocardiographic data: in vitro and in vivo validation". J AmCollCardiol2000;35:230.
- Binder TM, Moertl D, Mundigler G, Rehak G, Franke M, Delle-Karth G, et al. Stereolithographic biomodeling to create tangible hard copies of cardiac structures from echocardiographic data: in vitro and in vivo validation. J Am Coll Cardiol. 2000;35:230–7.
- Boneva R.S., Botto L.D., Moore C.A., Yang Q., Correa A. and Erickson J.D. : "Mortality associated with congenital heart defects in the United States". Circulation 2001; 103: 2376.
- Burkhardt BEU, Brown NK, Carberry JE, et al. Creating three dimensional models of the right ventricular outflow tract: infuence of contrast, sequence, operator, and threshold. Int Journal CardiovascImaging2019;35:2067-76.

- Boneva R.S., Botto L.D., Moore C.A., Yang Q., Correa A. and Erickson J.D. : "Mortality associated with congenital heart defects in the United States". Circulation 2001; 103: 2376.
- Brown K.L., Ridout D.A., Goldman A.P., Hoskote A. and Penny D.J. : "Risk factors for long intensive care unit stay after cardiopulmonary bypass in children". Crit Care Med 2003; 31: 28.
- Chaowu Y., Hua L. and Xin S. : "Three-dimensional printing as an aid in transcatheter closure of secundum atrial septal defect with rim deficiency: in vitro trial occlusion based on a personalized heart model". Circulation 2016; 133: e608. Chepelev
- L, Wake N, Ryan J, et al. Radiological Society of North America (RSNA) 3D printing Special Interest Group (SIG): guidelines for medical 3D printing and appropriateness for clinical scenarios. 3D Print Med 2018;4:1-38.
- Cheung DY, Duan B, Butcher JT. Current progress in tissue engineering of heart valves: multiscale problems, multiscale solutions. Expert Opin Biol Ther. 2015;15(8):1155–72.
- Costello J.P., Olivieri L.J., Su L.et al. : "Incorporating threedimensional printing into a simulation-based congenital heart disease and critical care training curriculum for resident physicians". Congenit Heart Dis 2015; 10: 185.
- Costello JP, Olivieri LJ, Su L, Krieger A, Alfares F, Thabit O, et al. Incorporating three-dimensional printing into a simulation-based congenital heart disease and critical care training curriculum for resident physicians. Congenit Heart Dis. 2015;10(2):185–90.
- Dearani J.A., Connolly H.M., Martinez R., Fontanet H. and Webb G.D. : "Caring for adults with congenital cardiac disease: successes and challenges for 2007 and beyond". Cardiol Young 2007;17:87.
- Erikssen G., Liestøl K., Seem E.et al. "Achievements in congenital heart defect surgery: a prospective, 40-year study of 7038 patients". Circulation 2015; 131: 337.
- Fan Y., Kwok K.W., Zhang Y. and Cheung G. : "Threedimensional printing for planning occlusion procedure for a double-lobed left atrial appendage". Circ Cardiovasc Interv 2016;9:e003561
- Fan Y, Yang F, Cheung GSH, et al. Device sizing guided by echocardiography-based three-dimensional printing is associated with superior outcome after percutaneous left atrial appendage occlusion. J Am Soc Echocardiogr 2019;32:708-19.
- Farooqi KM, Sengupta PP. Echocardiography and threedimensional printing: sound ideas to touch a heart. J Am Soc Echocardiogra.2015;28(4):398–404.
- Farooqi KM, Cooper C, Chelliah A, et al. 3D printing and heart failure: the present and the future. JACC Heart Fail 2019;7:132-42.
- Fleming M., Smith S. and Slaunwhite J. :"Investigating interpersonal competencies of cardiac surgery teams". Can J Surg 2006;49:22.
- Franklin RC, et al. Report from the international society for nomenclature of paediatric and congenital heart disease: creation of a visual encyclopedia illustrating the terms and definitions of the international pediatric and congenital cardiac code. World J PediatrCongenitHeartSurg.2010;1(3):300–13.
- Gosnell J., Pietila T., Samuel B.P., Kurup H.K.N., Haw M.P. and Vettukattil J.J. : "Integration of computed tomography and three-dimensional echocardiography for hybrid threedimensional printing in congenital heart disease". J Digit Imaging 2016; 29: 665.
- Grant E.K. and Olivieri L.J. : "The role of 3-D heart models in planning and executing interventional procedures". Can J Cardiol2017; 33: 1074.
- Hadeed K., Dulac Y. and Acar P. : "Three-dimensional printing of a complex CHD to plan surgical repair". Cardiol Young 2016; 26: 1432.
- Han F, Rapacchi S, Khan S, Ayad I, Salusky I, Gabriel S, et al. Four-dimensional, multiphase, steady-state imaging with contrast enhancement (MUSIC) in the heart: a feasibility study in children. MagnResonMed.2015;74(4):1042–9
- Hermsen J.L., Burke T.M., Seslar S.P.et al. : "Scan, plan, print, practice, perform: Development and use of a patientspecific 3-dimensional printed model in adult cardiac surgery". J Thorac CardiovascSurg2017;153:132.
- Hu A., Wilson T., Ladak H., Haase P. and Fung K. : "Threedimensional educational computer model of the larynx: voicing a new direction". Arch Otolaryngol Head Neck Surg 2009; 135: 677.
- Iriart X, Ciobotaru V, Martin C, et al. Role of cardiac imaging and three-dimensional printing in percutaneous appendage closure. Arch CardiovascDis2018;111:411-20.
- Jacobs C.A. and Lin A.Y. : "A new classification of threedimensional printing technologies: systematic review of threedimensional printing for patient-specific craniomaxillofacial surgery". Plast Reconstr Surg 2017;139:1211
- Jonas R.A. : "Training fellows in paediatric cardiac surgery". Cardiol Young2016;26:1474.
- Kang SL, Benson L. Recent advances in cardiac catheterization for congenitalheartdisease.F1000Res2018;7:1-13.
- Kapur K.K. and Garg N. :"Echocardiography derived threedimensional printing of normal and abnormal mitral annuli". Ann CardAnaesth2014;17:283.
- Khairy P., Ionescu-Ittu R., Mackie A.S., Abrahamowicz M., Pilote L. and Marelli A.J. : "Changing mortality in congenital heart disease". J AmCollCardiol2010;56:1149.
- Kim MS, Hansgen AR, Carroll JD. Use of rapid prototypingin the care of patients with structural heart disease. Trends Cardiovasc Med. 2008;18(6):210–6.
- Kirklin J.W., Blackstone E.H., Tchervenkov C.I. and Castaneda A.R. : "Clinical outcomes after the arterial switch operation for transposition: patient, support, procedural, and institutional risk factors. Congenital Heart Surgeons Society". Circulation 1992; 86: 1501.
- Kolli K.K., Min J.K., Ha S., Soohoo H. and Xiong G. : "Effect of varying hemodynamic and vascular conditions on fractional flow reserve: an in vitro study". J Am Heart Assoc 2016; 5. e003634–14.
- Kossivas F, Angeli S, Kafouris D, Patrickios CS, Tzagarakis V, Constantinides C. MRI-based morphological modeling, synthesis and characterization of cardiac tissuemimicking materials. Biomed Mater. 2012;7(3):035006
- Kurup HK, Samuel BP, Vettukattil JJ. Hybrid 3D printing: a game-changer in personalized cardiac medicine? Expert Rev Cardiovasc Ther.2015;13(12):1281–4.
- Lee J.M., Sing S.L., Tan E. and Yeong W.Y. : "Bioprinting in cardiovascular tissue engineering: a review". Int J Bioprinting 2016; 2: 27.
- Lee W., Debasitis J.C., Lee V.K.et al. : "Multi-layered culture of human skin fibroblasts and keratinocytes through three-dimensional freeform fabrication". Biomaterials 2009; 30: 1587.
- Ma XJ, Tao L, Chen X, Li W, Peng ZY, Chen Y, et al. Clinical application of three-dimensional reconstruction and rapid prototyping technology of multislice spiral computed tomography angiography for the repair of ventricular septal defect of tetralogy of Fallot. Genet Mol Res. 2015;14(1):1301–9

- Mahle W.T., Spray T.L., Wernovsky G., Gaynor J.W. and Clark B.J. : "Survival after reconstructive surgery for hypoplastic left heart syndrome". Circulation 2000; 102 Suppl 3: III136.
- Matsubara D, Kataoka K, Takahashi H, Minami T, Yamagata T. A patient-specific hollow three-dimensional model for simulating percutaneous occlusion of patent ductus arteriosus: Its clinical usefulness. International Heart Journal 2019;60:100-7.
- Matsumoto JS, Morris JM, Foley TA, Williamson EE, Leng S, McGee KP, et al. Three-dimensional physical modeling: applications and experience at mayo clinic. Radiographics. 2015;35(7):1989–2006.
- Mitsouras D, Liacouras P, Imanzadeh A, Giannopoulos AA, Cai T, Kumamaru KK, et al. Medical 3D printing for the radiologist. Radiographics. 2015;35(7):1965–88.
- Mitsouras D. and Liacouras P.C. : 3D Printing Technologies, Vol. 3 . Cham, Switzerland: Springer International Publishing 2017.
- Moons P., Bovijn L., Budts W., Belmans A. and Gewillig M. : "Temporal trends in survival to adulthood among patients born with congenital heart disease from 1970 to 1992 in Belgium". Circulation 2010; 122: 2264.
- Moore T., Madriago E.J., Renteria E.S.et al. : "Co-registration of 3D echo and MR data to create physical models of congenital heart malformations". J Cardiovasc Magn Resonan 2015; 17: P198.
- Mottl-Link S, Boettger T, Krueger JJ, Rietdorf U, Schnackenburg B, Ewert P, et al. Images in cardiovascular medicine. Cast of complex congenital heartmalformation in a living patient. Circulation. 2005;112:e356–7.
- Ngan E.M., Rebeyka I.M., Ross D.B.et al. : "The rapid prototyping of anatomic models in pulmonary atresia". J Thorac Cardiovasc Surg 2006; 132: 264.
- Ngan EM, Rebeyka IM, Ross DB, Hirji M, Wolfaardt JF, Seelaus R, et al. The rapid prototyping of anatomic models in pulmonary atresia. J Thorac Cardiovasc Surg. 2006;132:264–9.
- Noecker A.M., Chen J.-F., Zhou Q.et al. : "Development of patient-specific three-dimensional pediatric cardiac models". ASAIO J 2006; 52: 349.
- O'Neill B., Wang D.D., Pantelic M.et al. : "Transcatheter caval valve implantation using multimodality imaging". J Am Coll Cardiol Img 2015; 8: 221.
- Olivieri L., Krieger A., Chen M.Y., Kim P. and Kanter J.P. : "3D heart model guides complex stent angioplasty of pulmonary venous baffle obstruction in a Mustard repair of D-TGA". Int J Cardiol 2014; 172: e297.
- Olivieri LJ, Krieger A, Loke YH, et al. Three-dimensional printing of intracardiac defects from three-dimensional echocardiographic images: feasibility and relative accuracy. J Am Soc Echocardiogr 2015;28:392-7.
- Poterucha J.T., Foley T.A. and Taggart N.W. : "Percutaneous pulmonary valve implantation in a native outflow tract". J Am Coll CardiolIntv2014;7:e151..
- Qian Z, Wang K, Liu S, et al. Quantitative prediction of paravalvular leak in transcatheter aortic valve replacement based on tissue-mimicking 3D Printing. JACC Cardiovasc Imaging 2017;10:719-31.
- Rapid Prototyping in Cardiac Disease . Edited by Farooqi K.M. . Cham, Switzerland: Springer International Publishing2017.
- Rehder R., Abd-El-Barr M., Hooten K., Weinstock P., Madsen J.R. and Cohen A.R. : "The role of simulation in neurosurgery". Childs NervSyst2016;32:43..
- Ripley B., Kelil T., Cheezum M.K.et al. : "3D printing based on cardiac CT assists anatomic visualization prior to transcatheter aortic valve replacement". J Cardiovasc Comput Tomogr 2016; 10: 28.
- Saeed O., Farooqi K.M. and Jorde U.P. : Assessment of ventricular assist device placement and function. In: Rapid Prototyping in Cardiac Disease . Edited by Farooqi K.M. . Cham, Switzerland: Springer InternationalPublishing2017:133
- Samuel B.P., Pinto C., Pietila T. and Vettukattil J.J. : "Ultrasound-derived three-dimensional printing in congenital heart disease". J Digit Imaging2014;28:459.
- Samuel BP, Pinto C, Pietila T, Vettukattil JJ. Ultrasound-derived three-dimensional printing in congenital heart disease. J Digit Imaging.2015;28(4):459–61.
- Tack P., Victor J., Gemmel P. and Annemans L. : "3D-printing techniques in a medical setting: a systematic literature review". BiomedEngOnline2016;15: 115.
- U, Wolf I, Schnackenburg B, Ewert P, Huebler M, et al. The practical clinical value of three-dimensional models of complex congenitally malformed hearts. J Thorac Cardiovasc Surg. 2009;138(3):571–80
- Valverde I, Gomez G, Coserria JF, Suarez-Mejias C, Uribe S, Sotelo J, et al. 3D printed models for planning endovascular stenting in transverse aortic arch hypoplasia. Catheter Cardiovasc Interv. 2015;85(6):1006–12
- Warnes C.A., Bhatt A.B., Daniels C.J., Gillam L.D. and Stout K.K. : "COCATS 4 Task Force 14: training in the care of adult patients with congenital heart disease". J Am Coll Cardiol 2015; 65: 1887.
- Yoo S.-J., Thabit O., Kim E.K.et al. : "3D printing in medicine of congenital heart diseases". 3D Printing Med 2016; 2: 1
- Zopf D.A., Hollister S.J., Nelson M.E., Ohye R.G. and Green G.E. : "Bioresorbable airway splint created with a threedimensional printer". N Engl J Med 2013; 368: 2043.

38 Nano-technology Innovations in Pediatric Cardiology A Comprehensive Review

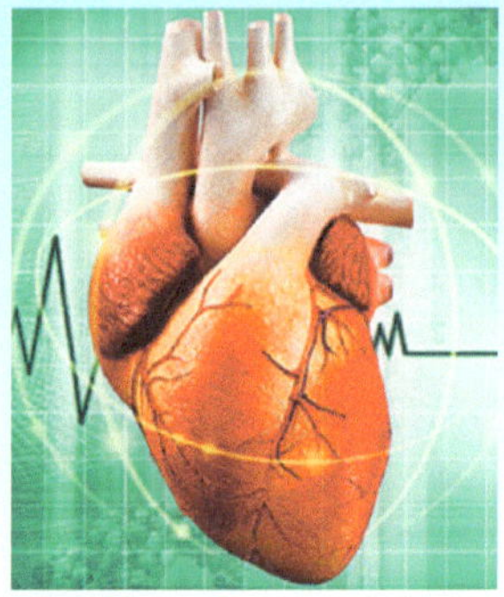

Nanotechnologies have significantly enhanced patient care by advancing the fields of biotechnology, medicine, and pharmaceuticals. These technologies have streamlined various healthcare processes, encompassing diagnosis, therapeutic interventions, and ongoing patient monitoring. An ongoing effort is being made to innovate and develop new nanomaterials to improve disease diagnosis and treatments. This innovation seeks to ensure that medical practices become more personalized, cost-effective, and safe, enhancing their potency, accuracy, and duration .The future of nanotechnology hinges on selecting appropriate nanomaterials while mitigating potential adverse effects. Like all medical products, nano-based products must undergo rigorous risk evaluations before clinical and commercial approval to minimize potential risks to human health and the environment. A comprehensive life cycle assessment is crucial to determine their usage's long-term sustainability and safety .

Nanotechnology constitutes a relatively new area of science, encompassing the investigation of nanoparticles and nanomaterials with dimensions less than 100 nm, which have unique advantages such as increased surface area, tunable physicochemical properties, and the ability to encapsulate various therapeutic agents . The European Medicines Agency defines nanomedicine as implementing nanotechnology in different medical domains, from prevention and diagnosis to targeted therapeutic interventions .

Several types of nanoparticles are available, and some of them have been explored in human subjects, including polymer-based (e.g., dendrimers, micelles, nanogels, drug conjugates), lipid-based (liposomes, exosomes, solid lipid nanoparticles), non-polymeric (e.g., nanotubes, nanodiamonds, metallic nanoparticles) and nanocrystalline nanoparticles .

Lipid-based nanoparticles, such as liposomes and lipid nanoparticles, have gained prominence for drug delivery in cardiovascular diseases. Liposomes can encapsulate hydrophobic and hydrophilic drugs, providing a versatile platform for controlled release.

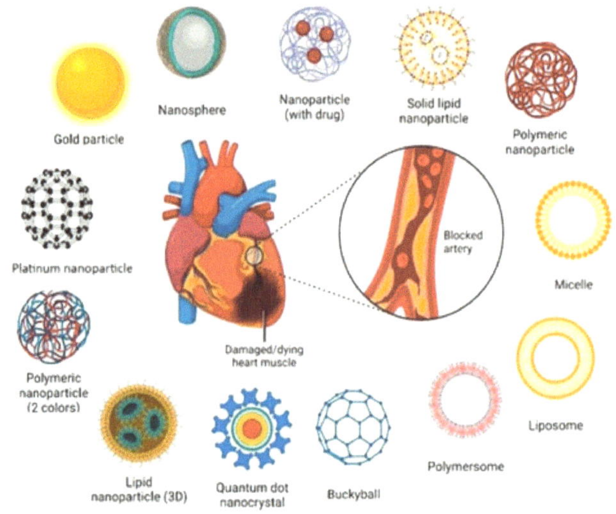

Fig. 38.1 Potential useful nanoparticles in cardiovascular diseases. Created with Biorender.com.

These nanoparticles enhance drug stability, improve pharmacokinetics, and reduce systemic toxicity . Polymeric nanoparticles, including dendrimers and micelles, offer customizable structures for cardiovascular drug delivery . Dendrimers exhibit a highly branched architecture, enabling precise control over drug release kinetics . Micelles, composed of amphiphilic polymers, enhance drug solubility and circulation time, leading to improved therapeutic outcomes .Inorganic nanoparticles, such as gold and silica nanoparticles, are utilized for their unique optical and magnetic properties. Gold nanoparticles serve as contrast agents in cardiovascular imaging, enabling precise detection of lesions and monitoring of treatment responses .Silica nanoparticles, with their porous structure, facilitate controlled drug release and targeted therapy . Magnetic nanoparticles, often based on iron oxide, provide a platform for targeted drug delivery and imaging guided by external magnetic fields. These nanoparticles enable site-specific drug release, enhancing drug concentration at the desired cardiovascular site while minimizing systemic exposure . Carbon-based nanoparticles, including carbon nanotubes and graphene, have shown potential in cardiovascular applications . Their high surface area and unique electronic properties make them suitable for drug delivery and imaging. However, concerns regarding biocompatibility and long-term safety necessitate further research .

Although nanoparticles have proved efficient in various biomedical areas, extensive clinical applicability is relatively limited. Some key factors that might perpetuate clinical translation reluctance are safety and toxicity concerns, unclear definitions and physical properties of nanoparticles, cost–efficiency ratios, and ambiguous regulatory guidelines .Also, other concerns regarding the biocompatibility of nanoparticles, pharmacokinetic and pharmacodynamic proprieties, and manufacturing process issues should be addressed when implementing nanomedicine in clinical practice .

Nanoparticle safety concerns are driven mainly by physical properties, such as size and shape, solubility, agglomeration state, and surface area . Concerning the link between size and safety, one study documented that only small gold nanoparticles (1.4 nm) were toxic, in comparison to bigger nanoparticles (15 nm) which were not . Nevertheless, technological progress has continuously improved the safety profile of nanoparticles in the last few years. Recently, Sani et al. emphasized that, even at present, small nanoparticles remain the most controversial regarding safety . However, nanotechnology implementation in clinical practice is trending upwards, as many products have been approved for use in adults and even in children .

Severe acute respiratory syndrome coronavirus 2 (SARS-CoV-2) vaccines (Pfizer-BioNTech, Moderna, Cambridge, MA, USA) represent one of the most extensive utilizations of nanoparticles in humans .Nevertheless, nanoparticles encompass far more than SARS-CoV-2 vaccines. In recent decades, the Food and Drug Administration (FDA) has approved an impressive arsenal of nanoparticles for different clinical applications . Consequently, nanoparticles have the potential to be used to manage various types of cancer, infections, transthyretin-mediated amyloidosis, multiple sclerosis, anemia (including patients with chronic kidney disease), and autoimmune, inflammatory, and metabolic disorders .Moreover, the FDA has approved some nanoparticles for administration in pediatric patients. In this regard, sodium ferric gluconate can be used in children ≥6 years old with end-stage kidney disease (ESKD) on hemodialysis for anemia correction due to iron deficiency .Octocog alfa is a lipid-based nanoparticle loaded with human coagulation factor VIII and has been approved for hemophilia A therapy irrespective of patients' age . Elixophyllin is a crystalline nanoparticle containing theophylline and has been approved for chronic asthma treatment and other conditions associated with airflow limitation . Also, nanoparticles could be used for cancer therapy in children. Mepact, a lipid-based nanoparticle loaded with mifamurtide, is indicated in patients with osteosarcoma in the postoperative setting, combined with other adjunctive therapies .

This review seeks to critically assess the current advancements in nanotechnology within cardiology and pediatric cardiology. We aim to investigate the benefits and limitations of nanomedicine in treating cardiovascular disorders, thereby setting the stage for future research and the development of clinical guidelines in this rapidly evolving sector.

Methodology

We conducted an extensive literature search across multiple databases, including PubMed, Embase, and ScienceDirect, employing the following search terms: "nanotechnology", "cardiology", "pediatric cardiology", "children", "cardiovascular", and "pediatric patients". The inclusion criteria encompassed the following key elements: articles available as full texts, studies published within the last 20 years (from 2003 onwards), clearly indicating the type of nanotechnology utilized and its relevance to either cardiology or pediatric cardiology, as well as articles presented in English. We considered various studies, including clinical, preclinical, animal research, literature reviews, and ongoing clinical trials. Additionally, we examined the reference lists of the included articles to identify further relevant studies. Exclusion criteria encompassed single case reports, letters to the editor, and studies available only in abstract form.

Our search revealed 74 potential articles. After removing duplicates and articles not meeting the inclusion criteria, 58 records were left for further analysis. The selection process involved a two-step evaluation conducted independently by two authors. In the first step, titles and abstracts were screened to determine eligibility. Subsequently, all studies meeting the inclusion criteria progressed to the second step, where the full texts of articles were thoroughly examined.

Notably, within this analysis, approximately a quarter of studies prioritized safety assessments of the proposed methods involving nanotechnologies, while the majority reported favorable efficacy outcomes.

Nanotechnology Imaging

Unstable atherosclerosis plaques are rich in macrophages. A novel imaging nanoparticle method involves tracing the metabolic activity of these macrophages by glucose analog uptake, specifically fluorine-labeled 2-deoxy-D-glucose (FDG) uptake. Then, positron emission tomography is employed to describe the state of the suspected atherosclerotic artery. Unstable plaques are additionally characterized by a significant population of apoptotic cells, detectable via the utilization of annexin labeled with radionuclides .The next step in vascular imaging is to detect the dysfunctional endothelium before the plaque is formed. This can be achieved by targeting VCAM-1 . E-selectin or P-selectin

Imaging can also be extrapolated to the electrical activity of the heart. In this regard, Shimozawa and colleagues have shown that cardiomyocyte electrical connectivity encompasses not only gap junctions and intercalated disks but also implicatesmechano- sensitive cardiac sodium channels. Employing real-time confocal imaging, they demonstrated that intercalated disks were flexible and varied in length during action potential propagation from one cardiomyocyte to another, leading to mechanical stress that activates cardiac sodium channels.

Nanomaterial-based noninvasive molecular imaging employs magnetic resonance imaging, optical imaging, nuclear scintigraphy, photoacoustic imaging, single photon emission computed tomography, optical coherence tomography/infrared luminescence, and X-ray-excited luminescence. These methods employ iron oxide, gadolinium, polylactide polycarboxybetaine or metal oxide-peptide amphiphile micelles as effective nanoparticles for imaging atherosclerotic plaque thrombosis. P selectin is overexpressed in inflamed endothelial cells. Nanoparticles composed of fucoidan and a thermolysin-hydrolyzed protamine peptide can be combined with magnetic resonance imaging to identify these endothelial cells. Dual-contrast iron oxide nanoparticles can be used as MRI contrast agents. Vulnerable atherosclerotic plaques can easily be identified using 18F-fluorodeoxyglucose (18F-FDG)-based positron emission tomography (PET), but this method lacks specificity .

Myocardial Ischemia

Heart failure is a preeminent global healthcare concern, ranking as the leading cause of mortality worldwide. Its etiology encompasses various factors, including cardiomyopathies, congenital cardiac anomalies, hypertension, valvular lesions, myocarditis, arrhythmias, drug-induced effects, neuromuscular disorders, and ischemic heart disease. Among adults, ischemic heart disease overwhelmingly predominates as the main precipitating factor of heart failure. Furthermore, ischemic heart disease imposes a substantial burden on public health, significantly increasing morbidity and mortality (even in the absence of heart failure).The early detection of myocardial ischemia is crucial in clinical practice. Established biomarkers such as cardiac troponins, myoglobin, and creatine kinase MB are employed to identify ischemic events within the bloodstream. However, these biomarkers are characterized by initially low peripheral blood concentrations. A promising step forward lies in the integration of biosensors and nanotechnology. Several laboratory methodologies can be enlisted for this purpose,includingelectrochemistry,chemiluminescence,el ectrochemiluminescence, photo electrochemistry, fluorescent assays, cyclic voltammetry, electrochemical impedance spectroscopy, Lateral Flow Immunosensors, Lateral Flow assays, and differential pulse voltammetry.Coronary atherosclerosis, the underlying pathology responsible for myocardial ischemia, may be effectively addressed through nanotechnologies. Several release systems (polyethylene glycol (PEG), poly lactic-co-glycolic acid (PLGA), or poly(d-lactic acid) are nowadays available to deliver anti-inflammatory molecules such as Ac2-26 peptide and interleukin-10 cytokine to the atherosclerotic plaque. Foam cell formation can also be inhibited using macromolecules by suppressing macrophage scavenger receptors using sugar-based amphiphilic macromolecules However, several aspects still need to be addressed, such as the potential proinflammatory effect of such technologies via fibrinogen conformational change induction

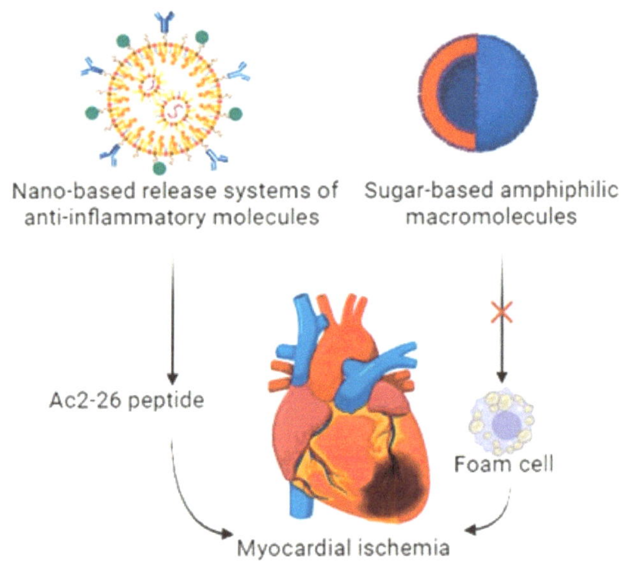

Fig.38.2 Potential application of nanoparticles in myocardial ischemia. Created with Biorender.com.

Another way to attempt reperfusion is to transplant nanomaterials (aligned nanofibrillar scaffolds) impregnated with stromal vascular fraction cells. This method proved superior to phosphate buffer saline administration in a mouse model .Furthermore, another alternative for reperfusion exists: vessel grafts with anthracene-grafted styrene-block-butadiene block-styrene, which proved to be a promising vascular tissue-engineering alternative in a recent study .When using conventional stents for coronary angioplasty, there is an early risk of thrombosis and a delayed risk of restenosis. These risks could be reduced by inserting nitric oxide-producing stents. This can be achieved using nitric oxide-releasing or nitric oxide-generating coatings for stents. Drug-eluting stents represent a notable advancement over bare metal stents for maintaining vessel patency. However, they remain susceptible to late thrombosis as a result of drug depletion . Nitric oxide donors serve as vehicles for the controlled delivery of nitric oxide, releasing it selectively in targeted regions for a finite duration of time . Nitric oxide donors include S-nitroso-N-acetylpenicillamine (SNAP) and N-diazeniumdiolates (NONOates.

Gene therapy has been proposed as a solution to the limited nitric oxide donation time problem. This can be achieved either by transfection of autologous adipose-derived stem cells (ASCs) or differentiated endothelial-like cells. or by using iNOS-encoding adeno-associated virus serotype 2 (AAV2) vectors .

Myocardial repair is also thought to be achievable using nanotechnology in the future. One study showed optimistic results by using human induced pluripotent stem cell-derived cardiomyocytes (hiPSC-CMs) cultured in a three-dimensional micro-environment, conjugated with an aligned polycaprolactone (PCL)-gelatin coaxial nanofiber patch fabricated using electrospinning. An alternative strategy involves tagging fresh cardiomyocytes with magnetic nanoparticles and immobilizing them by applying a localized magnetic field.Nevertheless, cell therapy is not exempt from associated risks, and its potential arrhythmic impact is under thorough investigation . One alternative is synthesizing patient-specific cardiomyocytes from stem cells . but they might be subject to immune rejection.Considering the substantial presence of fibrin within infarcted myocardial tissue, it is postulated to constitute an auspicious candidate for precisely targeting patient-specific therapeutic cardiomyocytes or alternative modalities for cardiac regeneration therapy, provided such interventions are administered promptly. Nonetheless, fibrin formation is not restricted exclusively to the infarcted region, presenting a significant drawback in this approach. More selective molecular targets include myosin, angiotensin II type 1 receptor, and phosphatidylserine .

While myocardial repair following an acute ischemic episode holds utmost significance, it is equally imperative to detect the onset of ischemia promptly. One way to achieve this is the detection of cardiac troponin I using a multi-functional DNA on Au nanocrystal-modified indium-tin-oxide substrate using an electrochemical method .

Myocarditis

Accurate diagnosis is pivotal for effective myocarditis management. Nanoparticles, including superparamagnetic iron oxide nanoparticles (SPIONs) and quantum dots, have demonstrated considerable potential as contrast agents for imaging modalities such as magnetic resonance imaging (MRI) and fluorescence imaging [68]. These nanomaterials enhance sensitivity and specificity, allowing for early detection and precise localization of inflammatory lesions in the myocardium .

Nanoparticles designed for targeted drug delivery present a paradigm shift in myocarditis therapeutics. Functionalized nanocarriers can deliver anti-inflammatory agents directly to the inflamed myocardium, minimizing systemic side effects. Toita et al. proposed a bioinspired anti-inflammatory nanomedicine conjugated with protein G that target proinflammatory cells, such as macrophages . This targeted approach is promising for improving treatment efficacy and reducing adverse effects on healthy tissues.

In animal models, Li et al. showed that using nano-alpha-linolenic acid in mice with viral-induced myocarditis improved their survival rate in a dose-dependent manner, but further research in humans is needed to replicate and extend these results .

Aneurysms

Aneurysms are a rare but serious condition requiring innovative approaches. Nanotechnology, operating at the nanoscale, offers a unique tool for precise diagnosis and treatment. Currently, most results are based on animal models, and few clinical trials have been conducted. In rodent studies, targeted nanoparticles showed promising results in abdominal aortic aneurysms.This represents a groundbreaking approach to enhancing the efficacy of pharmacological interventions while minimizing systemic side effects. Functionalized nanocarriers can deliver therapeutic agents directly to the aneurysm site, improving drug concentration and reducing off-target effects. This approach holds great promise for pediatric patients, where precise drug delivery is crucial for minimizing adverse effects on developing organs. However, surgical and endovascular treatment remains the preferred strategy to address these cases .

Collaborative efforts between researchers and clinicians are essential for establishing guidelines and standards for nanotechnological interventions in pediatric populations. However, nanotechnology holds immense potential for revolutionizing children's diagnosis and the treatment of aneurysms. Integrating nanomaterials into imaging, monitoring, drug delivery, and surgical guidance opens new avenues for personalized and minimally invasive interventions. Further research is required to address challenges related to biocompatibility, safety, and ethical considerations, paving the way to translating these exciting advancements into clinical practice.

Dilated Cardiomyopathies

Patients with dilated cardiomyopathy can benefit from pacing that bypasses scar tissue, which can be accomplished by using thread-like carbon nanotube fibers with high electrical conductivity . Attempts have also been made to treat cardiomyopathies by inducing the formation of new mature cardiomyocytes.. but the results were unsatisfactory. In some studies, attempts were made to inject several types of bone marrow-derived cells into dilated cardiomyopathy hearts, but severe side effects such as arrhythmia or tumors arose .Other authors attempted to transform fibroblasts into contractile cardiomyocytes. by using cardiac-specific transcription factors or mitochondrial RNA to induce cardiomyocyte regeneration and proliferation. Growth factors have been linked to nanoparticles and delivered to the heart to induce neovascularization . but this method is not yet used in clinical practice.

Pulmonary Hypertension

Pulmonary hypertension in children poses a significant challenge due to its complex pathophysiology and limited therapeutic options. Nanotechnology has emerged as a promising frontier for innovative and targeted interventions. In mice, Marulanda et al. proposed an intravenous delivery system for lung-targeted nanofibers, aiming to decrease pulmonary hypertension . Their results showed promising perspectives, especially for specific proteins overexpressed in this condition, such as the receptor for advanced glycation end-products (REGE).

Endothelial dysfunction and vasoconstriction are hallmarks of pediatric pulmonary hypertension. Nanoparticles can be engineered to release vasodilatory agents specifically in the pulmonary vasculature. Recently, Elbardisy et al. reported that aerosolized dilutable nanoemulsions of tadalafil showed a favorable safety profile in both in vitro and in vivo toxicity studies .This targeted approach holds promise for improving blood flow and alleviating symptoms in children with pulmonary hypertension .

Children with pulmonary hypertension can benefit from bosentan nanoparticle treatment, which increases the bioavailability of the molecule by several times . Akagi et al used a rat model to study beraprost nanoparticles for pulmonary hypertension treatment, with favorable results. Pulmonary arterial smooth muscle cell proliferation was effectively inhibited by using imatinib nanoparticles .Promising results were also obtained using fasudil . nuclear factor kappa B or pitvastatin nanoparticles While nanotechnology holds great promise in pediatric pulmonary hypertension management, challenges such as regulatory approval, scalability, and long-term safety must be addressed. The safe integration of nanotechnology into pediatric treatmentrequires rigorous evaluation of biocompatibility and potential long-term effects. Furthermore, developing biodegradable nanocarriers addresses concerns about long-term retention and potential toxicity

Vascular Tissue Engineering

Pediatric cardiology would highly benefit from manufacturing biological conduits; however, nowadays, science faces serious challenges in modeling compact structures. We are still in the era of monolayer cell groups, but a biological conduit or synthetic valves that would have the capability of growing at the same pace as the host body would signify a great leap forward. These conduits would have to be lined with endothelial cells. Golden et al have taken steps toward obtaining a network of narrow (6 μm) channels. The next step was seeding endothelial cells in this network. Moving on to three-dimensional structures, they met geometrical issues: corners of such structures impair blood flow and result in asymmetrical parietal stress. Their work was carried on by Borenstein et al., who obtained semicircular cross-sections and improved blood flow at bifurcations. Chrobak et al used a needle-collagen technique to obtain a tube network lined with endothelial cells that could be perfused with insignificant leakage.

Skardal et al. attempted to manufacture a bioartificial vessel-like graft by culturing microfilaments that fused together. Suri et al. used hyaluronic acid and a digital mirror device to fabricate layered structures, while Duan et al. used an ultraviolet-led module to manufacture artificial valves with a similar geometry to biological valves.

The application of nanomedicine in coronary artery bypass grafting (CABG) represents a significant stride in enhancing the efficacy and safety of this crucial cardiac procedure. Nanotechnology in CABG focuses on improving graft materials and enhancing post-surgical healing and integration.

Nanoscale modifications of graft surfaces can promote better endothelialization, reducing the risk of thrombosis and improving long-term patency rates Furthermore, nanomaterials can be engineered to deliver therapeutic agents directly to the graft site, aiding in the suppression of local inflammation and the prevention of neointimal hyperplasia, a common cause of graft failure. This targeted delivery system allows for a more efficient use of drugs, potentially reducing systemic side effects.

Additionally, nanoscale imaging agents can provide surgeons with enhanced visualization during procedures, ensuring more precise graft placement. As research advances, the integration of nanomedicine in CABG is poised to revolutionize the approach to coronary artery disease treatment, offering patients improved outcomes and quicker recoveries .

Nanomedical processes in cardiac repair, particularly for nerve regeneration, involve advanced materials and techniques that mimic the heart's extracellular matrix. These nanoscale innovations, such as electrically conductive nanomaterials and nanofibers, provide crucial support for the growth and healing of cardiac nerves. They can also deliver growth factors and other regenerative molecules directly to the damaged cardiac tissue. This integration of nanotechnology with regenerative medicine, like stem cell therapy, enhances the effectiveness of cardiac repair, aiming to restore the heart's normal function and electrical connectivity after injury. As this field is still developing, ongoing research is crucial for realizing the full potential of these nanomedical strategies in heart health .

Congenital Heart Disease

Congenital heart diseases are another field where coated nanotechnology devices can be used. Percutaneous closures offer several advantages over surgical thoracotomies, such as avoiding cardiopulmonary bypass, avoiding sternotomies, and potentially lowering postgraduate complications.

Closing different types of cardiac malformation (atrial septal defect, ventricular septal defect, patent ductus arteriosus, patent foramen ovale, etc.) may require cardiac devices. Most modern cardiac devices that undergo percutaneous closure are made of nitinol, an alloy of nickel and titanium. Nickel has been shown to leak from nitinol-containing occluders in previous studies. The mean serum nickel levels after Amplatzer device implantation rose significantly within 24 h of implantation and remained elevated until 1 month after implantation before gradually decreasing to baseline levels. In patients with ASD, Burian et al. also found that nickel levels rose significantly after implantation of a nickel device in serum and urine; nickel levels in serum increased up to fivefold after the 6-week post-closure period, and nickel levels returned to baseline levels after 4 to 6 months. After implanting the Amplatzer occluder, serum nickel levels rose dramatically, peaking at three months after implantation, and slowly dropping back to baseline during follow-up There is a risk of nickel allergy associated with the release of the nickel with time in some cases of these devices.The transcatheter closure of cardiac shunts has been associated with systemic adverse effects of nickel allergy, including pericarditis and migraine headaches. It may be necessary to surgically explant the device in patients with nickel allergy and severe refractory symptoms.To prevent nickel allergy, some companies have developed nanotechnologies to coat the devices with nanoparticles of platinum, bioceramic, or polymers (parylene) to prevent nitinol externalization .

Recent advancements in cardiac repair have shone a spotlight on the potential of extracellular matrix (ECM)-based cardiac patches .These patches, engineered to mimic the natural ECM of the heart, have emerged as a promising therapeutic strategy for repairing damaged myocardial tissue. The ECM, a complex network of proteins and polysaccharides, provides essential structural and biochemical support to cells. By replicating this environment, ECM-based patches facilitate the integration and proliferation of cardiac cells, thereby aiding in the regeneration of injured myocardial regions . A key attribute of these cardiac patches is their ability to provide a conducive microenvironment for the recruitment and maturation of cardiomyocytes and vascular cells, which is essential for restoring heart function. This is particularly significant in conditions like myocardial infarction, where the loss of viable heart tissue leads to compromised cardiac function. The application of ECM-based patches in such scenarios has shown promising results in promoting angiogenesis and myocardial regeneration

Moreover, the biocompatibility and biodegradability of these patches align well with the body's natural healing processes, minimizing the risk of adverse immune responses. This compatibility is crucial for ensuring the long-term success of cardiac repair and regeneration therapies. Ongoing research is focused on enhancing the mechanical properties and bioactivity of these patches to better mimic the native cardiac tissue, thus improving their therapeutic efficacy . Overall, ECM-based cardiac patches represent a significant leap forward in regenerative medicine. By leveraging the innate properties of the extracellular matrix, they offer a sophisticated approach to cardiac repair, with the potential to significantly improve outcomes for patients with heart diseases

The development of sirolimus or paclitaxel drug-eluting stents (DESs) has revolutionized coronary intervention by reducing intimal growth. In addition to their indication for myocardial ischemia, off-label DESs are used in pediatric cardiology with good results as palliation in hybrid interventions for hypoplastic left heart syndrome or different forms of pulmonary atresia in infants with duct-dependent circulation. Neonates with duct-dependent pulmonary circulation can benefit from ductalstents instead of Blalock–Taussig shunts. DESs are also preferred in children because they maintain a longer duct patency than bare-metal stents. However, DESs contain paclitaxel or sirolimus, which may cause concern for neonates regarding their immunosuppressive effects, especially if more than one stent is used or one longer than 22 mm. A study by Sivakumar et al. evaluated the increasing levels of sirolimus after stent implantation in neonates with pulmonary duct-dependent circulation.

Immunosuppressive sirolimus levels ranged from 5 to 15 ng/mL, and this was not surpassed whether one or two stents were used.

Conclusions

In this comprehensive narrative review, we have explored the landscape of nanotechnology advancements in cardiovascular medicine and pediatric cardiology. Nanomedicine, encompassing a diverse array of nanoparticles and nanomaterials, has emerged as a promising frontier in medical science. Despite initial reservations and concerns, substantial progress has been made, leading to the approval and utilization of various nanotechnology-based interventions in adult and pediatric patients. Myocardial ischemia, a critical concern in cardiology, has seen innovative approaches involving nanomaterials, including drug-eluting stents, nitric oxide donors, and magnetic nanoparticle-tagged cardiomyocytes. These developments hold immense potential for improving patient outcomes, particularly in the early detection and treatment of ischemic events. Nanotechnology has also revolutionized imaging techniques, enabling the noninvasive assessment of vascular and cardiac structures. Concerning pediatric cardiology, creating biological conduits, synthetic valves, and bioartificial vessel-like grafts represents a future research direction for addressing congenital heart defects. Moreover, nanotechnology-based treatments have shown potential in mitigating conditions such as dilated cardiomyopathy and pulmonary hypertension in children, thereby expanding therapeutic options for this vulnerable population. These findings lay the foundation for continued research and the development of guidelines to optimize the clinical utility of nanomedicine in cardiology.

Summary

(1) Background: Nanomedicine, incorporating various nanoparticles and nanomaterials, offers significant potential in medical practice. Its clinical adoption, however, faces challenges like safety concerns, regulatory hurdles, and biocompatibility issues. Despite these, recent advancements have led to the approval of many nanotechnology-based products, including those for pediatric use. (2) Methods: Our approach included reviewing clinical, preclinical, and animal studies, as well as literature reviews from the past two decades and ongoing trials. (3) Results: Nanotechnology has introduced innovative solutions in cardiovascular care, particularly in managing myocardial ischemia. Key developments include drug-eluting stents, nitric oxide-releasing coatings, and the use of magnetic nanoparticles in cardiomyocyte transplantation. These advancements are pivotal for early detection and treatment. In cardiovascular imaging, nanotechnology enables noninvasive assessments. In pediatric cardiology, it holds promise in assisting the development of biological conduits, synthetic valves, and bioartificial grafts for congenital heart defects, and offers new treatments for conditions like dilated cardiomyopathy and pulmonary hypertension. (4) Conclusions: Nanomedicine presents groundbreaking solutions for cardiovascular diseases in both adults and children. It has the potential to transform cardiac care, from enhancing myocardial ischemia treatment and imaging techniques to addressing congenital heart issues. Further research and guideline development are crucial for optimizing its clinical application and revolutionizing patient care.

Bibliography And Acknowledgement

- Abdellatif, A.A.H.; Alsowinea, A. Approved and marketed nanoparticles for disease targeting and applications in COVID-19. Nanotechnol. Rev. 2021, 10, 1941–1977. [Google Scholar] [CrossRef]
- Abdel-Mageed, H.M.; AbuelEzz, N.Z.; Radwan, R.A.; Mohamed, S.A. Nanoparticles in nanomedicine: A comprehensive updated review on current status, challenges and emerging opportunities. J. Microencapsul. 2021, 38, 414–436. [Google Scholar] [CrossRef]
- Babapulle, M.N.; Eisenberg, M.J. Coated stents for the prevention of restenosis: Part I. Circulation 2002, 106, 2734–2740. [Google Scholar] [CrossRef] [PubMed]
- Behfar, A.; Crespo-Diaz, R.; Terzic, A.; Gersh, B.J. Cell therapy for cardiac repair--lessons from clinical trials. Nat. Rev. Cardiol. 2014, 11, 232–246. [Google Scholar] [CrossRef] [PubMed]
- Bhatt, A.; Bates, M.J.; Marcu, C.B.; Matheny, R.G.; Carabello, B.A.; Yin, K.; Boyd, W.D. Second-generation extracellular matrix patch for epicardial infarct repair. J. Cardiothorac. Surg. 2023, 18, 255. [Google Scholar] [CrossRef
- Cassani, M.; Fernandes, S.; Vrbsky, J.; Ergir, E.; Cavalieri, F.; Forte, G. Combining Nanomaterials and Developmental Pathways to Design New Treatments for Cardiac Regeneration: The Pulsing Heart of Advanced Therapies. Front. Bioeng. Biotechnol. 2020, 8, 323. [Google Scholar] [CrossRef]

- Chen, L.; Nakano, K.; Kimura, S.; Matoba, T.; Iwata, E.; Miyagawa, M.; Tsujimoto, H.; Nagaoka, K.; Kishimoto, J.; Sunagawa, K.; et al. Nanoparticle-mediated delivery of pitavastatin into lungs ameliorates the development and induces regression of monocrotaline-induced pulmonary artery hypertension. Hypertension 2011, 57, 343–350. [Google Scholar] [CrossRef] [PubMed]
- Chnari, E.; Nikitczuk, J.S.; Wang, J.; Uhrich, K.E.; Moghe, P.V. Engineered polymeric nanoparticles for receptor-targeted blockage of oxidized low density lipoprotein uptake and atherogenesis in macrophages. Biomacromolecules 2006, 7, 1796–1805. [Google Scholar] [CrossRef]
- De Saint-Hubert, M.; Bauwens, M.; Deckers, N.; Drummen, M.; Douma, K.; Granton, P.; Hendrikx, G.; Kusters, D.; Bucerius, J.; Reutelingsperger, C.P.; et al. In vivo molecular imaging of apoptosis and necrosis in atherosclerotic plaques using microSPECT-CT and microPET-CT imaging. Mol. Imaging Biol. 2014, 16, 246–254. [Google Scholar] [CrossRef]
- Duan, B.; Kapetanovic, E.; Hockaday, L.A.; Butcher, J.T. Three-dimensional printed trileaflet valve conduits using biological hydrogels and human valve interstitial cells. Acta Biomater. 2014, 10, 1836–1846. [Google Scholar] [CrossRef]
- Eisen, A.H.; Bacal, H.L. Clinical evaluation of a theophylline solution (Elixophyllin) in children with bronchial asthma. Can. Med. Assoc. J. 1962, 86, 444–446. [Google Scholar] [PubMed]
  Falk, J.; Williams, M. No Limit yet for Carbon Nanotube Fibers. Rice News 2020, 17, 1–4. [Google Scholar]
- Farjadian, F.; Ghasemi, A.; Gohari, O.; Roointan, A.; Karimi, M.; Hamblin, M.R. Nanopharmaceuticals and nanomedicines currently on the market: Challenges and opportunities. Nanomedicine 2019, 14, 93–126. [Google Scholar] [CrossRef]
  Gao, F.; Kataoka, M.; Liu, N.; Liang, T.; Huang, Z.P.; Gu, F.;
- Ding, J.; Liu, J.; Zhang, F.; Ma, Q.; et al. Therapeutic role of miR-19a/19b in cardiac regeneration and protection from myocardial infarction. Nat. Commun. 2019, 10, 1802. [Google Scholar] [CrossRef]
  Gupta, V.; Gupta, N.; Shaik, I.H.; Mehvar, R.; McMurtry, I.F.;
- Oka, M.; Nozik-Grayck, E.; Komatsu, M.; Ahsan, F. Liposomal fasudil, a rho-kinase inhibitor, for prolonged pulmonary preferential vasodilation in pulmonary arterial hypertension. J. Control. Release Off. J. Control. Release Soc. 2013, 167, 189–199. [Google Scholar] [CrossRef]
- Hanafy, N.A.N.; El-Kemary, M.; Leporatti, S. Micelles Structure Development as a Strategy to Improve Smart Cancer Therapy. Cancers 2018, 10, 238. [Google Scholar] [CrossRef] [PubMed]
- Isomi, M.; Sadahiro, T.; Ieda, M. Progress and Challenge of Cardiac Regeneration to Treat Heart Failure. J. Cardiol. 2019, 73, 97–101. [Google Scholar] [CrossRef]
- Jacobin-Valat, M.J.; Deramchia, K.; Mornet, S.; Hagemeyer, C.E.; Bonetto, S.; Robert, R.; Biran, M.; Massot, P.; Miraux, S.; Sanchez, S.; et al. MRI of inducible P-selectin expression in human activated platelets involved in the early stages of atherosclerosis. NMR Biomed. 2011, 24, 413–424. [Google Scholar] [CrossRef]
- Kamaly, N.; Fredman, G.; Fojas, J.J.; Subramanian, M.; Choi, W.I.; Zepeda, K.; Vilos, C.; Yu, M.; Gadde, S.; Wu, J.; et al. Targeted Interleukin-10 Nanotherapeutics Developed with a Microfluidic Chip Enhance Resolution of Inflammation in Advanced Atherosclerosis. ACS Nano 2016, 10, 5280–5292. [Google Scholar] [CrossRef]
- Lee, J.M.; Yoon, T.J.; Cho, Y.S. Recent developments in nanoparticle-based siRNA delivery for cancer therapy. BioMed Res. Int. 2013, 2013, 782041. [Google Scholar] [CrossRef] [PubMed]
- Ma, X.; Hibbert, B.; Dhaliwal, B.; Seibert, T.; Chen, Y.X.; Zhao, X.; O'Brien, E.R. Delayed re-endothelialization with rapamycin-coated stents is rescued by the addition of a glycogen synthase kinase-3beta inhibitor. Cardiovasc. Res. 2010, 86, 338–345. [Google Scholar] [CrossRef] [PubMed
- Naqvi, S.; Panghal, A.; Flora, S.J.S. Nanotechnology: A Promising Approach for Delivery of Neuroprotective Drugs. Front. Neurosci. 2020, 14, 494. [Google Scholar] [CrossRef]
- Pan, Y.; Neuss, S.; Leifert, A.; Fischler, M.; Wen, F.; Simon, U.; Schmid, G.; Brandau, W.; Jahnen-Dechent, W. Size-dependent cytotoxicity of gold nanoparticles. Small 2007, 3, 1941–1949. [Google Scholar] [CrossRef]
- Qiu, J.; Liu, X.J.; You, B.A.; Ren, N.; Liu, H. Application of Nanomaterials in Stem Cell-Based Therapeutics for Cardiac Repair and Regeneration. Small 2023, 19, e2206487. [Google Scholar] [CrossRef]
- Rao, J.; Pan Bei, H.; Yang, Y.; Liu, Y.; Lin, H.; Zhao, X. Nitric Oxide-Producing Cardiovascular Stent Coatings for Prevention of Thrombosis and Restenosis. Front. Bioeng. Biotechnol. 2020, 8, 578. [Google Scholar] [CrossRef] [PubMed]
- Sharma, V.; DeShazo, R.A.; Skidmore, C.R.; Glotzbach, J.P.; Koliopoulou, A.; Javan, H.; McKellar, S.H.; Powell, D.L.;
- Selzman, C.H. Surgical explantation of atrial septal closure devices for refractory nickel allergy symptoms. J. Thorac. Cardiovasc. Surg. 2020, 160, 502–509.e501. [Google Scholar] [CrossRef] [PubMed]
- Tan, J.; Bai, J.; Yan, Z. An Aligned Patterned Biomimetic Elastic Membrane Has a Potential as Vascular Tissue Engineering Material. Front. Bioeng. Biotechnol. 2020, 8, 704. [Google
- Vandergriff, A.C.; Hensley, T.M.; Henry, E.T.; Shen, D.; Anthony, S.; Zhang, J.; Cheng, K. Magnetic targeting of cardiosphere-derived stem cells with ferumoxytol nanoparticles for treating rats with myocardial infarction. Biomaterials 2014, 35, 8528–8539. [Google Scholar] [CrossRef] [PubMed]
- Varna, M.; Xuan, H.V.; Fort, E. Gold nanoparticles in cardiovascular imaging. Wiley Interdiscip. Rev. Nanomed. Nanobiotechnol. 2018, 10, e1470. [Google Scholar] [CrossRef]
- Wang, D.K.; Rahimi, M.; Filgueira, C.S. Nanotechnology applications for cardiovascular disease treatment: Current and future perspectives. Nanomed. Nanotechnol. Biol. Med. 2021, 34, 102387. [Google Scholar] [CrossRef] [PubMed]
- Wolfram, J.; Zhu, M.; Yang, Y.; Shen, J.; Gentile, E.; Paolino, D.; Fresta, M.; Nie, G.; Chen, C.; Shen, H.; et al. Safety of Nanoparticles in Medicine. Curr. Drug Targets 2015, 16, 1671–1681. [Google Scholar] [CrossRef]
- Yang, F.; Xue, J.; Wang, G.; Diao, Q. Nanoparticle-based drug delivery systems for the treatment of cardiovascular diseases. Front. Pharmacol. 2022, 13, 999404. [Google Scholar] [CrossRef]
- Yasin, J.T.; Wallace, A.N.; Madaelil, T.P.; Osbun, J.W.; Moran, C.J.; Cross, D.T.; Limbrick, D.D.; Zipfel, G.J.; Dacey, R.G.; Kansagra, A.P. Treatment of pediatric intracranial aneurysms: Case series and meta-analysis. J. Neurointerventional Surg. 2019, 11, 257–264. [Google Scholar] [CrossRef]
- Yin, L.; Zhang, K.; Sun, Y.; Liu, Z. Nanoparticle-Assisted Diagnosis and Treatment for Abdominal Aortic Aneurysm. Front. Med. 2021, 8, 665846. [Google Scholar] [CrossRef]

39

Advances in the Prenatal Management of Fetal Cardiac Disease

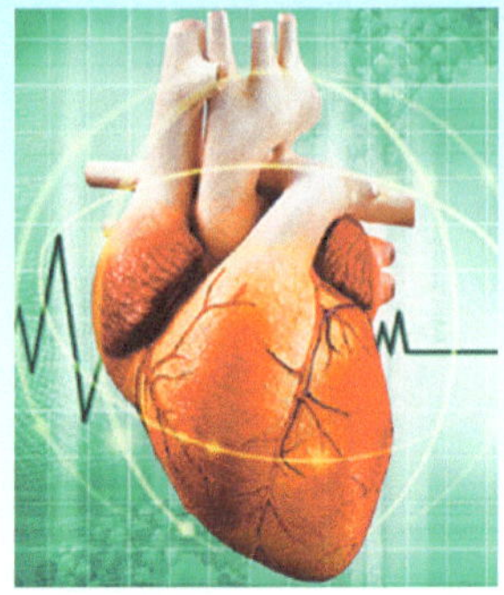

Among various congenital malformations diagnosed in utero, heart defects are one of the most common anomalies detected on prenatal ultrasound .Fetal cardiac screening between 18–22 weeks of gestation is the standard of care, specifically in high risk pregnancy ,however, first trimester imaging is being offered by some centers. Over the last few decades, our ability to detect various congenital heart defects has improved tremendously, secondary to improvement in ultrasound machines, curvilinear probes, three-dimensional and 4D ultrasound etcetera. These advances in fetal imaging, better understanding of the medical pharmacokinetics and the impact of medications on fetal growth, as well as advances in prenatal transcatheter intervention, have allowed us to take steps towards performing various non-invasive and invasive fetal cardiac interventions.

Although advances in fetal imaging have contributed greatly to our ability to intervene prenatally, prenatal approaches to treat cardiac disease date back to 1975, when Eibschitz et al. reported the use of propranolol to treat fetal ventricular tachycardia .In 1991, Maxwell et al. reported the first two cases of balloon valvuloplasty of the aortic valve to treat fetuses with critical aortic stenosis .The role of fetal cardiac therapies vary from the non-invasive medical management of arrhythmias, to performing palliative procedures to allow fetuses to be delivered closer to term and/or improve survival probability in the fetuses who are at risk for fetal/neonatal demise.

Diagnosis and Management of Fetal Arrhythmia

Fetal arrhythmia can be broadly classified in two broad categories, namely, fetal bradycardia or fetal tachyarrhythmias. Using M-mode echocardiography and spectral Doppler, it is possible to evaluate sequential motion of atria and ventricle and thus evaluate the mechanism of arrhythmia

Fetal Bradycardia

Fetal bradycardia can be classified as sinus bradycardia, bradycardia in the setting of long QT Syndrome and bradycardia in the setting of atrioventricular dissociation.

The management of fetal bradycardia depends on the cause of bradycardia as well as the ventricular rate and presence or absence of hydropic changes. Fetal sinus bradycardia is defined as the fetal ventricular rate of 110 beats per minute or less in the setting of 1:1 atrioventricular association .

Bradyarrhythmias can occur from atrioventricular block from congenital abnormality of the atrioventricular node with congenital heart disease such as congenitally corrected transposition of the great arteries, heterotaxy syndrome or from channelopathies, including long QT mutations . Acquired fetal bradyarrhythmias can occur from maternal antibodies to Ro (SS-A) and La (SS-B). Fetal bradycardia can be observed with blocked atrial premature complexes as well. In the setting of persistent fetal bradycardia, the potential consequences include fetal hydrops or fetal cardiomyopathy. In the current era, various transplacental treatment options for immune-mediated atrioventricular block include the administration of fluorinated steroids such as dexamethasone, hydroxychloroquine and/or sympathomimetic agents .More recently, there has been a spate of literature reporting the use of immunomodulatory therapies to prevent either the development or progression of the atrioventricular block to the complete atrioventricular block. Jaeggi et al. evaluated role of dexamethasone and beta-stimulation in 37 fetuses (25.6 +/− 5.2 gestational weeks) with complete heart blocks. In their study, 21 fetuses treated with dexamethasone were to found to have an improved one-year survival of 90%, compared with 46% without glucocorticoid therapy (P 0.02). In another study, Costedoat-Chalumeau et al. reported adverse events associated with use of dexamethasone.

This study evaluated 13 pregnancies in 7 mothers with a history of prior babies with congenital heart blocks associated with maternal anti-SSA/Ro antibodies. In their experience, six pregnancies in which women were treated with dexamethasone (4–5 mg/day) had adverse outcomes, including spontaneous abortion (N:2), stillbirths (N:2) and two live births with intrauterine growth restriction and mild adrenal insufficiency

A prior multicenter open-label study by Friedman et al. evaluated the role of IVIG in preventing the progression to second- or third-degree heart block with a small sample size, and demonstrated no benefit of IVIG to prevent the recurrence of heart block or reduce maternal antibody titers .

Carpenter et al. presented their experience in 1986 with fetal ventricular pacing for hydrops secondary to the complete atrioventricular block . There are various ongoing animal studies evaluating the use of percutaneously implantable fetal pacemaker with mixed results .

Fetal Tachyarrhythmias

Fetal tachycardia was first described by Hayman et al. in 1930 Fetal tachycardia is defined as a fetal heart rate greater than 180–200 beats per minute. Fetal tachyarrhythmias include supraventricular tachycardia (SVT) and atrial flutter, and ventricular tachyarrhythmia. The treatment for tachyarrhythmias primarily depends on the underlying mechanism for tachyarrhythmias. Various treatment options include transplacental therapy with antiarrhythmic such as digoxin, sotalol, amiodarone and flecainide.In cases of severe hydrops, transplacental therapy is known to be less effective. There are case reports on the use of intraperitoneal and intra-amniotic amiodarone injections in the successful treatment of fetal atrial flutter

Table 39.1 An overview of fetal cardiac procedures.

Overview of Fetal Cardiac Procedures		
Fetal cardiac interventions	Congenital heart disease	• Aortic stenosis: Balloon valvuloplasty • Pulmonary stenosis: Balloon valvuloplasty Restrictive atrial septum: HLHS, D-TGA: Atrial septoplasty or atrial stent placement
Other interventions	Fetal arrhythmia	Transplacental treatment: Antiarrhythmic medications (digoxin, sotalol, flecainide or a combination); immunomodulator (intravenous immunoglobulin, steroids); sympathomimetic agents
	Congestive heart failure	• Amnioreduction • Pericardiocentesis Medical management—Digoxin
	Twin-twin transfusion syndrome	• Amnioreduction Endoscopic laser ablation

Legend: HLHS: hypoplastic left heart syndrome; D-TGA: dextro-transposition of the great arteries; TTS: twin–twin transfusion syndrome.

Table 39.2 An overview of fetal cardiac diagnostic work-up.

	Summary of Fetal Cardiac Diagnostic Work-Up
Congenital heart disease	Fetal echocardiogram Fetal MRI
Fetal arrhythmia Other	Fetal magnetocardiogram (FMCG)
	Fetal hyperoxia testing

Pharmacological Approach to Treatment of Intracardiac Rhabdomyomas

With the advances in fetal echocardiographic techniques, prenatal detection of cardiac tumors has enabled us to use transplacental pharmacotherapy to treat cardiac rhabdomyoma.Recent reports have highlighted the transplacental use of the mechanistic target of rapamycin (m-TOR) inhibitors such as sirolimus in the treatment of fetal rhabdomyomas causing outflow obstruction The results reported appear to be promising; however, there are no larger scale trial data to recommend routine use at this time.

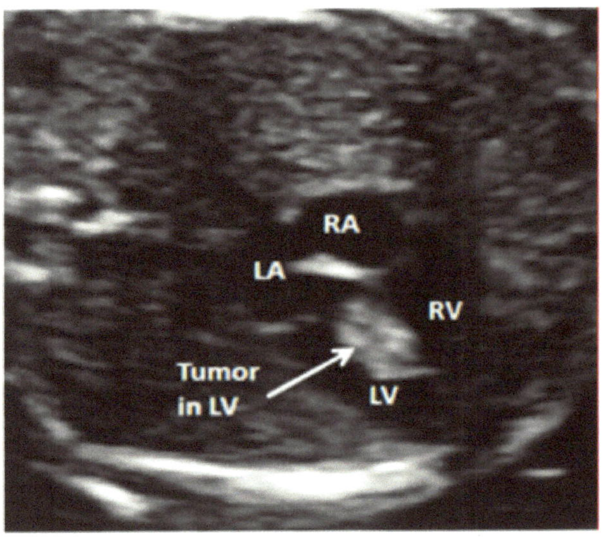

Fig. 39.3 An intracardiac tumor attached to the ventricular septum as observed on four chamber view—LA, left atrium; RA, right atrium; LV, left ventricle; RV, right ventricle.

Maternal Hyperoxia Therapy

Maternal hyperoxia therapy represents another frontier in fetal cardiac therapy. The role of maternal hyperoxygenation in fetuses with Hypoplastic Left Heart Syndrome (HLHS) has been matter of ongoing investigation. Various authors have proposed the role of maternal hyperoxygenation in increasing the fetal pO2 leading to an increase in pulmonary venous blood flow . Increased pulmonary flow can in turn cause increased flow through fetal mitral and aortic valve and thus can have a potential role in "recruiting" the hypoplastic left ventricle.

Apart from potentially therapeutic effects, maternal hyperoxygenation can aid in the identification of fetuses with a lower degree of prenatal pulmonary vasoreactivity, thus identifying those with significant pulmonary vascular disease to predict a need for immediate postnatal intervention .

In a murine model, hyperoxia therapy demonstrated the reduction of excess trabeculation and muscular ventricular septal defects and improved the organization of coronary vasculature in genetically modified mice. A small study of 24 mothers with fetuses known to have CHD demonstrated a variable response to hyperoxygenation on cerebral tissue oxygenation . The authors admit that the small sample size limits the conclusions gleaned from the study, but transplacental oxygen delivery may represent a promising intervention for fetuses with complex CHD. You et al. demonstrated improvement in cerebral blood oxygenation, particularly in fetuses with a single ventricle physiology in a small sample of 30 fetuses. In a study including 43 fetuses, differential response based on the cardiac lesion, with an improved middle cerebral artery pulsatility index in response to maternal hyperoxygenation in patients with d-TGA, but not to a significant extent in cases with left- or right-sided obstructive lesions, was demonstrated .

As our understanding regarding maternal hyperoxia therapy is still evolving, its role and treatment protocols are variable. A systematic review of the current literature by Co-Vu et al. found that most protocols used 8 L with 100% oxygen by a non-rebreather at a mean gestational age of 33.4 weeks . The duration of therapy ranges from 10 min in a single session to 3–4 h per day

Percutaneous Fetal Cardiac Interventions

Use of percutaneous transcatheter fetal intervention is used in a few congenital heart diseases. In 1991, Maxwell et al. reported the first two cases of balloon valvuloplasty of the aortic valve to treat fetuses with critical aortic stenosis . The specific examples include hypoplastic left heart syndrome (HLHS) patients with restrictive septum, HLHS patients with severe aortic valve stenosis, pulmonary atresia with intact ventricular septum, critical pulmonary stenosis and fetal hydrops with pericardial effusion .

As our learning curve as well as expertise increases, the outcomes of fetal intervention have demonstrated varying levels of success . Larger registries have offered insight into the success of fetal intervention. The International Fetal Cardiac Intervention Registry, which included multicenter data from 18 institutions from January 2001 through June 2014, reports varying success..Of a total of 370 cases of various cardiac disease, fetal intervention did not impact survival to discharge . One of the key findings in the registry was the role of fetal cardiac intervention in achieving biventricular repair after birth. In fetuses with a diagnosis of aortic stenosis or evolving HLHS who underwent fetal cardiac intervention, twice as many were discharged with biventricular circulation HLHS with restrictive or intact atrial septum is another area of interest for fetal cardiac intervention. The goal of fetal intervention is to decrease left atrial pressure creating a non-restrictive atrial level shunt. The procedure of choice varies per institute and commonly involves atrial septoplasty or atrial stent placement . In the International Fetal Cardiac Intervention Registry by Moon-Grady et al., 37 fetuses with HLHS underwent atrial septum intervention. A total of 24 out of 37 fetuses had successful intervention with 22/37 live births. However, mortality in the newborn period remained high and only 37 percent (14/17) survived to discharge. In another report by Jantzen et al. from same registry, the rate of procedural success was 85% (N:23/27) for septoplasty and 65% for atrial stent placement (N:13/20) The procedure-related fetal demise was 13% and survival was poor, with aggregate intervened and control fetuses with survival to discharge of 35% . For cases with documented follow-up, fetuses with an unrestricted foramen ovale at birth had a markedly improved survival relative to cases without intervention .

On the contrary, the intervention for pulmonary atresia with intact ventricular septum and critical pulmonary stenosis demonstrates less success. Among 84 cases, fetal complications were reported in 55% of cases including death and delayed fetal loss .

However, among successful cases, the measurement of the tricuspid valve increased on successive imaging with a higher percentage of biventricular function compared to non-intervened fetuses Complications of fetal interventions are relatively common and are often severe, including fetal hemodynamic instability manifesting as ventricular dysfunction and bradycardia . An evaluation of 83 fetuses undergoing fetal intervention demonstrated hemodynamic instability in 45% of cases. This was notably associated with ventricular distortion and one case of hemopericardium [36]. Though poorly understood, it is hypothesized that this may be due to a ventricular reflex or secondary to impaired cardiac output due to ventricular distortion. Improved understanding of fetal hemodynamics and electrophysiology may minimize this risk in the future. Several targets to improve the success of fetal cardiac intervention have been identified. Among these are laser technology for septal ablation, endoscopy to directly visualize the area of intervention, intraperitoneal imaging to improve visualization and miniaturization of catheters in order to enable intervention earlier in gestation than is currently possible .

Fetal cardiac intervention is technically challenging, and the learning curve is rather steep [38]. Using sheep as a model organism, a cardiac intervention team demonstrated significant reduction in the time required to position a needle tip at the aortic root, suggesting that simulation and repetition can improve technical aptitude . For this reason, it has been suggested that single center commitment to a large-volume fetal intervention program may be the best approach to standardize the approach to these interventions and permit sufficient volume to develop technical proficiency. Additional research in sheep models has evaluated the prospect of cardiac bypass for fetal intervention. Currently, this area is limited by significant morbidity due to placental dysfunction . However, novel devices, including the Tiny Pump, have demonstrated limited success . Though fetuses deteriorated after bypass on the TinyPump, the rate of compromise was slower than on a roller head pump [40]. Though clearly, further research is required, the prospect of fetal cardiac intervention on a bypass may be a reality in the decades to come. Currently, the surgical community has not been impacted by fetal intervention in dramatic ways. However, as the field expands it is anticipated that physiologic changes in utero may change the approach to surgical intervention in such fetuses . Further research must also target the long-term outcomesof fetal intervention, including neurodevelopment. One such study reports developmental delay in patients undergoing fetal aortic valvuloplasty, at a rate similar to patients with HLHS without intervention . Interestingly, biventricular physiology was not associated with better neurodevelopmental outcomes.The success of fetal intervention is dependent on technical factors including vascular access, fetal positioning and cardiac anatomy.

These factors likely contribute to the relatively high risk of such interventions and associated fetal and maternal morbidity and mortality. Further, investigation into the genetic and molecular basis of congenital heart disease and emerging technology including stem cell research, nanotechnology and personalized medicine may allow for further advances in fetal cardiac intervention . Proper case identification is imperative to assure the safety of the mother and the fetus, alike, as well as to allow for optimal results . This includes a thorough echocardiographic interrogation and assessment of fetal life Importantly, fetal interventions have also demonstrated safety in mothers, with single center studies reporting no major maternal complications related to fetal cardiac interventions . Among a series of 113 mothers, only one major complication, a placental abruption, was reported . No mothers required intensive care and only two required tocolysis. Importantly, 89% of deliveries were at term . As individual centers further develop their experience and expertise, multicenter and international collaboration is imperative to share best practices and advance the field for the benefit of all.

Conclusions

Whether pharmacologic or percutaneous, our understanding as well as the outcome for approaching congenital heart disease in the fetus has advanced by leaps and bounds. Developments in fetal imaging have improved the diagnosis and characterization of congenital heart disease in utero. However, there continues to be a need for larger studies and more experience in this highly challenging field. Collaboration between various centers to have a more uniform approach for pharmacologic intervention and a few nationalized centers with high volume for percutaneous intervention will help to achieve optimal outcomes. As these approaches increase in utilization, such collaboration may allow for the sharing of best practices and generation of guidelines to support widespread utilization. Future research aiming to improve the understanding of fetal hemodynamics and advanced embryology may direct the development of novel interventions. In addition, the expansion of pharmaceutical approaches and application in larger populations may broaden horizons for non-interventional therapies.

Abstract

Advances in the field have improved the prenatal management of cardiovascular diseases over the past few decades; however, there remains considerable challenges in the approach towards patient selection as well as the applicability of available therapies. This review aims to discuss the current knowledge, outcomes and challenges for prenatal intervention for congenital heart disease.

Bibliography And Acknowledgement

- American College of Obstetricians and Gynecologists ACOG Practice Bulletin No. 106: Intrapartum Fetal Heart Rate Monitoring: Nomenclature, Interpretation, and General Management Principles. Obstet. Gynecol. 2009;114:192–202. doi: 10.1097/AOG.0b013e3181aef106. [PubMed] [CrossRef] [Google Scholar]
- Bacha E.A. Impact of Fetal Cardiac Intervention on Congenital Heart Surgery. Semin. Thorac. Cardiovasc. Surg. Pediatric Card. Surg. Annual. 2011;14:35–37. doi: 10.1053/j.pcsu.2011.01.003. [PubMed] [CrossRef] [Google Scholar]
- Barnes B.T., Procaccini D., Crino J., Blakemore K., Sekar P., Sagaser K.G., Jelin A.C., Gaur L. Maternal Sirolimus Therapy for Fetal Cardiac Rhabdomyomas. N. Engl. J. Med. 2018;378:1844–1845. doi: 10.1056/NEJMc1800352. [PMC free article] [PubMed] [CrossRef] [Google Scholar]
- Carpenter R.J., Strasburger J.F., Garson A., Smith R.T., Deter R.L., Engelhardt H.T. Fetal ventricular pacing for hydrops secondary to complete atrioventricular block. J. Am. Coll. Cardiol. 1986;8:1434–1436. doi: 10.1016/S0735-1097(86)80319-9. [PubMed] [CrossRef] [Google Scholar]
- Donofrio M.T., Schidlow D.N. Prenatal Maternal Hyperoxygenation Testing and Implications for Critical Care Delivery Planning among Fetuses with Congenital Heart Disease: Early Experience. Am. J. Perinatol. 2017;35:16–23. doi: 10.1055/s-0037-1603991. [PubMed] [CrossRef] [Google Scholar]
- Doll C.F., Pereira N.J., Hashimi M.S., Grindrod T.J., Alkassis F.F., Cai L.X., Milovanovic U., Sandino A.I., Kasahara H. Gestational intermittent hyperoxia rescues murine genetic congenital heart disease in part. Sci. Rep. 2021;11:1–9. doi: 10.1038/s41598-021-85569-9. [PMC free article] [PubMed]
- Eibschitz I., Abinader E., Klein A., Sharf M. Intrauterine diagnosis and control of fetal ventricular arrhythmia during labor. Am. J.Obstet.Gynecol.1975;122:597–600.doi 10.1016/0002-9378(75)90056-3. [PubMed] [CrossRef] [Google
- Emery S.P., Kreutzer J., McCaffrey F.M., Sherman F.S., Simhan H.N., Keller B.B. The Learning Curve for a Fetal Cardiac Intervention Team. Minim. Invasive Surg. 2010;2010:674185. doi: 10.1155/2010/674185. [PMC free article] [PubMed] [CrossRef]
- Friedman D.M., Kim M.Y., Copel J.A., Llanos C., Davis C., Buyon J.P. Prospective evaluation of fetuses with autoimmune-associated congenital heart block followed in the PR Interval and Dexamethasone Evaluation (PRIDE) Study. Am. J.Cardiol.2009;103:1102–1106.doi:10.1016j.amjcard.2008.12.027. [PMC free article] [PubMed] [CrossRef] [Google Scholar]
- Guseh S.H., Friedman K.G., Wilkins-Haug L.E. Fetal cardiac intervention—Perspectives from a single center. Prenat. Diagn. 2019;40:415–423. doi: 10.1002/pd.5631. [PubMed] [CrossRef]
- Hogan W.J., Grinenco S., Armstrong A., Devlieger R., Dangel J., Ferrer Q., Frommelt M., Galindo A., Gardiner H., Gelehrter S., et al. Fetal Cardiac Intervention for Pulmonary Atresia with Intact Ventricular Sep-tum: International Fetal Cardiac Intervention Registry. Fetal Diagn. Ther. 2020;47:731–739. doi: 10.1159/000508045. [PubMed]
- Hogan W.J., Moon-Grady A.J., Zhao Y., Cresalia N.M., Nawaytou H., Quezada E., Brook M., McQuillen P., Peyvandi S. Fetal cerebrovascular response to maternal hyperoxygenation in congenital heart disease: Effect of cardiac physiology. Ultrasound Obstet. Gynecol. 2020;57:769–775. doi: 10.1002/uog.22024.

- International Society of Ultrasound in Obstetrics and Gynecology. Carvalho J., Allan L., Chaoui R., Copel J., DeVore G., Hecher K., Lee W., Munoz H., Paladini D., et al. ISUOG Practice Guidelines (updated): Sonographic screening examination of the fetal heart. Ultrasound Obstet. Gynecol. 2013;41:348–359. doi: 10.1002/uog.12403. [PubMed] [CrossRef] [Google Scholar]
- Jaeggi E.T., Fouron J.-C., Silverman E.D., Ryan G., Smallhorn J., Hornberger L.K. Transplacental Fetal Treatment Improves the Outcome of Prenatally Diagnosed Complete Atrioventricular Block Without Structural Heart Disease. Circulation. 2004;110:1542–1548.doi: 10.1161/01.CIR.0000142046.58632.3A. [PubMed] [CrossRef] [Google Scholar]
- Kang S.-L., Jaeggi E., Ryan G., Chaturvedi R.R. An Overview of Contemporary Outcomes in Fetal Cardiac Intervention: A Case for High-Volume Superspecialization? Pediatr. Cardiol. 2020;41:479–485. doi: 10.1007/s00246-020-02294-2. [PubMed] [CrossRef] [Google Scholar]
- Kohl T. Chronic Intermittent Materno-Fetal Hyperoxygenation in Late Gestation May Improve on Hypoplastic Cardiovascular Structures Associated with Cardiac Malformations in Human Fetuses. Pediatr. Cardiol. 2009;31:250–263. doi: 10.1007/s00246-009-9600-5. [PMC free article] [PubMed] [CrossRef] [Google Scholar]
- Laraja K., Sadhwani A., Tworetzky W., Marshall A.C., Gauvreau K., Freud L., Hass C., Dunbar-Masterson C., Ware J., Lafranchi T., et al. Neurodevelopmental Outcome in Children after Fetal Cardiac Intervention for Aortic Stenosis with Evolving Hypoplastic Left Heart Syndrome. J. Pediatr. 2017;184:130–136.e4. doi: 10.1016/j.jpeds.2017.01.034. [PMC free article] [PubMed] [CrossRef] [Google Scholar]
- Lee F.-T., Marini D., Seed M., Sun L. Maternal hyperoxygenation in congenital heart disease. Transl. Pediatr. 2021;10:2197–2209. doi: 10.21037/tp-20-226. [PMC free article] [PubMed] [CrossRef] [Google Scholar]
- Lin P.-H., Wu H.-H., Tsai H.-D., Hsieh C.T.-C. Successful treatment of atrial flutter by repeated intraperitoneal and intra-amniotic injections of amiodarone in a fetus with hydrops. Taiwan. J.Obstet.Gynecol.2016;55:434–436.doi:10.1016/j.tjog.2016.04.022. [PubMed] [CrossRef] [Google Scholar]
- Maxwell D., Allan L., Tynan M.J. Balloon dilatation of the aortic valve in the fetus: A report of two cases. Heart. 1991;65:256–258. doi: 10.1136/hrt.65.5.256. [PMC free article] [PubMed] [CrossRef]
- McElhinney D.B., Tworetzky W., Lock J.E. Current Status of Fetal Cardiac Intervention. Circulation. 2010;121:1256–1263. doi: 10.1161/CIRCULATIONAHA.109.870246. [PMC free article] [PubMed] [CrossRef] [Google Scholar]
- Moon-Grady A.J., Morris S.A., Belfort M., Chmait R., Dangel J., Devlieger R., Emery S., Frommelt M., Galindo A., Gelehrter S., et al. International Fetal Cardiac Intervention Registry: A Worldwide Collaborative Description and Preliminary Outcomes. JACC. 2015;66:388–399. doi: 10.1016/j.jacc.2015.05.037. [PubMed]
- Ozawa Y., Asakai H., Shiraga K., Shindo T., Hirata Y., Hirata Y., Inuzuka R. Cardiac Rhythm Disturbances in Heterotaxy Syndrome. Pediatr. Cardiol. 2019;40:909–913. doi: 10.1007/s00246-019-02087-2. [PubMed] [CrossRef] [Google Scholar]

- Ozawa Y., Asakai H., Shiraga K., Shindo T., Hirata Y., Hirata Y., Inuzuka R. Cardiac Rhythm Disturbances in Heterotaxy Syndrome. Pediatr. Cardiol. 2019;40:909–913. doi: 10.1007/s00246-019-02087-2. [PubMed] [CrossRef] [Google Scholar]

- Park H., Chang C.S., Choi S.-J., Oh S.-Y., Roh C.-R. Sirolimus therapy for fetal cardiac rhabdomyoma in a pregnant woman with tuberous sclerosis. Obstet. Gynecol. Sci. 2019;62:280–284. doi: 10.5468/ogs.2019.62.4.280. [PMC free article] [PubMed]
- Peyvandi S., Xu D., Wang Y., Hogan W., Moon-Grady A., Barkovich A.J., Glenn O., McQuillen P., Liu J. Fetal Cerebral Oxygenation Is Impaired in Congenital Heart Disease and Shows Variable Response to Maternal Hyperoxia. J. Am. Heart Assoc. 2021;10:e018777. doi: 10.1161/JAHA.120.018777. [PMC free article] [PubMed] [CrossRef] [Google Scholar]
- Rasanen J., Wood D.C., Debbs R.H., Cohen J., Weiner S., Huhta J.C. Reactivity of the Human Fetal Pulmonary Circulation to Maternal Hyperoxygenation Increases During the Second Half of Pregnancy: A randomized study. Circulation. 1998;97:257–262.
- Rebizant B., Koleśnik A., Grzyb A., Chaberek K., Sękowska A., Witwicki J., Szymkiewicz-Dangel J., Dębska M. Fetal Cardiac Interventions—Are They Safe for the Mothers? J. Clin. Med. 2021;10:851. doi: 10.3390/jcm10040851. [PMC free article] [PubMed] [CrossRef] [Google Scholar]
- Rooth G., Huch A., Huch R. Guidelines for the use of fetal monitoring. Int. J. Gynecol. 1987;25:159. [Google Scholar]
Schidlow D.N., Freud L., Friedman K., Tworetzky W. Fetal interventions for structural heart disease. Echocardiography. 2017;34:1834–1841. doi: 10.1111/echo.13667. [PubMed] [CrossRef] [Google Scholar]
- Sebastian V.A., Ferro G., Kagawa H., Nasirov T., Maeda K., Ferrier W.T., Takatani S., Riemer R.K., Hanley F.L., Reddy V.M. Fetal cardiac intervention: Improved results of fetal cardiac bypass in immature fetuses using the TinyPump device. J. Thorac. Cardiovasc. Surg. 2013;145:1460–1464. doi: 10.1016/j.jtcvs.2012.08.014. [PubMed] [CrossRef] [Google Scholar]
- Szwast A., Tian Z., McCann M., Donaghue D., Rychik J. Vasoreactive Response to Maternal Hyperoxygenation in the Fetus with Hypoplastic Left Heart Syndrome. Circ. Cardiovasc. Imaging. 2010;3:172–178. doi: 10.1161/CIRCIMAGING.109.848432. [PMC free article] [PubMed] [CrossRef] [Google Scholar]
- Todros T., Capuzzo E., Gaglioti P. Prenatal diagnosis of congenital anomalies. Images Paediatr. Cardiol. 2001;3:3–18. [PMC free article] [PubMed] [Google Scholar]
- Tunks R.D., Clowse M.E., Miller S.G., Brancazio L.R., Barker P.C. Maternal autoantibody levels in congenital heart block and potential prophylaxis with antiinflammatory agents. Am. J. Obs. Gynecol. 2013;208:64.e1–64.e7. doi: 10.1016/j.ajog.2012.09.020. [PubMed] [CrossRef] [Google Scholar]
- Van Aerschot I., Rosenblatt J., Boudjemline Y. Fetal cardiac interventions: Myths and facts. Arch. Cardiovasc. Dis-Ease. 2012;105:366–372. doi: 10.1016/j.acvd.2012.01.011. [PubMed] [CrossRef] [Google Scholar]
- Van den Heuvel F., Bink-Boelkens M.T., du Marchie Sarvaas G.J., Berger R.M. Drug management of fetal tachyarrhythmias: Are we ready for a systematic and evidence-based approach? Pacing Clin. Electrophysiol. 2008;31((Suppl. 1)):S54–S57. doi: 10.1111/j.1540-8159.2008.00958.x. [PubMed] [CrossRef] [Google Scholar]
- Wohlmuth C., Tulzer G., Arzt W., Gitter R., Wertaschnigg D. Maternal aspects of fetal cardiac intervention. Ultrasound Obstet. Gynecol. 2014;44:532–537. doi: 10.1002/uog.13438. [PubMed]
- You W., Andescavage N.N., Kapse K., Donofrio M.T., Jacobs M., Limperopoulos C. Hemodynamic Responses of the Placenta and Brain to Maternal Hyperoxia in Fe-tuses with Congenital Heart Disease by Using Blood Oxygen–Level Dependent MRI. Radiology. 2020;294:141–148. doi: 10.1148/radiol.2019190751. [PMC free article] [PubMed] [CrossRef] [Google Scholar]
- Zhou L., Vest A.N., Chmait R.H., Bar-Cohen Y., Pruetz J., Silka M., Zheng K., Peck R., Loeb G.E. A percutaneously implantable fetal pacemaker. Annu. Int. Conf. IEEE Eng. Med. Biol. Soc. 2014;2014:4459–4463. doi: 10.1109/embc.2014.6944614. [PMC free article] [PubMed] [CrossRef] [Google Scholar

40 Tropical Diseases Affecting Cardiovascular System

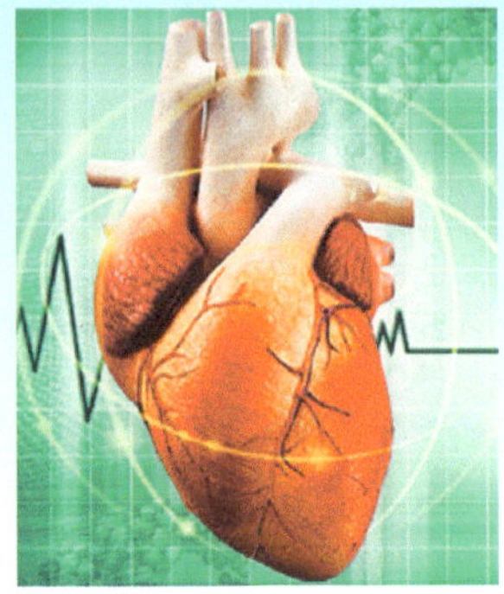

DEFINITION OF TROPICAL DISEASE

A tropical disease is any illness that is most common or only occurs (endemic) in tropical or subtropical areas. Beyond location, many have little in common with each other. They are caused by a variety of factors, including viruses, bacteria, protozoa and parasitic worms (nematodes and trematodes). Some frequently cause no symptoms, while others are severe and may become fatal. The routes of transmission also range widely and include insect bites, contaminated water and food, and direct contact with an infected person.The tropics are defined by geography and climate.

They are the areas between the Tropic of Cancer and the Tropic of Capricorn (23.5 degrees of latitude north and south of the equator, respectively). In the Western Hemisphere, this includes much of the Caribbean and Mexico, Central America and much of South America. Also considered tropical are Africa between the Sahara Desert and South Africa, southern Asia, much of India, northern Australia and many of the island nations in the western Pacific Ocean. These areas have high temperatures and humidity throughout the year. Seasons are marked more by changes in rainfall than other conditions.

The subtropics are the climatic region between tropical and temperate areas. Unlike the tropics, they do not occur within defined latitudes.The reasons these diseases are geographically limited vary. Some can not develop outside the environmental conditions (e.g. temperature, humidity) provided by tropical and subtropical climates. Others require specific animal hosts that occur within this limited range. Certain diseases once had broader ranges but have been eliminated. Many of the countries in the tropics are developing nations and may not be able to afford the sanitation and medical programs required to eliminate these diseases.

The tropical diseases are largely absent naturally or as a result of eradication programs in the developed countries and other industrialized nations. Outbreaks in these countries are often linked to immigrants or travelers returning from areas where the diseases are endemic. They may occur sporadically, but are often limited by seasonal climate changes.

Types and Differences of Tropical Disease

The tropics include portions of nearly every continent and some of the world's most populous countries. The number of diseases endemic to such a large area with so many people is difficult to estimate. To better understand them, they may be categorized by the organisms. They have a more complex structure, including a nucleus (the core of a cell containing chromosomes) and are often classified within the animal kingdom. Some may infect humans and cause disease. In the tropics, these diseases include:

Cardiac Involvement in Infectious Diseases

Evidence of cardiac affection in the infectious fevers may be of several different types:

1. There may be histological evidence of myocarditis in autopsied patients, in whom the cardiac diagnosis mayor may not have been suspected during life. The incidence of myocarditis in such an autopsy series would be unduly high, since patients with myocarditis are more likely to die.
2. The diagnosis of myocarditis may be based on ECG abnormalities. It is doubtful whether T wave or ST segment changes alone justify a diagnosis of myocarditis, since there is evidence that such changes can be caused by pyrexia, electrolyte imbalance or other physiological disturbances.
3. One may find definite or presumptive clinical signs of cardiac affection, such as pericardial rub, cardiac dilatation, gallop rhythm, muffling of the first heart sound, or tachycardia out of proportion to the fever. There may be ECG abnormalities such as gross conduction defects and serious arrhythmias. These

signs of carditis are superimposed and perhaps over shadowed by the other clinical manifestations of the infectious disease itself. Unexpected sudden death occurring during the course of an infectious disease is usually presumed to be due to myocarditis.

4. There is a group of cases in which pericarditis or myocarditis is apparently "idiopathic" or "isolated" with no overt involvement of any other system. Only during this last decade has it been realised that certain viruses are responsible for some of these cases

2.Infections and infestations.

Bacterial Infections

Diphtheria

Acute myocarditis is said to complicate 10 to 25% of all cases of diphtheria, the incidence varying fromepidemic to epidemic. Histologically fatty degeneration and necrosis of the cardiac muscle fibres are seen at the end of the first week and beginning, of the second week of the illness; interstitial inflammatory changes consisting of edema and cellular infiltrations are seen later in the second week. Fibroblasts and granulation tissue then appear and scar tissue is well formed after 3 weeks.

The clinical picture of myocarditis conforms with pathological evidence that myocarditis does not occur very early in the course of the disease. Thus cough, cyanosis and tachycardia during the first few days of the illness are usually due to the respiratory obstruction caused b the diphtheritic membrane and surrounding edema.

True cardiac manifestations usually appear at the end of the first week or during the second week, but occasionally after several weeks, particularly in cutaneous diphtheria. The onset of myocarditis in a child with diphtheria may be heralded by bradycardia. When present, a slow pulse rate mayor may not be due to A.V. heart block. Gallop rhythm, mufHing of the first heart sound, tic-tac rhythm and cardiac enlargement are other signs of myocarditis.The classical manifestation of of congestive heart failure such as orthopnea,hepatomegaly, pitting edema and engorged veins are the exception rather than rule. Severe diphtheritic myocarditis manifests as "cardiogenic shock" with a small thready pulse, vomiting, abdominal pain, marked apathy and severe,4 arterial hypotension.

Electrocardiography is very useful in diagnosing myocarditis and assessing its severity, especially if serial tracings are taken. The earliest change may be slight sagging of the ST segment, and the commonest abnormality is flattening or inversion of the T wave, usually in several leads. More ominous, though less frequent, are the disturbances of impulse conduction. These include

1. First, second and third degrees of atrio-ventricular block
2. Intraventricular conduction defects, including bundle branch block. If complete heart block or complete hundle branch block is present, the mortality is from 70 to 100%.

Partial defects of conduction carry a somewhat better prognosis, and normal conduction is usually restored within a week (Figs 47.1 and 47.2).

Other rare cardiac complications of diphtheria are:

1. Arrhythmias such as extrasystoles, nodal rhythm, paroxysmal tachycardias, atrial flutter and fibrillation, and ventricular fibrillation.
2. Intracardiac thrombi may form which embolise to the brain, the lungs or the extremeties, causing hemiplegia, hemoptysis or gangrene of a limb respectively.

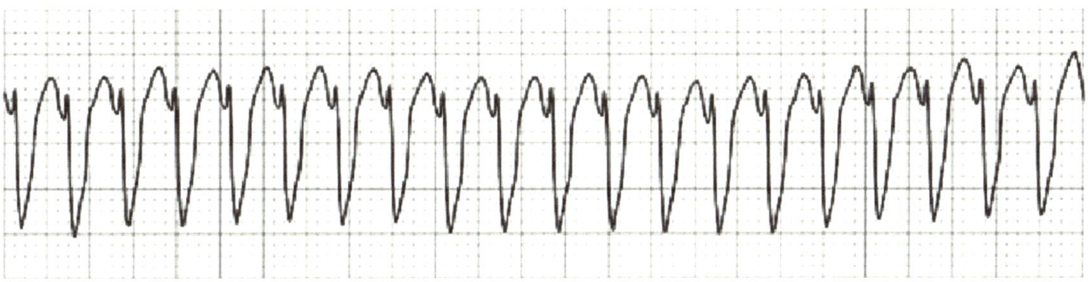

Fig. 40.1: *Graph showing ventricular tachycardia: Broad QRS complexes with no visible P waves*

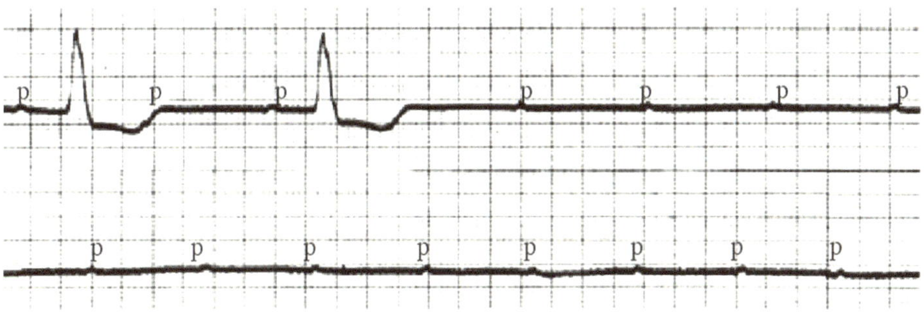

Fig. 40.2: *Graph showing extreme form of bradycardia in complete heat block in a patient who presented with stoke-Adam attacks*

3. A true bacterial endocarditis due to the diphtheria (Klebs Loeffler) bacillus has been reported.
4. Tachycardia at rest may persist for many weeks.

Prognosis

Acute myocarditis accounts for 60% of all deaths due to diphtheria. It has been estimated that the overall mortality of diphtheritic myocarditis is between 50 and 60%, being almost 100% in infants, 50% between 2 and 10 years and 25% in adults. In fatal cases death usually occurs in the first 2 weeks of the illness. It is controversial as to whether diphtheritic myocarditis ever results in permanent cardiac damage in the form of cardiac enlargement or complete heart block. Long term follow-up studies have not shown any such persisting heart damage in individuals who have suffered from severe diphtheria in the past.

Treatment

Therapy is mainly that of diphtheria ihself with antitoxin and penicillin.Patients recovering from diphtheritic myocarditis require a longer period of bed rest than uncomplicated cases of diphtheria. Digitalis is indicated unless heart block is present.

Pneumonia (Figs 47.3 and 47.4)

In pre-antibiotic days, pneumococcal endo-carditis to complicate 4% of all cases of lobar pneumonia. Local spread of the pneumococcus to the pericardium from the contiguous lung or pleura was also not uncommon. Acute peripheral circulatory failure is well known as a preterminal but potentially reversible complication of lobar pneumonia. Non-specific ECG changes in the T wave and ST segment were frequently found. Pneumonia often causes rapid deterioration in patients with pre-existing heart disease, especially in children suffering from congenital heart with left-to-right shunts and in adults with mitral stenosis. Unfortunately such patients are particularly prone to intercurrent respiratory infections.

Typhoid fever: Very rarely a typhoid endocarditis, pericarditis or interstitial myocarditis can occur, although non-specific T wave changes and prolongation of the P-R interval are frequently observed.

Meningococcal Infection: Meningococci can cause acute bacterial endocarditis, which is often overshadowed by the concomitant meningitis. Other rarely reported cardiac involvement in bacterial infections include pericarditis, endocarditis or myocarditis caused by brucellosis, leptospirosis or salmonellosis.

Virus Infections

Poliomyelitis: Myocardial involvement has been found in 40 to 90% of autopsied cases. Microscopically a is seen with focal collections of inflammatory cells in the interstitial tissue. The poliomyelitis virus has been isolated from the heart in fatal cases.

Electrocardiographic: Changes have varied from 15 to 45% in different series. These changes include prolonged PR interval, ST segment deviations, flattening or inversion of the T waves and prolonged QT interval. About two-thirds of patients develop hypertension, between the third and seventh days. Subsequently the blood pressure falls and almost always reaches normal at the end of two weeks. It is extremely unusual for the hypertension to persist. Viral involvement of the hypothalamus and arterial hypoxia (due to hypoventilation) may be important in the pathogenesis of hypertension. Hypertension particularly occurs in bulbar poliomyelitis (Figs 47.5 and 47.6).

A shock-like state is also seen in bulbar poliomyelitis, partly due to the myocarditis and partly to destruction of vasomotor centres in the brain sten. It is usually accompanied

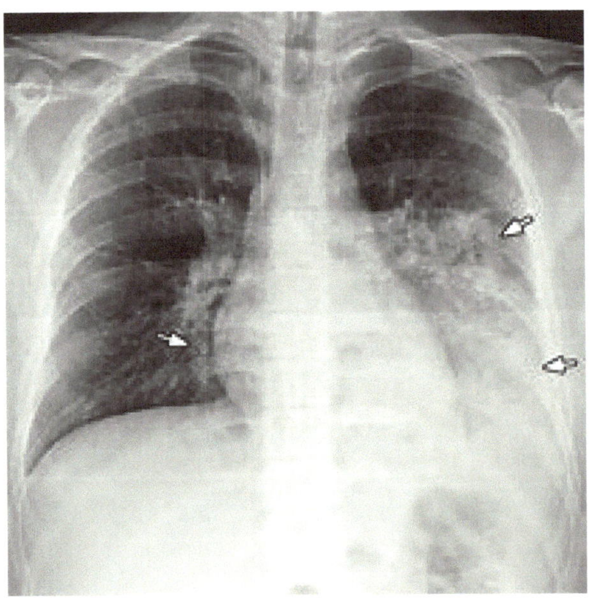

Fig. 40.3: *X-ray chest PA view showing left lung pneumonia with pulmonary arterial hypertension and acute right heart failure in one year old child with post measles infection*

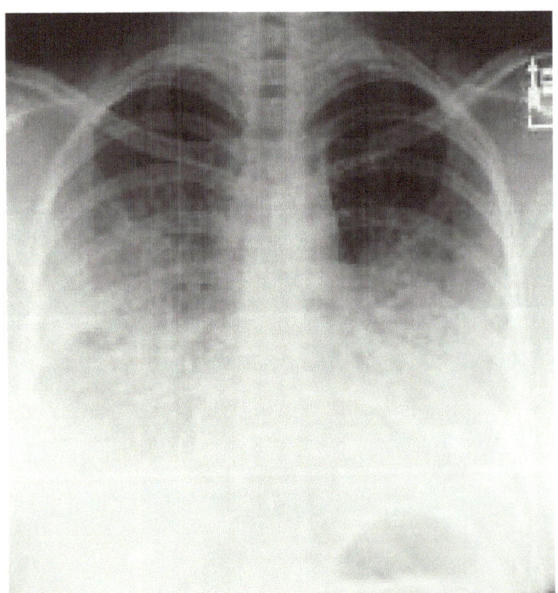

Fig. 40.4: *X-ray chest PA view showing bilateral widespread broncho-pneumonia with congestine heart failure in 2yrs old child with pneumococcal infection*

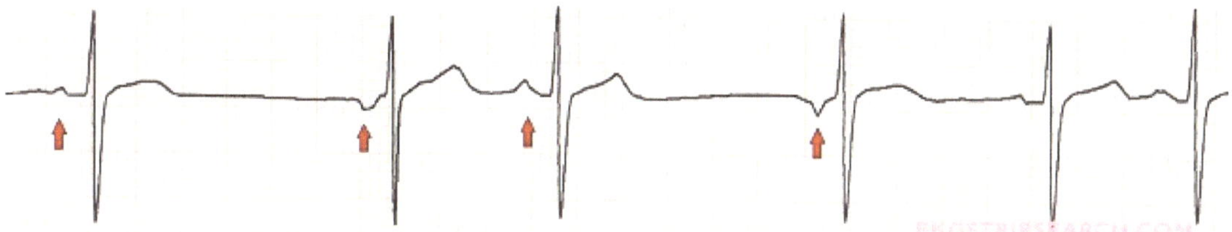

Fig. 40.5: *ECG showing varying P wave morphology and P-R interval as a part of wandering pacemaker in 6yrs old boy with Coxsackie virus B myopericarditis*

by hyper-pyrexia and tachycardia. Pulmonary edema is often seen in the terminal stage. Inhalation of 100% oxygen or its administration by positive pressure may be valuable in such cases. Digitalis is indicated when hypertension and myocarditis are both present.

Measles: Non-specific ECG changes occur in 20% of children suffering from measels. Measels myocarditis and pericarditis have been reported.

Influenza: During the influenza pandemic which swept the earth 16 years ago, caused by the Asian Virus (Type A), myocarditis was frequently demonstrated at autopsy.

Myocarditis has been diagnosed clinically in children who have serological evidence of a recent influenza virus infection. The clinical picture was characterised by fever, a transient skin rash and severe congestive heart failure of sudden onset. The cardiac failure did not improve with routine measures, but responded dramatically to corticosteroids.

Mumps: Non-specific ECG changes are observed in 5 to 15% of all patients affected by epidemic parotitis. However, mumps myocarditis severe enough to cause death is extremely rare, though it undoubtedly occurs.

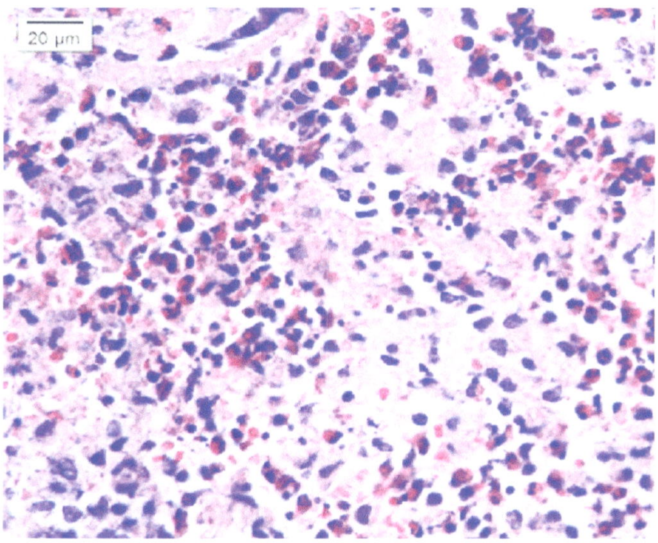

Fig. 47.6: *An endomyocardial biopsy specimen showed remarkable eosinophilic cell infiltration at the interstitium of the myocardium and necrosis of the myocardium. This findings were compatible with eosinophilic myocarditis (Hematoxylin and Eosin staining, ×200).*

Coxsackie virus carditis: Much interest has been aroused in recent years by the frequent implication of Coxsackie virus group B as a cause of myocarditis and pericarditis in both children and adults. It tends to occur in epidemics; outbreaks have been reported from Germany, Australia, South Africa and North America.

Infants are commonly affected. Clinically here is a sudden onset of malaise and the infant goes off feeds; three tto 10 days later high fever develops with marked tachycardia, respiratory distress, cyanosis, cardiac dilatation, gallop rhythm and hepato-splenomegaly. In severe cases, signs of aseptic meningitis or encephalomyelitis may coexist. The patient usually dies in a few days or rapidly recovers. In reported cases there has been a history of upper respiratory infections in the mother during the last weeks of pregnancy. Infection of neonatal infants with Coxsackie B virus is believed to take place either transplacentally or by the oral route after birth.

In suspected cases, the diagnosis of Coxsackie virus is made by isolating it from blood, faces, or throat and by demonstrating a rising titre of neutralising antibodies in the patients' blood.

Other Viral Infections

Viral myocarditis has also been reported in association with infection by ECHO viruses, adenoviruses, varicella, psittacosis, dengue, epidemic encephalits, herpes zoster, rabies and lymphocytic choriomeningitis. In addition there is an encephalo-myocarditis family of viruses which have been shown to cause encephalitis and myocarditis in

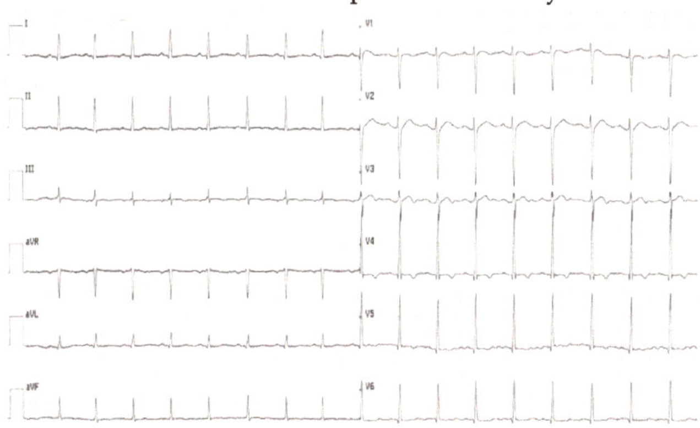

Fig.40.7: *ECG of a patient with viral infection . Electrocardiogram showing sinus tachycardia with T-wave inversion in V4 and flat T in V5 - V6 and in the limb leads.*

experimental animals, particularly in monkeys. There is also strong evidence of their potential pathogenecity in man. The theory has often been put forward that many cases of cardiomyopathy are really the end-result or burnt-out stage of viral myocarditis. Until recently this supposition was merely a speculation not substantiated by actual proof, but recently workers in Europe and America have accumulated an impressive array of virological and autopsy evidence demonstrating that endocardial fibroelastosis is an aftermath of viral myocarditis probably caused by the Coxsackie virus.

Very little is known of the prevalence of cardiac involvement in viral infections in India. Facilities for viral studies and research are extremely limited in this country. There is much scope for investigation as to whether some cases of so-called idiopathic cardiomyopathy, idiopathic myocarditis or idiopathic pericarditis are in fact related to a preceding viral infection.

Cardiac Involvement in Parasitic Diseases

Human parasitic infections are ubiquitous and affect a substantial number of individuals worldwide. Protozoan and helminth parasites can lead to a wide array of clinical manifestations during their migration inside the human body or when they reach their end organ of infection. Moreover, some parasitic infections are associated with significant morbidity and mortality in areas of high endemicity

The heart and the lungs are the thoracic organs more frequently affected by parasitic infections. The involvement of the heart may be part of a more generalized illness, as is the case with human African trypanosomiasis (HAT). In other situations, parasitic infections may have more direct effects on various structures of the heart (myocardium, pericardium, endocardium, or the cardiac vasculature). The involvement of the myocardium may lead to myocarditis or different types of cardiomyopathies (i.e. dilated or restrictive). When the pericardium is affected, it may lead to pericarditis, pericardial effusion, cardiac tamponade, or constrictive pericarditis. Some parasitic infections, such as schistosomiasis, may cause pulmonary hypertension in many developing tropical and subtropical settings. Latent parasitic infections may also reactivate and manifest as systemic disease, often ultimately affecting the heart, in immunosuppressive states such as organ transplantation, the use of immunosuppressive agents, or HIV/AIDS. Due to growing migration, population displacement, and travel, clinicians anywhere around the globe must be aware of the potential cardiac manifestations of parasitic diseases. In this regard, Chagas' cardiomyopathy is the hallmark of a disease that is currently considered a global parasitic disease.

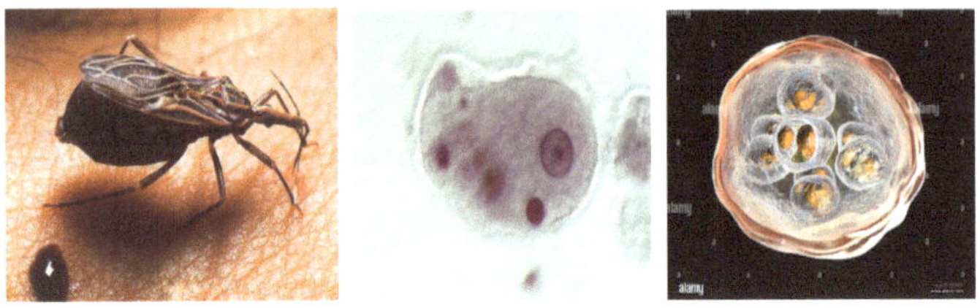

Fig.47.8:Photographic features of three parasites involving heart disease (from left to right)are American trypanosomiasis,Amoebiasis and Echinococcus

Table 40.1: *Parasitic diseases affecting the heart*

Myocarditis	American trypanosomiasis African trypanosomiasis Visceral larva migrans Toxoplasmosis Trichinella spiralis Amoebiasis Echinococcus
Cardiomyopathy	Chagas' disease Toxoplasmosis
Pericarditis	Amoebiasis African trypanosomiasis Chagas disease' Toxoplasmosis Echinococcus

In this review, we present an overview of the most frequently identified parasitic infections that affect the heart. For each topic we present a discussion of the epidemiology, pathogenesis, clinical manifestations, and treatment

PARASITES THAT PREFERENTIALLY INVOLVE THE MYOCARDIUM OR CAUSE PANCARDITIS

Trypanosomes

Trypanosoma Cruzi (Chagas' Disease)

Chagas' disease, also known as American trypanosomiasis, is a zoonotic tropical disease caused by the flagellate protozoan parasite *Trypanosoma cruzi*. Most infections occur through vector-borne transmission by triatomine insects in areas of endemicity but can also occur through blood transfusion or organ transplantation, vertically from mother to infant, and, more rarely, by ingestion of food or liquid contaminated with *T. cruzi* or accidents among laboratory

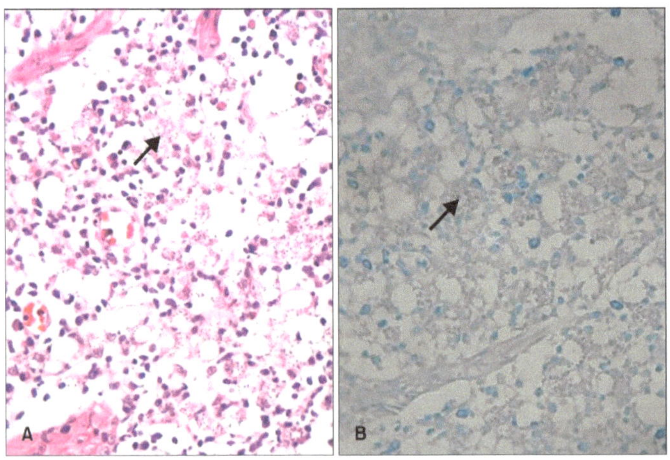

Fig.40.9: Histopathological findings show numerous Leishman-Donovan bodies (arrows) in the cytoplasm of macrophages (A: H&E stain, ×400; B: Giemsa stain, ×400).

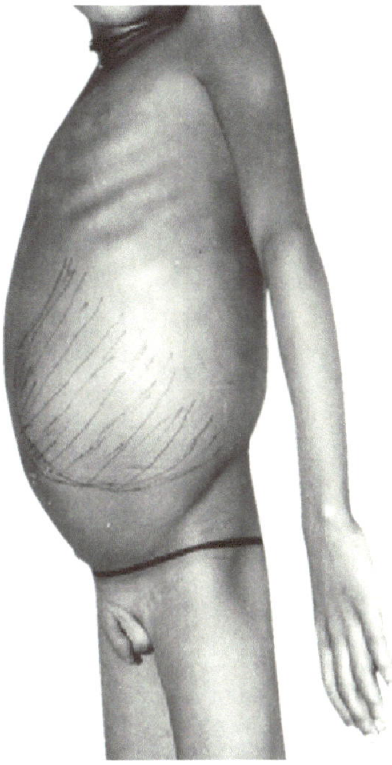

Fig. 47.10: *Showing tropical splenomegaly (marked))in a young patient with chronic recurrent malaria*

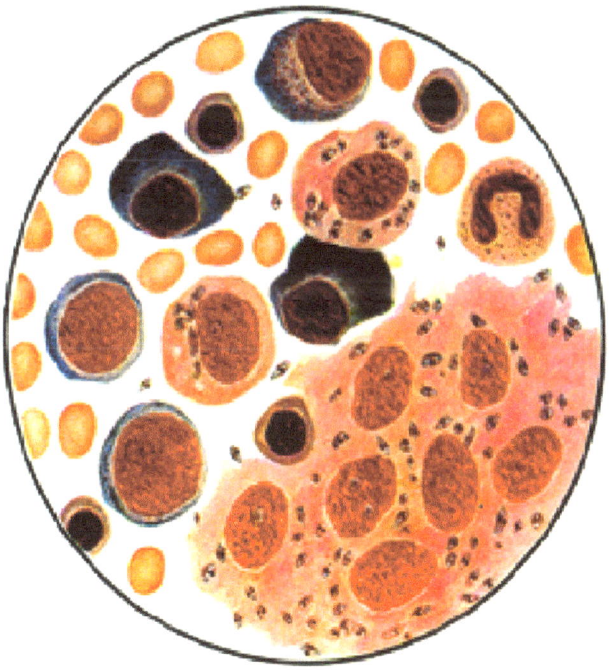

Fig. 40.11: *Microphotograph showing Sternal aspirate in visceral leishmaniasis in which there is hyperplasia of reticulo-histiocystic elements,which contain great numbers of leishmania parasites*

personnel who work with live parasites). Vector-borne transmission involves the transmission of the infective form of the parasite (the metacyclic trypomastigotes) to humans by the excreta of the triatomine insect through mucous membranes or through breaks in the skin. Trypomastigotes then invade local host cells, where they differentiate into amastigotes and multiply within the cell. When the cell is swollen with amastigotes, they transform back into trypomastigotes by growing flagellae. The trypomastigotes lyse the cells, invade adjacent tissues, and spread via the lymphatics and bloodstream to distant sites. The cycle is completed when a reduviid bug becomes infected by ingesting blood from an infected host A minority of patients will develop an acute syndrome of 4 to 8 weeks' duration, which invariably involves prolonged fever in addition to a variable constellation of symptoms, which include inflammation at the portal of entry, subcutaneous edema (localized or generalized), lymphadenopathy, hepatosplenomegaly, myocarditis, and, more rarely, meningoencephalitis The manifestations of the acute phase resolve spontaneously for the vast majority of individuals even if the infection is not treated with an antiparasitic drug. About 60 to 70% of these patients will never develop clinically apparent diseases. They remain asymptomatic and infected life long, being recognized only if serological tests are performed (the so-called indeterminate form of chronic Chagas' disease). Roughly 30 to 40% of infected patients will subsequently develop the cardiac and/or digestive (megaesophagus and megacolon) form of chronic Chagas' disease, usually 10 to 30 years after the initial infection

Epidemiology

Trypanosoma cruzi is endemic in South America, Central America, and parts of North America (Southern United States and Mexico). Historically, the disease disproportionately affected the poor because the transmission of *T. cruzi* infection occurred mainly in rural areas where humans live in poor-quality houses and in close contact with potential vectors. However, rural-to-urban and international migrations have changed the epidemiology of Chagas' disease, affecting periurban areas, urban areas, areas of endemicity, and areas of nonendemicity alike As a result of these dynamic changes in the population and the coordinated efforts of countries where disease is endemic to interrupt vectorial and transfusional transmission, the prevalence and incidence of the disease are constantly changing. In the 1980s the overall prevalence of *T. cruzi* infection was estimated to reach 17 million cases in 18 countries where disease is endemic, with 100 million people at risk Multinational vector control programs and compulsory blood bank screening achieved enormous success in the 1990s, decreasing the incidence of new infections (700,000 cases per year in 1983) by 70% and the number of annual deaths by approximately 50% for the whole continent and eradicating the transmission of *T. cruzi* by the main domiciliary vector species, *Triatoma infestans*, from three of the countries where *T. cruzi* is endemic (Uruguay in 1997, Chile in 1999, and Brazil in 2006) According to the most recent estimates, there are currently 7.6 million people infected with *T. cruzi* in Latin America Although precise figures documenting the total burden of cardiac involvement with *T. cruzi* are not available, it can be assumed that 20 to 30% of the 7.6 million infected individuals are or will potentially be developing chronic

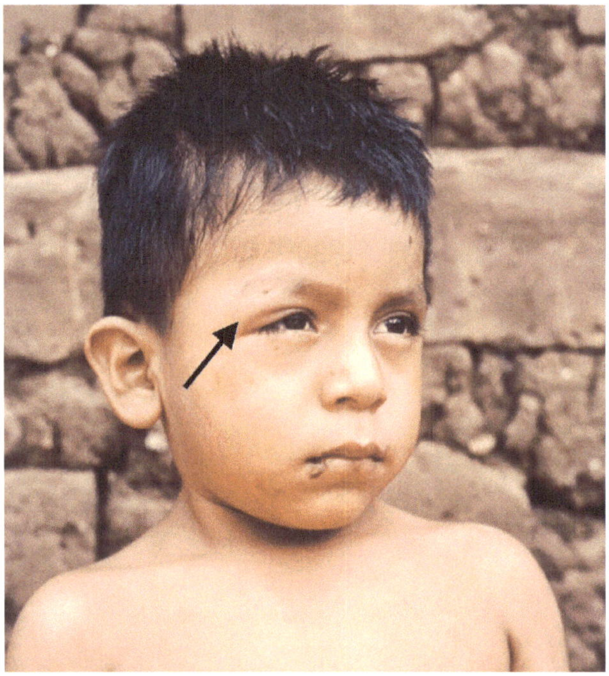

Fig. 40.12: *A young child showing swelling of right eye as one of the manifestations of the acute phase of chagas disease (Romana" sign)*

cardiac lesions. Chagas' cardiomyopathy, in turn, is thought to represent the principal cause of cardiac morbidity and mortality among young adults in countries where *T. cruzi* is endemic and has been estimated to result in at least 21,000 deaths each year,, Additionally, because of the constant influx of immigrants from countries where the disease is endemic, Chagas' disease is becoming an important health issue in North America (United States and Canada) and many parts of Europe, where a growing number of individuals are suspected to be infected (e.g. 300,000 individuals in the United States and 48,000 to 67,000 individuals in Spain

Pathology and Pathophysiology of Acute Myocarditis and Chronic Cardiomyopathy

Initially, the abundance of parasites associated with the acute phase of *T. cruzi* infection argued in favor of the parasite's direct implication in the tissue damage and myocarditis observed during this stage of the disease. Shortly afterwards, a demonstration of myocytolysis of nonparasitized cardiomyocytes led to the implication of parasite-directed cellular immune-mediated inflammatory damage. This immune-mediated damage, associated with large numbers of amastigotes in cardiac myocytes, translates into the hyaline degeneration of muscle fibers, the coagulation necrosis of myocytes and surrounding tissues, as well as the involvement of the epicardium and pericardium. Cellular and, possibly, humoral immune responses elicited by the parasite eventually control the acute infection but fail to completely eliminate the parasite. A variably long asymptomatic phase then ensues, where factors such as the parasite strain, the parasite load during the acute phase, the quality of the immune response, and the presence or absence of reinfection all might influence the course of chronic disease). Regarding the pathogenesis of the interstitial fibrosis, myocytolysis, and ongoing lymphocytic infiltration observed for the chronic phase of Chagas' disease, the paucity of parasites in cardiac tissue probably reflects the use of insensitive histological techniques in past decades. In recent years, more powerful and sensitive methods of parasite detection, such as immunohistochemistry and PCR, have demonstrated a higher frequency of *T. cruzi* antigens or parasite DNA in chronic lesions). The spectrum of outcomes for patients infected with *T. cruzi* is varied and probably stems from intrinsic genetic differences of both the parasite and the host and perhaps even the likelihood of ongoing infection in areas where the disease is highly endemic. Evidence exists for multiple hypotheses to explain the etiology of chronic cardiac lesions that implicate the parasite directly, the immune reaction to the parasite, and autoimmunity elicited either directly by the parasite (mimicry) or indirectly (bystander activation). The products of these lesions are various degrees of necrosis, neuronal damage, microvascular damage, and fibrosis. The contributing role of each mechanism to the pathogenesis of Chagas' cardiomyopathy is a whole other topic of debate.

There is evidence for both functional and anatomical parasympathetic neuronal damage in Chagasic patients Patients with Chagas' disease lack the tonic inhibitory parasympathetic action on the sinus node and, thus, the chronotropic mechanism to respond to changes in blood pressure or venous return. Neuronal loss is thought to occur during the acute stage of the disease; the extent of neuronal damage, however, does not correlate with disease stage Therefore, despite possible contributions of parasympathetic impairment to the impact of Chagas' heart disease (e.g. increasing vulnerability to malignant arrhythmias and sudden death or accentuating existing contraction abnormalities that can culminate in chamber dilatation), cardiac dysautonomia is unlikely to explain the main pathogenic mechanism underlying Chagas' cardiomyopathy.

In addition to the neuronal damage, microcirculatory changes leading to ischemia have also been implicated in the pathogenesis of chronic Chagas' cardiomyopathy. A diffuse collapse of intramyocardial arterioles in the hearts of chronically infected patients has been observed Occlusive platelet thrombi in small epicardial and intramural coronary arteries and increased production of cytokines and mediators that promote vasospasm and platelet aggregation have been demonstrated with experimental models of Chagas' disease, Clinically, despite consistently normal epicardial coronary arteries upon coronary angiography, reversible perfusion defects upon stress-induced myocardial perfusion scintigraphy that correlate with ischemia and abnormal coronary flow regulation have been shown for patients with chronic Chagas' cardiomyopathy.

As mentioned above, tissue damage caused directly by the parasite or, more likely, by the immune response elicited

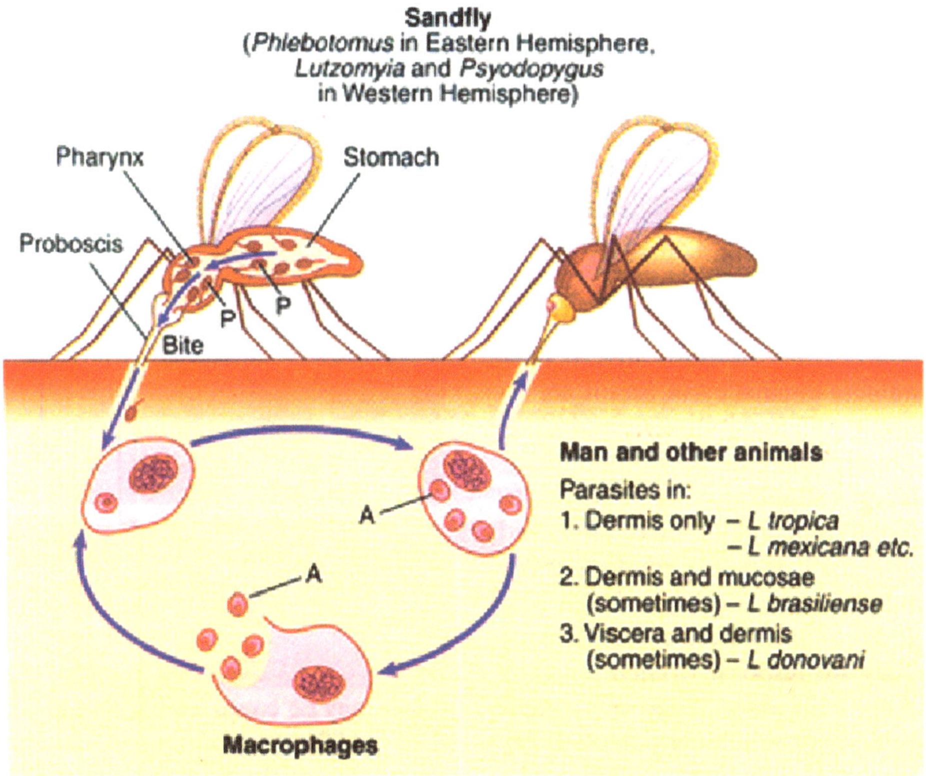

Fig. 40.13: *Showing how sand fly is busy introducing the organisms in human and other animals in the process of disease*

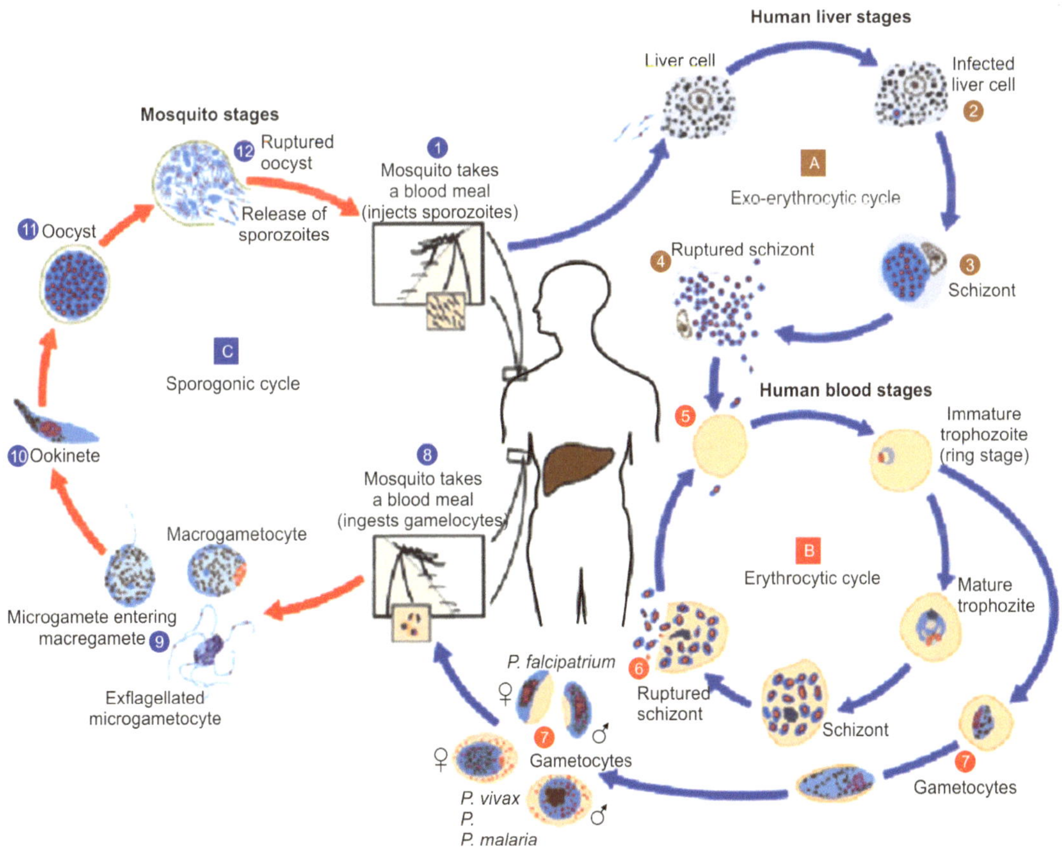

Fig. 40.14: *Showing life cycle of Trypanosoma cruzi in human body inthe causation of chaga's disease*

by it has been postulated to underlie and potentiate the aggression to cardiac myocytes and neurons. The inflammatory infiltrate in chronic Chagas' cardiomyopathy involves a predominance of macrophages, $CD8^+$ and $CD4^+$ lymphocytes (in a 2:1 ratio), and in some instances has been shown to correlate with more advanced stages of the disease. The persistence of parasites and antigens is thought to be involved in the recruitment of *T. cruzi*-specific $CD8^+$ T lymphocytes, which predominate in the myocardial infiltrate in cases of chronic Chagas' myocarditis. The cytokine profile associated with this myocarditis is also shifted toward Th1 cytokines, so elevated gamma interferon (IFN-ã) levels and decreased interleukin-10 (IL-10) levels may potentially perpetuate an existent, ongoing inflammatory process.However, the exact mechanism responsible for the turning point from immunoprotection to immune-mediated aggression leading to irreversible tissue damage remains elusive: not only is parasite persistence true for both symptomatic and asymptomatic patients, but the presence of the parasite in heart tissue does not always correlate with inflammation.

Autoimmunity has also been postulated to be a plausible etiology for the chronic myocarditis observed for *T. cruzi*-infected patients. Several *T. cruzi* antigens that cross-react with cardiac and noncardiac host components have been identified, but only some have been shown to have functional activity Among these, attention has focused on antibodies that cross-react with cardiac myosin and the immunodominant *T. cruzi* antigen B13 initially, because they were detected in 100% of patients with chronic Chagas' cardiomyopathy, in contrast to 14% of asymptomatic infected individuals and later because T-cell clones derived from lesions of patients with chronic Chagas' cardiomyopathy were found to be simultaneously reactive to cardiac myosin heavy chain and the B13 *T. cruzi* protein. Opponents of the molecular mimicry theory with specific relevance to anti-B13-cardiac myosin cross-reactive antibodies and derived cellular autoimmunity contend that these antibodies do not bind to intact myocytes, are not unique to *T. cruzi* infection, and are present in asymptomatic patients without heart lesions and that myosin autoimmunity is not essential for cardiac inflammation in experimental models. Arguing against autoimmunity developing as a result of parasite-specific immune responses, antigen exposure after tissue damage may also sensitize autoreactive T cells to self-antigens given a proinflammatory environment The question, therefore, is not whether autoimmunity is present but whether it is a primary cause of or merely a contributing factor to the pathogenesis of chronic Chagas' myocarditis. As proposed by Kierszenbaum, this question remains to be answered by experiments that prove a clear association between the development of similar cardiac lesions with the transfer of autoantibodies and/or autoreactive cells to susceptible hosts.

To synthesize, although the effects of both autonomic and microvascular disturbances in Chagas' cardiomyopathy may play an important role in potentiating and perpetuating cardiac muscle damage, persistent inflammation in the setting of continuous antigenic stimulation is perhaps the common pathway for tissue damage. Multiple mechanisms seem to explain this chronic inflammation (mainly antiparasite immunity and, possibly, autoimmunity), which are not necessarily mutually exclusive. The course of progression to chronic Chagas' cardiomyopathy and other forms of the disease was suggested to be related to genetic properties of both the host and the parasite. However, the molecular mechanisms underlying tissue tropism and the initial trigger or determinant of the course of chronic disease are not yet known.

Table 40.2: *Hallmarks of chronic Chagas' cardiomyopathy*[a]

Hallmark of CCC
Arrhythmias
Ventricular extrasystoles
Nonsustained and sustained ventricular tachycardia
Bradyarrhythmias
Ventricular fibrillation
Atrial fibrillation/flutter
Conduction abnormalities
Sick sinus syndrome
Complete and incomplete right bundle branch block
Left anterior fascicle block
Bifascicular and trifascicular blocks
1st, 2nd and 3rd degree AV blocks
Thromboembolic phenomena
Brain (most frequent)
Lungs, kidneys, spleen
Cardiac failure
Diastolic dysfunction initially
Isolated left heart failure in the early stage of cardiac
Decompensation
Biventricular with a predominance of right-sided failure in

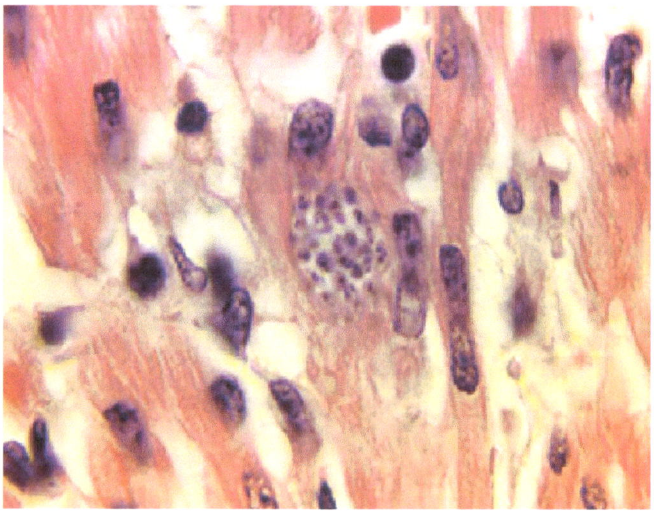

Fig. 40.15: *Photomicrograph of stained Trypanosoma cruzifound in the myocardium of the patient with chaga's disease*

Clinical Manifestations of Heart Involvement

a. *Myocarditis during the acute phase*: Acute myocarditis as evidenced by autopsy studies probably happens in close to 100% of patients with acute Chagas' disease However, there is an enormous discrepancy between autopsy findings and clinical data: first because acute infection is asymptomatic for approximately 90 to 95% of cases and second because even for symptomatic patients, acute Chagasic myocarditis is diagnosed for only 1 to 40% of them findings upon cardiac auscultation may include tachycardia (not always proportional to the degree of fever), cardiac murmurs, and muffled heart sounds. The principal electrocardiographic (ECG) alterations are first-degree atrioventricular (AV) block, low Q-R-S (Q-R-S interval of the ECG) voltage, and primary T-wave changes. A chest radiograph may show variable degrees of cardiomegaly, and pericardial effusion is the most frequently reported echocardiographic abnormality. Death in the acute phase occurs occasionally (for 5 to 10% of symptomatic patients) as a result of congestive heart failure (due to severe myocarditis) and/or meningoencephalitis. After the acute phase most patients return to a normal or near-normal myocardial status, but some patients (30%) then chronically develop fibrosing myocarditis.

Among immunosuppressed hosts such as HIV-infected individuals and transplant recipients, reactivation of infection and *de novo* infection (including transmission with transplanted organs among transplant patients) have been reported. With reactivation in HIV-positive patients, myocarditis has been reported for up to 45% of cases. Reactivation of Chagas' disease among heart transplant patients has been estimated to occur in approximately 30% of cases however, not all these cases are accompanied by florid symptoms or diagnosed by endomyocardial biopsy, and therefore, the true incidence of myocarditis with reactivation is difficult to estimate. Acute *T. cruzi* infection can also result as a consequence of donor-related transmission, which has been reported after kidney, heart, liver, and multiorgan transplants Involvement in this setting can range from asymptomatic parasitemia that easily responds to treatment without further complications to severe, fulminant disease despite therapy (including death directly attributable to Chagasic myocarditis In congenitally infected infants, the most common symptoms, which may be apparent at birth or develop within weeks after delivery, are hipotonicity, fever, hepatosplenomegaly, and anemia. Other findings include prematurity and low birth weight). *In utero* infections are also associated with abortion and placentitis. Serious manifestations, including myocarditis, meningoencephalitis, and pneumonitis, are uncommon but carry a high risk of death

b. *Chronic Chagas' cardiomyopathy*: Cardiac involvement is the most frequent and most severe manifestation of chronic Chagas' disease Transition from the indeterminate form to the cardiac form of chronic Chagas' disease is usually manifested by the appearance of ECG changes such as incomplete or complete right bundle branch block (RBBB), left anterior fascicular block (LAFB), minimal ST-T (ST-to-T interval of the ECG) changes, and monomorphic premature ventricular contractions (PVCs), mostly in asymptomatic or oligosymptomatic patients As the disease advances, associated intraventricular conduction defects (usually RBBB with LAFB), polymorphic PVCs bradyarrhythmias, high-grade atrioventricular blocks, Q waves, nonsustained or sustained ventricular tachycardia, and, ultimately, atrial flutter or fibrillation may ensue Symptoms like

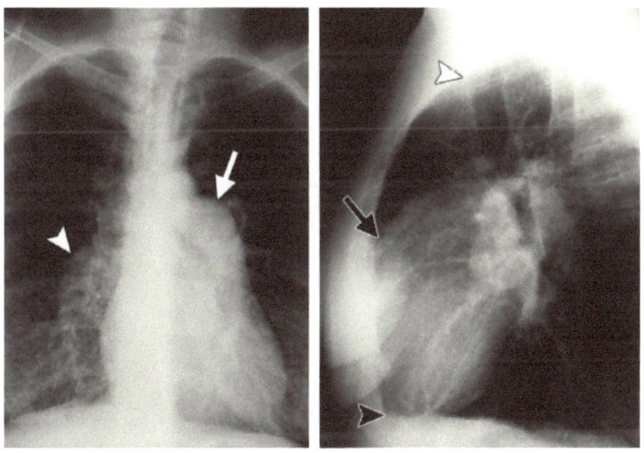

a. b.

Fig.40.16: *Radiographic findings of pulmonary hypertension. (a) Frontal chest radiograph shows a prominent main pulmonary artery (arrow), dilated right interlobar artery (arrowhead), and pruning of peripheral pulmonary vascularity. (b) Lateral chest radiograph shows filling of the retrosternal airspace (arrow), a result of right ventricular dilatation. The right ventricle is in contact with more than one-third of the distance from the sternodiaphragmatic angle (black arrowhead) to the point where the trachea meets the sternum (white arrowhead). n patient with chagas disease*

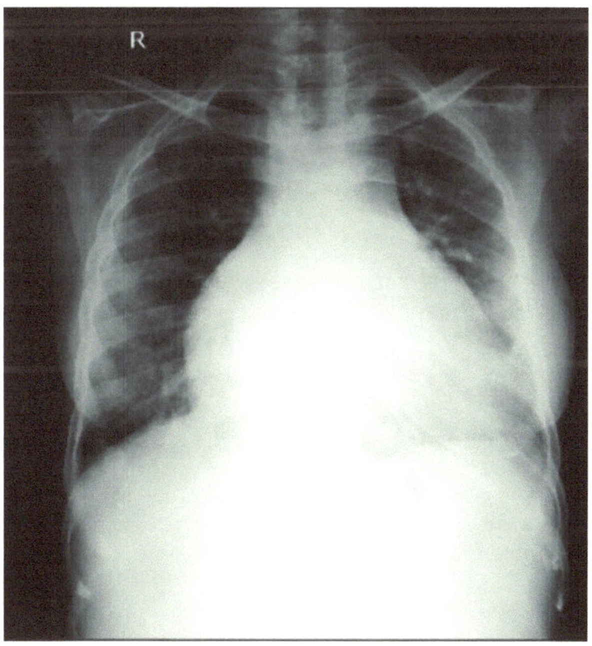

Fig. 40.17: *Showing chest X-ray PA view cardiomegaly in patient with chagas disease*

palpitations, atypical chest pain, presyncope, syncope, dyspnea upon exertion, and edema are usually observed throughout the course of chronic Chagas' cardiomyopathy (CCC). Findings upon physical examination vary according to the stage of the disease and the presence of conduction system abnormalities. These findings include cardiac rhythm irregularities, a displaced point of maximal impulse, gallop rhythms, a loud second heart sound implying pulmonary hypertension, mitral or tricuspid regurgitation murmurs, an increase in the systemic venous pressure with liver enlargement and edema, and a borderline low systolic blood pressure with a reduced radial pulse implying systolic dysfunction Upon echocardiogram, diastolic dysfunction usually precedes systolic dysfunction, potentially allowing the early detection of cardiac involvement in Chagas' disease (Characteristic echocardiographic findings include apical aneurysms (Fig. which are reported for 8.5 to 55% of cases (depending on the stage of the disease and the method of detection, i.e. if postmortem or at echocardiography or angiography); segmental left ventricular (LV) contractile abnormalities (more commonly at the posteroinferior wall); and reduced LV systolic function Echocardiographic evidence of impaired LV function, as characterized by increased LV systolic dimension, reduced LV ejection fraction, or the presence of segmental or global LV wall motion abnormality and/or an LV aneurysm, is the most common and consistent independent predictor of death Other important clinical and noninvasive adverse prognostic indicators, which not surprisingly reflect and parallel the degree of myocardial dysfunction, include advanced functional class (New York Heart Association [NYHA] classification III/IV), cardiomegaly, and nonsustained ventricular tachycardia upon 24-h ECG monitoring .

The clinical course of CCC is diverse and difficult to predict, with some patients remaining asymptomatic life long despite electrocardiographic and/or echocardiographic evidence of the disease, some presenting with signs, symptoms, and complications of progressive heart failure or advanced cardiac arrhythmias, and others dying unexpectedly without prior symptoms.Currently, several staging systems are available. These staging systems can help to identify patients at different degrees of risk, facilitate choices among treatment alternatives, and aid patient counseling. Most systems classify patients into four or five stages based on their functional capacity, ECG findings, and the presence or absence of heart enlargement and/or systolic dysfunction upon echocardiogram. The progression of disease to more advanced stages has been estimated to occur for 10% of patients over a follow-up period of 3 to 10 years.Another important aspect of staging is derived from its prognostic information: the rate of mortality for individuals at early stages of CCC is not

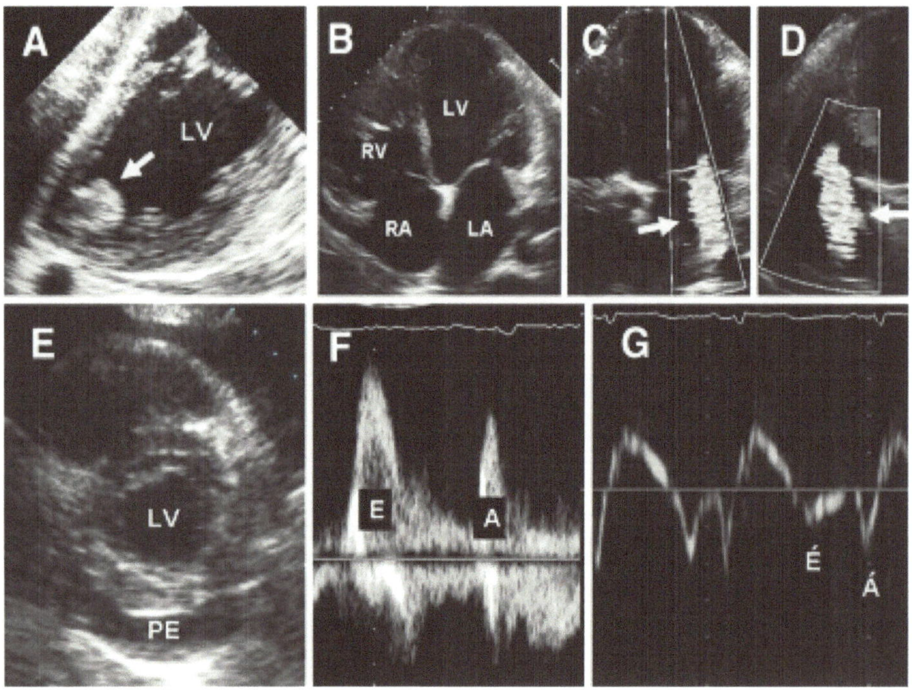

Fig. 40.18(A to G): *(A) Transesophageal echocardiography demonstrating an apical aneurysm containing a large, round, and protruding thrombus (arrow). (B to D), Transthoracic apical 4-chamber views of the heart showing dilated cardiac chambers (B), and functional mitral (C) and tricuspid (D) regurgitation (arrows). (E), Parasternal short-axis view of the heart showing a large pericardial effusion (PE). (F and G), Transmitral pulsed-Doppler (F) and lateral annulus tissue Doppler (G) demonstrating apparently normal peak early (E) and late (A) transmitral velocities, E/A ratio, and E-wave deceleration time (F) but abnormal early (E?) and late (A?) velocities (G) consistent with advanced diastolic dysfunctionin a patient with Chagas Disease LA, left atrium; LV, left ventricle; PE, pericardial effusion; RA, right atrium*

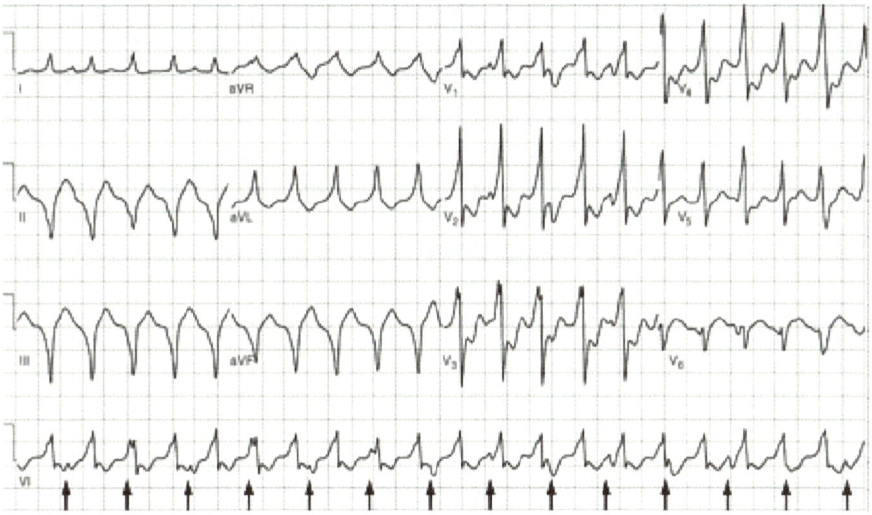

Fig. 40.19: *ECG showing AV dissociation (arrows mark P waves), wide QRS >200 ms, superior frontal plane axis, slurring of the initial portion of the QRS, and large S wave in V6—all clues to the diagnosis of ventricular tachycardia. in a patient with chaga's myocarditis*

significantly different from that of the general population). However, the life expectancy of patients with symptomatic and advanced CCC stages (involving systolic dysfunction and/or cardiomegaly) is less than 30% at 5 years and their overall prognosis is worse than that of patients with dilated cardiomyopathies of other etiologies Systemic and pulmonary embolisms arising from mural thrombi in the cardiac chambers are relatively Although the brain is by far the most common clinically recognized site of embolisms (followed by limbs and lungs), at necropsy, embolisms are found more frequently in the lungs, kidneys, and spleen. Chagas' disease is an independent risk factor for stroke in areas where the disease is endemic. Mortality in CCC is due to sudden cardiac arrest in 55 to 65% of patients, congestive heart failure in 25 to 30% of patients, and thromboembolic phenomena in 10 to 15% of patients.

Diagnosis

Diagnosis of acute Chagas' myocarditis relies on the demonstration of the parasite and/or anti-*T. cruzi* IgM in a patient with the correct epidemiological background and clinical picture. IgM serology assays are not widely available in developing countries and not standardized, so diagnosis is usually performed by visualizing the trypomastigotes in fresh blood smears, thick drop preparations, or buffy coat smears The level of parasitemia diminishes to almost undetectable levels by the 6th to 10th weeks of infection, making parasite identification in peripheral blood extremely difficult at this time Diagnosis could also be attempted by hemoculture on specialized medium (which has improved sensitivity over direct examination) or xenodiagnosis (which involves detecting the parasite by infecting laboratory-reared triatomine bugs directly or indirectly with the patient's blood. However, even considering only congenital Chagas' disease, hemoculture is rarely performed for the diagnosis of acute infection since it requires a specialized laboratory and trained personnel and is usually not widely available. Indirect parasitological tests are of limited value in the diagnosis of acute Chagas' disease, as they can take more than 1 month to obtain results (retarding the beginning of trypanocidal therapy).

A diagnosis of CCC should be suspected for young or middle-aged patients who present with a segmental or dilated cardiomyopathy of unknown etiology if within areas of endemicity or within the right epidemiological context. It should be remembered that CCC presents years after the initial infection, and therefore, patients who migrated to areas where the disease is not endemic are still at risk of developing cardiac compromise. Given the low and probably intermittent parasitemia in the chronic phase, diagnosis relies on serological methods by detecting IgG that binds to *T. cruzi* antigens Enzyme-linked immunosorbent assay (ELISA), indirect immunofluorescence (IIF), and indirect hemagglutination (IHA) methods are most commonly employed Two positive tests using any of the three conventional techniques are recommended for a final diagnosis. Identification of the parasite by hemoculture or xenodiagnosis in the chronic phase of the disease is hampered by the low sensitivity of the methods, which is dependent directly on the level of parasitemia. However, these methods may have a role in confirming the diagnosis in rare cases of serologically doubtful results or in evaluating treatment failures at specialized centers.

PCR-based methods using one of two target sequences (the variable region of the minicircle kinetoplast DNA and a 195-bp reiterated DNA sequence of the parasite) have achieved higher sensitivities than those of xenodiagnosis and hemoculture). The major problems with PCR-based techniques are the lack of standardization and commercial availability of assays for *T. cruzi*, the high level of complexity required, and the reliance of their sensitivity on the level of parasitemia (which is low, by definition, in chronic disease PCR is therefore still considered among

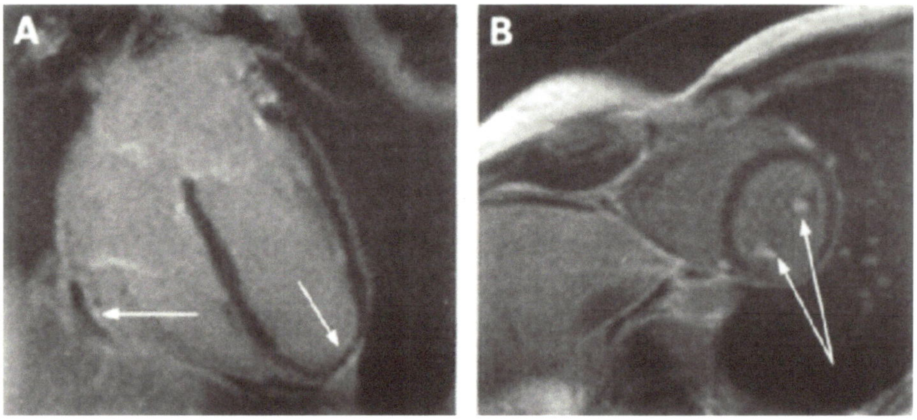

Fig. 40.20: *Showing Contrast-enhanced magnetic resonance imaging of endomyocardial fibrosis secondary to Bancroftian filariasis. The left ventricle has an elongated appearance and there is a small posterior mitral valve leaflet with two regurgitant jets into a normal left atrium. Delayed imaging performed 10 minutes after intravenous contrast injection (0.2 mmol/ kg Gd-DTPA) showed subendocardial hyperenhancement of the left ventricular apex, both papillary muscles and the basal right ventricle (panels A and B). Contrast-enhallfed magnetic resonance imaging has noninvasively confirmed endomyocardial fibrosis as a complication of filariasis. In addition, this case is an example of non-ischaemic subendocardial delayed hyperenhancemen. A midnight blood sample was checked for microfilaria and identified as Wuchereria bancrofti. At echocardiography there was mild mitral regurgitation and pulmonary hypertension. At cardiac catheterisation the left ventricular ejectionfraction was 65%, the end-diastolic pressure was raised and coronary arteries normal. Right ventricular endomyocardial biopsy showedendocardial and interstitial fibrosis. The diagnosis of filariasis with hypereosinophilia complicated by endomyocardial fibrosis was made.He was treated with ivermectin and mebendazole with steroid cover and lisinopril. The patient made an excellent recovery with gradual normalisation of the eosinophil count. At follow-up she remains clinically stable and echocardiography has shown no change III left ventricular ejection fraction or mitral regurgitation*

nonconventional methods and is recommended only as an adjunct in specialized centers to confirm parasitemia in congenital *T. cruzi* infection (since in this context, its sensitivity seems to be greater than that of microscopic examination) or for the evaluation of antiparasitic drug therapy. However, a single or even repeated negative posttreatment PCR results do not necessarily mean parasitological cure. The negative results are indicative only of the absence of parasite DNA at those moments. The value of PCR lies mainly in the positive results that they yield, which usually reflect treatment failure Whether assessments of parasite load by quantitative real-time PCR will correlate with the impact of trypanocidal treatment on parasitological cure or resistance, as well as on disease evolution, should be a matter for further investigation.

The initial evaluation of the newly diagnosed patient with chronic *T. cruzi* infection includes a complete medical history and physical examination and a resting 12-lead electrocardiogram. Asymptomatic patients with a normal ECG have a favorable prognosis and should be followed up only annually or biannually. Patients with ECG changes consistent with CCC should undergo a routine cardiac evaluation, including ambulatory 24-h Holter monitoring (complemented with an exercise test whenever possible) to detect arrhythmias and assess functional capacity, chest radiography and two-dimensional (2D) echocardiography to assess ventricular function, and other cardiologic tests as indicated, Based on the results of these tests, it is possible to stratify individual patients by risk and implement appropriate therapy

Treatment and Preventive Measures

a. *Etiological treatment*: Only two drugs, benznidazole and nifurtimox, are recommended for the treatment of Chagas' disease Of the two, benznidazole (a nitroimidazole derivative) has been more extensively investigated in clinical studies and is better tolerated overall. Adverse reactions such as generalized or sometimes localized allergic dermatitis occur in approximately 20 to 30% of patients and consist of pruritic and nonbullous polymorphous erythematous rashes, often followed by desquamation Severe exfoliative dermatitis can occur and should lead to a prompt discontinuation of treatment Another adverse effect that occurs in approximately 5 to 10% of patients, most commonly late in the treatment course, is a dose-dependent peripheral sensitive neuropathy affecting mainly the distal parts of the lower limbs; it also should prompt the cessation of treatment. Rare serious adverse events include leukopenia with granulocytopenia or agranulocytosis (sometimes followed by fever and tonsillitis) and thrombocytopenic purpura. Additional reported side effects include nausea, vomiting, anorexia, weight loss, insomnia, loss of taste, and onycholysis. Nifurtimox, a nitrofuran compound, has been associated with gastrointestinal side effects in 30 to 70% of patients as well as central and peripheral nervous system toxicity. Both compounds are better tolerated by children, allowing increased dosage regimens. Children should be treated with 10 mg/kg of body weight of benznidazole per day in two divided doses for 30 to 90 days or 15 to 20 mg/kg of nifurtimox per day in four divided doses for 90 to 120 days. Adults should be treated with 5 to 7 mg/kg of benznidazole per day in two divided doses for 30 to 60 days or 8 to 10 mg/kg of nifurtimox per day in three to four divided doses for 90 to 120 days.

Treatment has been recommended for all cases of acute and congenital infection, reactivated infection, and early chronic Chagas' disease (particularly children/adolescents ^{3}18 years of age) based on evidence of the shortening of the disease's clinical course, cure of infection, or reduction in numbers of parasites. For infected adults without advanced cardiomyopathy up to the age of 50 years, etiological treatment should generally also be offered. The rationale for these recommendations stems from evidence of a slowing of the progression of cardiomyopathy.In a recent observational trial, 566 chronically infected adults (30 to 50 years of age) without heart failure were assigned, in alternating sequences, to benznidazole or no treatment After a median follow-up period of 9.8 years, fewer treated patients had a progression of disease or developed ECG abnormalities. Negative seroconversion was more frequent for treated patients. Another recently published controlled study, including 111 patients (17 to 46 years of age) with chronic Chagas' disease and a normal electrocardiogram, showed similar favorable results with benznidazole over a mean follow-up period of 21 years For those patients over the age of 50 years, etiological treatment is considered optional because of the lack of any available data. A multicenter, randomized, placebo-controlled trial of benznidazole enrolling 3,000 patients with mild to moderate CCC who were 18 to 75 years of age is currently under way and should help clarify treatment decisions for this population.

In contrast, etiological treatment is contraindicated during pregnancy and for patients with severe renal or hepatic insufficiency, and it should generally not be offered to patients with advanced Chagasic cardiomyopathy or megaesophagus with significant impairment of swallowing. A more controversial issue is prophylactic treatment for transplant patients: some authors have recommended it for patients with Chagasic cardiomyopathy who undergo cardiac transplantation to prevent disease reactivation.while others recommend it for all infected donors pretransplant and for their respective recipients posttransplant. For chronic Chagas' disease, cure is documented when previously positive serological tests are negative, usually years or decades after treatment.

b. *Symptomatic treatment*: Medical treatment of heart failure for patients with CCC should follow specific treatments targeted at each stage according to current guidelines for heart failure of other etiologies An important exception is the use of beta blockers, which should be used with caution for CCC due to a higher incidence of atrioventricular conduction defects and associated bradyarrhythmias. Cardiac transplantation has been performed with good results for patients with advanced CCC but may not be available or accessible in all countries where this disease is endemic. Although not tested in randomized controlled clinical trials, amiodarone has been associated with a survival advantage in case-control studies among patients with ventricular tachycardia and has therefore been proposed for the management of patients with sustained and nonsustained ventricular tachycardia. However, treatment with amiodarone has been associated with pulmonary, cardiac, thyroid, liver, ocular, skin, central nervous system (CNS), and genitourinary toxicities, so treatment needs to be individualized Pacemaker implantation is the recommended treatment for severe bradyarrhythmias and advanced conduction abnormalities. The roles of cardioverter-defibrillator implantation and cardiac resynchronization, however, are not well established for CCC.Finally, anticoagulation has been advocated for patients with atrial fibrillation, previous thromboembolic phenomena, or an LV aneurysm with thrombus

c. *Preventive measures*: Most *T. cruzi* infections can be prevented by decreasing vectorial transmission, improving blood product screening, and detecting and treating transplacental transmission. Multinational programs involving countries where the disease is endemic have achieved enormous success in decreasing both the prevalence and incidence of Chagas' disease by following several operational stages. The tools for interrupting transmission are based on the implementation of vector control activities such as insecticide spraying, housing improvements, and education as well as the strengthening of the implementation of policy for use and screening of blood products for transfusion. Since the end of January 2007, the American Red Cross and other blood collection agencies in the United States began screening blood donations for antibodies to *T. cruzi* donations with the approved ELISA (referred to as universal testing). All initially reactive donations are retested in duplicate by using the same screening test; donations testing repeatedly reactive undergo confirmatory testing by the radioimmunoprecipitation assay (RIPA) Continued surveillance is also important to consolidate and maintain the success achieved.

For persons traveling to areas of endemicity, compliance with general food and water precautions is advised to prevent the extremely rare occurrence of food-borne Chagas' disease. More importantly, travelers should avoid sleeping in poorly constructed houses or else consider sleeping in insecticide-impregnated bed nets. However, the protective efficacy of insecticide-treated materials in reducing Chagas' disease transmission and eliminating the vector population has yet to be demonstrated. Finally, no vaccine for Chagas' disease is available.

Other Parasites

Toxoplasmosis

Epidemiology

Toxoplasma gondii is a worldwide zoonosis capable of causing several distinct clinical syndromes in immuno-

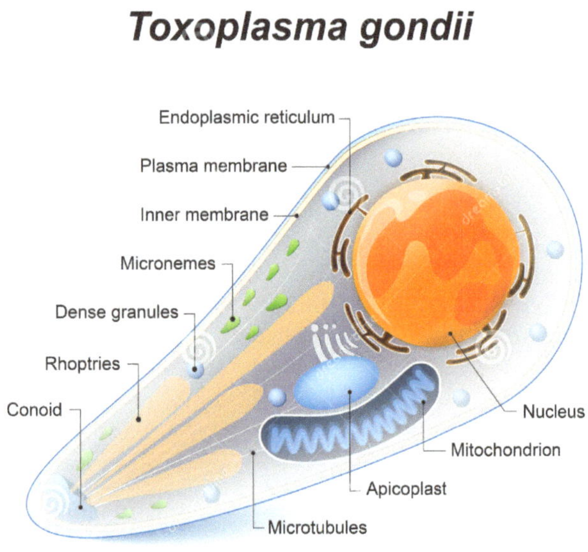

Fig. 40.21: *showing morphological interior features of Toxoplasma gondii*

competent and immunocompromised individuals. *T. gondii* is a parasite of members of the cat family, with humans and other warm-blooded animals serving as intermediate hosts.Humans become infected by either the eating of undercooked meat, ingestion of contaminated water, fecal-oral transmission from feline feces, congenitally through transplacental transmission, blood transfusion, or

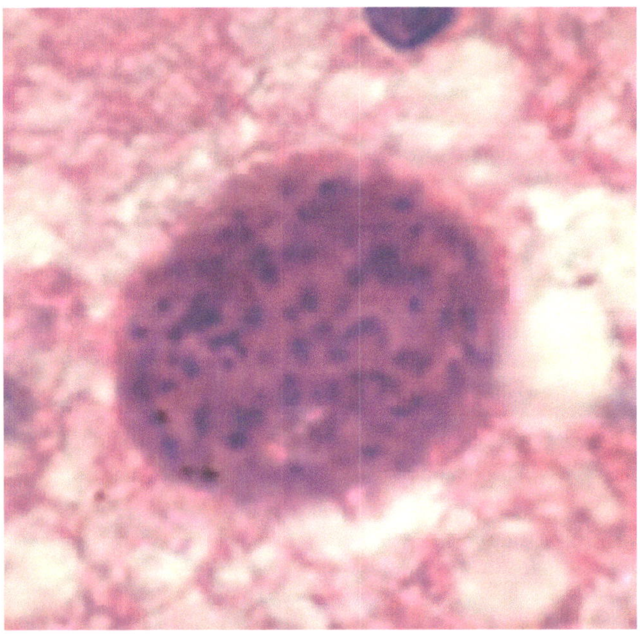

Fig. 40.22: *Cysts of Toxoplasma gondii usually range in size from 5–50 μm in diameter. Cysts are usually spherical in the brain but more elongated in cardiac and skeletal muscles. They may be found in various sites throughout the body of the host, but are most common in the brain and skeletal and cardiac muscles*

transplantation. Meat for human consumption is not routinely inspected for *T. gondii* infection in the United States or elsewhere in the world.Human-to-human transmission does not occur, with the exception of mother-to-fetus transmission. The incidence of *T. gondii* antibodies increases with increasing age but does not vary between sexes. The prevalences of antibody titers vary considerably among geographic regions and within a given population. The overall seroprevalence among adolescents and adults in the United States was found to be 22.5%, with a seroprevalence among women of childbearing age (15 to 44 years) of 15%, using specimens collected by the third National Health and Nutrition Examination Survey (NHANES III) between 1988 and 1994.In the United States, *T. gondii* seropositivity among HIV-infected individuals varies from 10% to 45% and correlates with seropositivity in the non-HIV-infected population. In Western Europe and Africa, the seroprevalence among HIV-infected populations is approximately 50% to 78%

Pathophysiology

Toxoplasma gondii multiplies intracellularly at the site of invasion and may spread to distant organs by the invasion of lymphatics and blood. Tissue cyst formation occurs within the first week of infection and is responsible for latent infection. *T. gondii* resides intracellularly in phagosomes within macrophages and myocardial cells The parasite is propelled by an actin-myosin-dependent gliding-motility mechanism and establishes intracellular vacuoles. This remodeling prevents lysosome fusion, which leads to the intracellular survival of the parasite The immune competency of the individual is the determining factor in the recrudescence of latent infection. Immunity in the immunocompetent individual persists for life. T cells, macrophages, and type 1 cytokines are crucial for the control of *T. gondii* infection. Defective production of IFN-© and interleukin-12, possibly mediated by CD40 ligand, may play a role in the lack of containment of the infection. Cytokine stimulation of macrophage production of reactive nitrogen intermediates was hypothesized to assist in the host control of established infection Both host and parasitic genetics appear to be important for disease pathogenesis. Associations of HLA-DQ3 with the development of toxoplasmic encephalitis and the possible protective role of HLA-DQ1 suggest that host genetic factors contribute to the development of disease. In addition, population genetic analysis of *T. gondii* suggests clonal expansion, which may identify clinically relevant biological differences

Clinical manifestations

The clinical expression of toxoplasmosis depends on the level of immunity in the human host In immunocompetent patients, acute toxoplasmosis is most often asymptomatic, but latent infection can persist for life. Latent infection is due to cyst formation and may subsequently reactivate in immunocompromised persons. Among these populations, toxoplasmosis often presents in the form of encephalitis or chorioretinitis. Myocarditis has rarely been reported as a manifestation of acute toxoplasmosis. This manifestation may occur in isolation or as part of a broader clinical spectrum of illness. Pericardial effusion, constrictive pericarditis, arrhythmias, and congestive heart failure in patients with *T. gondii* myocarditis have been described. In patients with AIDS, the heart is the second most commonly affected organ after the brain.Prevalences vary according to various studies, and diagnosis is usually made postmortem since cardiac involvement is usually clinically silent or dominated by CNS manifestations.Approximately 12 to 22% of AIDS patients had evidence of endomyocardial involvement by *T. gondii* at autopsy. The prevalence of cardiac toxoplasmosis confirmed at autopsy in the era of highly active antiretroviral therapy has been reported to be less than 10% *Toxoplasma gondii*-associated myocarditis can also occur in transplant patients due either to reactivation or to *de novo* infection from a seropositive donor to a seronegative recipient. Indeed, toxoplasmosis is the most commonly reported parasitic disease occurring after heart transplantation and may simulate organ rejection. Disseminated toxoplasmosis with associated myocarditis can lead to a fatal outcome if no prior prophylaxis is given to transplant patients.The prevention of toxoplasmosis relies on the serological screening of donors and recipients before transplantation to identify patients at a higher risk of toxoplasmosis, i.e. seropositive hematopoietic stem cell transplant recipients and mismatched (seropositive donor/ seronegative recipients) solid-organ transplant recipients. Prevention in those patients presently relies on prophylaxis, usually with cotrimoxazole

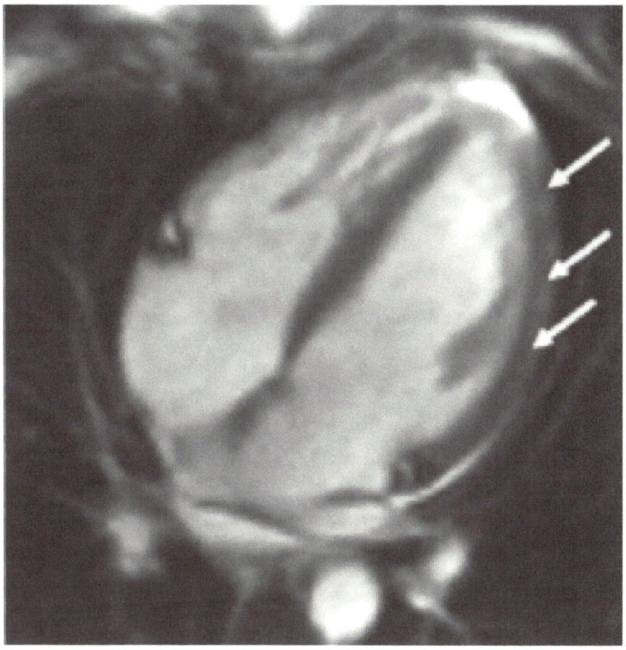

Fig. 47.23: *Cardiac MRI. Delayed-enhancement sequences performed after perfusion of gadolinium demonstrated a diffuse lumpy subepicardial enhancement (white arrows)in a patient with toxoplasminosis causing Acute Myopericarditis*

Diagnosis

Test essentially rules out prior or recent infection of an immunocompetent host IgM antibodies may persist for years after infection and should not be used as the sole diagnostic criteria for recent infection.Antibody avidity testing has proven very useful as a.

The diagnosis of toxoplasmosis relies on serology or the identification of tachyzoites in myocardial tissue. There is considerable variation in the sensitivities and specificities of commercially available serological assays. IgG antibodies appear early, peak within 6 months of infection, and remain detectable for life. A negative IgG antibody marker of the timing of infection. The presence of a high avidity indicates that the infection occurred at least 3 to 5 months earlier. This test is most helpful during pregnancy, where additional evaluation and treatment depend on the timing of infection relative to pregnancy.No single serological test is sufficient to support the diagnosis of acute or chronic toxoplasmosis, and the use of a reference laboratory is often required. Patients may have slight lymphocytosis, and hepatic transaminase levels may be slightly elevated. Otherwise, laboratory findings are not specific. Kean and Grocott first described a toxoplasmosis-like cysts in the myocardium in 1945, and Adams subsequently described fluctuating S-T (S-to-T interval tracing of the ECG) changes in a 15-year-old boy with glandular-type toxoplasmosis. Endomyocardial biopsy has successfully identified the organism in heart transplant patients. Although uncommonly reported, the benefit of early and specific diagnosis with endomyocardial biopsy in the setting of heart transplantation likely outweighs the potential risks. Local necrosis with edema and an inflammatory infiltrate upon biopsy are typical.Myocardial abscesses have also been reported; however, abscesses are not common pathological features of toxoplasmosis Parasites may also be detected by using DNA amplification techniques. The sensitivity with whole blood or buffy coat is 15% to 85% and appears most valuable for disseminated disease Performance characteristics vary by the timing of testing in relation to therapy, gene target, primers, and sample preparation. PCR has been reported to diagnose *Toxoplasma* more frequently than histology of cardiac biopsy specimen samples in the transplant setting.PCR assays can be valuable in making this difficult diagnosis, and reference laboratories with experience with these assays should be utilized.

Treatment

The treatment of choice is based on a combination of pyrimethamine and sulfadiazine or pyrimethamine and clindamycin. Leucovorin should be given to all patients taking pyrimethamine. Combinations of pyrimethamine and azithromycin or atovaquone may be considered for patients intolerant to other regimens based on data from immunosuppressed patients. The combination of prime-thamine and sulfadiazine is also a first-line treatment regimen during pregnancy. However, alternatives exist for those concerned about potential toxicity and teratogenicity, and treatment choice is influenced by the duration of pregnancy and documentation of fetal infection. Serological

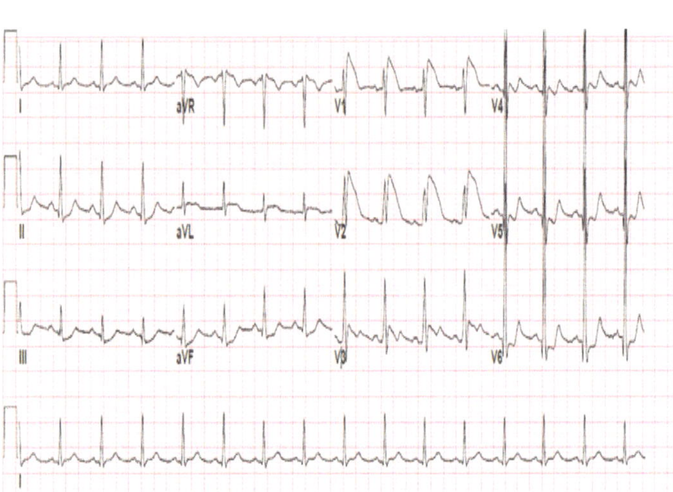

Fig. 47.24: *ECG pattern characterized by coved ST-segment elevation followed by T-wave inversions in V1 and V2. indicating myocarditis caused by Trichinella spiralis*

screening of organ donors and recipients before transplantation allows the identification of patients at the highest risk of toxoplasmosis and provision of prophylaxis for these individuals. The optimal schedule for the provision of trimethoprim (TMP)-sulfamethoxazole (SMZ) prophylaxis in the transplant setting has not been defined; however, this drug is often administered daily or three times a week. Prevention is important for seronegative pregnant women and immunodeficient patients. Prevention is accomplished through physician-patient education and prophylaxis prescription, where appropriate. Educational efforts should focus on the avoidance of contact with materials potentially contaminated with cat feces, the use of gloves when handling cat litter or gardening, washing of hands thoroughly after contact with raw meat, cooking of meat until "well done," and washing of fruits and vegetables before consumption.

Cysticercosis

Epidemiology

Cysticercosis is a consequence of the ingestion of the eggs of the pork tapeworm *Taenia solium*. Cerebral cysticercosis is considered the most serious complication. The condition can also present as ocular, spinal, cutaneous, muscular, or cardiac lesions The prevalence of cysticercosis varies in countries where cysticercosis is endemic and is often increased in regions where pigs are raised and sanitary conditions are lacking. Few cases are acquired in the United States, and travel to areas of endemicity may pose a small risk to travelers.

Pathophysiology

Following egg ingestion, oncospheres invade the bowel wall and disseminate to the brain, striated muscles, and other tissues. Cysticerci can remain quiescent for many years in a state of immune tolerance. Poorly understood metacestode-elaborated substances divert the complement pathway and inhibit normal cellular immune responses, including macrophage function and lymphocyte proliferation. The ability of the cyst to moderate the host immune response may be lost with time.

Clinical Manifestations

Clinical manifestations often develop at the time of cyst degeneration. The trigger for this event is unknown. The myocardial inflammatory response is variable, resulting in granuloma formation and fibrosis, which subsequently leads to arrhythmias and conduction abnormalities either spontaneously or during treatment Cardiac involvement in cysticercosis was thought to be rare, but autopsy studies have shown a prevalence of 20 to 25% in patients with concomitant documented neurocysticercosis. Cardiac cysticercosis is often asymptomatic and discovered during cardiac surgery or at autopsy. Cysticerci are usually multiple and randomly distributed in cardiac tissues, including the subpericardium, subendocardium, and myocardium. Rarely, a single cardiac cyst may be present.

Diagnosis

The diagnosis is based on suggestive epidemiology and serology. The extent of diagnostic evaluation depends on the severity of clinical presentation. Routine blood tests may reveal marked peripheral eosinophilia only in the case of a leaking cyst. The sensitivity and specificity of serology vary with the site and stage of infection. An enzyme-linked immunoelectrotransfer blot assay is the test of choice for the detection of antibodies. PCR-based tests have an emerging role in the epidemiological investigation of taeniasis and are available for the diagnosis of cysticercosis. Most individuals with cysticercosis do not have viable *T. solium* in their intestines. Echocardiography may play some role in identifying cardiac cysts and occasionally identifies cardiac cysts consistent with cysticercosis upon routine screening for other purposes. Cardiac magnetic resonance imaging (MRI) may also demonstrate cystic lesions, which are hypointense on T1-weighted images and hyperintense on T2-weighted images. Rounded scolices, when seen, are of intermediate to low signal intensity on T2-weighted images and of intermediate to hyperintense signal intensity within the low-signal fluid on T1-weighted images.

Treatment

Patients with extraneural cysticercosis should be evaluated with brain imaging for possible neurocysticercosis. Asymptomatic extraneural cysts may not require specific surgical or antihelminthic therapy. The role of albendazole and praziquantel or surgery in cardiac cysticercosis is unclear and has not been directly investigated; however, these therapies are likely to be effective given their efficacy at other sites. Adjunctive corticosteroids are sometimes administered during therapy for neurocysticercosis. The potential benefit of decreasing treatment-related inflammation in cardiac cysticercosis has not been defined but remains theoretically possible.

Trichinellosis

Epidemiology

Trichinellosis is caused by the nematode *Trichinella spiralis* and other *Trichinella* species and is common worldwide. Humans become infected when eating undercooked meat contaminated with cysts of *Trichinella* larvae. Approximately 15 cases of trichinellosis are reported annually in the United States.Wild carnivorous animals perpetuate infections in a sylvatic cycle, and wild-game meat is emerging as a source of infection.

Pathogenesis

Trichinella larvae excyst and cross the small intestine, where they travel through lymphatics and the bloodstream until finally encysting in striated muscle tissue. The striated muscle cell is induced to transform into a nurse cell, which supports the long-term viability of the encysted larvae The process of encystment and nurse cell formation is unique to skeletal muscle and does not take place within the heart. *Trichinella spiralis*-associated myocarditis is not caused by the direct larval invasion of the myocardium with encystation but is likely induced by an eosinophil-enriched inflammatory response resulting in eosinophilic myocarditis similar to the pathogenic process associated with tropical endomyocardial fibrosis. Some patients with trichinellosis develop organ-specific autoantibodies, whose role in pathogenesis remains unclear.

Clinical Manifestations

The clinical picture of trichinellosis is proportional to the number of larvae ingested and manifests with two clinical stages: the intestinal stage and the muscular stage). Larval migration into the muscles can cause periorbital and facial edema; subungal, conjunctival, and retinal hemorrhages; myalgias; weakness; and fever. The tropism of *T. spiralis* for striated muscle may involve the myocardium in 21 to 75% of infected patients.Myocarditis is a consequence of migrating larvae and the resulting inflammatory response and typically occurs in the third week of infection. Trichinosis myocarditis may initially manifest with chest pain and mimic an acute myocardial infarction.Reports suggest that ECG evidence of myocardial involvement may be found for up to 75% of patients. Complications such cardiac arrhythmias are considered the most common cause of death associated with trichinellosis.In addition, pericardial effusions have also been reported during *T. spiralis* infection.

Diagnosis

The clinical suspicion of trichinellosis is based on suggestive epidemiology associated with the typical clinical presentation and the presence of eosinophilia during the second to fourth week of the muscle stage. There is no direct relationship between the severity of eosinophilia and clinical course. Confirmation is based on serology and muscle biopsy specimens. Serology is generally reliable and first becomes positive about 3 weeks after infection. Antibody levels may remain positive for longer than a year after clinical resolution. For patients without obvious myocardial involvement, some researchers have recommended screening with troponin to detect asymptomatic myocarditis.The finding of larvae in a muscle biopsy specimen provides a definitive diagnosis; however, biopsy is rarely necessary. ECG findings are considered nonspecific. In a study of 154 cases of trichinellosis, 56% of the patients had ECG abnormalities, most commonly nonspecific repolarization changes, without an association with poor prognosis.One study reported pericardial effusion as the most common cardiac manifestation of trichinosis, affecting 10% of patients.Cardiac MRI may provide supportive evidence of myocardial involvement, although the MRI findings are not specific to trichinellosis.

Treatment

Treatment consists of the administration of albendazole or mebendazole in conjunction with steroids for severe cases. Although albendazole and mebendazole are relatively contraindicated in pregnancy, both have been used in patients without adverse fetal effects Adjunctive steroids are commonly utilized for 10 to 15 days.

PARASITES THAT OCCASIONALLY INVOLVE THE PERICARDIUM

Entamoeba Histolytica

Epidemiology

Amebic pericarditis is caused by the protozoon *Entamoeba histolytica*, which is transmitted by the fecal-oral route. It has a worldwide distribution but is found mainly in developing countries in the tropics. In the United States, amebiasis is seen in immigrants and travelers returning from countries where the disease is endemic.Following malaria and schistosomiasis, amebiasis is the third most common cause of parasitic death. Particular high-risk groups include children, pregnant women, and malnourished individuals.Invasive amebiasis may be more common among HIV/AIDS patients, prompting some to call for routine HIV testing of those diagnosed with the disease.

Pathophysiology

The ability of *Entamoeba histolytica* to invade tissues distinguishes it from the morphologically identical *Entamoeba dispar*. The parasite causes acute inflammation and ulceration of the colonic mucosa. Adherence to colonic epithelial cells using the Gal/GalNAc lectin is essential for amebic survival and pathogenicity.Mucosal IgA immunity to this lectin has been associated with protection from *Entamoeba* infection and disease in Bangladeshi children. The trophozoite utilizes the secretion of proteinases for the dissolution of the extracellular matrix and the formation of amebepores resulting in target cell cytolysis, among other mechanisms, to establish its pathogenic niche.

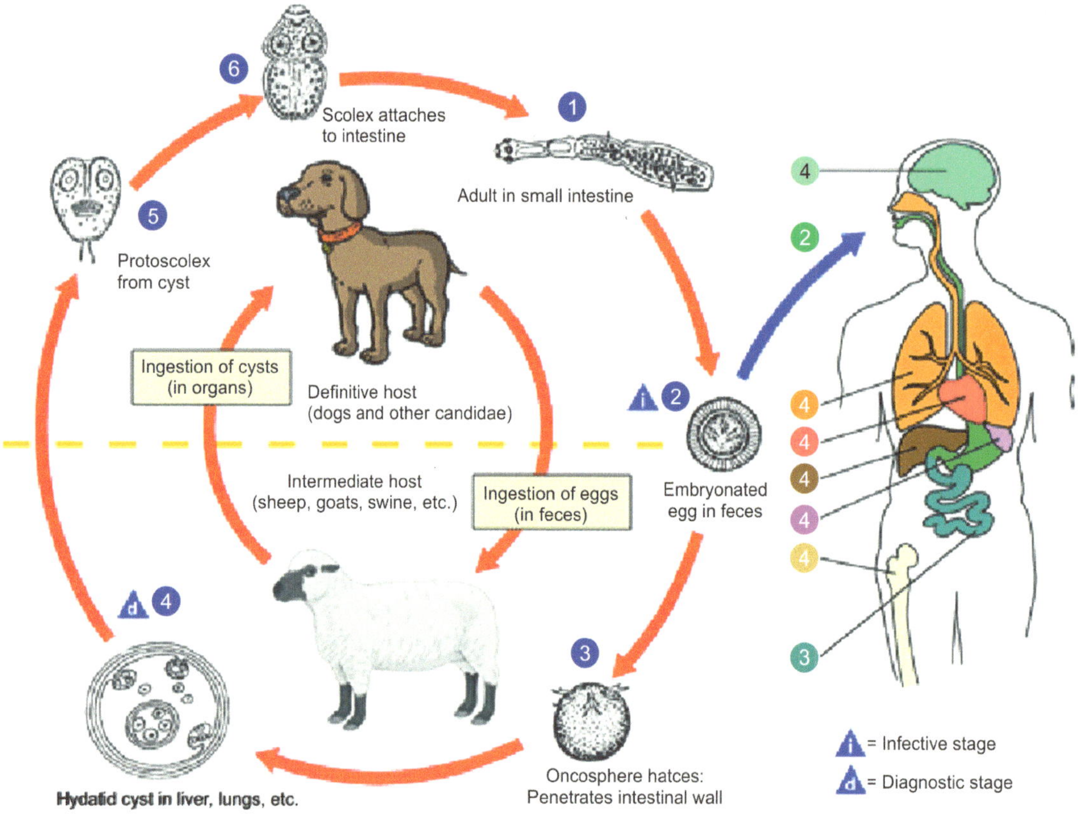

Fig. 40.25: *Diagram showing life cycle of a echinococcus parasite*

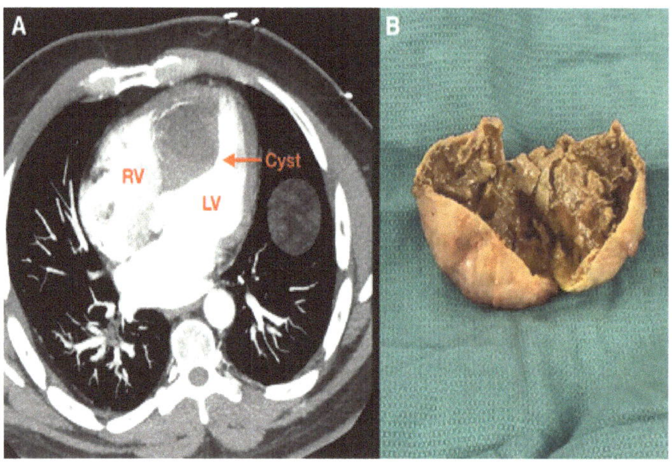

Fig.47.26: *Intracardiac echinococcal cyst. A, Computed tomographic angiogram shows an intracardiac mass within the interventricular septum between the right ventricle (RV) and the left ventricle (LV). B, Surgically excised echinococcal cyst with calcified shell and necrotic material inside.*

Clinical Manifestations

Extraintestinal amebic disease is localized mainly to the liver.The involvement of the pericardium is very rare but is a serious complication of amebiasis.Amebic pericarditis may present as either a pericardial rub with electrocardiographic changes associated with an abscess of the left lobe or purulent pericarditis from the perforation of the abscess into the pericardium.Amebic abscesses in the right lobe of the liver have also been reported to communicate with the pericardium.The presenting clinical syndrome is usually one of two forms: (i) sudden onset as cardiac tamponade with chest pain, shortness of breath, and shock or (ii) progressive effusion with a slower course to develop fever, dyspnea, and pain.Amebic pericarditis has been more frequently described for pediatric populations in which the association of concomitant intestinal amebiasis may be as high as 20%

Diagnosis

Diagnosis is usually established by serology, which has a sensitivity of about 90%.Infection with *E. histolytica* results in the development of antibodies, while infection with *E. dispar* does not. Positive serology does not distinguish between acute and past infections. For this reason, serum antigen tests are often used to complement diagnosis. The galactose lectin serum antigen is present in 75% of individuals with amebic liver abscesses. Peripheral eosinophilia is not particularly common Stool microscopy has limited value for the diagnosis of extraintestinal amebiasis. Amebic cysts or trophozoites are detected in the stool only 15 to 33% of the time In addition, the presence of amebic cysts or trophozoites determined by stool microscopy does not definitively indicate that the extraintestinal focus is secondary to the identified intestinal parasite because both pathogenic and nonpathogenic *Entamoeba* may be present in the gut. However, an ELISA method can differentiate pathogenic from nonpathogenic *Entamoeba* in stool samples. DNA amplification techniques for the rapid and specific identification of *E. histolytica* are in development. Aspirated pus is usually sterile, and diagnosis should not be excluded based on its gross characteristics. Given the limitations of serology in the diagnosis of invasive amebiasis, PCR-based diagnostic methods have become an invaluable sensitive and specific tool for the diagnosis of intestinal and extraintestinal amebiasis and are available from many reference laboratories. The suppurative feature of amebic pericarditis may also cause it to be confused with tuberculous pericarditis. A distinguishing factor between tuberculous pericarditis and amebic pericarditis is that there is a predominance of neutrophils in patients with amebiasis. Imaging with chest computed tomography (CT) and echocardiography can be useful given the potential to demonstrate a liver abscess in continuity with the pericardium and fluid within the pericardial sac, with or without the fistulous tract.

Treatment

The treatment of pericardial amebiasis requires a combination of surgical drainage and metronidazole. Metronidazole should be given three times daily for 7 to 10 days. Clinical improvement is expected within 48 to 72 h. If clinical improvement does not occur, bacterial superinfection should be considered and treated if found, and metronidazole therapy may be prolonged. Metronidazole resistance has not been reported.Treatment with a luminal agent to is required following therapy with metronidazole, even if prior stool examination was negative.

Echinococcosis

Epidemiology

Human infection with the metacestode form of one of the four species of the tapeworm *Echinococcus* (*E. granulosus*, *E. multilocularis*, *E. vogeli*, or *E. oligarthrus*) may result in echinococcal disease.*Echinococcus* species have a worldwide distribution. *Echinococcus granulosus* causes cystic echinococcosis, the form most frequently encountered. Humans become accidental intermediate hosts when they ingest eggs from the feces of infected dogs or other canids. Direct transmission from human to human does not occur. Pathophysiology.

After the ingestion of the eggs by an intermediate host, the eggs hatch and release oncospheres, which cross the small intestine and spread to encyst in various visceral organs. Both humoral and cellular immune responses to the presence of the oncospheres and metacestodes develop. The parasite evades the host immune response by using a number of mechanisms, including the cyst-laminated cuticle as a barrier to host cells, polyclonal activation of lymphocytes by parasite soluble antigens, and depression of host cell immune responses.For instance, chronic stimulation of the host by cyst fluid antigens leads to increased levels of specific IgG4 production, which is suggestive of host response immunomodulation. Th1 cell activation appears critical for protective immunity, while a Th2 response is correlated with progressive disease.

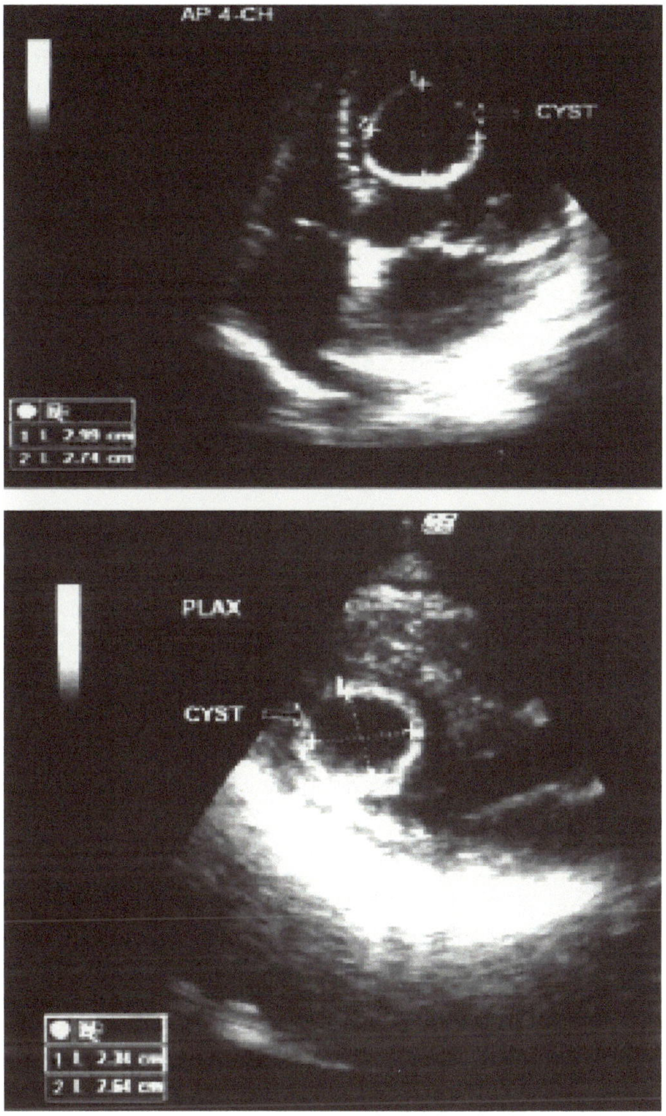

Fig. 40.27: *Upper and lower panels Showing left ventricular Myocardial invasion by Echinococcosis (Hydatid Cyst Disease)as marked by circle*

Clinical Manifestations

Hydatid cysts develop over months to years. Most of them will remain asymptomatic, but some of them become large enough to cause symptoms. Echinococcal disease is often diagnosed as an incidental finding during imaging for other reasons. Cysts are located mainly in the liver and the lung, and only 10% can occur in the rest of the body.Cardiac hydatid cysts have been described for 0.5 to 3% of echinococcosis cases and are usually univesicular Clinical presentations of cardiac echinococcosis include arrhythmias, myocardial infarction, cardiac tamponade, pulmonary hypertension syncope, purulent pericarditis, and sudden cardiac death. Isolated cardiac hydatid cysts without liver involvement are uncommon Hydatid cysts can even mimic ST segment elevation myocardial infarction upon electrocardiography. Most cases of pericardial echinococcosis may be due to spread from an initial location at the liver dome. Rarely, an atrial or ventricular thrombus may mimic a hydatid cyst.

Diagnosis (Figs 47.25 and 47.26)

Diagnosis relies on positive serological testing and radiographic findings.The sensitivity and specificity of serology in those patients with liver involvement are greater than 80% but less sensitive when echinococcal disease is isolated at other sites. Children and pregnant women more often have negative serology than other populations.The identification of antigens in cyst fluid or serum may also assist in diagnosis. Fewer than 15% of cases have peripheral eosinophilia. DNA amplifications tests are not currently available outside the research setting. Echocardiography is the most appropriate imaging test to evaluate potential myocardial or pericardial hydatid cysts. CT imaging and MRI may also demonstrate specific signs, including the calcification of the cysts' walls, the presence of daughter cysts, and membrane detachment.

Treatment

The drug of choice for the treatment of echinococcosis is albendazole or mebendazole. Mebendazole is usually continued for 3 to 6 months. Albendazole is preferred and is also used for 3 to 6 months.Antiparasitic therapy should be started at least 4 days before surgery and be continued for at least 1 month (albendazole) or 3 months (mebendazole) after surgery. Surgery, when feasible, is the most common form of treatment of echinococcosis. According to the WHO, surgery is not recommended for pregnant women, those with multiple or difficult-to-access cysts, or patients with dead or totally calcified cysts. Asymptomatic cysts, if heavily calcified and presumed nonviable, may be monitored without specific therapy. The routine use of a protoscolicidal agent during surgery is not necessary.The puncture, aspiration, injection, and respiration (PAIR) technique is an option for inoperable cysts. Patients should be on antiparasitic therapy prior to this procedure to reduce the risk of cyst dissemination. The response to specific therapy may be monitored with serology and imaging.

MISCELLANEOUS SYNDROMES

Schistosomiasis

Myocardial or pericardial involvement by *Schistosoma* species is a rare event and is due to the accumulation of *Schistosoma* eggs, which induce a local granulomatous response. However, chronic schistosomiasis may lead to severe liver fibrosis secondary to hepatosplenic involvement. This process involving portal hypertension may produce a hepatopulmonary syndrome manifested as dyspnea upon exertion, right ventricular hypertrophy, and, ultimately, *cor pulmonale*. In addition, endothelial damage to the pulmonary circulation results from the shunting of *Schistosoma* eggs through portosystemic shunts. The ability of *Schistosoma mansoni* to survive during its residence in the pulmonary circulation is due to molecular masking by coating with ABO blood group glycolipids and major histocompatibility complex (MHC) molecules derived from the human host. *Schistosoma*-induced pulmonary hypertension carries a grave prognosis since it usually denotes an advanced stage of hepatosplenic schistosomiasis. Thrombosis *in situ*, particularly of the right pulmonary artery, as well as cardiac arrhythmias and sudden cardiac death syndromes may occur.The treatment of schistosomiasis (all species) is praziquantel or, alternatively, oxamniquine for *S. mansoni*.

Myocarditis Associated with *Naegleria fowleri*

Naegleria fowleri is a free-living amoeba, which is well known to cause an acute, purulent, primary amoebic meningoencephalitis (PAM), often in previously healthy young individuals with a recent history of water-sport activity in rivers, lakes, or ponds.The disease process is usually confined to the central nervous system. One report in the literature, which reexamined an earlier case report of disseminated amebiasis, provided evidence of possible disseminated *N. fowleri*. Several authors have described the pathological recognition of PAM-associated diffuse or focal myocarditis. In the reported cases of associated myocarditis, clinical cardiac manifestations have been nearly universally absent. Additionally, amoebas have not been found in the heart tissue, making causal conclusions speculative. The diagnosis of PAM, when made premortem, is typically accomplished by direct wet-mount examination of the cerebral spinal fluid for trophozoite forms. *Naegleria fowleri* can be grown on agar plates coated with Gram-negative bacteria. Serological tests are not useful in the acute clinical setting given the delay in the mounting of a detectable immune response. A real-time PCR assay has been developed for *N. fowleri* identification and could become useful for fast laboratory diagnosis of PAM.To date, there are no reports of the use of this assay on myocardial specimens. Additionally, PCR-based diagnosis has been evaluated with formalin-fixed and paraffin-embedded brain sections. Amphotericin B remains the backbone of PAM therapy, and *N. fowleri* is highly susceptible to this drug *in vitro*. Successful therapy has been rare, and when reported, amphotericin B is usually part of the therapy. In a mouse model of PAM, azithromycin and amphotericin B have demonstrated synergistic success and may hold promise as combination therapy.

Zoonotic Filariasis

Dirofilaria immitis, a common parasite of dogs and other canids, is prevalent in many areas of the world and can occasionally affect humans. In the dog, the parasite undergoes its early development in the subcutaneous tissues for about 3 months before migrating to the right side of the heart. Once deposited by a mosquito vector, the adult worms live in vascular beds and can induce myocarditis. Although adult *D. immitis* worms have been found in the heart and major vessels of humans at autopsy on several occasions.the usual finding is for immature worms to be located in partially or completely occluded small pulmonary arteries, where the obstruction has produced a distal pneumonitis followed by granuloma formation, resulting in a well-circumscribed coin lesion containing the parasite.These lesions are usually identified in asymptomatic individuals undergoing routine chest radiographs. No worms have been identified by echocardiography or angiography during premortem evaluation. Other filarial species, such as lymphatic-dwelling human filariae (*Wuchereria* spp. and *Brugia* spp.), may also be identified as pulmonary nodules.The occurrence of severe, and occasionally lethal, myocardial involvement that often occurs in dogs and other canids has not been described for humans.

Tropical Pulmonary Eosinophilia

Tropical pulmonary eosinophilia is a syndrome caused by a hypersensitivity response to microfilariae of the lymphatic-dwelling filariae *Wuchereria bancrofti* and *Brugia malayi* This process, manifested as chronic pulmonary infiltrates with eosinophilia, may result in permanent deficits in pulmonary function.Clinical symptoms usually include cough, dyspnea, and nocturnal wheezing. Eosinophils located in the lung, as a response to the presence of filariae in the pulmonary circulation, degranulate and lead to the production of toxic oxygen radicals that contribute to a chronic pulmonary inflammatory process.These restrictive pulmonary function deficits may result in pulmonary hypertension that subsequently contributes to *cor pulmonale*. The treatment of choice recommended by the WHO is the oral antifilarial drug diethylcarbamazine (DEC) for 3 weeks.

ENDOMYOCARDIAL FIBROSIS

Endomyocardial fibrosis (EMF) is an idiopathic disorder of the tropical and subtropical regions of the world that is characterized by the development of restrictive cardiomyopathy.

The nosology of EMF coincides with some related disorders. EMF is sometimes considered part of a spectrum of a single disease process that includes Löffler endocarditis (nontropical eosinophilic endomyocardial fibrosis or fibroplastic parietal endocarditis with eosinophilia).

Tropical EMF and Löffler endocarditis should be distinguished from endocardial fibroelastosis, which is characterized by cartilaginous thickening of the mural endocardium, chiefly of the left ventricle. This disease is most common in the first 2 years of life and, in some patients, appears to be an inherited disorder that is associated with congenital cardiac malformations.

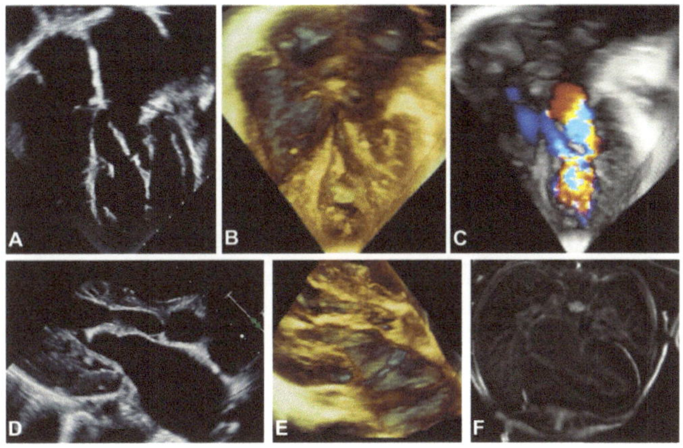

Fig 40.28: Echocardiographic apical 4-chamber view (A–C), parasternal long axis (D,E) and MRI (F) imaging before EFE resection. 2D (A,D) and 3D (B,C,E) echocardiography showing hyperechogenic thickening of the endocardium on atrial, mitral valve, LV and LVOT level consistent with generalized EFE in the left sided structures of the heart is shown. Severe dilation of the left atrium can be noted. (C) Severe turbulences are detected by color Doppler in all left sided structures affected by EFE as compared to physiological color Doppler appearance in the right sided structures of the heart that are not affected by EFE. (F) Late gadolinium enhancement on endocardial level encapsulating all structures of the left atrium and ventricle is depicted.

Pathophysiology

In EMF, the underlying process produces patchy fibrosis of the endocardial surface of the heart, leading to reduced compliance and, ultimately, restrictive physiology as the endomyocardial surface becomes more generally involved. Endocardial fibrosis principally involves the inflow tracts of the right and left ventricles and may affect the atrioventricular valves, leading to tricuspid and mitral regurgitation.

The earliest changes of EMF are not well described because most patients do not present with symptoms until relatively late in the clinical course. Olsen described 3 phases of EMF. The first phase involves eosinophilic infiltration of the myocardium with necrosis of the subendocardium and a pathologic picture consistent with acute myocarditis. This is reportedly present in the first 5 weeks of the illness. The second stage, typically observed after 10 months, is associated with thrombus formation over the initial lesions, with a decrement in the amount of inflammatory activity present. Ultimately, after several years of disease activity, the fibrotic phase is reached, when the endocardium is replaced by collagenous fibrosis. Extensive calcification is rarely associated with fibrosis. This pathomorphologic schema is not observed uniformly and has not been consistently supported by other investigators.

The etiology of EMF remains unclear. Hypotheses include infectious, inflammatory, and nutritional processes. EMF is frequently associated with concomitant parasitic infections (e.g. helminths) and their attendant eosinophilia, although the role of parasitic infections and/or the eosinophil remains speculative. The development of EMF as a sequela to toxoplasma-related myocarditis has also been described, as has a relationship of malarial infection to development of EMF. However, no specific organism has been consistently associated with EMF.

The role of the eosinophil in the pathogenesis of EMF is controversial. Whether the eosinophil actually induces myocardial necrosis and subsequent fibrosis or is attracted to the endocardial surface as a result of the initial insult is unknown. The eosinophil is not present as frequently in cases of tropical EMF as in Löffler endocarditis; thus, the role of the eosinophil in the tropical disease is likely less significant.

EMF is most frequently observed in the socially disadvantaged and in children and young women. These groups frequently have malnutrition, and in regions of sub-Saharan Africa where the disease is most prevalent, the typical diet is high in a tuber called cassava, which contains relatively high concentrations of the rare earth element cerium (Ce). The combination of high Ce levels and hypomagnesemia has been shown to produce EMF-like lesions in laboratory animals. A familial tendency has rarely been noted in Uganda and Zambia.

Incidence

EMF is rarely encountered in patients who have not traveled from the subtropical regions of Africa and tropical and subtropical regions elsewhere in the world, including areas in India and South America that are within 15° of the equator. Löffler endocarditis (also called nontropical eosinophilic endocarditis) is a related condition that is observed in the United States and is considered by some authors to be a different stage of a similar process related to eosinophilia.

EMF occurs primarily in the subtropical regions of Africa but is also encountered in tropical and subtropical regions elsewhere in the world, including areas in India and South America that are within 15° of the equator.

More than 90% of reported cases of EMF have occurred in geographic locations that are within 15° of the equator. In equatorial African nations, such as Nigeria, EMF is the fourth most common cause of cardiac disease in adults, and EMF accounts for 22% of cases of heart failure in Nigerian children. EMF is the most common type of restrictive cardiomyopathy in tropical countries.

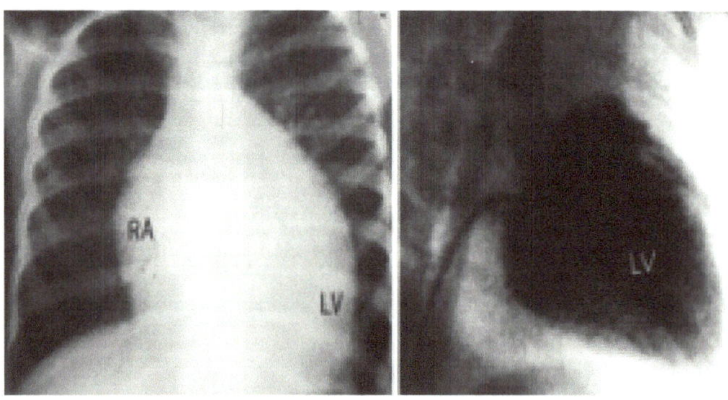

Fig. 40.29: *Photograph X-ray chest PA view (left) showing diffuse cardiomegaly with congested lung fieldsand hugely dilated and akinetic LV as seen on LV angiography (Right) in a young patient with endocardial fibroelastosis*

Mortality/Morbidity

The overall prognosis of patients with EMF is poor and depends on the extent and distribution of disease within the various chambers and valves of the heart.

Most patients have extensive disease at the time of presentation; therefore, survival after diagnosis is relatively brief. In one study, 95% of a group of patients had died at 2 years. In a second study, 44% of patients died within 1 year after the onset of symptoms, and another 40% of patients died 1–3 years after onset. EMF is most commonly reported in individuals living in Nigeria and Uganda. Women of reproductive age and children are more commonly affected than men.

Age Distribution

EMF is not generally observed in children younger than 4 years, although the typical pathology for EMF has recently been described in a 4-month-old infant with left ventricular inflow tract obstruction. The people most commonly affected are older children (aged 5–15 y) and young adults, but cases have been reported in individuals aged 70 years.

History

Typically, endomyocardial fibrosis (EMF) has an insidious onset, and symptoms relate to the specific chambers and valves where the disease is most extensive. When right ventricular involvement or tricuspid regurgitation predominates, lower extremity swelling, increasing abdominal girth, and nausea may be expected.With left ventricular involvement, dyspnea is the predominant symptom, especially exertional dyspnea. Additionally, fatigue, paroxysmal nocturnal dyspnea, and orthopnea may be present.

Thromboembolic complications may occur in EMF. Rarely, patients may present early in the course of the

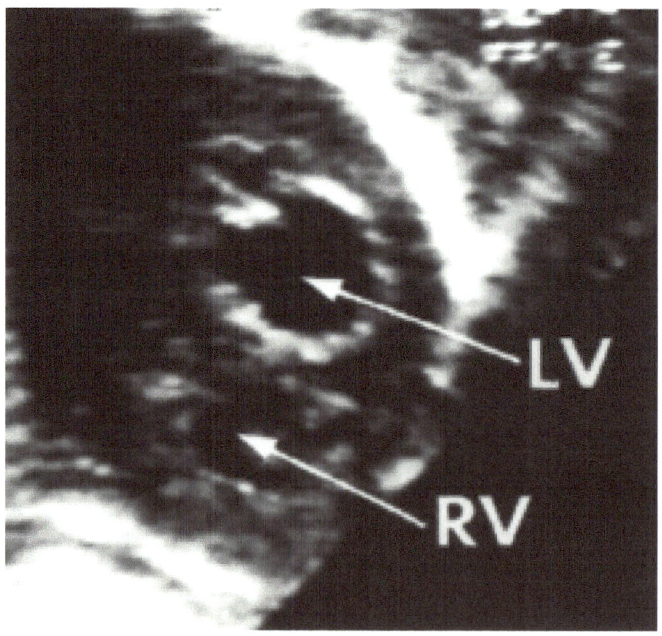

Fig. 40.30: *Echocardiogaph showing dilated LV as compared to right ventricle(RV) in patient with endocardial fibroelastosis*

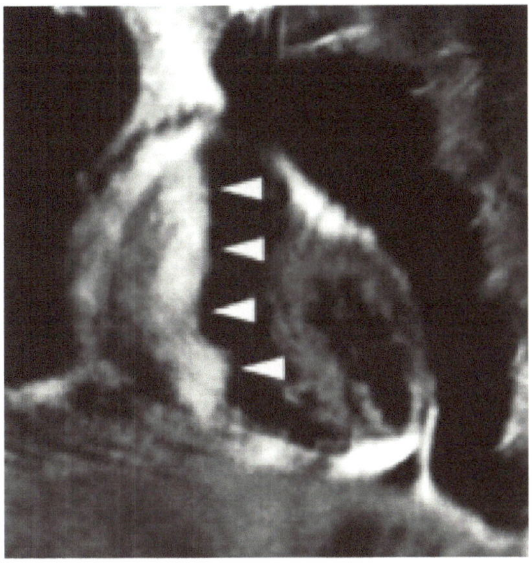

Fig. 40.31: *T1-weighted MR images after administration of gadopentetate dimeglumine show homogeneous enhancement of right ventricular mass (arrowheads). Mass is attached to free wall of right ventricle, extending from lateral tricuspid valve annulus to right ventricular outflow tract without involvement of apical portion. Mass protrudes toward right ventricular cavity with broad base on right ventricular free wall. Signal intensity of mass was intermediate on T1-weighted images and high on T2-weighted images (not shown). Note dilatation of right atrium*

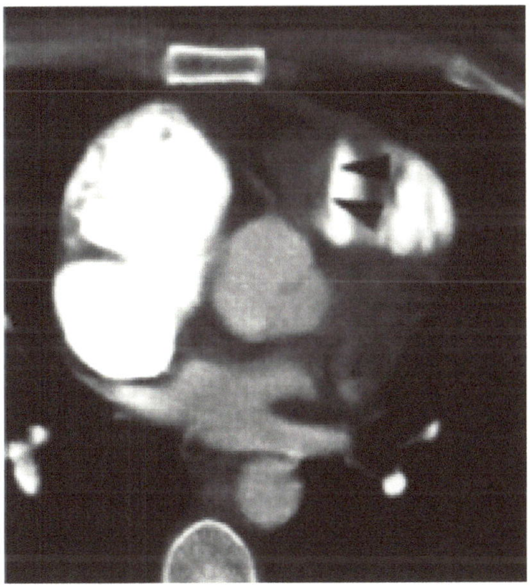

Fig. 40.32: *Follow-up contrast-enhanced CT scans obtained 3 years after A and B reveal larger right ventricular mass (arrowheads), contributing to stenosis of right ventricular outflow tract. Mass shows homogeneous low attenuation, probably because CT was performed during arterial phase of contrast enhancement. Size of right atrium has also increased*

disease with an acute febrile illness with symptoms of cardiac insufficiency mimicking myocarditis. Recently, anginalike chest pain and syncope were reported in a patient with EMF involving the left ventricle.

Physical

Physical findings are also dependent on the extent and distribution of disease.In those with right ventricular involvement, jugular venous pressure elevation, ascites, and edema may be present. The presence of ascites may appear out of proportion to the amount of peripheral edema. This may occur because of the co-comitant presence of a protein-losing enteropathy and subsequent hypoalbuminemia. Patients with tricuspid regurgitation may have giant V waves observed in the jugular venous pulsations. A third or fourth heart sound and tachycardia may be present. Signs of pulmonary congestion are present in patients with left-sided disease.

Causes

A specific single etiology of EMF has not been established. Suggested potential causes include the following:

Infectious causes

Parasites (e.g. helminths)
Protozoans (e.g. toxoplasmosis, malaria)

- Inflammatory causes - Eosinophilia
- Nutritional causes
  - General malnutrition
  - High-tuber diet
  - Ce toxicity
  - Hypomagnesemia**on 4 of 9**
- Other Problems to be Considered
  - Anthracycline toxicity
  - Carcinoid heart disease
  - Drug-induced cardiotoxicity (e.g. serotonin, methysergide, ergotamine, mercurial agents, busulfan) \
- Fabry disease
- Fatty infiltration
- Gaucher disease
- Glycogen storage disease
- Hurler disease
- Idiopathic cardiomyopathy
- Metastatic cancers
- Radiation
- Rheumatic heart disease
- Occasionally, a masslike lesion seen in endomyocardial fibrosis masquerades as an intracardiac tumor.

Lab Studies

Complete blood cell count may show anemia and eosinophilia.

Imaging Studies

Chest Radiography

The cardiac silhouette in endomyocardial fibrosis (EMF) may be normal in size, and generalized cardiomegalyis unusual because the ventricles are not typically dilated.

The roentgenographic image may exhibit significant enlargement of the atria, and significant right atrial enlargement creates a cardiac silhouette in the shape of the African continent, which is a specific heart shadow sign that has been termed the heart of Africa.

Echocardiography

Echocardiography is a useful tool when making the diagnosis of EMF and has been demonstrated to successfully differentiate EMF and other processes such as rheumatic heart disease and congenital heart disease.The presence and location of fibrosis as determined by echocardiography correlates well with autopsy findings. Findings include thickening of the inferior and basal left ventricular wall, apical obliteration, thrombi adherent to endocardial surface, mitral regurgitation, and tricuspid regurgitation. A pericardial effusion is frequently present and may be large. While parameters of diastolic function by Doppler echocardiography tend to correlate with the functional status of the patient, because most patients present with later stages of EMF, a restrictive filling pattern in the left ventricular outflow tract is most common.

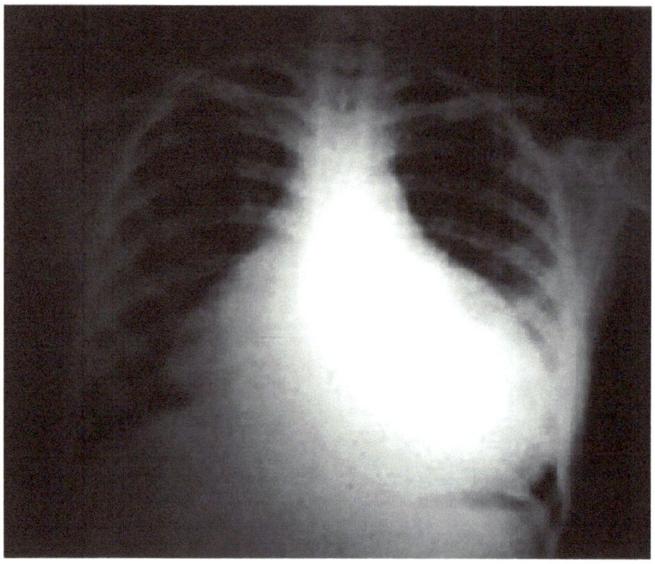

Fig. 40.33: *Photograph of X-ray chest PA showing cardiomegaly in a young child with endomyocardial fibrosis*

Recently, decreased flow propagation velocity (Vp) has been demonstrated in a large percentage of patients with EMF.Color-flow imaging frequently exhibits tricuspid and mitral regurgitation. Spectral Doppler analysis of tricuspid regurgitation frequently reflects an increased pulmonary artery systolic pressure.

Angiography (Fig. 47.29)

Traditionally, angiography has been considered the criterion standard when making the diagnosis of EMF.

Left and right ventriculography exhibits distortion of chamber morphology by fibrosis and obliteration and variable degrees of mitral and tricuspid regurgitation.

The mushroom sign has been used to describe the shape of the affected ventricle when the apex is obliterated completely by fibrosis.

Electron Beam Computed Tomography Scanning

Features of EMF observed with this modality were described in the mid 1990s.The fibrotic process is delineated as a band of low attenuation within the endocardium. Obliteration of the apex and inflow tract, when present, is also demonstrated This method reportedly assists in distinguishing EMF from constrictive pericarditis (Fig. 47.32).

Cardiovascular Magnetic Resonance Imaging

Recently, the use of cardiovascular magnetic resonance imaging has been shown to demonstrate obliterative

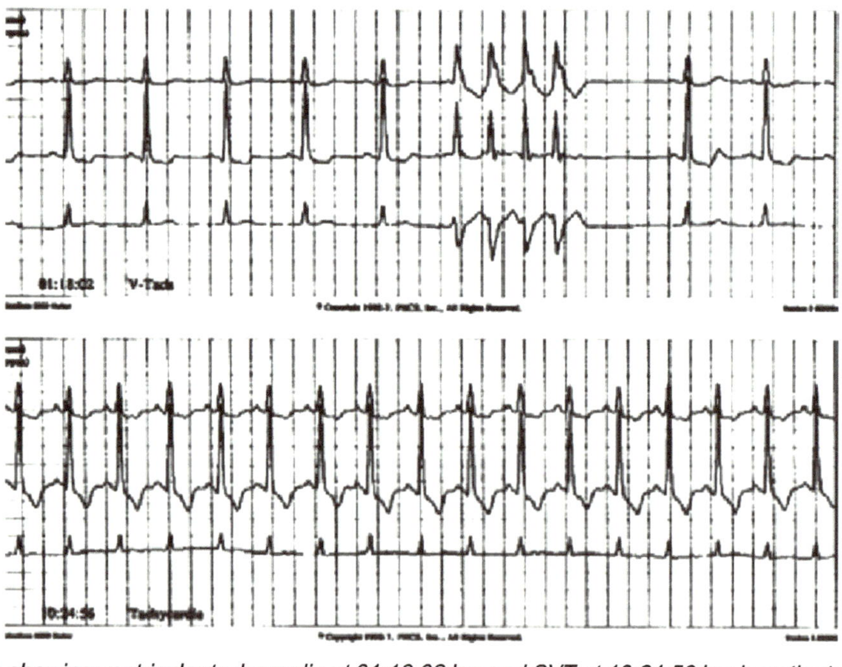

Fig. 40.34: *Holter graph showing ventricular tachycardia at 01;18;02 hrs and SVT at 10;24;56 hrs in patient with recurrent palpitation as a result of EFE*

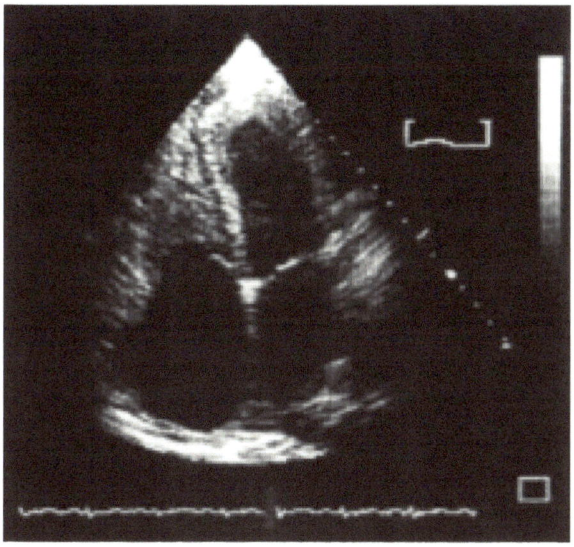

Fig. 40.35: *Apical four chamber echocardiographic image from an individual with cardiomyopathy associated with hypereosinophilic syndrom showing soft tissue thrombus deposition within the left and right ventricular apices. Right atrial deposition is also present*

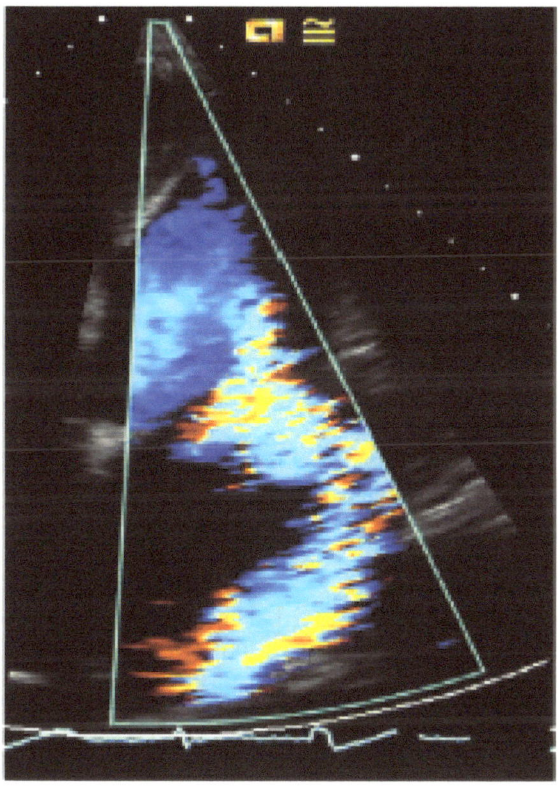

Fig. 40.36: *Colour-Doppler imaging from the same patient as in Figure 10 showing the extent of mitral regurgitation. Calculated regurgitant volume 35 mL (moderate)*

changes in the ventricles, atrial dilation, and regurgitant atrioventricular valve lesions in patients with EMF.

However, the use of contrast-enhanced imaging was not able to demonstrate fibrosis within the ventricles of these patients (Fig. 47.31).

Other Tests

Electrocardiography

Atrial fibrillation Low QRS voltage First-degree atrioventricular block in up to 44% of patients Incomplete right bundle-branch block in up to 30% of patients Left atrial enlargement.

Procedures

Cardiac catheterization likely exhibits hemodynamic findings consistent with restrictive cardiomyopathy. Findings from endomyocardial biopsy may be diagnostic, but this procedure is typically not needed.

Biopsy findings may be nondiagnostic when the disease is patchy and sampling sites do not correlate with areas of disease. Because biopsy (especially from the left ventricle) carries some risk, reserve the use of this technique until other diagnostic approaches have been used.

Histologic findings: The heart size is not usually enlarged in EMF. The ventricular cavities are frequently laden with thrombi and, in severe cases, may be nearly totally obliterated by endocardial thickening and thrombosis. The histologic findings of EMF are characterized by reactive fibrosis associated with a selective increase in type I collagen deposition, subendocardial infarction and fibrosis, and thrombus formation. Additionally, specific features of other diseases, such as those associated with hemochromatosis or glycogen storage disease, are notably absent.

Medical Care

In general, the response to medical therapy is poor and unproven. Because most patients with endomyocardial fibrosis (EMF) present long after any possible period of early active myocarditis may have existed, little, if any, role exists for immunosuppressive therapy as is used in some patients with Löffler disease.

Symptomatic therapy with diuretics has been shown to be useful, but digoxin, afterload reducers, and beta-blockers

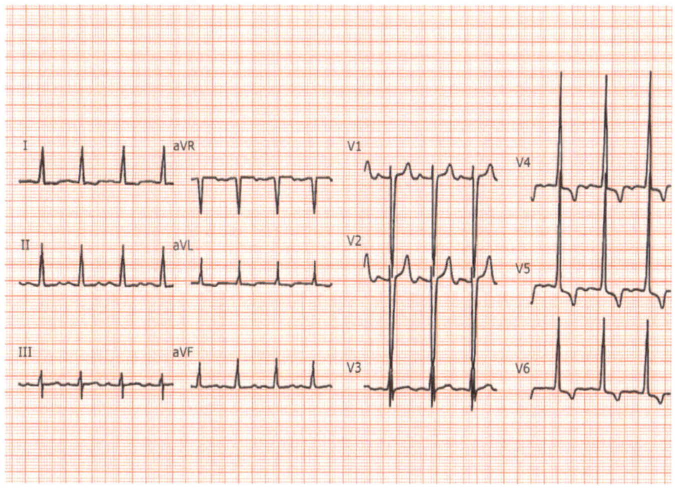

Fig. 40.37: *ECG showing tall R waves in Left precordial leads with T wave inversion in leads 11,111 aVF,V5 and V6with voltage criteria of left ventricular hypertrophy in patient with endocardial fibroelastosis*

have little role in EMF. For patients with severe symptoms, consider surgical therapy because the prognosis for these patients with continued medical therapy alone is dismal. Because the rate of thromboembolism is low among patients with EMF and the patient population affected is not typically compliant with anticoagulation regimens, most authors do not recommend anticoagulant therapy.

Surgical Care

Surgical therapy by endocardial decortication seems to be beneficial for many patients with advanced disease who are in functional-therapeutic class III or IV. The operative mortality rate is high (15–20%), but successful surgery has a clear benefit on symptoms and seems to favorably affect survival as well. The most commonly used approach is endocardiectomy, combined with mitral and/or tricuspid repair or replacement (when indicated), using a midline thoracotomy and cardiopulmonary bypass.

Depending on the location of the disease (right or left ventricle, apex or inflow tract), a transapical or transventricular approach can be used. Because a well-defined plane of cleavage usually exists between the endocardium and myocardium, endocardiectomy is most frequently feasible.Because the myocardium is not usually affected, the severe hemodynamic derangement associated with EMF is relieved with successful resection of the endocardium. Common postoperative complications include low cardiac output, heart block, and ventricular arrhythmias.

Diet

No specific diet is recommended for this condition. No activity restrictions are recommended because activity restrictions have not been proven to alter the prognosis of this condition, and no specific activity has

ENDOCARDIAL FIBROELASTOSIS (EFE)

The term endocardial fibroelastosis (EFE) was introduced by Weinberg and Himmelfarb in 1943. EFE refers to a pronounced, diffuse thickening of the ventricular endocardium and presents as unexplained heart failure in infants and children. The disease can be primary or secondary to various congenital heart diseases, most notably hypoplastic left heart syndrome, aortic stenosis, or atresia. The 2 pathologic forms of primary EFE include dilated, which is most common, and contracted. Primary EFE is not associated with any significant structural anomaly of the heart. Secondary EFE is associated with other congenital heart diseases. Once regarded as a common cause of unexplained heart failure, EFE is now considered rare.

Pathophysiology

EFE is characterized by diffuse endocardial thickening and myocardial dysfunction. The endocardial thickening is believed to be caused by persistent and increased wall tension in the ventricles, possibly secondary to damaged myocardium, mitral regurgitation, or both. However, EFE changes are progressive with age. The disease is usually sporadic, but familial cases have been reported (10%). Observations that favor a viral etiology include a clinical presentation similar to that of chronic myocarditis, findings of myocarditis or myocardial fibrosis in affected patients, a higher incidence following epidemics of coxsackievirus B infection, demonstration of persistent viral infection with molecular studies, and experimental production of the disease in animal models by viral infections of the myocardium. A phenotypic resemblance to dilated cardiomyopathy has been noted. Dilated EFE is characterized by a markedly enlarged globular heart, mainly involving the left ventricle (LV) and left atrium (LA). The LV endocardium is opaque, glistening, milky white, and diffusely thickened to about 1–2 mm. The thickening is most marked in the outflow tract. Papillary muscles arise more superiorly on the ventricular wall with thickened and shortened chordae tendineae, the characteristic rolled-free edge of mitral leaflets. Papillary muscles and trabeculae carneae are flattened and partially incorporated in the fibrotic process, giving a smooth appearance to the lining of the cavity; thus, the papillary muscles exert an undesirable lateral traction on the chordae tendineae and mitral cusps, leading to faulty leaflet opposition.

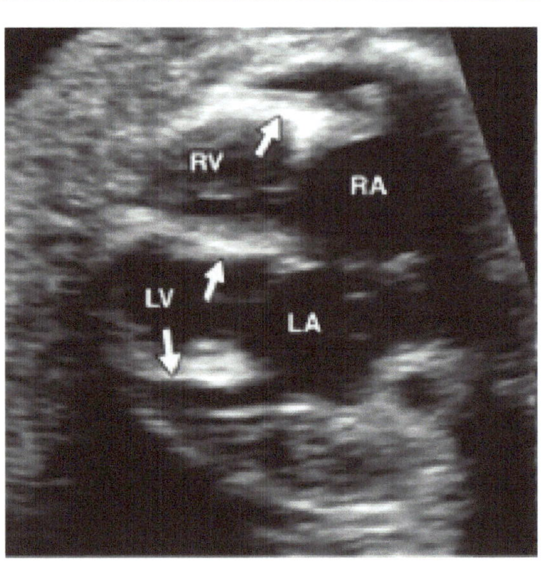

Fig. 40.38: Endocardial fibroelastosis. Four-chamber views show increased echogenicty (arrows) within myocardium of left ventricle (LV) and right ventricle (RV) in patient with endocardial fibroelastosis. LA = left atrium, RA = right atrium

Although the endocardium is thickened, the ventricular wall (myocardium) thickness is within the reference range. Endocardial thickening extends to the LA, right ventricle, and right atrium. Microthrombi may adhere to the endocardium. The right ventricle is anteriorly displaced to the right, and its cavity is usually flattened. The pulmonary artery may be enlarged, but the aorta and coronary arteries appear normal in caliber. In approximately 50% of patients, the mitral and aortic valves are involved, often producing marked deformity and either valvar regurgitation or stenosis.

The less common contracted type of primary EFE is associated with a relatively hypoplastic or normal LV size. The right and left atria and the right ventricle are markedly enlarged and hypertrophied, with minimal or no endocardial sclerosis. An early event in fetal life is believed to result in dilated EFE, which later morphoses into a contracted type. This suggests that the dilated type could appear as 2 different diseases while remaining a single disease. Secondary EFE, associated with cardiac malformations, is attributed to the cardiac hypertrophy and consequent imbalance in the myocardial oxygen supply-demand relationship. Resultant fibroelastotic thickening is often focal and less severe.

Acute congestive heart failure (CHF) becomes progressive CHF that results in death within weeks, usually within the first 6 months of life. In a subgroup of individuals who survive from a few months to several years, a more chronic course is common. Such patients respond to medications used to treat CHF. A variable cyclical clinical course ensues, with CHF recurrences related to respiratory or other intercurrent infections or to progression of disease. Remissions can occur with intensification of medical therapy.

History

Symptoms include feeding difficulty, excessive sweating, breathlessness, ·failure to thrive, and wheezing. Onset may acute enough to produce cardiogenic shock or sudden death; it is a recognized cause of sudden death in infancy.

- Approximately 20% of patients have a history of frequent or recent respiratory tract infections.
- Episodes of severe sudden abdominal pain may indicate coronary insufficiency.

The contracted form of endocardial fibroelastosis (EFE) presents with features of left-sided obstructive disease and acute LV failure. EFE is one of the recognized causes of nonimmune hydrops fetalis.

Physical

- EFE manifests as the classic features of heart failure. Tachypnea during feeding and grunting respirations with subcostal or intercostal retractions have been reported. Fine expiratory wheezes or rales in the lung bases are common. The following may be present upon admission:
  - Pallor
  - Peripheral cyanosis
  - Fever
  - Leukocytosis
  - Anemia
  - Rash

Thromboembolic episodes may lead to sudden death, myocardial infarction, cerebrovascular events, or even pulmonary embolism. The usual physical findings are as follows:

Cardiomegaly with normal-to-faint first and second heart sounds, a gallop rhythm with an audible third heart sound, apical pansystolic murmur of mitral regurgitation, and hepatosplenomegaly.

Clinically detectable pleural or pericardial effusions (rare)

Causes

Possible causative factors include intrauterine viral infection (mumps, coxsackievirus B), subendocardial ischemia, impaired lymphatic drainage of the heart, and systemic carnitine deficiency. Using polymerase chain reaction (PCR) analysis, Ni et al reported that the mumps viral genome persisted in the myocardium of children with EFE; however, this requires further study.·The authors suggested cause and effect and speculated that the disease disappeared after the initiation of the measles-mumps-rubella (MMR) vaccination.

- Nine patients with familial EFE were reported in 4 families, and inheritance patterns included X-linked recessive, autosomal dominant, and autosomal recessive.

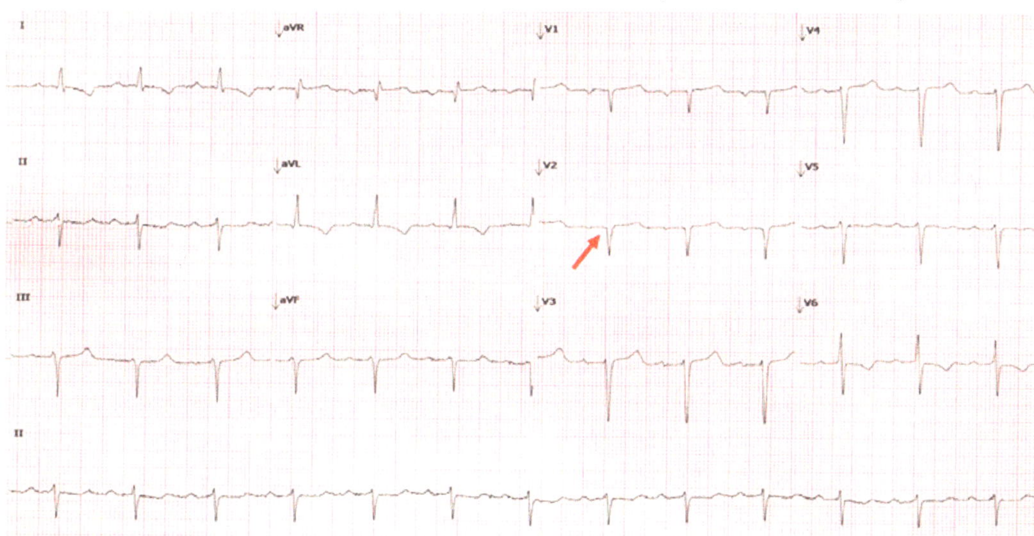

Fig. 40.39: *Electrocardiogram (ECG) from a patient with confirmed wild-type transthyretin amyloidosis with a 'pseudo-infarction' pattern (arrow). Also notable is the lack of ECG low-voltage despite the presence of severe concentric left ventricular hypertrophy on echocardiography*

- Recently, mutation of the gene *G4.5* (tafazzin) has been associated with familial X-linked EFE and Barth syndrome and has been reported to result in morphologic changes in the fetal heart as early as 18 weeks' gestation. Dilated (primary) EFE occurs when the heart is otherwise normal and no other cause of unexplained heart failure, including systemic carnitine deficiency, is demonstrable. Dilated EFE (secondary) is associated with aortic stenosis or atresia and includes coarctation of the aorta, ventricular septal defect, anomalous origin of left coronary artery from the pulmonary artery, myocardial injury from any cause, and metabolic or carnitine deficiency. Contracted EFE (secondary) is associated with hypoplastic left heart syndrome.

Lab Studies

Blood Tests Include the following:

- Serum electrolyte levels
- BUN and creatinine levels
- CBC count
- Blood culture tests indicated for management of acute episodes
- Autoantibody profile including anti-Ro and anti-La

Imaging Studies

Chest radiography: Cardiomegaly and cardiothoracic ratios exceed 0.65 in 50% of patients. CE is present in some patients at birth. In others, the heart size is normal during the first few weeks to the first few months of life, but CE subsequently develops.

The shape of the cardiac silhouette varies, although it is often globular. Pulmonary venous congestion is common. Left lower lobe atelectasis secondary to dilated LA is found in 25% of patients.

Echocardiography

LA and LV Dimensions are Increased

LV, septal, and posterior wall (PW) excursions are reduced The ejection fraction (EF) is reduced. Mitral valve (MV) motion is abnormal. Echogenicity along the endocardium of the LV (diagnostic clue) is dense.

Suggestive indicators include increased endocardial echo brightness and globular shape of the LV. The echocardiograph may depict a normalization of the shortening fraction and the LV dimensions when the clinical condition improves following medical therapy.

A varying degree of mitral regurgitation is common.

Fetal Echocardiography

This is a valuable tool for early identification, particularly of the secondary type.

One of the congenital malformations (e.g. aortic stenosis) is often demonstrated at the initial study. The EFE becomes obvious in repeat studies.

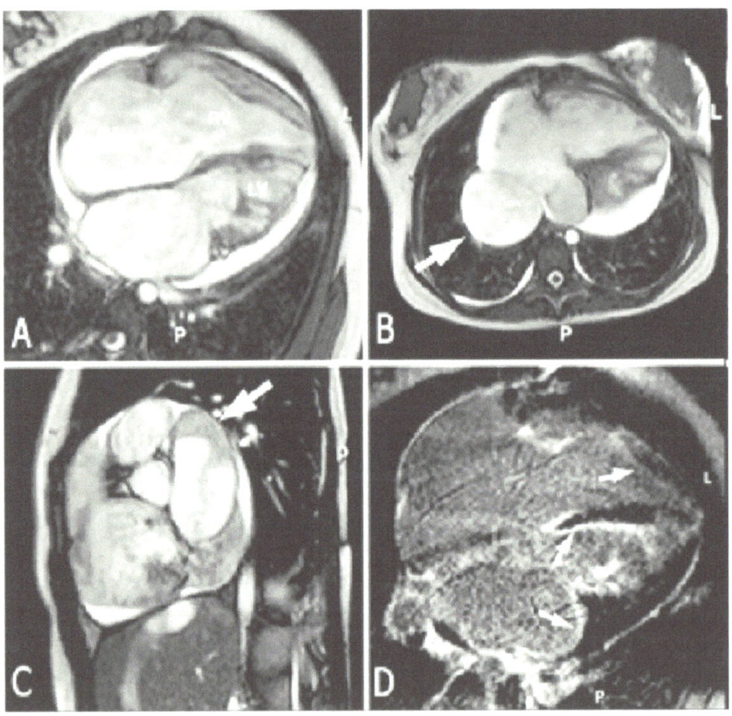

Fig. 40.40: *(A) Four-chamber cine image demonstrating biatrial dilation, right ventricular hypertrophy, a small left ventricular cavity and pericardial effusion. (B) Cine image demonstrating dilation of the inferior vena cava (arrow). (C) Short-axis cine image demonstrating thrombus (arrow) extending from the left atrial appendage into the left atrium. (D) Four-chamber late gadolinium hyperenhancement image demonstrating high-signal intensity in the atrial and ventricular endocardium (arrows)in a patient with EFE . L Left; LA Left atrium; LV Left ventricle; P Posterior; RA Right atrium; RV Right ventricle*

- Recently, electron beam CT has been reported to be useful in the early diagnosis of EFE because of its demonstration of calcification and fibrosis of the ventricles, especially at the apex.
- **Myocardial delayed-enhancement MRI has been reported to assist in delineation of the extent of endocardial fibroelastosis (Fig. 47.40).**

Other Tests

The 24-hour Holter ECG is **useful in documenting ambient arrhythmias.**

Electrocardiography: Tall R waves, deep Q waves, and T-wave inversion or flattening in the left precordial or inferior lead have been reported. Findings depict LV hypertrophy in more than 75% of patients. In the first few weeks of life, right axis deviation and isolated right ventricular hypertrophy are more common. Pulmonary hypertension may develop in patients who survive for a long period and appears as biventricular hypertrophy on electrocardiography. Patterns of left, right, or biatrial enlargement are evident in 50% of patients. Conduction or rhythm abnormalities include Wolff-Parkinson-White syndrome, left bundle branch block, supraventricular and ventricular arrhythmias, and varying degrees of atrioventricular block. Low-voltage tracings in the initial stage of heart failure and in the terminal phase are noted in 5% of patients. Occasionally, an infarct pattern appears, pointing to extensive myocardial fibrosis and necrosis (Fig. 47.39).

Procedures

Cardiac catheterization: Cardiac chambers and pulmonary arteries contain elevated pressures consistent with heart failure. Generally, systolic pulmonary artery pressure is not more than 50% of systemic pressure. Marked pulmonary hypertension may be seen in older children.

The constrictive type of EFE is rare and is associated with a left-sided atrioventricular obstructive pattern, with very high LA pressures from an early age. A diastolic gradient can be detected across the MV. Pulmonary artery pressure is elevated and often reaches systemic levels in this type of EFE.

Postcatheterization precautions include hemorrhage, vascular disruption after balloon dilation, pain, nausea and vomiting, and arterial or venous obstruction due to thrombosis or spasm.

Complications may include blood vessel rupture, tachyarrhythmias, bradyarrhythmias, and vascular occlusion. Angiocardiographic findings

- Marked dilation of the LV cavity
- Reduced EF with little or no LV wall thickening
- Dyskinetic LV contraction
- Mitral regurgitation (common)

In the contracted type, dilated right ventricle, right atrium, and pulmonary artery with slow clearance of the contrast from the left side of the heart.

Digital subtraction angiography **may demonstrate** an avascular rim between the opacified LV cavity and the ventricular walls perfused by the coronary arteries. The contrast void rim can be identified even in ordinary cineangiographic films. In cases in which the diagnosis is unclear, myocardial biopsy can be helpful.

Medical Care

The treatment of endocardial fibroelastosis (EFE) is essentially the same as that of chronic cardiac failure; its acute exacerbations are often precipitated by respiratory infections. Early and prolonged treatment with digoxin is suggested. Continue therapy for several years after the symptoms disappear; cessation of drug administration may result in acute cardiac failure, even when heart size has returned to normal.

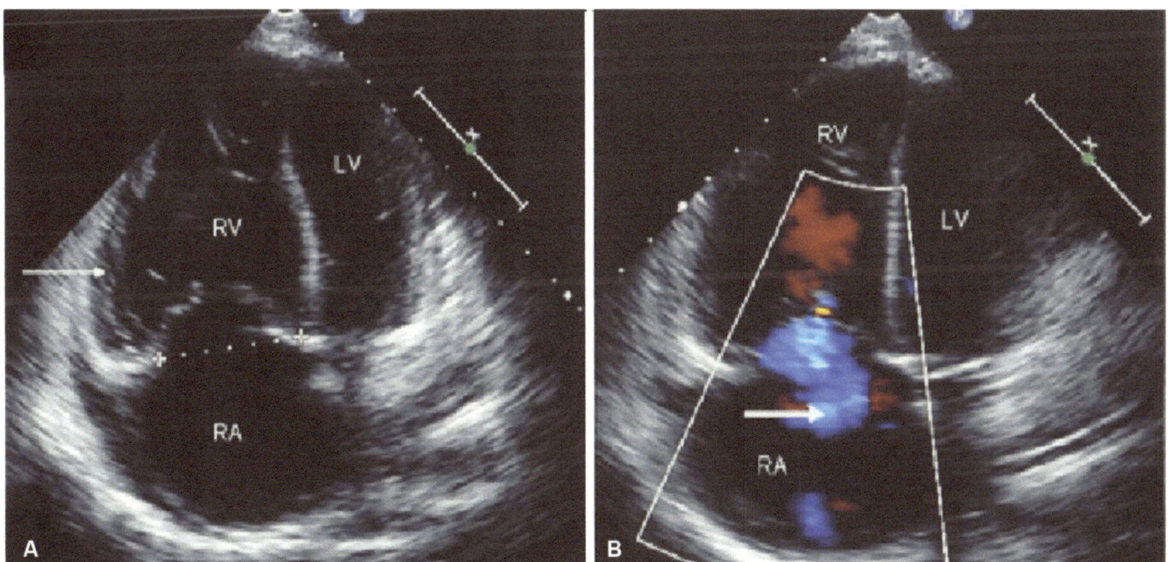

Fig. 40.41: *(A) Apical four chamber view shows right heart chamber dilatation and right ventricular hypertrophy (arrow) (B) Showing tricuspid regurgitation in color Doppler mode of echocardiography*

Other measures for acute failure and exacerbations of failure may be required, and precipitating factors, such as infection and anemia, require attention. Anticoagulation may be required in the presence of thromboembolic complications. Case reports in the literature cite resolution of antenatally diagnosed EFE associated with positive anti-Ro and anti-La antibodies with corticosteroid therapy.

Surgical Care

Both pericardial poudrage and MV replacement have had disappointing results.

Cardiac transplantation may be recommended for patients with end-stage disease.

Medication

If the patient is asymptomatic and his or her heart size is normal, provide early, adequate, and prolonged therapy with digitalis and diuretics for at least 2–3 years, with gradual discontinuation.

Early and prolonged treatment with digoxin is suggested. Anticoagulants may be required in the presence of thromboembolic complications.

Antibiotics for endocarditis prophylaxis are administered to patients with certain cardiac conditions, such as endocardial fibroelastosis, before procedures that may cause bacteremia are performed. Complications

- Resistant cardiac failure
- Recurrent chest infections
- Severe failure to thrive
- Cardiac cirrhosis
- Cerebral, coronary, and pulmonary thromboembolism

Persistent collapse of left lower lobe or entire left lung prognosis

Primary endocardial fibroelastosis (EFE) prognosis is relatively poor, although the condition is not universally fatal. The prognosis is worse if onset of heart failure occurs earlier.

CONGESTIVE HEART FAILURE

Acute CHF becomes progressive CHF and terminates in death within weeks, usually within the first 6 months of life.In patients who survive from a few months to several years, a more chronic course is common. Such patients respond to medications for CHF. A variable cyclical clinical course ensues, with CHF recurrence related to respiratory or other intercurrent infections or to progression of disease. Remissions can occur through intensification of medical therapy.

Progressive CHF causes deteriorating conditions that lead to death in one third of patients. One third of the patients survive and may experience persistent symptoms or show residual ECG abnormalities or evidence of cardiomegaly. Some believe that approximately one third of patients completely recover, although others are skeptical.

Early diagnosis and prompt persistent administration of digitalis may result in clinical improvement and reversion of the ECG and CE to normal.

Poor prognostic signs of CHF include (1) presentation in the newborn period and (2) recurrent episodes of CHF despite adequate therapy, especially if episodes recur more than 6 months after initial onset of symptoms.

CARDIOVASCULAR SYSTEM IN HIV

Cardiovascular manifestations of HIV infection have been observed for more than 15 years and finally prospective data substantiates this association.1 Studies published over the past 2–3 years have tracked the incidence and course of HIV infection in relation to cardiac illness in both children and adults. These recent studies show that subclinical echocardiographic abnormalities independently predict adverse outcomes and identify high risk groups to target for early intervention and treatment. The introduction of highly active antiretroviral therapy (HAART) regimens has significantly modified the course of HIV disease, with longer survival rates and improvement of life quality in HIV infected subjects expected. However, early data raised concerns about HAART being associated with an increase in both peripheral and coronary arterial diseases.

Understanding the effects of HAART on the cardiovascular system is only possible by understanding the effects of HIV co-infections first. HAART is only available to a minority of HIV infected individuals worldwide and studies before HAART remain globally applicable. UNAIDS estimates that 36.1 million people were living with HIV infection at the end of the year 2000. If 8–10% of patients develop symptomatic heart failure over a 2–5 year period, then three million cases of HIV related heart failure will have presented in that time period. 2 Dilated cardiomyopathy, coronary artery disease, endocarditis, and pericardial effusion related to HIV infection will be reviewed here (Figs 47.48, 47.49).

DILATED CARDIOMYOPATHY

HIV disease is recognised as an important cause of dilated cardiomyopathy, with a prevalence reported at 3.6% among cardiomyopathy patients, increasing as patients with HIV infection live longer. Compared to patients with idiopathic dilated cardiomyopathy, those with HIV infection and dilated cardiomyopathy have greatly reduced survival and a hazard ratio of death of 4.0.3 The importance of cardiac dysfunction is demonstrated by a reported median survival to AIDS related death which is 101 days in patients with left ventricular dysfunction and 472 days in patients with a normal heart by echocardiography at similar infection stage.

Myocarditis still represents the best studied cause of dilated cardiomyopathy in HIV disease. HIV virions appear to infect myocardial cells in patchy distributions4 without a clear direct association between HIV and cardiac myocyte dysfunction. It is unclear how virus enters CD4 receptor negative cells such as myocytes. Reservoir cells (for example, dendritic cells) may play a pathogenic role in the interaction between HIV and the myocyte and in the activation of multifunctional cytokines that contribute to

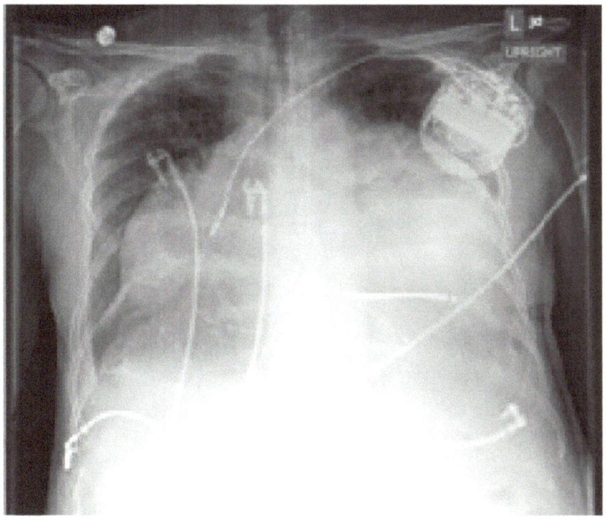

Fig. 40.42: *X-ray chest PA view shows grossly dilated heart with implanted pacemaker in patient with dilated cardiomyopathy in HIV infection*

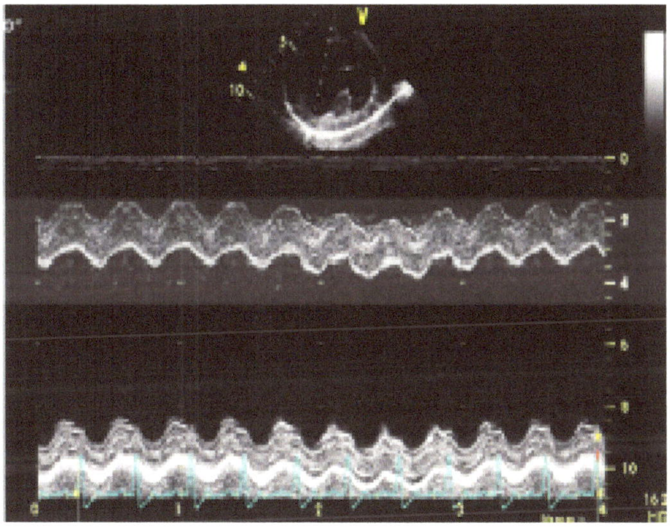

Fig. 40.43: *M-Mode Echo scan shows dilated LV cavity in dilated cardiomyopathy in HIV infection*

progressive and late tissue damage. Asymptomatic left ventricular dysfunction and increased left ventricular mass independently predict accelerated mortality in both adults and children infected with HIV. Treatment for dilated cardiomyopathy associated with HIV infection is generally similar to treatment for non-ischaemic cardiomyopathy. Angiotensin converting enzyme inhibitors are recommended based on general heart failure studies, but may be poorly tolerated because of low systemic vascular resistance from diarrhoeal disease, infection, or dehydration. No studies have investigated the efficacy of specific therapeutic regimens, including HAART, other than intravenous immunoglobulin. The apparent efficacy of immunoglobulin treatment may be the result of immunoglobulins inhibiting cardiac autoantibodies by competing for Fc receptors or dampening the secretion or effects of cytokines and cellular growth factors.

Encephalopathy influences negatively the clinical course of dilated cardiomyopathy in HIV disease. HIV may persist in reservoir cells in the myocardium and the cerebral cortex even after antiretroviral treatment. The reservoir cells may hold HIV-1 on their surfaces for extended time periods and may chronically release cytotoxic cytokines (tumour necrosis factor-(TNF), interleukin-6 (IL-6), endothelin-1 (ET-1)) contributing to progressive and late tissue damage in both systems independently of HAART.

CORONARY ARTERY DISEASE

Accelerated coronary artery disease in HIV infected patients may result from atherogenesis stimulated by virus infected monocyte–macrophages, possibly caused by altered leucocyte adhesion or arteritis.10 Coronary artery disease is observed with increasing frequency among HIV patients receiving protease inhibitors in the ambit of HAART. Despite the clinical benefits of protease inhibitors, complications such as lipodystrophy, insulin resistance, and high concentrations of low density lipoprotein and triglycerides have been described in up to 60% of patients treated with HAART regimens. In 10–20% of patients, these alterations of metabolism have severe manifestations. Effects of pre-existing cardiovascular risk factors combined with atherogenic effects of current drug treatments for HIV infection appear to result in an increase in acute coronary syndromes, even in young HIV infected individuals. It may be important to consider traditional coronary risk profiles and to alter those that can be modified in the evaluation and continued treatment of patients for HAART. Diet and exercise should not be overlooked, because both can be effective in managing these complications without causing further side effects. Fibric acid derivatives and statins can lower HIV associated cholesterol and triglyceride concentrations, although further data are needed on interactions between statins and protease inhibitors.

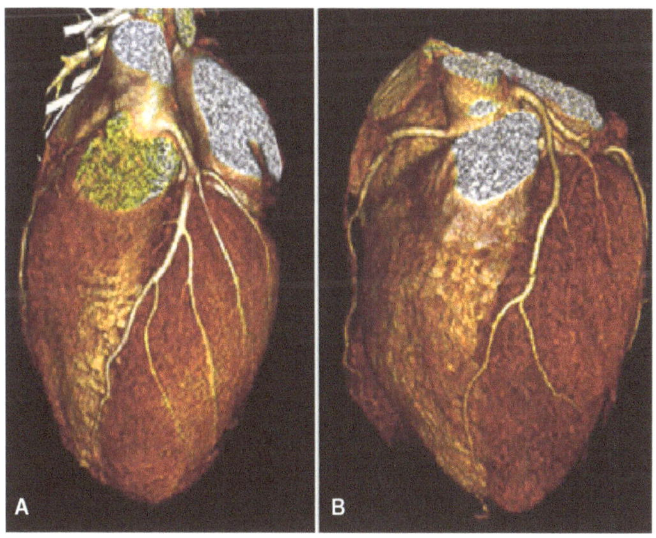

Fig. 40.44: *Multislice CT reconstructions of (a) a control heart and (b) a heart affected by DCM in HIV infection showing marked epicardial coronary artery mismatch for left ventricular mass and side-branch reduction. Abbreviation: DCM, dilated cardiomyopathy*

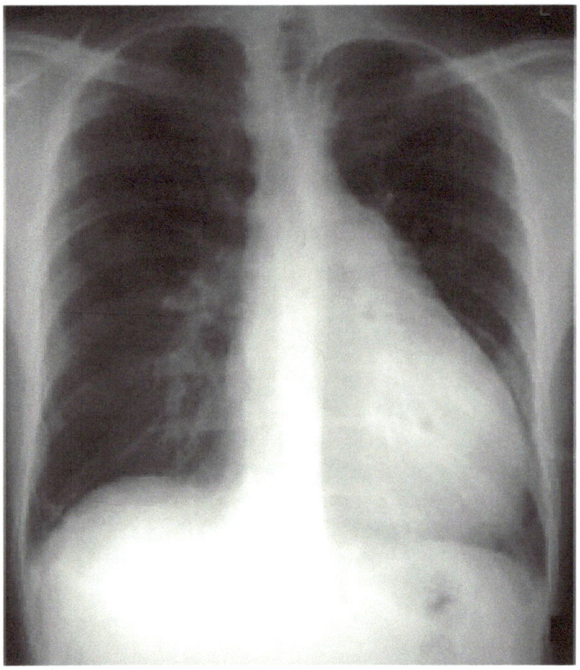

Fig. 40.45: *Chest radiograph of a patient with primary pulmonary hypertension. Note the enlarged proximal pulmonary arteries*

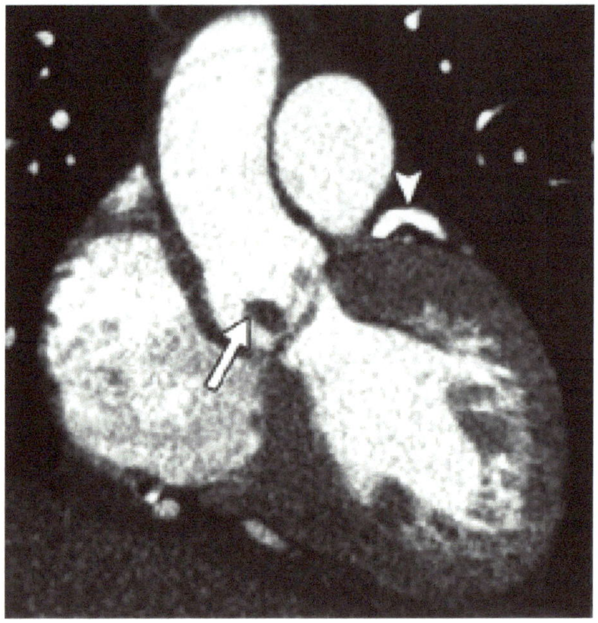

Fig. 40.46: *A patient with HIV infection, endocarditis, and coronary artery disease who had history of IV drug abuse and highly active antiretroviral therapy. Coronal multiplanar reformatted contrast-enhanced CT image shows vegetation (arrow) adjacent to aortic valve and calcified plaques (arrowhead) in left anterior descending artery (LAD)*

Lovastatin should be avoided in patients receiving concomitant drugs that may potentiate skeletal muscle toxicity with this agent. Hypoglycaemic agents may have some role in managing glucose abnormalities, although troglitazone cannot be recommended for fat abnormalities alone and metformin may cause lactic acidosis. Perhaps a better understanding of protease inhibitors' effects on lipid and metabolic pathways will lead to a new generation of drug treatments without metabolic alterations. This understanding may also lead to new treatments for dyslipidaemias and alterations of metabolism unrelated to HIV infection.

HIV Associated Pulmonary Hypertension and Right Ventricular Dysfunction

The incidence of HIV associated pulmonary hypertension is estimated to be 1/200, much higher than the 1/200 000 found in the general population. Primary pulmonary hypertension is estimated to occur in about 0.5% of hospitalized AIDS patients and is a cause of severe cardiac impairment with associated cor pulmonale and death.[1] The pathogenesis is multifactorial and poorly understood. HIV may cause endothelial damage and mediator related

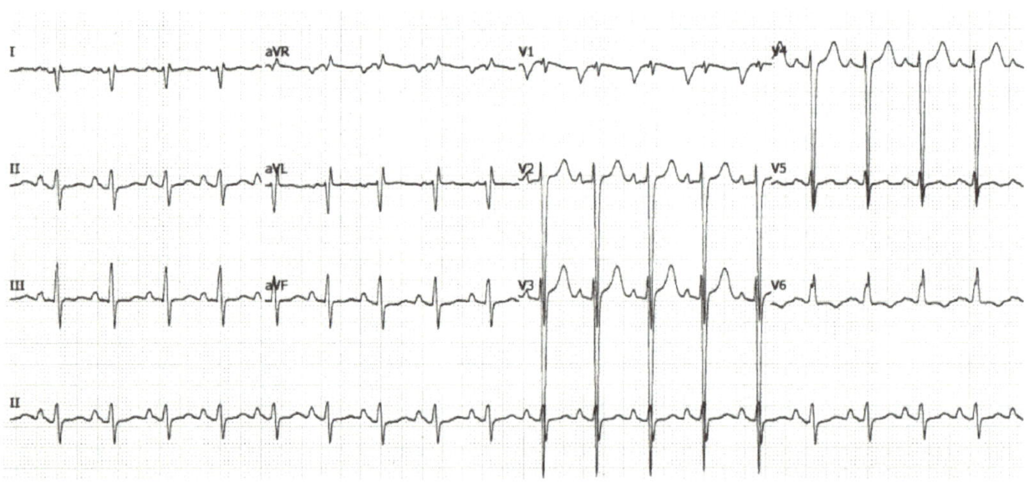

Fig. 40.47: *Showing dilated cardiomyopathyas seen in HIV infection * There is marked LVH (S wave in V2 > 35 mm) with dominant S waves in V1-4 * Right axis deviation suggests associated right ventricular hypertrophy (i.e. biventricular enlargement).* There is evidence of left atrial enlargement (deep, wide terminal portion of the P wave in V1).* There are peaked P waves in lead II suggestive of right atrial hypertrophy (not quite 2.5mm in height)*

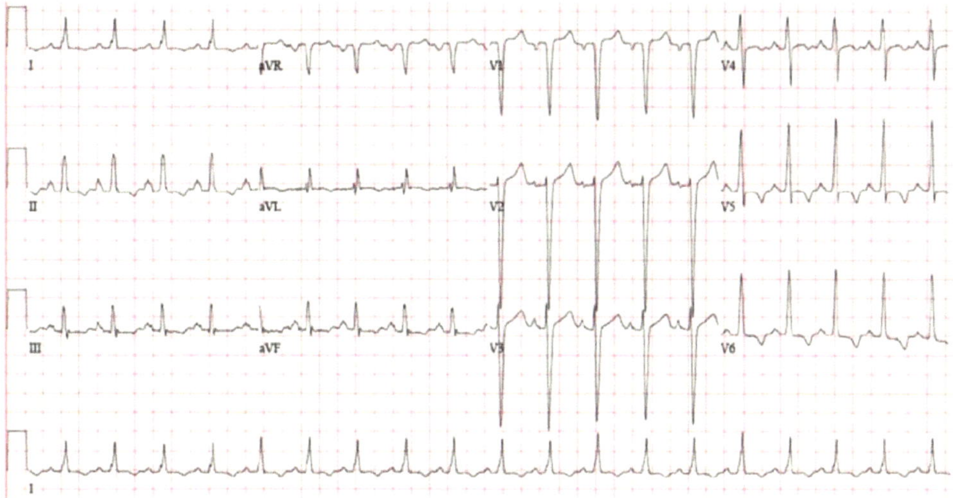

Fig. 40.48: *Showing dilated cardiomyopathyas seen in HIV infection * There is marked LVH (S wave in V2 > 35 mm) with dominant S waves in V1-4 .There is evidence of left atrial enlargement (deep, wide terminal portion of the P wave in V1).* There are peaked P waves in lead II suggestive of right atrial hypertrophy (not quite 2.5mm in height).*

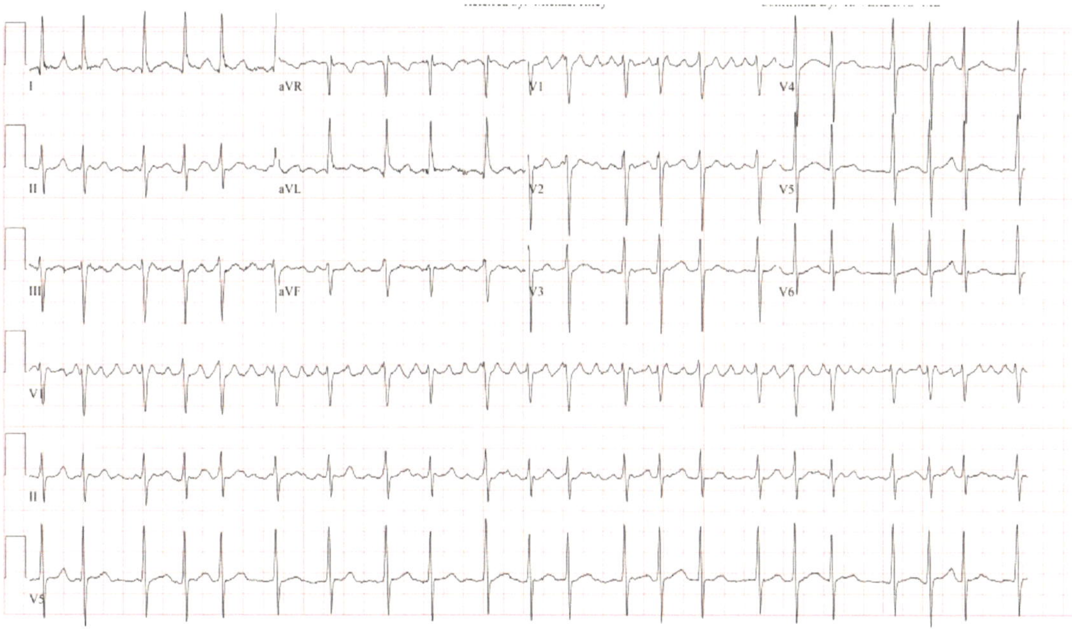

Fig. 40.49: *Atrial fibrillation with fast ventricular rate in dilated cardiomyopathy in HIV infection*

vasoconstriction through stimulation by the envelope glycoprotein, including direct release and pulmonary vasoconstrictor effects of ET-1, IL-6 and TNF-?. HIV is frequently identified in alveolar macrophages on histology. These macrophages release TNF, oxide anions, and proteolytic enzymes in response to infection. Effects of HAART on pulmonary artery endothelial cells are unknown.

Endocarditis (Fig. 47.46)

The prevalence of infective endocarditis in HIV infected patients is similar to that of patients of similar behaviour risk—that is, intravenous drug use.1 Estimates of endocarditis occurrence vary from 6.3–34% of HIV infected patients who use intravenous drugs. Right sided valves are predominantly affected. Patients with and without HIV generally have similar presentation and survival rates from infective endocarditis. However, patients with late stage HIV disease have higher mortality from infective endocarditis than do asymptomatic HIV infected patients. As the autoimmune response to bacterial endocarditis is often largely responsible for associated valvar destruction, HIV infected patients may have an altered course. For example, HIV infected patients have a higher risk of developing salmonella endocarditis than immuno-competent patients because they are more likely to develop

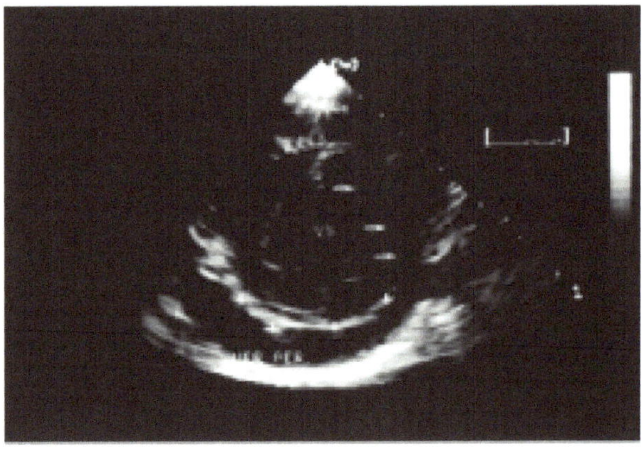

Fig. 40.50: *Circumferential pericardial effusion (arrows) in HIV infected patients induced Mycobacterium avium intracellulare infection (parasternal short axis view)*

salmonella bacteraemia during salmonella infection. However, they respond better to antibiotic treatment and may be less likely to sustain valvar damage because of impaired immune function.

Necropsy finding of Candida albicans endocarditis in an AIDS intravenous heroin users. Note the thrombotic formation on the closing edge of the posterior leaflet of the tricuspid valve (arrow) going down to the right ventricular cavity and involving the chordae tendineae.

Pericardial Effusion

The prevalence of pericardial effusion in asymptomatic HIV infected patients is estimated at 22%.15 Pericardial effusion in HIV disease may be related to opportunistic infections or to malignacy, but most often a clear aetiology is not found. The effusion may be part of a generalized serous effusive process also involving pleural and peritoneal surfaces. This "capillary leak" syndrome is likely related to enhanced cytokine expression in the later stages of HIV disease. Pericardial effusion spontaneously resolves in up to 42% of patients. Mortality remains increased in HIV infected patients who develop an effusion, even if the effusion resolves over time. Pericardiocentesis is currently recommended only in large or poorly tolerated effusions, for diagnostic evaluation of systemic illness, or in the presence of cardiac tamponade. The effects of HAART on pericardial effusion are largely unexplored.

Circumferential pericardial effusion (arrows) in HIV infected patients induced Mycobacterium avium intracellulare infection (parasternal short axis view).

Conclusions

Cardiovascular complications of HIV infection are generally late disease manifestations. Often symptoms of congestive heart failure or pericardial effusion in HIV infected patients are non-specific and may be attributed to generalized illness or co-infection. Echocardiographic screening non-invasively and accurately aids diagnosis during any change in clinical status and directs treatment. Patients will usually respond to early treatment for left ventricular dysfunction and increased left ventricular mass. Treatment based on these findings may prolong the quality and duration of life, and direct further patient evaluation. The role of the cardiologist in the evaluation and treatment of patients with HIV infection should therefore be expanded to include patients who are being evaluated for or who are receiving HAART regimens, especially those with underlying cardiovascular risk. HIV associated heart disease may be an important model for aetiologic mechanisms of dilated cardiomyopathy with important implications in non-HIV related cardiovascular diseases. The role of infection and inflammation in many other cardiovascular diseases is beginning to be recognized, and discovering the molecular mechanisms of HIV related heart disease may provide the basis for rational therapeutic strategies and improved care.

PROTEIN ENERGY MALNUTRITION; (PEM)

The World Health Organization defines malnutrition as the cellular imbalance between supply of nutrients and energy and the body's demand for them to ensure growth, maintenance, and specific functions." Malnutrition is globally the most important risk factor for illness and death, contributing to more than half of deaths in children worldwide. Protein-energy malnutrition (PEM), first described in the 1920s, is observed most frequently in developing countries but has been described with increasing frequency in hospitalized and chronically ill children in the United States.

Kwashiorkor and marasmus are 2 forms of PEM that have been described. The distinction between the 2 foms of PEM is based on the presence (kwashiorkor) ereas kwashiorkor represents a dysadaptation to starvation-

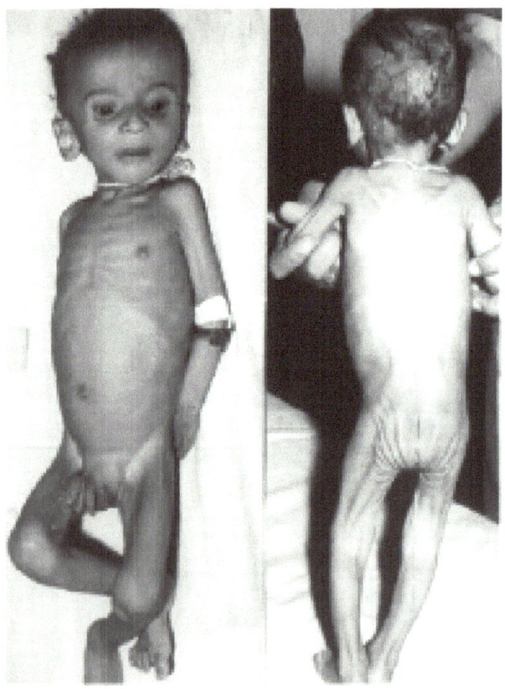

Fig. 40.51: *Showing stunted physical growth, anemia waisting of musclesand loss of subcutaneous fat in a 2 yrs old child with marasmus type of PEM*

ntries, while deficiencies of vitamin C, B, and D have improved in recent years. Micronutrient deficiencies and protein and calorie deficiencies must be addressed for optimal growth and development to be attained in these individuals.

Pathophysiology

Malnutrition affects virtually every organ system. Dietary protein is needed to provide amino acids for synthesis of body proteins and other compounds that have a variety of functional roles. Energy is essential for all biochemical and physiologic functions in the body. Furthermore, micronutrients are essential in many metabolic functions in the body as components and cofactors in enzymatic processes.

In addition to the impairment of physical growth and of cognitive and other physiologic functions, immune response changes occur early in the course of significant malnutrition in a child. These immune response changes correlate with poor outcomes and mimic the changed es observed in children with acquired immune deficiency syndrome (AIDS). Loss of delayed hypersensitivity, fewer T lymphocytes, impaired lymphocyte response, impaired phagocytosis secondary to decreased complement and certain cytokines, and decreased secretory immunoglobulin A (IgA) are some changes that may occur. These immune changes predispose children to severe and chronic infections, most commonly, infectious diarrhea, which further compromises nutrition causing anorexia, decreased nutrient absorption, increased metabolic needs, and direct nutrient losses.

Early studies of malnourished children showed changes in the developing brain, including, a slowed rate of growth of the brain, lower brain weight, thinner cerebral cortex, decreased number of neurons, insufficient myelinization,

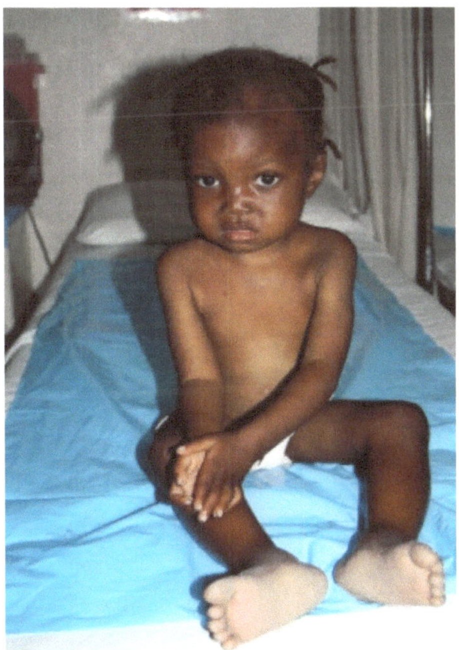

Fig. 40.52: *Showing generalised edema anemia, puffiness of face and stunted physical growth in a 2yrs old child with Kwashiorkor*

and changes in the dendritic spines. More recently, neuroimaging studies have found severe alterations in the dendritic spine apparatus of cortical neurons in infants with severe protein-calorie malnutritary hyperaldosteronism.

Mortality/Morbidity than 5 years in developing countries and contributes indirectly to over half the deaths in childhood worldwide-ent of immunologic functions in these children mimics those observed in children wcal childhood infections. ·Children who are chronically malnourished exhibit behavioral changes, including irritability, apathy and decreased social responsiveness, anxiety, and attention deficits. In addition, infants and young children who have malnutrition frequently demonstrate developmental delay or permanent cognitive deficits. The degree of delay and deficit depends on the severity and duration of nutritional compromise and the age at which malnutrition occurs. In general, nutritional insults at younger ages will have worse outcomes.

Although death from malnutrition in the United States is rare, in developing countries, more than 50% of the 10 million deaths each year are either directly or indirectly secondary to malnutrition in children younger than 5 years.

Age

Children are most vulnerable to the effects of malnutrition in infancy and early childhood. Premature infants have special nutritional needs that are not met with traditional feeding recommendations; they require fortified human milk or specially designed preterm formula until later in infancy. Children are susceptible to malnutrition for differing reasons. During adolescence, self-imposed dietary restrictions contribute to the incidence of nutritional deficiencies.

History

- Clinical signs and symptoms of PEM include the following:
- Poor weight gain
- Slowing of linear growth
- *Behavioral changes:* Irritability, apathy, decreased social responsiveness, anxiety, and attention deficits.

Clinical signs and symptoms of micronutrient deficiencies: Some of the clinical signs and symptoms of specific micronutrient deficiencies may closely resemble those observed in PEM. Deficiencies of micronutrients, including vitamins, minerals, and trace elements have been well described. The most common and clinically significant deficiencies include the following:

- *Iron:* Fatigue, anemia, decreased cognitive function, headache, glossitis, and nail changes
- *Iodine:* Goiter, developmental delay, and mental retardation
- **Vitamin D:** Poor growth, rickets, and hypocalcemia Vitamin A - Night blindness, xerophthalmia, poor growth, and hair changes
- **Folate:** Glossitis, anemia (megaloblastic), and neural tube defects (in fetuses of women without folate supplementation)

- *Zinc:* Anemia, dwarfism, hepatosplenomegaly, hyperpigmentation and hypogonadism, acrodermatitis enteropathica, diminished immune response, poor wound healing

Physical

- Physical findings that are associated with PEM include the following:
  Decreased subcutaneous tissue: Areas that are most affected are the legs, arms, buttocks, and face.
- *Edema:* Areas that are most affected are the distal extremities and anasarca [generalized edema].
- Oral changes
- Cheilosis
- Angular stomatitis
- Papillar atrophy
- Abdominal findings
- Abdominal distension secondary to poor abdominal musculature
- Hepatomegaly secondary to fatty infiltration
- Skin changes
- Dry peeling skin with raw exposed areas
- Hyperpigmented plaques over areas of trauma
- *Nail changes:* Nails become fissured or ridged.
- *Hair changes:* Hair is thin, sparse, brittle, easily pulled out, and turns a dull brown or reddish color

Causes

- Inadequate food intake is the most common cause of malnutrition worldwide. In developing countries, inadequate food intake is secondary to insufficient or inappropriate food supplies or early cessation of breastfeeding. In some areas, cultural and religious food customs may play a role. Inadequate sanitation further endangers children by increasing the risk of infectious diseases that increase nutritional losses and alters metabolic demands.
- In developed countries, inadequate food intake is a less common cause of malnutrition. Instead, diseases and, in particular, chronic illnesses play an important role in the etiology of malnutrition. Children with chronic illness are at risk for nutritional problems for several reasons, including the following:
- Children with chronic illnesses frequently have anorexia, which leads to inadequate food intake.
- Increased inflammatory burden and increased metabolic demands can increase caloric need.
- Any chronic illness that involves the liver or small bowel affects nutrition adversely by impairing digestive and absorptive functions.
- Chronic illnesses that commonly are associated with nutritional deficiencies include the following:
- Cystic fibrosis
- Chronic renal failure
- Childhood malignancies
- Congenital heart disease
- Neuromuscular diseases
- Chronic inflammatory bowel diseases
- In addition, the following conditions place children at significant risk for the development of nutritional deficiencies:
- Prematurity
- Developmental delay
- In utero toxin exposure (i.e. fetal alcohol exposure)
- Children with multiple food allergies present a special nutritional challenge because of severe dietary restrictions. Patients with active allergic symptoms may have increased calorie and protein needs.

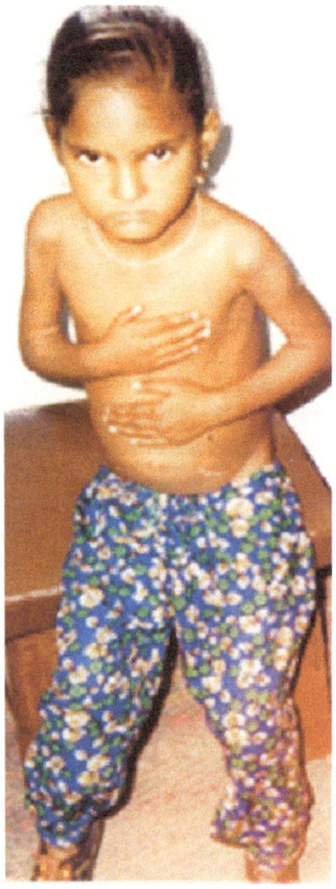

Fig. 40.53: *Stunted physical growth, anemia edema feet and dyscolouration of hair in a 6 yrs old child with Kwashiorkor*

Lab Studies

- The most helpful laboratory studies in assessing the nutritional status of a child are hematological studies and laboratory studies evaluating protein status.
- Hematological studies should include a complete blood count (CBC) with red blood cell indices and a peripheral smear. This could also help exclude anemias from nutritional deficiencies such as iron, folate, and vitamin B-12 deficiencies.
- Measures of protein nutritional status include serum albumin, retinol-binding protein, prealbumin, transferrin, creatinine, and BUN levels. Retinol-binding protein, prealbumin, and transferrin determinations are much better short-term indicators of protein status than albumin. However, in the field, a better measure of long-term malnutrition is serum albumin because of its longer half-life.
- Additional diagnostic evaluation
- In children who have a history of adequate food intake and signs/symptoms of malnutrition, focus on identifying the cause of malnutrition. Perform laboratory studies based on information from a complete history and physical examination.

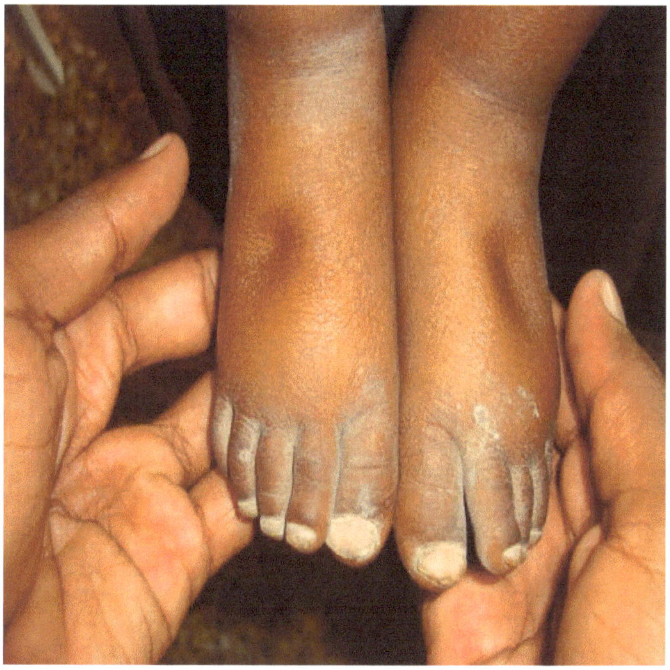

Fig. 40.54: *Showing edema of legs and feet with mixed picture of malnutrition in older boy with chronic wet beri -beri who was suffering from malabsorption syndrome*

- Initial diagnostic laboratory studies include a CBC, sedimentation rate, serum electrolytes, and urinalysis and culture. Stool specimens should be obtained if the child has a history of abnormal stools or stooling patterns or if the family uses an unreliable or questionable source of water.
- Additional studies may focus on thyroid functions or sweat chloride tests, particularly if height velocity is abnormal. Further diagnostic studies should be determined as dictated by the history and physical examination. For example, lab tests evaluating renal function, such as phosphorus and calcium, should be obtained in the presence of renal symptoms. Children with suspected liver disease should have triglyceride and vitamin levels obtained, while zinc levels should be obtained in patients with chronic diarrhea.
- Celiac serology is a useful screening test and should be considered, especially if there is a family history of celiac disease or if other autoimmune diseases, such as type I diabetes mellitus, are present.
- Other tests
- Practical nutritional assessment
- Complete history, including a detailed dietary history
- Growth measurements, **including weight and length/** height; head circumference in children younger than 3 years
- Complete physical examination·

Sensitive measures of nutritional status

- Height-for-age or weight-for-height measurements greater than 2 standard deviations below the mean for age
- Height-for-age or weight-for-height measurements more than 2 standard deviations less than the mean for age
- Height-for-age measurements **less than 95% of expected value**
- Weight-for-height measurements less than 90% of expected value
- Less than 5 cm/y of growth in children older than 2 years
- Body mass index (BMI) (although not established by the CDC as a criteria for failure to thrive)

Treatment

Medical Care

Following evaluation of the child's nutritional status and identification of the underlying etiology of the malnutrition, dietary intervention in collaboration with a dietitian or other nutritional professionals should be initiated. Children with edema must be assessed carefully for actual nutritional status because edema may mask the severity of malnutrition. Children with chronic malnutrition may require caloric intakes more than 120–150 kcal/kg/d to achieve appropriate weight gain. The formula for determining adequate caloric intake is: kcal/kg = (RDA for age X ideal weight)/actual weight

- Additionally, any micronutrient deficiencies must be corrected for the child to attain appropriate growth and development. Most children with mild malnutrition respond to increased oral caloric intake and supplementation with vitamin, iron, and folate supplements. The requirement for increased protein is met typically by increasing the food intake, which, in turn, increases both protein and caloric intake. Adequacy of intake is determined by monitoring weight gain.
- In mild-to-moderate cases of malnutrition, initial assessment and nutritional intervention may be done in the outpatient setting. A patient with malnutrition may require hospitalization based on the severity and instability of the clinical situation. Hospitalization of patients with suspected malnutrition secondary to neglect allows observation of the interactions between parent/caregiver and child and documentation of actual intake and feeding difficulties. It may also be warranted in cases where dehydration and acidosis complicate the clinical picture. In moderate-to-severe cases of malnutrition, enteral supplementation via tube feedings may be necessary.

BERI- BERI

In 1630 a Dutch physician, Jacobus Bonitus, observed in Java, "a very troublesome affliction, called by the inhabitants Beri-beri (which means sheep), those, whom this same disease attacks, with their knees shaking and the legs raised up, walk like sheep."

In the last 100 years, the cause of beriberi was determined to be deficiency of thiamine (vitamin B1), a water-soluble and heat-labile vitamin required for carbohydrate metabolism. Thiamine is essential for most vertebrates and some microorganisms. Beriberi has 2 main forms in humans, depending on the system of maximum involvement: wet beriberi (edematous cardiovascular

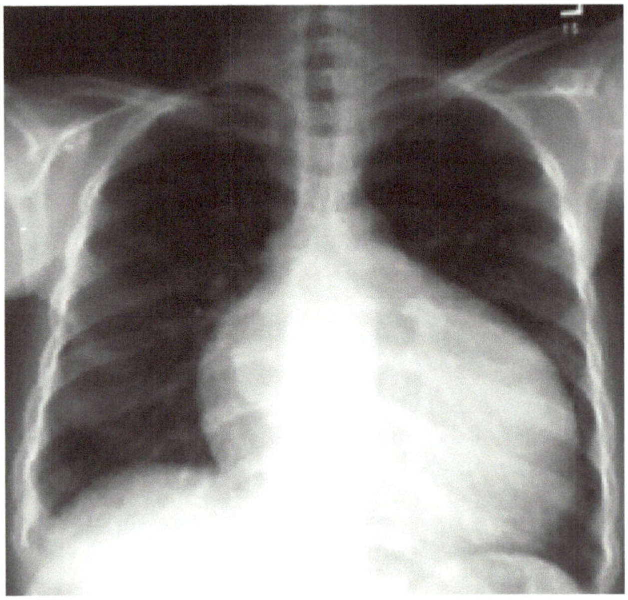

Fig. 40.55: *Showing cardiomegaly in -wet beri-beri (B1, thiamin deficiency)*

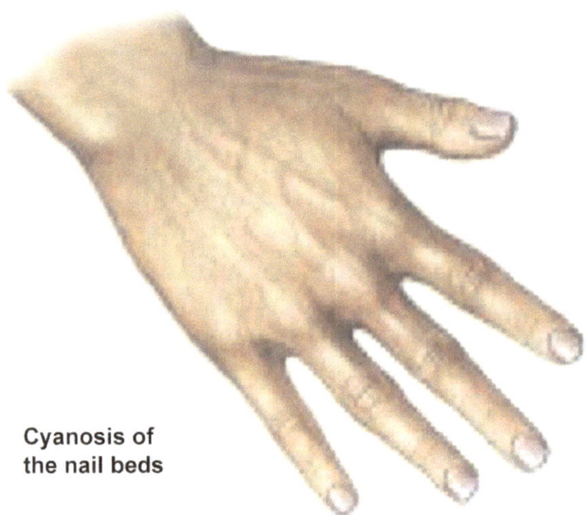

Fig. 40.56: *Cyanosis in hand nails in beri beri disease*

dysfunction) and dry beriberi (multifocal peripheral and/or central neurologic dysfunction). Often times, patients present with features of both.

How a single vitamin deficiency can have such diverse patterns of presentation is not fully understood. Possible explanations include the coexistence of other vitamin or dietary deficiencies; simultaneous comorbidities, simultaneous stressors, or both; individual genetic differences among the various enzymes that have thiamine as their cofactor; and variations in tissue stores or turnover of the vitamin.

In the Western world, beriberi is usually seen in patients in defined situations outside of the normal protective measures of modern society. Also, unusual physiologic conditions in which beriberi could have been predicted are recognized. Finally, chance circumstances in which thiamine deficiency is fully unanticipated are also recognized. Dietary thiamine deficiency can be caused by an overall poor nutritional intake, by dietary customs that rely heavily on inadequate food sources (e.g. milled rice), and, rarely, by consuming foods that contain thiaminases or antithiamine compounds. A cohort at particularly high risk are individuals with alcoholism with poor nutrition because alcohol also impairs thiamine absorption.

In 1998, the Institute of Medicine of the National Academies published the recommended dietary intake of thiamine and other B vitamins for males and females (from infants to the elderly). Also, a comprehensive monograph on beriberi was commissioned by the World Health Organization; it recommends that the term beriberi be replaced by thiamine deficiency. For more information regarding the cardiovascular and neurologic manifestations encountered in adult patients,

Pathophysiology

Thiamine mainly functions as thiamine pyrophosphate (TPP), which serves as a prosthetic group or cofactor for several enzymes in carbohydrate metabolism. These enzymes all use thiamine's thiazole ring to activate and transfer a 2-carbon unit (aldehyde). They catalyze decarboxylation of pyruvate, ketoglutarate, and the transketolation reaction in the pentose phosphate pathway. Thiamine is also believed to have a role in nerve conduction through the synthesis of acetylcholine. An impairment in the decarboxylation pathway causes a decrease in ATP (energy) synthesis. A reduction of transketolase activity compromises the hexose monophosphate shunt and yields decreases in nicotinamide adenine dinucleotide phosphate (NADPH) formation, in electron transport, and in ATP synthesis.[3]

Impaired energy production, increased manufacturing of free radicals, and possible *N*-methyl-D-aspartate (NMDA) receptor–mediated toxicity have been hypothesized to yield neuronal injury (dry beriberi). The exact biochemical defect responsible for the clinical manifestations of cardiac beriberi (wet beriberi) or its acute form, Shoshin beriberi (from the Japanese, meaning "sudden collapse"), is not yet fully elucidated. Cardiac dysfunction may simply be compromised by myocardial tissue edema and energy depletion.

Thiamine is not widely distributed in high concentrations; consequently, many foods are now routinely fortified with it. Rich natural sources include whole grains, lean pork, peas, spinach, and legumes. Very little thiamine is present in fats, oils, and refined sugars. It is destroyed by heat, pasteurization, and ionizing radiation. Freezing does not affect the bioavailability of thiamine; however, it is insoluble in alcohol. The risk of beriberi increases in individuals who consume a diet high in thiaminase rich foods (e.g. raw freshwater fish or shellfish, ferns), a diet high in antithiamine factors (e.g. tea, coffee, betel nuts), or both.

Deficiency of thiamine affects the cardiovascular, muscular, nervous, and GI systems. The body stores of

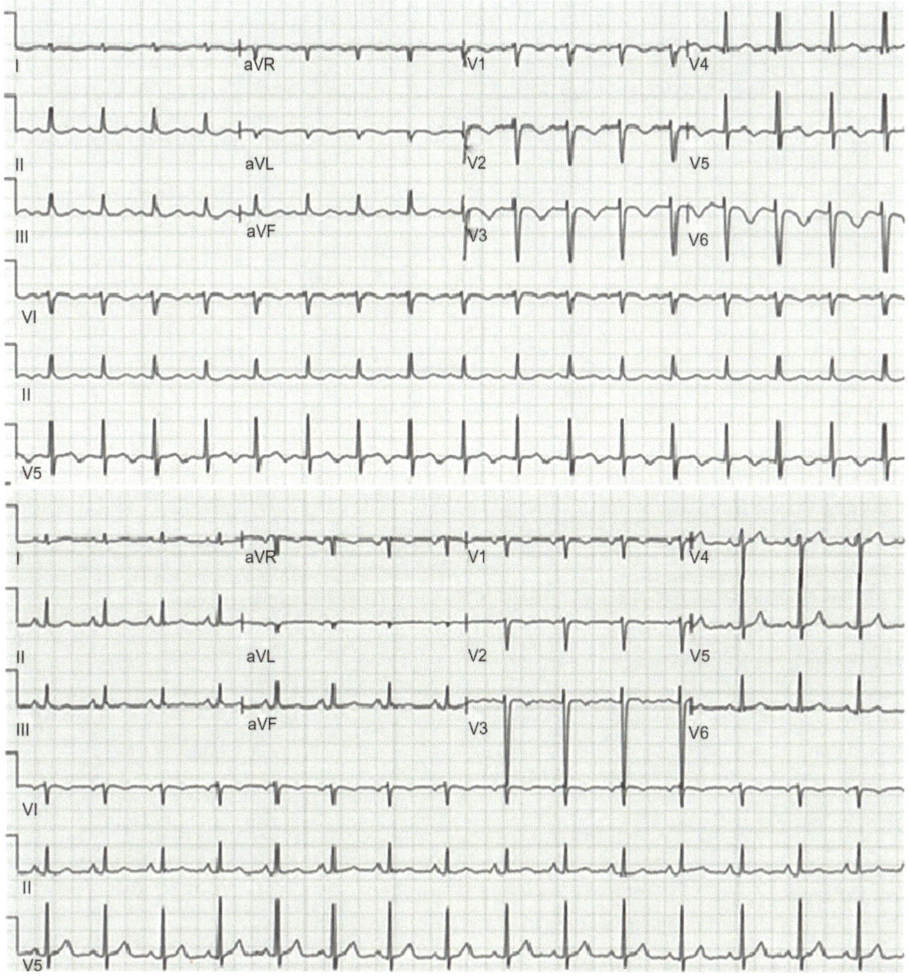

Fig. 40.57: *(Top) The electrocardiogram showed diffuse disturbances of repolarisation (ST-depression and negative T-wave). (Bottom) showed disappearance of changes after therapeutic doses of B1*

thiamine are minimal, and the duration of thiamine reserves is unknown. In one study, deficiency was detected after approximately 6 weeks without thiamine. In another study of healthy young men who consumed less than 0.2 mg of thiamine daily, urinary excretion of thiamine stopped within 18 days. Case studies have suggested that fatal deficiency can develop in as little as 3 weeks without thiamine intake. Despite the widespread fortification of many foods and infant formulas with thiamine, clinicians must remain aware of the signs and symptoms of beriberi, a life-threatening, but rapidly reversible, condition.

Mortality/Morbidity

Mortality is rare and is usually restricted to wet beriberi (cardiac) that goes undiagnosed for too long and, hence, can not be treated. Morbidity is also rare and is usually seen in dry beriberi (neurologic) that is treated so late in the course of the illness that some residual neurologic deficits remain. In both situations, the timely recognition of the signs and symptoms of beriberi can result in thiamine replacement, which rapidly reverses the cardiovascular and neurologic dysfunction.

The prevalence is highest in cultures that depend on a high proportion of their calories from foods that have poor thiamine content, such as milled rice.

Beriberi can affect both genders, although alcoholism (a major risk factor) is more prevalent in males.

Beriberi is predominantly observed in adults and infants aged 124 months (infantile beriberi).

Wet Beriberi

Clinical Examination

History

Thiamine deficiency has a wide range of clinical presentations. Although clinical overlap is common, the basic phenotypes are as follows:

This phenotype affects the cardiovascular system and is divided into acute and chronic forms.

- In acute wet beriberi or Shoshin beriberi, the predominant injury is to the heart, and rapid deterioration occurs because of the heart's inability to maintain function. Presenting symptoms include tachycardia, low diastolic pressure, cardiomegaly, pulmonary edema, and cyanosis.

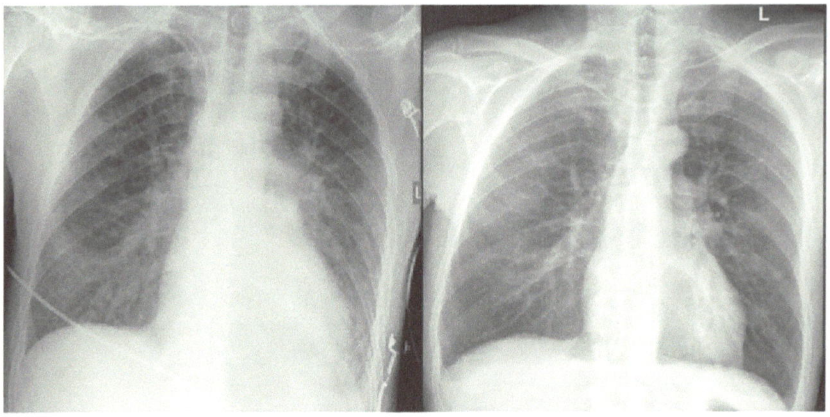

Fig. 40.58: *(Left X-ray chest PA view showed significant cardiomegaly due to heart failure . Right) showed normal sized heart after therapeutic doses of B1*

Wet beriberi is characterized by elevated lactic acid levels. This condition can be readily reversed with thiamine infusion, if administered early.

- **Chronic wet beriberi with high-output cardiac failure has 3 stages.**
  Initially, peripheral vasodilatation occurs, yielding high-output cardiac failure.
- Then, the progression of vasodilatation is perceived by the kidney as a relative loss of volume. The ensuing activation of the renin angiotensin system produces greater salt and water retention.
- Consequently, further fluid overload results in peripheral edema and pulmonary effusions.
  Cardiac overuse injury that occurs in the above setting results in tachycardia, hypertension, and chest pain.
- Thyrotoxicosis, a more common cause of high-output cardiac failure, is always among the differential diagnoses.

Dry Beriberi

- This phenotype affects the neuromuscular system.
- Polyneuritis and symmetric, ascending paralysis of the peripheral nerve systems predominate.
- The sensory system is affected first, followed by the motor and autonomic systems.
- Typically, tactile sensation is the first to be lost, followed by pain, and, finally, temperature.
- Paresthesia and hyperesthesia usually begin with the lower extremities and gradually involve the upper extremities and perioral area.
- Deep tendon reflexes are lost, calf muscles become painful, and foot drop and, eventually, wrist dropoccur.
- If untreated, progressive weakness, wasting of muscles, and, ultimately, complete paralysis occur.
- Encephalopathy is an alternative mode of presentation, with vomiting, disorientation, horizontal nystagmus,

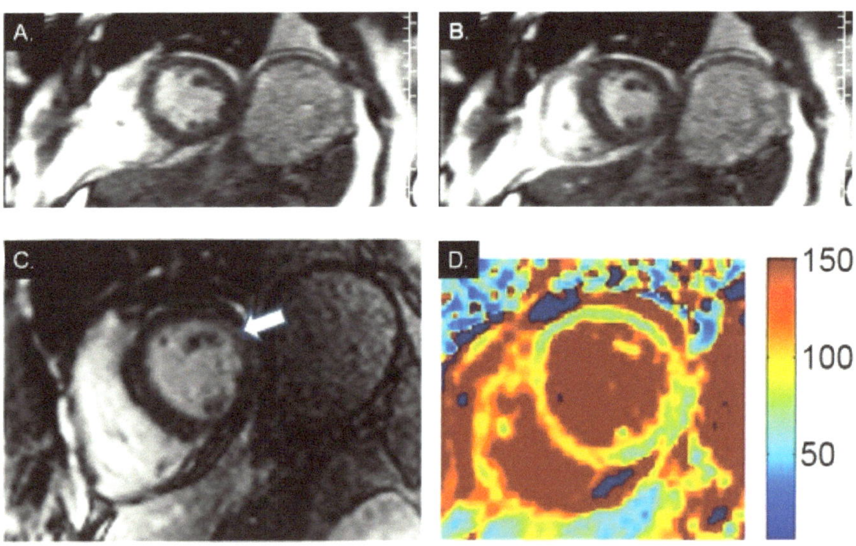

Fig. 40.59: *CMR findings in wet beriberi. End-diastolic (A) and end-systolic (B) frames from short axis cine imaging demonstrate global hypokinesis of the left ventricle. (C.) LGE image shows borderline hyperenhancement of the basal lateral wall (arrow). (D) T2 mapping demonstrates significantly elevated myocardial T2 values suggestive of diffuse edema in a patient with beri-beri heart disease*

palsies of the eye movements (ophthalmoplegia), ataxia, and progressive mental impairment.

- Korsakoff syndrome is a more ominous condition that usually precludes complete recovery. Confusion is followed by the loss of recent memory and confabulation, which is the creation of accounts of events to cover up the loss of memory.
- **Infantile thiamine deficiency**
  This occurs in various forms and typically affects breastfed infants whose mothers had beriberi.
- Early on, the infant is constipated, crying, restless, and has emesis. Three forms are recognized:

The pure cardiologic or pernicious form is common in infants aged 1–3 months. They present with cyanosis and features of acute cardiac failure. Infants usually die within 2–4 hours, but this type of deficiency responds very rapidly to thiamine.

The aphonic form is seen in infants aged 4–6 months. This milder form causes loss of voice due to paralysis of the vocal cords. The pseudomeningitic form is encountered in infants aged 7–9 months. It presents with clinical signs of meningitis, but cerebrospinal fluid findings exclude infection. Vomiting, sweating, and seizures may be present.

Wernicke-Korsakoff syndrome

- This is an autosomal recessive genetic disease seen most often in Europeans.
- Affected patients have transketolases that bind thiamine pyrophosphate 10 times less frequently than normal. Patients with Wernicke-Korsakoff are much more sensitive to less severe thiamine deficiency.
- This syndrome occurs most often in individuals with alcoholism who are malnourished. It is often precipitated by administration of glucose because excessive carbohydrate metabolism exacerbates a subclinical thiamine deficiency. Clinically, it combines features of both Wernicke encephalopathy and Korsakoff psychosis.

Subclinical Thiamine Deficiency

- This deficiency is seen in people with high carbohydrate intake and low thiamine intake.
- Other at-risk groups include those with increased thiamine requirements because of raised physiological or metabolic demands. Clinical scenarios include pregnancy and lactation, heavy physical exertion, intercurrent illness (e.g. cancer, liver diseases, infections, hyperthyroidism), and surgery.
- This deficiency is rarely encountered in patients with increased losses, such as those seen with dialysis, chronic diuretic use, and malabsorption.
- Symptoms are usually mild, with anorexia often the presenting symptom. Anorexia is regarded to be a protective phenomenon because continued intake of a high-carbohydrate diet could be detrimental.
- Other early symptoms include weakness, aching, burning sensation in the hands and feet, indigestion, irritability, and depression. After 6–8 weeks, the only objective signs at rest may be a slight fall in blood pressure and moderate weight loss. After 2-3 months, apathy and weakness become extreme and calf muscle tenderness develops. Also, loss of recent memory, confusion, ataxia, and, sometimes, persistent vomiting occur.
- Pediatric associations include growth restriction and sudden infant death syndrome (SIDS).

Causes

- Beriberi is caused by thiamine deficiency, which can be the result of different physiologic, dietary, and environmental factors. ·Frequently, more than one risk factor is present.

Lab Studies

- The most rapid, and thus the best diagnostic test in urgent situations, is observing a clinical response to administration of intravenous thiamine (few hours duration). The most reliable in vitro laboratory tests involve measurement of whole blood or erythrocyte transketolase activity. An enhancement of enzymatic activity from the in vitro addition of TPP is referred to as the TPP effect.
- An increase in the enzymatic activity of more than 15% strongly supports the diagnosis of thiamine deficiency.
- A depressed blood level of thiamine can be seen.
- Elevated measurements of the following substances are characteristically noted because their metabolism depends on enzymes that have thiamine as their cofactors:
- Pyruvate
- Alpha-ketoglutarate
- Lactate
- Glycosylate
- Physical

Wet Beriberi (cardiac)

- Edema
- Waxy skin
- Vomiting
- Widened pulse pressure
- Systolic flow murmur
- Gallop rhythm (third heart sound); best heard in left-lateral position during inspiration
- Jugular venous distension
- Tachycardia
- Cardiomegaly
- Pallor
- **ECG changes** (prolonged QT, T-wave inversion, low voltage)
- **Acute fulminant cardiovascular beriberi (Shoshin beriberi or occidental beriberi)**
- Breathlessness, cyanosis
- Wet crackles in lower lung fields
- Classic heart failure
- **Dry beriberi (paralytic or nervous)**
- Pallor
- Wasting
- Listlessness

- Tachycardia
- **Hepatomegaly**
- Symmetric peripheral neuropathy
- Symmetric paresthesias, especially of the distal extremities, with diminished touch sensation
- Weakness (starting with feet)
- Loss of ankle and knee reflexes
- Normal vibration and pain sensation
- Wernicke disease
- Irritability, forgetfulness
- Ataxia
- Mental confusion
- Nystagmus (horizontal more common than vertical)
- Ptosis
- Ophthalmoplegia
- Delirium
- Coma
- Korsakoff psychosis
- Retrograde amnesia
- Inability to learn
- Confabulation
- Wernicke-Korsakoff syndrome - Combined features of both Wernicke disease and

Korsakoff Psychosis

- Infantile beriberi
- Physical findings depend on the form but usually begin with nonspecific early findings, including the following:
- Fatigue
- Anorexia
- Headaches
- Irritability, fatigue
- The physical findings in acute cardiac infantile beriberi are similar to those found in Shoshin beriberi, often with cyanosis.

The physical findings in aphonic infantile beriberi include hoarseness that progresses to a complete loss of crying. The physical findings in pseudomeningeal infantile beriberi include nystagmus, muscle twitching, bulging fontanelle, convulsions and coma.

Additional investigations that have been proposed as diagnostic tests include the following:

- Urinary thiamine
- Thiamine metabolites (thiazole or pyrimidine)
- Methylglyoxal values
- Unexplained lactic acidosis that persists after fluid bolus should prompt consideration of beriberi.

Imaging Studies

- In infants, thiamine deficiency is characterized by involvement of the frontal lobes and basal ganglia, in addition to lesions present in the periaqueductal region, thalami, and the mammillary bodies that have been described in adults.
- MR spectroscopy (MRS) reveals a characteristic lactate peak.
- Other Tests
- Diffuse slowing of the EEG can be observed.

Procedures

- An intravenous push of thiamine is recommended in a deteriorating patient who has features suggestive of beriberi.

Histologic Findings

- The histologic lesions of wet beriberi have been reported to be due to degeneration of myelin in the muscular sheaths without inflammation.

Treatment

Medical Care

- Monitor patients with cardiac failure in an intensive care unit. Because beriberi often presents with other vitamin B deficiencies, administer a complete vitamin B complex. After the high-output state has been addressed with thiamine, patients can go into standard congestive heart failure and, thus, may require ongoing cardiology consultation, possibly remaining in an intensive care unit.

Consultations

- Cardiologic evaluation with 2-dimensional echocardiography is necessary.
- Essential for diagnosis and management of beriberi
- Reveals congestive heart failure and the poor ventricular function observed in beriberi
- Assists in cardiac dysfunction that remains after thiamine administration.
- Neurologic and psychiatric consultations are usually necessary. If dry beriberi has progressed, ongoing care is required.
  Nutritional consultation should be aimed at preventing a recurrence of the deficiency.
- For psychosocial causes, support counseling is essential to avoid recurrence. Specialized multidisciplinary teams are advisable for patients with chronic alcoholism to monitor their future course. Comprehensive follow-up programs are necessary to minimize recidivism in most cases of nutritional beriberi.

Diet

- Patients with lethargy, confusion, and severe heart failure need to be kept on a diet of nothing by mouth (NPO) to prevent aspiration.
- Dietary sources of thiamine must be emphasized along with ongoing supplementation.

ACTIVITY

Patients who present with congestive heart failure should have activity restricted.

The treatment of choice is thiamine hydrochloride (i.e. aneurine hydrochloride, vitamin B-1). In a prospective study of the safety of thiamine hydrochloride, Wrenn et al evaluated 989 patients (1070 doses of 100 mg). A total of 12 adverse reactions (1.1%) were reported. Minor reactions consisting of transient local irritation were observed in 11 patients (1.02%), and only one major reaction occurred (0.093%), consisting of generalized pruritus. Several thiamine derivatives (e.g. thiamine propyl disulfide [TPD], thiamine tetrahydrofurfuryl disulfide [TTFD]) have also been used to treat beriberi. These compounds are barely soluble in water. Even when orally administered, TPD and TTFD produce a higher thiamine level in the blood than thiamine hydrochloride.

If beriberi occurs in a breastfed infant, both the mother and child should be treated with thiamine. The physician should also be aware that thiamine deficiency can occur concurrently with other water soluble vitamin deficiencies.

Drug Vitamins

These agents are organic substances required by the body in small amounts for various metabolic processes. Vitamins may be synthesized in small or insufficient amounts in the body or may not be synthesized at all, thus requiring supplementation.

Complications

- GI complaints, including constipation and colicky abdominal pain
- Muscle wasting
- Vision or hearing impairment
- Complete paralysis
- Ataxia
- Profound loss of recent memory with active imagination
- Delirium
- **Death**

Prognosis

- In patients with wet beriberi, improvement is observed in the first 6–24 hours after thiamine administration.
- Cyanosis disappears.
- The heart rate reduces.
- The respiratory rate reduces.
- Diuresis and reduction in heart size may be apparent within 1–2 days.
- In patients with dry beriberi, the complete resolution of the peripheral neurologic symptoms can take weeks to months. ·In patients with Wernicke encephalopathy, the ocular symptoms resolve within hours to days, and the confusional state subsides in days to weeks. ·Korsakoff syndrome resolves over months, and residual deficits are often reported

RICKETS (VITAMIN D-DEFICIENCY)

Rickets is a disease of growing bone that is unique to children and adolescents. It is caused by a failure of osteoid to calcify in a growing person. Failure of osteoid to calcify in adults is called osteomalacia. Vitamin D deficiency rickets occurs when the metabolites of vitamin D are deficient. Less commonly, a dietary deficiency of calcium or phosphorus may also produce rickets. Vitamin D-3 (cholecalciferol) is formed in the skin from a derivative of cholesterol under the stimulus of ultraviolet-B light. Ultraviolet light or cod liver oil was the only significant source of vitamin D until early in the 20th century when ergosterol (vitamin D-2) was synthesized from irradiated plant steroids.

During the Industrial Revolution, rickets appeared in epidemic form in temperate zones where the pollution from factories blocked the sun's ultraviolet rays. Thus, rickets was probably the first childhood disease caused by environmental pollution.

Natural nutritional sources of vitamin D are limited primarily to fatty, ocean-going fish. In the United States, dairy milk is fortified with vitamin D (400 IU/L) Human milk contains little vitamin D, generally less than 20–40 IU/L. Therefore, infants who are breastfed are at risk for rickets, especially those who receive no oral supplementation and those who have darkly pigmented skin, which blocks penetration of ultraviolet light (Fig. 47.61).

Pathophysiology

Cholecalciferol (i.e. vitamin D-3) is formed in the skin from 5-dihydrotachysterol. This steroid undergoes hydroxylation in 2 steps. The first hydroxylation occurs at position 25 in the liver, producing calcidiol (25-hydroxycholecalciferol), which circulates in the plasma as the most abundant of the vitamin D metabolites and is thought to be a good indicator of overall vitamin D status. The second hydroxylation step occurs in the kidney at the 1 position, where it undergoes hydroxylation to the active metabolite calcitriol (1,25-dihydroxycholecalciferol). This cholecalciferol is not technically a vitamin but a hormone.

Calcitriol acts at 3 known sites to tightly regulate calcium metabolism. Calcitriol promotes absorption of calcium and phosphorus from the intestine, increases reabsorption of phosphate in the kidney, and acts on bone to release calcium and phosphate. Calcitriol may also directly facilitate calcification. These actions increase the concentrations of calcium and phosphorus in extracellular fluid. The increase of calcium and phosphorus in extracellular fluid, in turn, leads to the calcification of osteoid, primarily at the metaphyseal growing ends of bones but also throughout all osteoid in the skeleton. Parathyroid hormone facilitates the 1-hydroxylation step in vitamin D metabolism.

In the vitamin D deficiency state, hypocalcemia develops, which stimulates excess parathyroid hormone, which stimulates renal phosphorus loss, further reducing deposition of calcium in the bone. Excess parathyroid hormone also produces changes in the bone similar to those occurring in hyperparathyroidism. Early in the course of rickets, the calcium concentration in the serum decreases. After the parathyroid response, the calcium concentration usually returns to the reference range, though phosphorus levels remain low. Alkaline phosphatase, which is produced by overactive osteoblast cells, leaks to the extracellular fluids so that its concentration rises to anywhere from moderate elevation to very high levels.

Intestinal malabsorption of fat and diseases of the liver or kidney may produce the clinical and secondary biochemical picture of nutritional rickets. Anticonvulsant drugs (e.g. phenobarbital, phenytoin) accelerate metabolism of calcidiol, which may lead to insufficiency and rickets, particularly in children who are kept indoors in institutions.

Calcium and vitamin D intakes are low in infants who are fed vegan diets, particularly lactovegans, and monitoring of their vitamin D status is essential.[1]

Incidence

In the United States, vitamin D deficiency rickets does not occur in formula-fed infants because formula and milk sold in the United States contains 400 IU of vitamin D per liter.

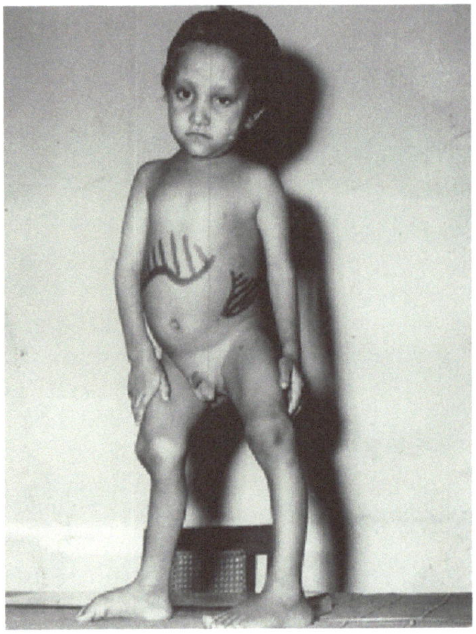

Fig. 40.60: *Showing bony deformities of lower legs with widening of the bony ends in a 6 yrs old boy with clinical ricket*

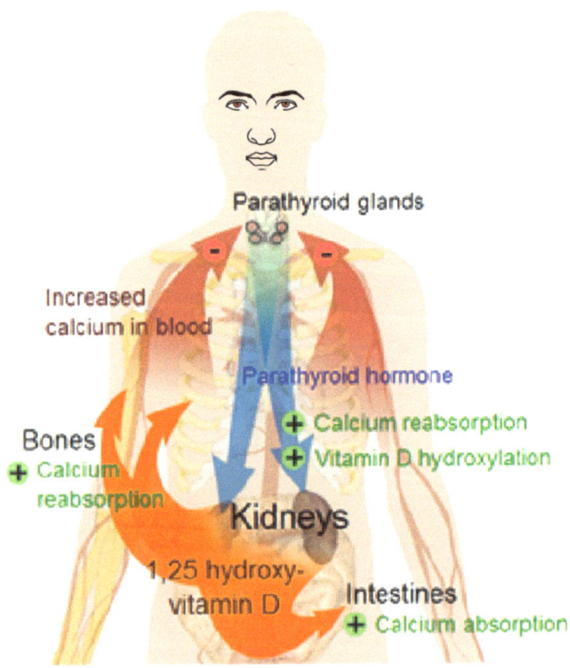

Fig. 40.61: *Calcium regulation from different organs of the body*

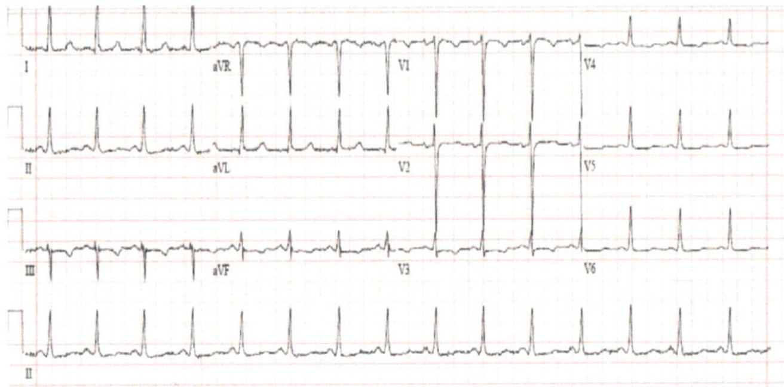

Fig. 40.62: Prolonged QTc (510 ms) due to hypocalcaem

Mortality/Morbidity

Skeletal deformity and short stature may occur. Severe rickets has been associated with respiratory failure in children, and resulting pelvic distortion in females may lead to problems with vaginal delivery later in life.

Race

Individuals with dark skin are at increased risk for vitamin D deficiency rickets.

Sex

No sexual predilection is noted.

Age

By definition, rickets is observed only in growing children, although the effects may be observed later in life.

History

- Generalized muscular hypotonia of an unknown mechanism is observed in most patients with clinical (as opposed to biochemical and radiographic) signs of rickets. Craniotabes manifests early in infants with vitamin D deficiency, although this feature may be normal in infants, especially for those born prematurely.
- If rickets occurs at a later age, thickening of the skull develops. This produces frontal bossing and delays the closure of the anterior fontanelle. In the long bones, laying down of uncalcified osteoid at the metaphases leads to spreading of those areas, producing knobby deformity, which is visualized on radiography as cupping and flaring of the metaphyses.
- Weight bearing produces deformities such as bowlegs and knock-knees.
- In the chest, knobby deformities results in the rachitic rosary along the costochondral junctions. The weakened ribs pulled by muscles also produce flaring over the

diaphragm, which is known as Harrison groove. The sternum may be pulled into a pigeon-breast deformity.

- In more severe instances in children older than 2 years, vertebral softening leads to kyphoscoliosis. The ends of the long bones demonstrate that same knobby thickening. At the ankle, palpation of the tibial malleolus gives the impression of a double epiphysis (Marfan sign). Because the softened long bones may bend, they may fracture one side of the cortex (i.e. greenstick fracture).

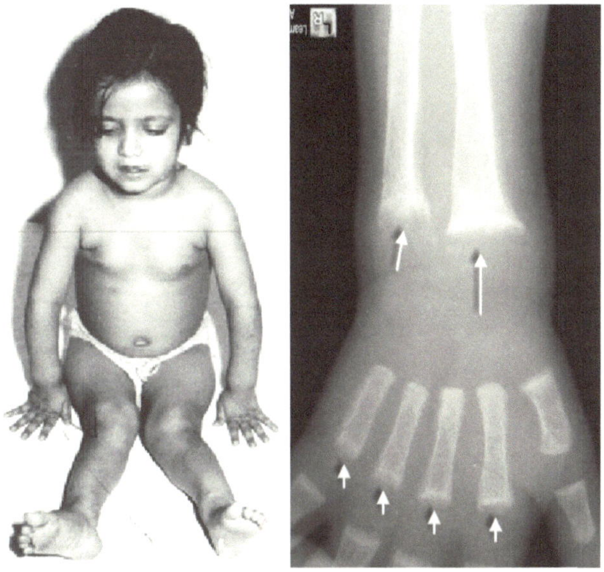

Fig. 40.63: *Showing bony deformities of lower legs with genu valgum(left) and radiological features of active ricket with cupping, fraying and increased distance between epiphysis and metaphysis in hand bone(right) in a 6 yrs old boy with clinical ricket*

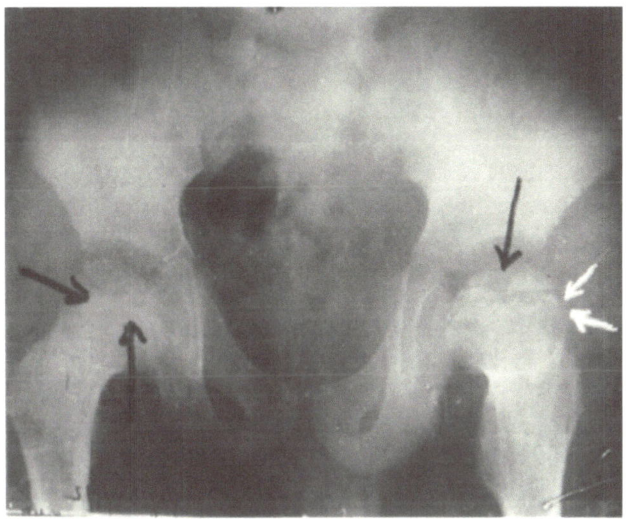

Fig. 40.64: *X-ray leg bones at the region of hip joints Showing bony deformities of bones with radiological features of active ricket with epiphysiseal dysgenesis and rarefaction (arrows) in a 10 yrs old boy with clinical ricket*

Lab Studies

- Early on in the disease course, the calcium (ionized fraction) is low; however it is often within the reference range at the time of diagnosis as parathyroid hormone levels increase.
- Calcidiol (25-hydroxy vitamin D) levels are low, and parathyroid hormone levels are elevated; however, determining calcidiol and parathyroid hormone levels is typically not necessary. Calcitriol levels maybe normal or elevated because of increased parathyroid activity.
- The phosphorus level is invariably low for age unless recent partial treatment or recent exposure to sunlight has occurred.
- Alkaline phosphatase levels are elevated.
- A generalized aminoaciduria occurs from the parathyroid activity; aminoaciduria does not occur in familial hypophosphatemia rickets (FHR).

Imaging Studies

- The best single radiographic view for infants and children younger than 3 years is an anterior view of the knee that reveals the metaphyseal end and epiphysis of the femur and tibia. This site is best because growth is most rapid in this location, thus the changes are accentuated.

The metaphyses exhibit widening and cupping because of their exaggerated normal concavity and irregular calcification. Because calcified osteoid is abundant, the provisional calcification zone of the metaphysis is much more distant from the calcification center of the epiphysis than is normal for age. Along the shaft, the uncalcified osteoid causes the periosteum to appear separated from the diaphysis. Generalized osteomalacia occurs (observed as osteopenia), with visible coarsening of trabeculae in contrast to the ground-glass osteopenia of scurvy.

Other Tests

- Serum measurements include calcium, phosphorus, alkaline phosphatase, parathyroid hormone, 25-hydroxy vitamin D, and 1,25-dihydroxyvitamin D.

Treatment

- Treatment for rickets may be gradually administered over several months or in a single-day dose of 15,000 mcg (600,000 U) of vitamin D.· If the gradual method is chosen, 125–250 mcg (5000–10,000 U) is given daily for 2–3 months until healing is well established and the alkaline phosphatase concentration is approaching the reference range. Because this method requires daily treatment, success depends on compliance.
- If the vitamin D dose is administered in a single day, it is usually divided into 4 or 6 oral doses. An intramuscular injection is also available. Vitamin D is well stored in the body and is gradually released over many weeks. Because both calcitriol and calcidiol have short half-lives, they are unsuitable; they would bypass the natural physiologic controls of vitamin D synthesis. The single-day therapy avoids problems with compliance and may be helpful in differentiating nutritional rickets from FHR. In nutritional

rickets, the phosphorous level rises in 96 hours and radiographic healing is visible in 6–7 days. Neither happens with FHR.

- If severe deformities have occurred, orthopedic correction may be required after healing. Most of the deformities correct with growth.

Drug Category: Vitamin D

Fat-soluble vitamin used to treat vitamin D deficiency or for prophylaxis of deficiency.

Drug: Cholecalciferol (Delta-D)

Description Vitamin D-3. 1 mg provides 40000IU vitamin D activity.

Pediatric dose: Single-day dose method: 15,000 mcg (600,000 U) PO qd divided in 4–6 doses for 1 dGradual method: 125–250 mcg (5000–10,000 U) qd for 2–3 month

Clinical Implications

The possibility of a causal link between vitamin D deficiency and cardiovascular disease is supported by biological plausibility, the demonstration of a temporal association, and the finding of a dose response between 25-OH D deficiency and risk. These data raise the possibility that treatment of vitamin D deficiency, via supplementation or lifestyle measures, could reduce cardiovascular risk. However, treatment strategies suggested by observational data are not always borne out by randomized trials, as evidenced by studies of hormone replacement therapy and B vitamins for homocysteine lowering. Problems related to the use of observational data include indication bias, confounding, and reverse causation. Several features of the study design suggest that the present data may be less susceptible to these problems. First, we used a direct, objective measure of vitamin D status (25-OH D levels) rather than relying on self-reported vitamin D intake or sunlight exposure. Second, 25-OH D levels were assessed on blood samples drawn at baseline, years before the acute cardiovascular events. Third, cardiovascular risk factors and comorbid diagnoses are well characterized in the Framingham Offspring cohort, which has been followed for >3 decades.

In small clinical trials, vitamin D supplementation has promoted reductions in blood pressure,[57,58] left ventricular hypertrophy,[59] and inflammatory cytokines.[60] On the other hand, Hsia and colleagues[61] recently reported that use of calcium and vitamin D supplements was not associated with a reduction in cardiovascular events in the Women's Health Initiative. These apparently discrepant findings could be attributable to several factors. First, the Women's Health Initiative was a fracture-prevention trial and was not designed to evaluate cardiovascular risk. Second, the dose of vitamin D in the treatment arm (400 IU/d) was far below the amount necessary to correct vitamin D deficiency (>800 IU/d) or doses used in previous cardiovascular studies. Third, patients in the placebo arm were allowed to take vitamin D supplements, which resulted in a mean consumption of vitamin D in the placebo arm of nearly 400 IU/d. Lastly, baseline 25-OH D levels were not measured in the Women's Health Initiative; thus, the trial did not address whether vitamin D supplementation benefited individuals with vitamin D deficiency, because enrollment was performed irrespective of vitamin D status. It is noteworthy that vitamin D did appear to reduce cardiovascular risk in obese individuals, who are prone to endogenous vitamin D deficiency, and also in those with multiple coronary risk factors.[61] The mean body mass index among individuals with vitamin D deficiency in the present study was >30 kg/m^2, in the overweight-to-obese range.

The present data, although observational, permit an assessment of cardiovascular risk across a broad range of baseline 25-OH D levels and could motivate additional prospective or interventional studies. Still, barriers to future trials of vitamin D for cardiovascular prevention exist. A primary prevention trial would require a very large sample and may be hampered by the perception that it would be unethical to randomize individuals with moderate vitamin D deficiency to placebo therapy. In this regard, additional observational studies could be used to identify surrogate end points or subgroups most likely to benefit from vitamin D supplementation, which may facilitate smaller trials.

Scurvy, (Deficiency of Vitamin C)

Scurvy, a state of dietary deficiency of vitamin C (ascorbic acid) is an ancient disease. Egyptians recorded its symptoms as early as 1550 BC. Scurvy was the scourge of the sea explorers of the Renaissance era (16th-18th centuries). In 1746, James Lind, a British naval surgeon, established the fact that oranges and lemons were effective in curing scurvy. The incidence of scurvy among the British sailors sharply declined upon routine provision of lemon juice on board. During the 19th century, people who experienced the Great Potato Famine, armies of the Crimean War and American Civil War, Arctic explorers, and California Gold Rush communities were prominent victims of "land" scurvy. Francis Glisson is credited with the earliest description of infantile scurvy. In 1650, Glisson observed the co-occurrence of scurvy in infants with rickets. After Glisson's description, infantile scurvy was not reported for another 200 years. By the end of the 19th century, infantile scurvy was readily recognized and frequently observed in Britain and the United States. The increased incidence of infantile scurvy during this era was attributed to the consumption of heated milk and proprietary foods deficient in vitamin C.

In 1912, Holst and Frolisch induced and cured scurvy in guinea pigs through dietary modification. Utilization of an animal model for induction and treatment of scurvy was a major advance. Soon, human experiments followed. In 1914, Alfred Hess, a pediatrician practicing at the Hebrew Asylum in New York, observed an increase in scurvy among the infants at the asylum. This increase in scurvy coincided with the introduction of pasteurized milk and exclusion of orange juice from the infants' diet (Fig. 47.65).

Modifying the infants' diet, with the provision of raw milk or orange juice or potatoes, Hess reversed the scurvy

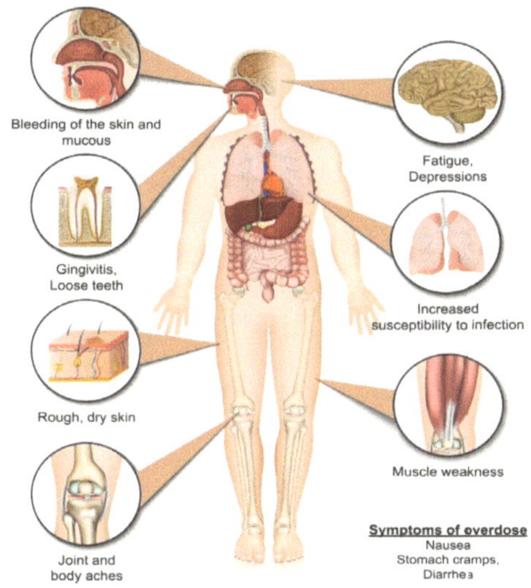

Fig. 40.65: Illustration shows deficiency signs of vit.C (Scurvy)

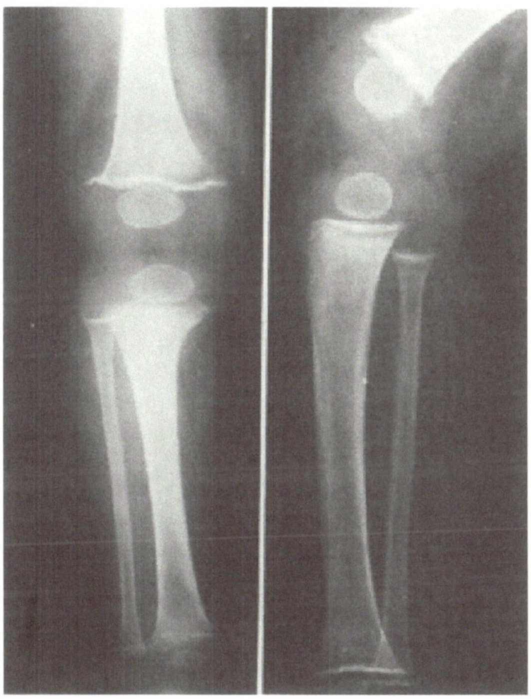

Fig. 40.66: *X-ray leg bones at the region of knee joint Showing white line of Frankel, corner sign and spur formation in a young child with scurvy*

and effected a cure. Hess had demonstrated that pasteurization results in the loss of vitamin C. He recommended the provision of fresh fruit or vegetable juice for the prevention of scurvy in infants fed on heated formulas. This practice of supplementing the diet of infants receiving heated formulas with fresh fruit or vegetable juices eventually led to the eradication of infantile scurvy in the United States.

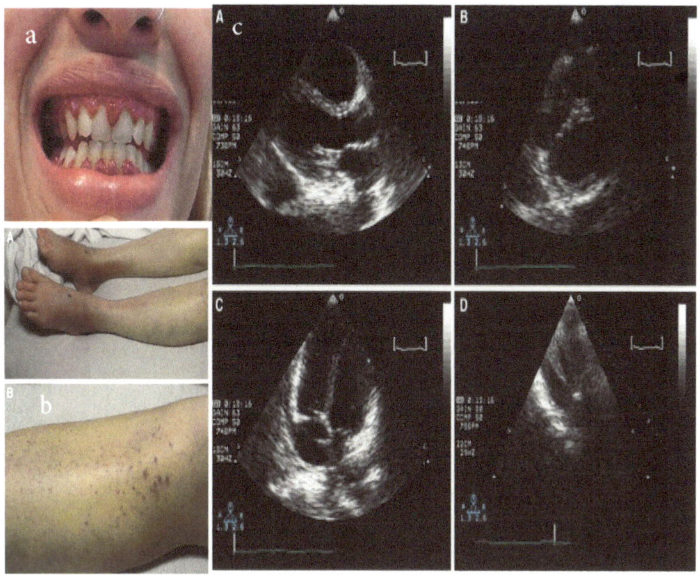

Fig. 40.67:(a) *Gingivalhypertrophy and bleeding,(b)The petechial rash spreading from the dorsal aspects of her feet up to her knees. (c) A, Long-axis view showing dilated right ventricle. B, Short-axis view—septal flattening indicating pulmonary hypertension. C, Four-chamber view showing right atrial and ventricular enlargement. D, Subcostal view showing dilated, noncollapsing inferior vena cava and hepatic vein.*

The human body lacks the ability to synthesize and make vitamin C and therefore depends on exogenous dietary sources to meet vitamin C needs. Consumption of fruits and vegetables or diets fortified with vitamin C are essential to avoid ascorbic acid deficiency. Even though scurvy is uncommon, it still occurs and can affect adults and children who have chronic dietary vitamin C deficiency.

Pathophysiology

Vitamin C is functionally most relevant for collagen synthesis, and a vitamin C deficiency results in impaired collagen synthesis. The typical pathologic manifestations of vitamin C deficiency are noted in collagen-containing tissues and in organs and tissues such as skin, cartilage, dentine, osteoid, and capillary blood vessels. Pathologic changes are a function of the rate of growth of the affected tissues; hence, the bone changes are often observed only in infants during periods of rapid bone growth.

Defective collagen synthesis leads to defective dentine formation, hemorrhaging into the gums, and loss of teeth. Hemorrhaging is a hallmark feature of scurvy and can occur in any organ. Hair follicles are one of the common sites of cutaneous bleeding.

Bone involvement is typical for infantile scurvy. The bony changes occur at the junction between the end of the diaphysis and growth cartilage. Osteoblasts fail to form osteoid (bone matrix), resulting in cessation of endochondral bone formation. Calcification of the growth cartilage at the end of the long bones continues, leading to the thickening of the growth plate. The typical invasion of the growth cartilage by the capillaries does not occur.

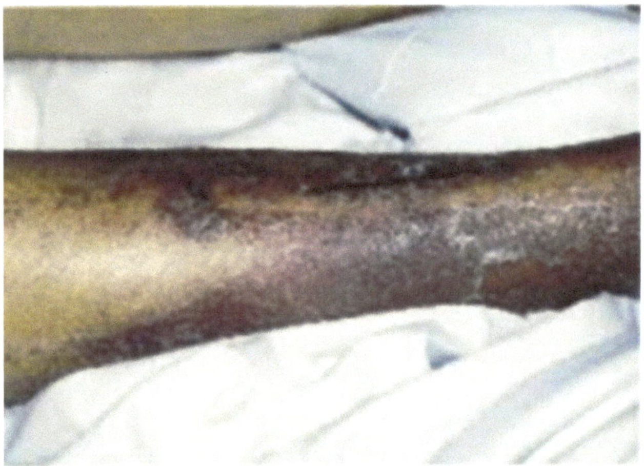

Fig. 40.68: *Lower extremity abnormalities in scurvy. In this patientxerosis is present, accompanied by ecchymoses and increasedpigmentation from repeated cutaneous hemorrhages. Alinear superficial wound covered with hemorrhagic crust has been cr present for an extended period, indicating impaired wound healing*

Preexisting bone becomes brittle and undergoes resorption at a normal rate, resulting in microscopic fractures of the spicules between the shaft and calcified cartilage. With these fractures, the periosteum becomes loosened, resulting in the classic subperiosteal hemorrhage at the ends of the long bones. Intra-articular hemorrhage is rare because the periosteal attachment to the growth plate is very firm.

Cardiovascular Diseases and Vit. C

Besides being essential for collagen synthesis, ascorbic acid is important for biosynthesis of carnitine and neurotransmitters and in hematopoiesis by promoting iron absorption.

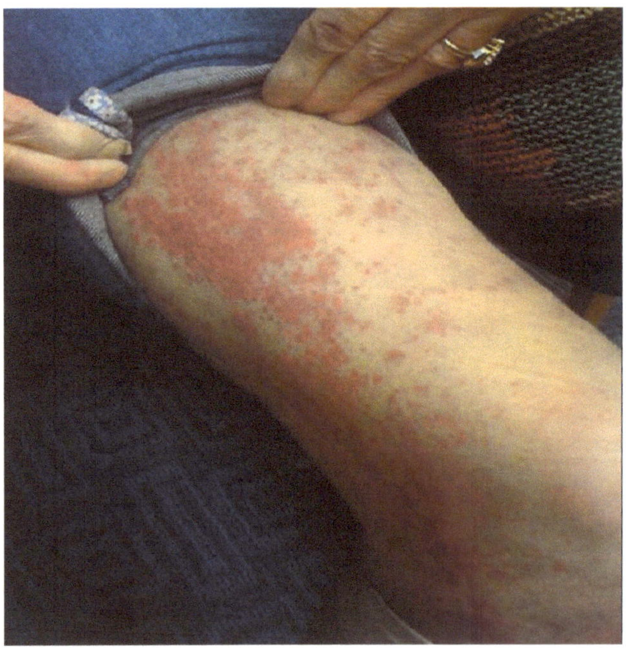

Fig. 40.69: *Perifollicular hemorrhage.in scurvy*

Those few species that fail to synthesize ascorbic acid (vitamin C) are prone to a form of ?heart disease? that is not prevalent in other species. The theory that Cardiovascular Disease (CVD) is related to a deficiency of vitamin C was first proposed by the Canadian physician G. C. Willis in 1953. He found that atherosclerotic plaques form over vitamin-C-starved vascular tissues in both guinea pigs and human beings. In 1989, after the discoveries of the Lp(a) cholesterol molecule (circa 1964) and its lysine binding sites (circa 1987), ***Linus Pauling and his associate Matthias Rath*** formulated a unified theory of heart disease and invented a cure. Vitamin C and lysine (and proline) in large amounts become Lp(a) binding inhibitors that restore vascular health and are patented to destroy atherosclerotic plaques.

Chronic scurvy: Heart disease is a misnomer; the underlying disease process reduces the supply of blood to the heart and other organs leading to angina ("heart amp"), heart attack and stroke. The disease is characterized by scab-like build-ups that grow on the walls of blood vessels. The correct terminology for this disease process is chronic scurvy, a slower form of the classic vitamin C deficiency disease.

The hypothesis that CVD is an ascorbic acid (vitamin C) deficiency disease was first conceived and tested in Canada. Willis devised a method of photographing plaques with X-rays and observed that atherosclerotic plaques were not uniformly distributed throughout the vascular system; rather these "blockages" are concentrated near the heart, where arteries are constantly bent or squeezed.

Another Canadian, Paterson, had found that the tissues of heart patients were generally depleted of vitamin C, and it was well known that vitamin C is required for strong and healthy arteries. Willis reasoned that only the mechanical stress caused by the pulse could explain the typical pattern of atherosclerosis. To Willis, the body was laying down plaque precisely where it was needed in order to stabilize the vascular system.

By the late 1980s, medical researchers had made several intriguing discoveries.

First came the discovery that heart disease begins with a lesion, a crack or stress fracture, in the arterial wall. The question became, and remains, as to the cause of these lesions in human beings since they do not arise in most other animals. Then a variant of the so-called "bad" LDL cholesterol called lipoprotein(a), or Lp(a) for short, was studied and found to be really bad. Lp(a) is sticky because of receptors on the surface of the molecule called lysine binding sites. Work that led to the 1987 Nobel prize in medicine discovered that lysine (and proline) binding sites cause the formation of atherosclerotic plaques. Then, Beisiegel et. al. in Germany examined plaques post mortem and found only Lp(a), not ordinary LDL cholesterol.

Lp(a) was the genetic difference between beings that suffer cardiovascular disease and those that do not. Lp(a) had evolved only in species that do not make their own vitamin C - e.g. humans and guinea pigs.

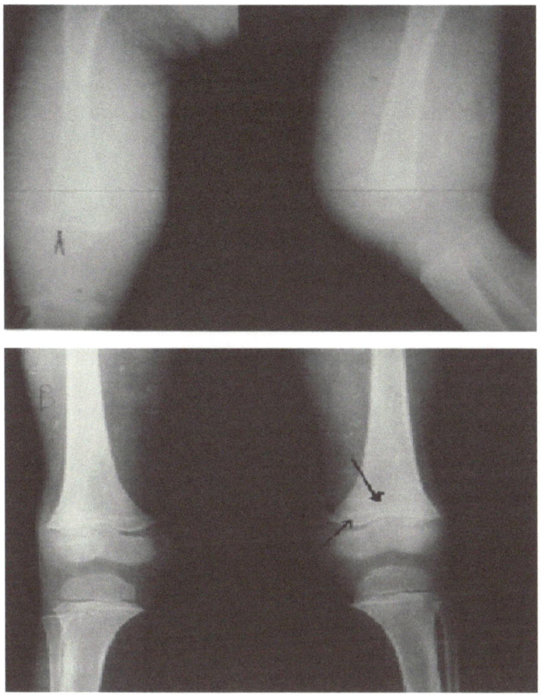

Fig. 40.70: *X-ray leg bones at the region of knee joint showing boggy swelling of the thigh (upper) rarefaction of the bones at metaphysis ans epiphysis with white line of Frankel (lower)in clinical scurvy*

Pauling and Rath repeated the earlier Willis experiments, but this time they monitored Lp(a). They discovered that it becomes elevated in guinea pigs deprived of vitamin C, but not in the controls. These experiments connected elevated-Lp(a) with low serum vitamin C. They realized that in most species, sufficient ascorbic acid will prevent stress fractures, but in those species that suffer chronic scurvy, Lp(a) had evolved to patch cracked blood vessels. As chronic scurvy progresses, the liver produces more Lp(a) molecules. As the number of Lp(a) molecules increases, they tend to deposit on top of existing plaque formations. When the healing process overshoots, the arteries narrow and the flow of blood is reduced.

This problem has a solution. The Lp(a) molecule has a finite number of lysine binding sites - points of attachment to lysine. Pauling?s invention - the cure for heart disease - is to increase the serum concentration of the amino acid lysine enough to make the Lp(a) unattractive. As more lysine enters the blood stream, the probability increases that floating Lp(a) molecules will bind with it (rather than with the patches of plaques growing on the arterial walls.) After all the Lp(a) molecule?s binding receptors are filled with the free lysine floating in the blood, the Lp(a) molecule becomes as harmless as ordinary LDL cholesterol.

Pauling and Rath called the substances that treat chronic scurvy and destroy existing plaques Lp(a) binding inhibitors. Vitamin C, to increase collagen production and to improve the health and strength of arteries, and lysine, to prevent and to dissolve Lp(a) plaques, are the primary binding inhibitors. These substances taken together are clinically effective.

Linus Pauling believed that chronic scurvy can be prevented with an orthomolecular daily intake of between 3,000 to 10,000 mg or more vitamin C. This amount approximates what the animals synthesize, and matching animal production is the reason Pauling ingested 18,000 mg daily.

Pauling and Rath's invention for destroying existing atherosclerotic plaques is the large amount of another essential nutrient, the amino acid lysine. Pauling filmed a video lecture in which he recommended that heart patients take between 2,000 and 6,000 mg of lysine daily with their vitamin C (more if serum Lp(a) is elevated). Neither vitamin C nor lysine have any known lethal dose.

The Lp(a) binding inhibitors become the Pauling Therapy for heart disease only at high dosages, between vitamin 3 to 18 g ascorbic acid and 3 to 6 g lysine. In his video, Pauling recounts the first cases where his high vitamin C and lysine therapy quickly resolved advanced cardiovascular disease in humans. The effect is so pronounced, and the inhibitors are so nontoxic, that Pauling doubted a clinical study was even necessary.

Recently, the amino acid proline was found to be an even more effective Lp(a) binding inhibitor than lysine in vitro. Adding between 5 and 2 g proline may be of significant additional benefit. When serum Lp(a) is elevated, Lp(a) binding inhibitors can profoundly interfere with the disease process. Binding inhibitor formulas that include proline have been documented to lower Lp(a) in six to 14 months. In cases where Lp(a) is not reduced, binding inhibitors become even more important to neutralize Lp(a) regardless of their effect on serum Lp(a).

Recently a reevaluation of the Framingham Heart study that Lp(a) and not ordinary LDL is highly predictive of CVD and Oxford found that elevated Lp(a) increases the risk of heart attack and stroke by 70%.

Incidence

Currently, scurvy occurs very rarely in the United States. Patients who are elderly or alcoholic and who subsist on diets devoid of fresh fruits and vegetables are vulnerable. Infants and children on restrictive diets because of medical, economic, or social reasons are at risk for scurvy. Occurrence of scurvy is uncommon in those younger than 7 months.

Global occurance

International occurrence is unknown. A case series from Thailand reviewed 28 cases of scurvy in infants and children (10 mo to 9 y and 7 mo; median age, 29 mo) hospitalized over a 7-year period (1995–2002) and noted prolonged consumption of heated milk (ultra-high temperature [UHT] milk) and inadequate intake of vegetables and fruits as the risk factors for the development of scurvy. Epidemic scurvy has been reported among refugee populations.

Mortality/Morbidity

Sudden death due to cardiac failure is reported in infants and adults.

- **Predominant morbidity is a result of hemorrhage into various tissues. Subperiosteal hemorrhage in the tibia and femur causes excruciating pain.**

Race

No racial predilection exists.

Sex

No sexual preponderance exists.

Age

Scurvy can occur at any age. Most cases of infantile scurvy occur when the infant is aged 6-24 months. Scurvy is uncommon in the neonatal period.

Clinical

History

Initial symptoms are nonspecific and include the following:

- Loss of appetite
- Peevishness
- Poor weight gain
- Diarrhea
- Tachypnea
- Fever
- Specific symptoms include the following:
- Irritability
- Pain and tenderness of the legs
- Pseudoparalysis
- Swelling over the long bones
- Hemorrhage·

Physical

The infant is apprehensive, anxious, and progressively irritable. Upon handling and changing of diapers, severe tenderness over the thighs is present. The excruciating pain results in pseudoparalysis. The infant assumes the frog leg posture (i.e. keeping hips and knees slightly flexed and externally rotated) for comfort.

- Hemorrhages of the gums usually involve the tissue around the upper incisors. The gums have a bluish-purple hue and feel spongy. Gum hemorrhage occurs only if teeth have erupted.
- Subperiosteal hemorrhage is a typical finding of infantile scurvy. The lower ends of the femur and tibia are the most frequently involved sites. The subperiosteal hemorrhage is often palpable and tender in the acute phase.
  Petechial hemorrhage of the skin and mucous membranes can occur. Rarely, hematuria, hematochezia, and melena are noted.
- Proptosis of the eyeball secondary to orbital hemorrhage is a sign of scurvy.
- Costochondral beading or scorbutic rosary is a common finding. The scorbutic rosary is distinguished from rickety rosary (which is knobby and nodular) by being more angular and having a step-off at the costochondral junction. The sternum is typically depressed.
- Low-grade fever, anemia, and poor wound healing are signs of scurvy.
- Hyperkeratosis, corkscrew hair, and sicca syndrome are typically observed in adult scurvy but rarely occur in infantile scurvy.

Causes

- Inadequate intake of vitamin C
- Long sea voyages (historically)
- Famines
- Food faddism
- Ignorance (e.g. boiling of fruit juices)
- Neglect (e.g. self-imposed restrictive diets in anorexia nervosa)
- Restrictive diets imposed by food allergies
- Neurodevelopmental disabilities associated with compromised oral intake of foods

Lab Studies

- Laboratory tests are usually not helpful to ascertain a diagnosis of scurvy. Presentation of an infant with the typical clinical and radiologic picture of scurvy, along with a supportive history of dietary deficiency of vitamin C, is often sufficient to diagnose infantile scurvy.
- Serum ascorbic acid levels
- A fasting serum ascorbic acid level greater than 0.6 mg/dL rules out scurvy.
- Serum ascorbic acid levels of 0.2 mg/dL or greater are considered nutritionally acceptable.
- Levels of 0.10–0.19 mg/dL are considered low.
- Levels less than 0.10 mg/dL are considered deficient. White blood cell ascorbic acid concentration is a more accurate measure of a vitamin C nutritional state.
- A level of zero indicates latent scurvy.
- Levels greater than 15 mg/dL reflect a state of nutritional adequacy.
- Levels of 8–15 mg/dL are considered low.
- Levels of 0–7 mg/dL reflect a state of deficiency.

Imaging Studies

- Radiologic findings in infantile scurvy are diagnostic. The characteristic radiologic changes occur at the growth cartilage-shaft junction of bones with rapid growth. The knee joint, wrist, and sternal ends of the ribs are typical sites of involvement.
- Radiologic diagnosis of scurvy is based on the following specific changes: In the early phase of scurvy, the cortex becomes thin and the trabecular structure of the medulla atrophies and develops a ground-glass appearance. The zone of provisional calcification becomes dense and widened, and this zone is referred to as the white line of Fränkel. The epiphysis also shows cortical thinning and the ground-glass appearance.
  As scurvy becomes advanced, a zone of rarefaction occurs at the metaphysis under the white line. The zone of

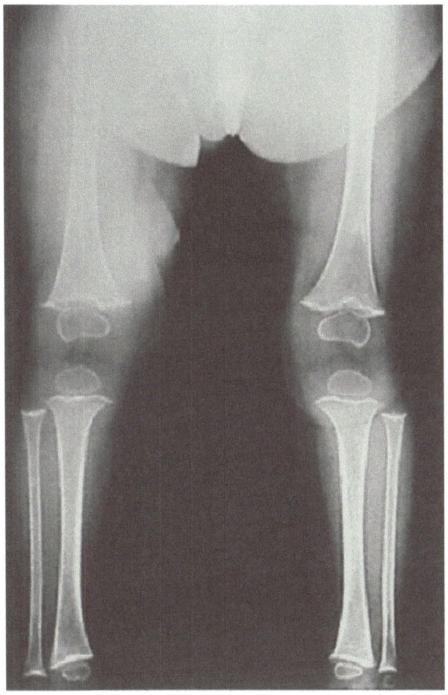

Fig. 47.71: *Radiograph of the lower extremities shows ground-glass osteopenia, a characteristic of scurvy*

rarefaction typically involves the lateral aspects of the white line, resulting in triangular defects called the corner sign of Park. This area has multiple microscopic fractures and may collapse with impaction of the calcified cartilage onto the shaft. The lateral aspect of the calcified cartilage can project as a spur. Subperiosteal hemorrhages are not visualized in the active phase. With healing, they become calcified and are readily observed.

Medical Care

- Vitamin C administered by mouth or the parenteral route is effective in curing infantile scurvy.
- Orange juice is an effective dietary remedy for curing infantile scurvy and was the standard treatment before the discovery of vitamin C.
- Upon instituting dietary or pharmacologic treatment, the clinical recovery is impressive. The appetite of the infant is recovered within 24–48 hours. The symptoms of irritability, fever, tenderness upon palpation, and hemorrhage generally resolve within 7 days.

Diet

A diet adequate in vitamin C can prevent the development of scurvy. The dietary requirements of vitamin C sufficient to prevent deficiency vary with the age of the individual. The following are the Food and Nutrition Board of the National Academy of Sciences, National Research Council's minimum recommended daily dietary allowances of vitamin C:

- Infants - 30–40 mg
- Children and adults - 45–60 mg
- Pregnant women – 70 mg
- Lactating mothers – 90–95 mg
- Food sources rich in vitamin C include the following:
- Citrus fruits
- Berries
- Cantaloupe
- Broccoli
- Cauliflower
- Cabbage
- Spinach
- Potatoes
- Tomatoes

Drug Therapy

Vitamins

Vitamins are organic substances required by the body in small amounts for various metabolic processes. Vitamins may be synthesized in small or insufficient amounts in the body or not synthesized at all, thus requiring supplementation. They are classified as either fat soluble or water soluble. Vitamins A, D, E, and K are fat soluble, whereas biotin, folic acid, niacin, pantothenic acid, B vitamins (i.e. B–1, B–2, B–6, B–12), and vitamin C are generally water soluble.

Vitamin deficiency may result from an inadequate diet, from increased requirements (e.g. pregnancy, lactation), or secondary to disease or drugs. Vitamin supplements are used clinically for the prevention and treatment of specific vitamin-deficiency states.

Drug: Ascorbic acid (Cecon, Ce-Vi-Sol, Dull-C)

Ascorbic acid (vitamin C) administered by mouth or parenterally effectively cures infantile and adult scurvy. Used by the body for collagen synthesis and tissue repai

Adult dose 100–200 mg PO q6h for 1 wk

Pediatric dose 25 mg PO q6h for 1 wk

Complications

- Scurvy, if left untreated, can be fatal and has been associated with sudden death.
- Lethargy, fatigue, and hemorrhagic manifestations of impaired collagen synthesis affecting oral, ophthalmic, musculoskeletal, cardiac, and gastrointestinal structures and functions may occur.
- Cerebral hemorrhage or hemopericardium are potential complications that may lead to death

Morbidity associated with hemorrhages depends on the site of involvement. Subperiosteal hemorrhages cause pain and tenderness resulting in pseudoparalysis. Loss of function at the site of the hemorrhage and anemia are typical sequelae of the hemorrhages observed in scurvy.

Prognosis

Typically, scurvy carries an excellent prognosis if diagnosed and treated appropriately.

ANEMIA AND HEART DISEASE

Blood is the body's delivery system. It carries oxygen and other nutrients around the body, delivering them to the cells that need them. At the same time, the blood picks up and takes away the waste products One of the most important things the blood does is carry oxygen from the lungs to every cell, of every muscle and organ. Without that oxygen, cells could not operate properly. Hemoglobin is the part of the red blood cells that carry the oxygen.

Anemia, one of the more common blood disorders, occurs when the number of healthy red blood cells decreases in the body. The disc-shaped red blood cells contain hemoglobin, a unique molecule that carries oxygen to the body's tissues

Anemia is a below-normal level of hemoglobin or hematocrit. Hemoglobin is the substance in red blood cells that carries oxygen to all parts of your body. Anemia can be temporary or it can be along-term disease/illness. People with mild anemia may not have any symptoms or may have only mild symptoms. People withsevere anemia can feel tired, get short of breath with activity, and have problems doing the things they usually do.

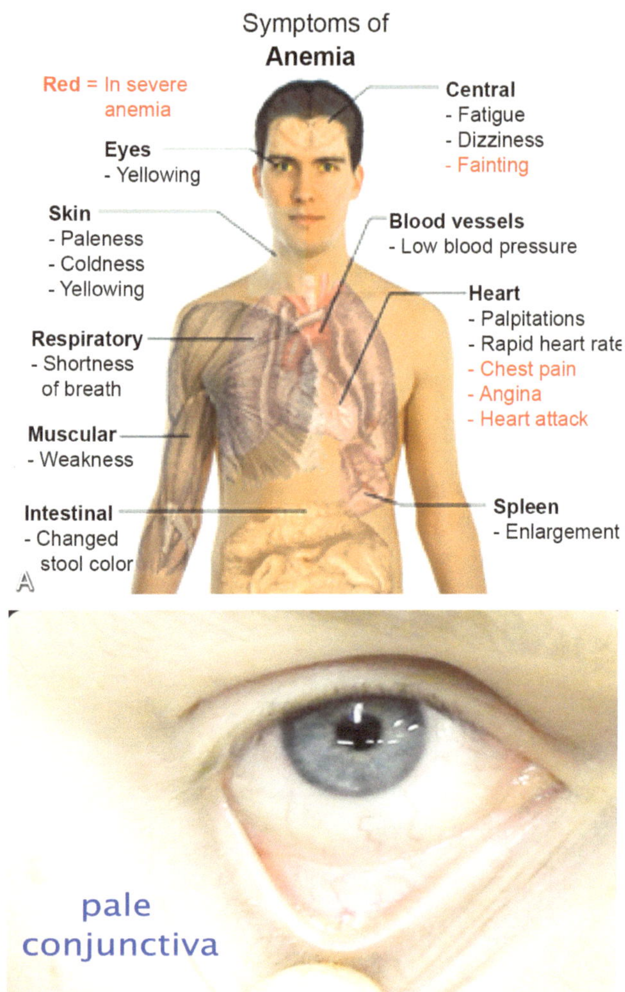

Fig. 47.72: *Examining of anemia by pulling down both the lower lids of the eyes for pallor*

Anemia Occurs Due to Various Reasons

Anemia occurs for different reasons

These include: increased destruction (break down) of red blood cells (RBCs) increased blood loss from the body inadequate production of red blood cells by the bone marrow.

In some cases anemia results from an inherited disorder, whereas in other cases the condition is caused by something in a person's environment, such as a nutritional problem, infection, or exposure to a drug or toxin.

How common is Anemia in people with heart disease? Many large studies have shown anemia is common in 17% to 48% of people with heart failure. One study showed that 43% of people who were hospitalized after a heart attack had anemia.

Relationship Between Anemia and Heart Disease

Anemia occurs when your body has a below-normal level of hemoglobin, which in turn prevents your body from getting enough oxygen. In certain cases, this lowers level of oxygen causes your heart to work harder. These effects on your heart can make you susceptible to heart disease or worsen existing heart disease.

What are the effects of untreated anemia in heart disease?

With anemia, the heart is forced to work harder to d liver oxygen-rich blood, yet does not receive enough oxygen to support the body's normal functions, resulting in extensive tissue damage and death.

Anemia can lead to severe chest pain because parts of the heart are not getting enough oxygen. As the heart works harder due to lack of oxygen, the muscles in the left lower chamber can get too thick. This can result in a condition called left ventricular hypertrophy, which can worsen heart disease and increase the chance of heartfailure.

In a study of people who initially had no heart disease, people with anemia were 41% more likely than those without anemia to have a heart attack, need an artery-clearing procedure, or die of heart disease within 6 years. Another study showed that anemia increases the chance of artery blockages in the arteries of the neck, a problem that can result in a stroke. The presence of anemia increases the death rate in people with heart failure and those who have had a heart attack. The death rate is especially high in anemic people with heart failure who also have kidney disease and/or diabetes.

These studies do not guarantee you will live longer if the anemia is corrected, but they do show how important it is to pay attention to anemia.

Signs and Symptoms of Anemia

Most people do not realize they are anemic until a blood test shows a low hemoglobin or hematocrit. Symptoms and signs usually develop when anemia is moderate to severe, and can include fatigue, weakness, pale skin, chest pain, dizziness, irritability, numbness or coldness in your hands and feet, trouble breathing, a fast heartbeat, and headache. It is important to see your doctor on a regular basis in order to be tested possible anemia.

The most common sign of iron deficiency and other types of nutritional anemia is mild paleness of the skin, along with decreased pinkness of the lips, the lining of the eyelids, and the nail beds. A friend or relative who sees your child only occasionally may be more likely to notice this than you because the changes usually happen so gradually.

Other Common Signs of Anemia may Include Irritability fatigue

Dizziness, lightheadedness, and a rapid heartbeat

Depending on the condition causing the anemia, other signs and symptoms may occur, such as jaundice (yellow-tinged skin), dark tea-colored urine, easy bruising or bleeding, and enlargement of the spleen or liver.

In many cases, doctors don't discover anemia until they run blood tests as part of a routine physical examination. A complete blood count (CBC) may indicate that there are fewer red blood cells than normal. Other diagnostic tests may include:

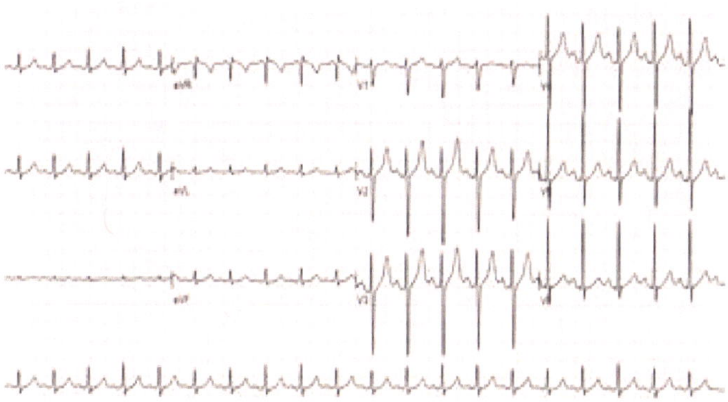

Fig. 40.73: *ECG Showing sinus tachycardia with heart rate of 125 beats/min in p a atient with severe* anemia.

Blood smear examination: Microscopic examination of red blood cells after blood is smeared on a glass slide can sometimes indicate the cause of the anemia.

Iron tests: These include total serum iron and ferritin tests, which can help to determine whether anemia is due to iron deficiency.

Hemoglobin electrophoresis: This test identifies various abnormal hemoglobin in the blood and is used to diagnose sickle cell anemia and the thalassemias.

Bone marrow aspiration and biopsy: This test can help determine whether cell production is happening normally in the bone marrow. It's the only way to diagnose aplastic anemia definitively and is also used if it is suspected that a disease affecting the bone marrow (such as leukemia) could be the cause for the anemia.

Normal Lab Values

Normal hemoglobin
>12 g/dL for women
>14 g/dL for men
Normal hematocrit
>36% for women
>42% for men

Treat of anemia: The treatment of anemia varies greatly depending on the type. Your physician will help you determine the best treatment options, such as diet modification, or nutritional supplements, or medication, if needed. Close communication with your doctor will ensure you will receive the best anemia treatment available. Treating anemia is not only vital to prevent the development of severe, possibly life-threatening complications, but to improve a patient's quality of life. Patients with serious illnesses such as CKD, diabetes, cancer, heart disease and rheumatoid arthritis are at the greatest risk for anemia

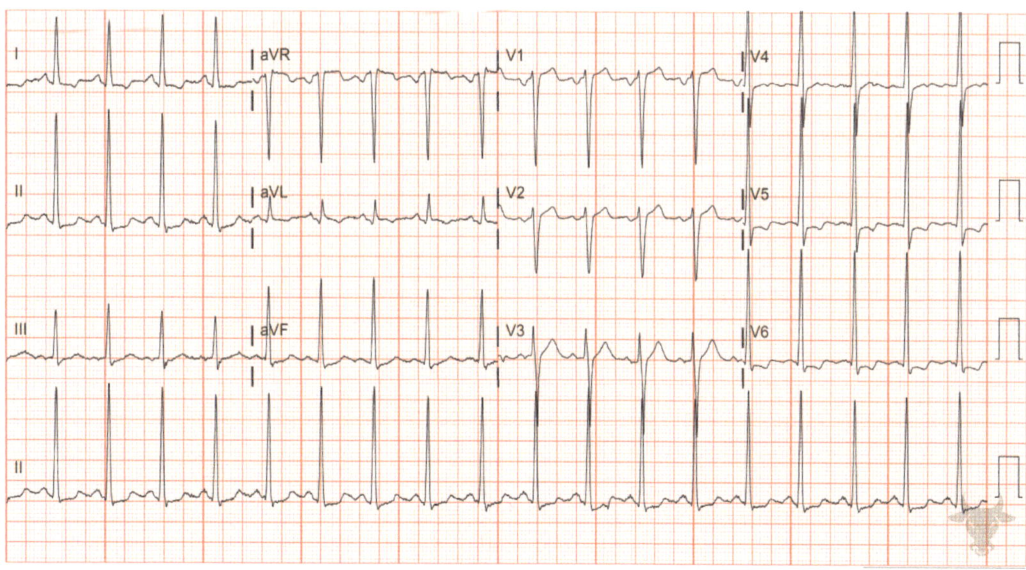

Fig. 40.74: *Left ventricular hypertrophy—12-lead ECG demonstrating NSR with LVH. The ST segment depression in the lateral leads (I, aVl, V5, and V6) is seen in approximately 70% of patients with electrocardiographic LVH; such a finding has been termed the "strain pattern." While this finding may represent altered repolarisation attributable to the presence of LVH, it may also be a manifestation of myocardial ischaemia*

Treatment is based on: your age, overall health, and medical history extent of the disease your tolerance for specific medications, procedures, or therapies expectations for the course of the disease your opinion or preference *Treatment may include:* Treatment of the causative disease vitamin and mineral supplements change in diet medication blood transfusion bone marrow transplant surgery (to remove the spleen, if related to hemolytic anemia) antibiotics (if an infection is the causative agent)

ACUTE RHEUMATIC FEVER

Rheumatic fever is an autoimmune inflammatory disease which may develop after a Group A streptococcal infection (such as strep throat or scarlet fever) and can involve the heart, joints, skin, and brain. It commonly appears in children ages 6 through 15

General Information

Rheumatic fever is common worldwide and responsible for many cases of damaged heart valves. In the Western countries, it became fairly rare since the 1960s, probably due to widespread use of antibiotics to treat streptococcus infections. While it is far less common in the United States since the beginning of the 20th century, there have been a few outbreaks since the 1980s. Although the disease seldom occurs, it is serious and has a mortality of 2–5%.

Rheumatic fever primarily affects children between ages 6 and 15 years and occurs approximately 20 days after strep throat or scarlet fever. In up to a third of cases, the underlying strep infection may not have caused any symptoms

The rate of development of rheumatic fever in individuals with untreated strep infection is estimated to be 3%. The incidence of recurrence with a subsequent untreated infection is substantially greater (about 50%). The rate of development is far lower in individuals who have received antibiotic treatment. Persons who have suffered a case of rheumatic fever have a tendency to develop flare-ups with repeated strep infections. The recurrence of rheumatic fever is relatively common in the absence of maintenance of low dose antibiotics, especially during the first three to five years after the first episode. Heart complications may be long-term and severe, particularly if valves are involved.

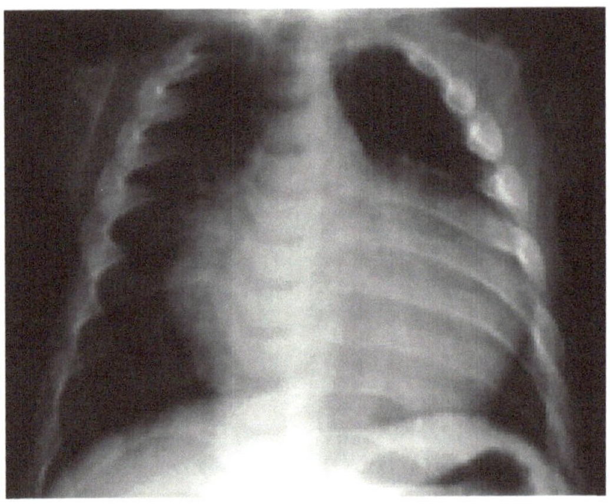

Fig. 40.75: *Chest X-ray PA view illustrating cardiomegaly in severe anemia in a child*

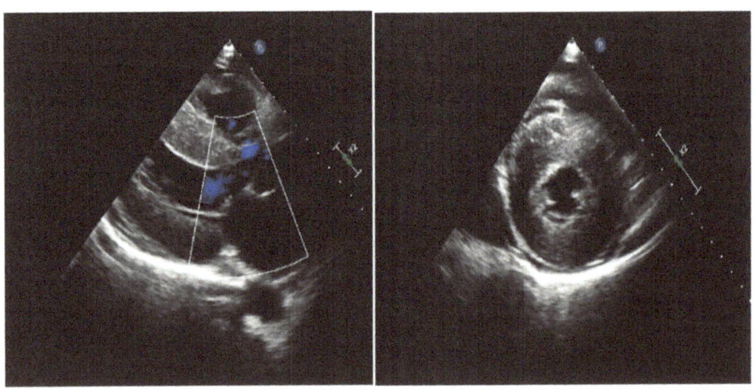

Fig. 40.76: (left) *Parasternal long axis view showing concentric left ventricular hypertrophy. Short axis view shows LVH in an adolescent with prolonged severe anemia (right)*

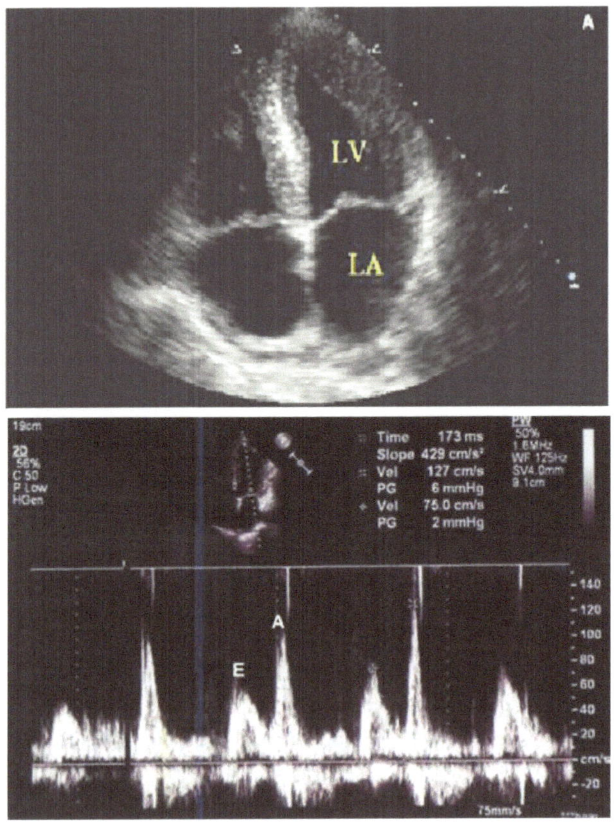

Fig. 40.77: *(Top) The apical 4-chamber view shows a thickened left ventricular wall and enlarged left atrium (LA).(Bottom) Doppler evaluation shows impaired early diastolic relaxation (E wave) and vigorous atrial contraction (A wave) resulting in an E/A ratio of less than 0.75, which signifies early reduced left ventricular compliance (B). A normal E/A ratio is greater than 1.5, since most of the diastolic filling occurs early in a compliant left ventricle with the atrial component contributing a smaller volume at a lower velocity in an adolescent with severe anemia (LV, left ventricle; LA, left atrium)*

Diagnosis: Modified Jones Criteria

T. Duckett Jones, MD, first published these criteria in 1944.[3] They have been periodically revised by the American Heart Association in collaboration with other groups. **Two major criteria, or one major and two minor criteria**, when there is also evidence of a previous strep infection, support the diagnosis of rheumatic fever. Exceptions are chorea and indolent carditis, each of which by itself can indicate rheumatic fever.

Major Criteria

The mnemonic JONES is often used to recall the major criteria

Joints *(Migratory polyarthritis):* A temporary migrating inflammation of the large joints, usually starting in the legs and migrating upwards

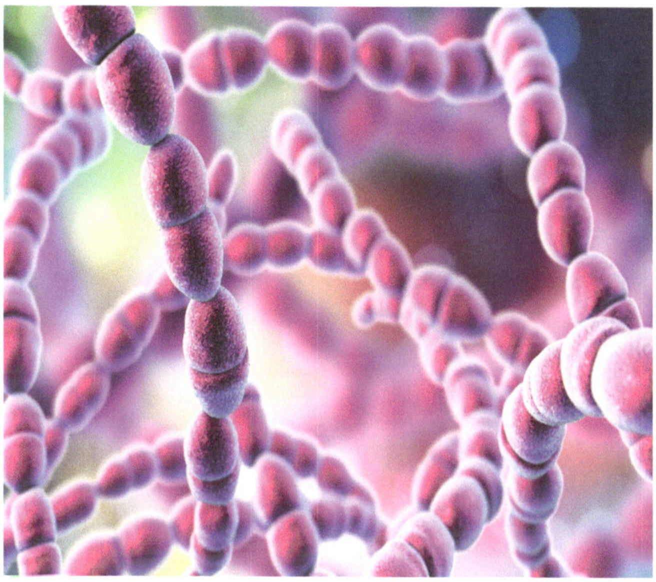

Fig. 40.78: *Electron micrograph of a chain of group A streptococci (type M-24) isolated during a rheumatic fever epidemic in a military population.*

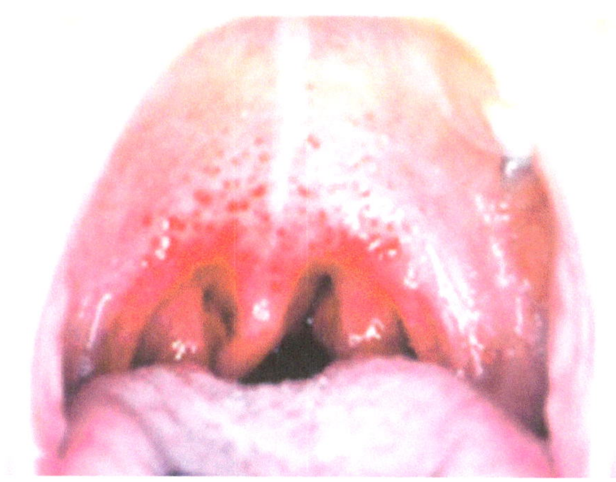

Fig. 40.79: *Showing acute throat infection with group A beta hemolytic streptococcoi*

O (carditis): Inflammation of the heart muscle which can manifest as congestive heart failure with shortness of breath, pericarditis with a rub, or a new heart murmur (Fig. 47.86).

Nodules *(subcutaneous nodules - a form of Aschoff bodies):* painless, firm collections of collagen fibers on the back of the wrist, the outside elbow, and the front of the knees. These now occur infrequently .

***Erythema marginatum*:** A long lasting rash that begins on the trunk or arms as macules and spreads outward to form a snakelike ring while clearing in the middle. This rash never starts on the face and is made worse with heat

Sydenham's Chorea

(St. Vitus' dance): A characteristic series of rapid movements without purpose of the face and arms. This can occur very late in the disease. an additional way to remember the major criteria is by the mnemonic: **C.A.N.C.ER**

- C: Carditis
- A: Arthritis
- N: Nodules (sub cutaneous)
- C: Chorea
- ER: ERythema Marginatum

Minor Criteria

Fever: Temperature elevation
Arthralgia: Joint pain without swelling
Laboratory abnormalities: Increased Erythrocyte sedimentation rate, increased C reactive protein, leukocytosis
Electrocardiogram abnormalities: A prolonged PR interval·
Evidence of Group A Strep infection: Positive culture for Group A Strep, elevated or rising Antistreptolysin O titre.
Previous rheumatic fever or inactive heart disease

Other Signs and Symptoms

- Abdominal pain
- Nosebleeds

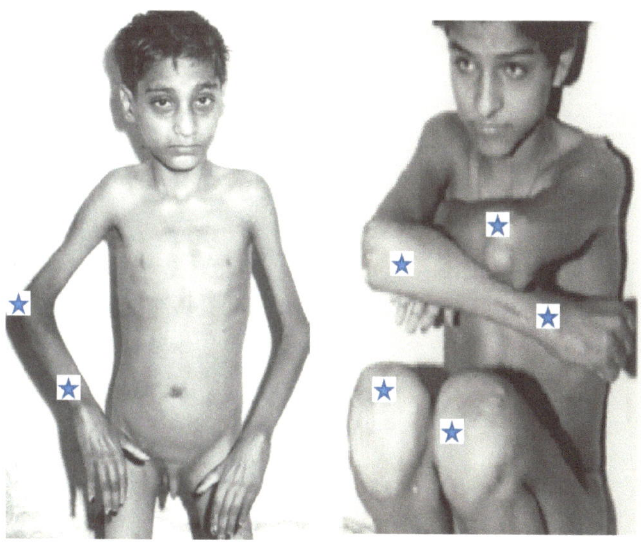

Fig. 40.80: *Showing subcutaneous nodules (arrows) over the writs,elbows ands finger in a young child with acute rheumatic fever*

Pathophysiology

Rheumatic fever is a systemic disease affecting the peri-arteriolar connective tissue and can occur after an untreated

A

B

C

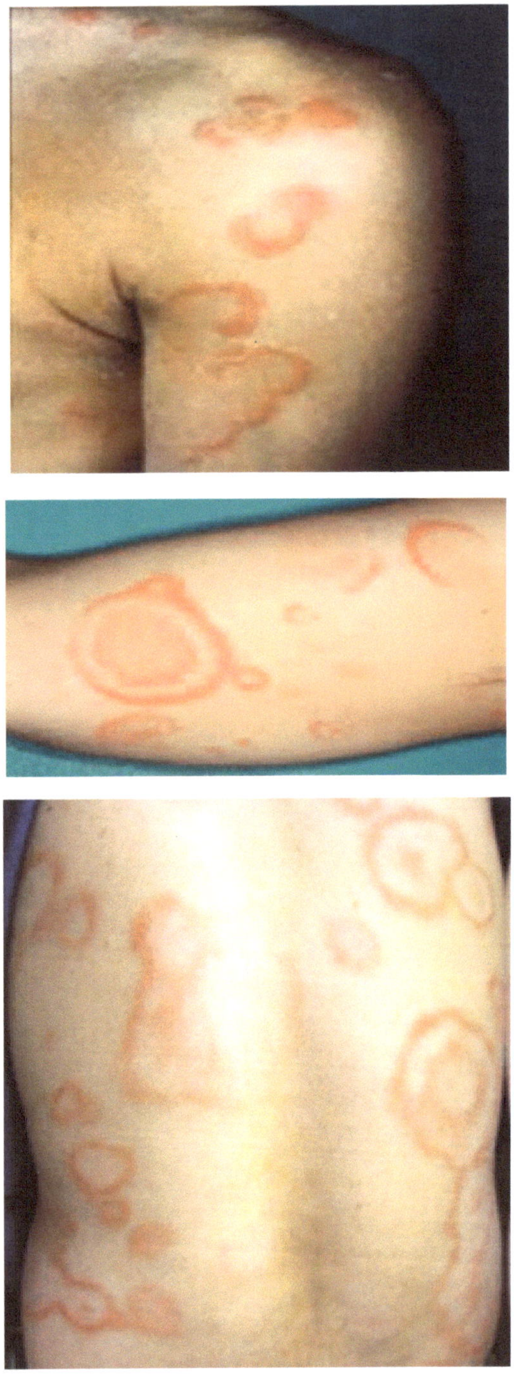

Fig. 40.81: *(A) shoulder and upper arm areas (B) Forearm and (C) back area Erythema marginatum. The rash is classically flat to slightly elevated, erythematous and annular (ring-like) in appearance*

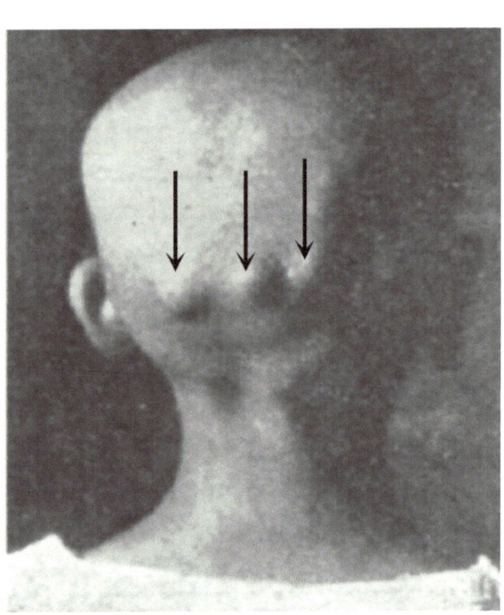

Fig. 40.82: *Rheumatic nodules over the occipit of a young child with acute rheumatic fever*

Group A streptococcal pharyngeal infection. It is believed to be caused by antibody cross-reactivity. This cross-reactivity is a Type II hypersensitivity reaction and is termed *molecular mimicry*. Usually, self reactive B cells remain anergic in the periphery without T cell co-stimulation. During a Strep. Infection activated antigen presenting cells such as macrophages present the bacterial antigen to helper T cells. Helper T cells subsequently activate B cells and induce the production of antibodies against the cell wall of Streptococcus. However the antibodies may also react against the myocardium and joints,[8] producing the symptoms of rheumatic fever. Group A *streptococcus pyogenes* has a cell wall composed of branched polymers which sometimes contain "*M proteins*" that are highly antigenic. The antibodies which the immune system generates against the "*M proteins*" may cross react with cardiac myofiber protein myosin[9] and smooth muscle cells of arteries, inducing cytokine release and tissue destruction. This inflammation occurs through direct attachment of complement and Fc receptor-mediated recruitment of neutrophils and macrophages. Characteristic Aschoff bodies, composed of swollen eosinophilic collagen surrounded by lymphocytes and macrophages can be seen on light microscopy. The larger macrophages may become Aschoff giant cells. Acute rheumatic valvular lesions may also involve a cell-mediated immunity reaction as these lesions predominantly contain T-helper cells and macrophages in acute RF, these lesions can be found in any layer of the heart and is hence called pancarditis. The inflammation may cause a serofibrinous pericardial exudates described as "bread-and-butter" pericarditis, which usually resolves without sequelae. Involvement of the endocardium typically results in fibrinoid necrosis and verrucae formation along the lines of closure of the left-sided heart valves. Warty projections arise from deposition, while subendothelial lesions may induce irregular thickenings called MacCallum plaques. Chronic rheumatic heart disease is characterized by repeated inflammation with fibrinous resolution. The cardinal anatomic changes of the valve include leaflet thickening, commissural fusion and shortening and thickening of the tendinous cords.

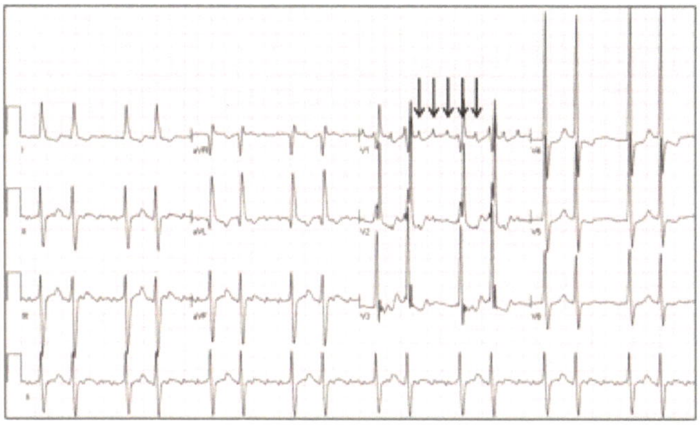

Fig.40.84: *ECG trace shows Multifocal atrial tachycardia in patient with acute rheumatic fever*

Treatment

The management of acute rheumatic fever is geared toward the reduction of inflammation with anti-inflammatory medications such as aspirin or corticosteroids. Individuals with positive cultures for strep throat should also be treated with antibiotics. Aspirin is the drug of choice and should be given at high doses of 100mg/kg/day. One should watch for side effects like gastritis, salicylate poisoning etc. Steroids are reserved for cases where there is evidence of involvement of heart. The use of steroids may prevent further scarring of tissue and may prevent development of sequelae such as Mitral stenosis. Monthly injections of Long acting Penicillin must be given for a period of 5 years in patients having one attack of Rheumatic fever. If there is evidence of carditis, the length of Penidure therapy may be up to 40 years. Another important cornerstone in treating rheumatic fever includes the continual use of low dose antibiotics (such as penicillin, sulfadiazine, or erythromycin) to prevent recurrence.

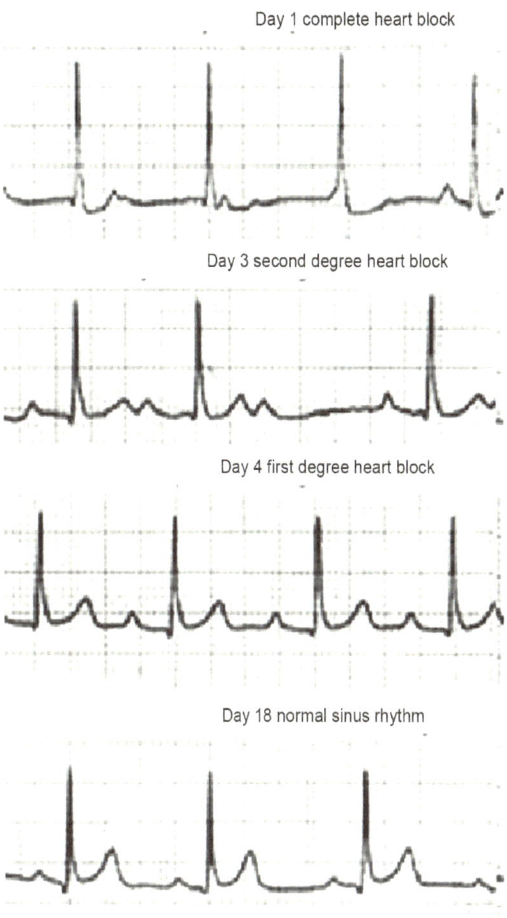

Fig. 40.85: *Showing regression of ECG changes from complete heart block to normal sinus rhythm in patient with ARF*

Infection

Patients with positive cultures for *streptococcus pyogenes* should be treated with penicillin as long as allergy is not present. This treatment will not alter the course of the acute disease.

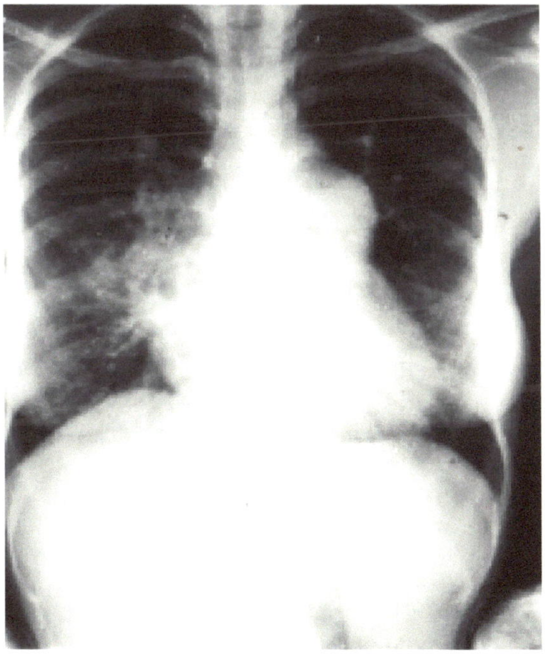

Fig. 40.83: *X-ray chest PA view showing cardiomegaly, prominent pulmonary artery due to acute on chronic rheumatic heart disease*

Inflammation

Patients with significant symptoms may require corticosteroids. Salicylates are useful for pain.

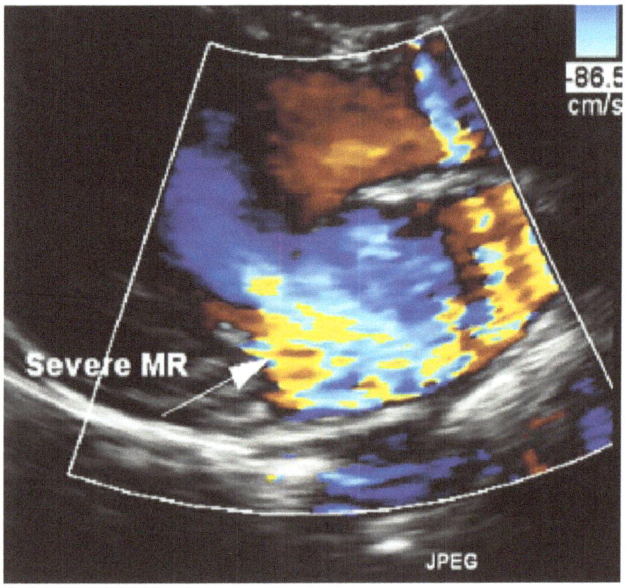

Fig. 40.86: *Color Doppler ecocardiography shows severe MR in patient with acute rheumatic fever*

Heart failure

Some patients develop significant carditis which manifests as congestive heart failure. This requires the usual treatment for heart failure: diuretics and digoxin. Unlike normal heart failure, rheumatic heart failure responds well to corticosteroids.

Prevention

Prevention of recurrence is achieved by eradicating the acute infection and prophylaxis with antibiotics. The American Heart Association recommends daily or monthly prophylaxis continue long-term, perhaps for life.

Nurses also have a role in prevention, primarily in screening school-aged children for sore throats that may be caused by Group A streptococci (especially Group A â Hemolytic Streptococcus pyogenes)

KAWASAKI DISEASE

Kawasaki disease, also known as lymph node syndrome, mucocutaneous node disease, infantile polyarteritis and Kawasaki syndrome, is a poorly understood self-limited vasculitis that affects many organs, including the skin and mucous membranes, lymph nodes, blood vessel walls, and the heart. It does not seem to be contagious. It was first described in 1967 by Dr. Tomisaku Kawasaki in Japan.

Incidence and Risk Factors

By far, the highest incidence of Kawasaki disease occurs in Japan (175 per 100,000), though its incidence in the United States is increasing. Kawasaki disease is predominantly a disease of young children, with 80% of patients younger than 5 years of age. Additional risk factors in the United States include Asian race and male sex. Approximately 2000 cases are identified in the United States each year.

Causes

The causative agent of Kawasaki disease is still unknown.[3] However, current etiological theories center primarily on immunological causes for the disease. Much research is being performed to discover a definitive toxin or antigenic substance, possibly a superantigen, that is the specific cause of the disease.

An unknown virus may play a role as an inciting factor as well. An association with ITPKC has been identified.

Presentation

The cardiac complications are, by far, the most important aspect of the disease. Kawasaki disease can cause vasculitic changes (inflammation of blood vessels) in the coronary arteries and subsequent coronary artery aneurysms. These aneurysms can lead to myocardial infarction (heart attack) even in young children. Overall, about 10–18% of children with Kawasaki disease develop coronary artery aneurysms Kawasaki syndrome and risk factors for coronary artery abnormalities: United States, 1994-2003. with much higher prevalence among patients who are not treated early in the course of illness. Kawasaki disease and rheumatic fever are most common causes of acquired heart disease among children in the United States.

Symptoms

Kawasaki disease often begins with a high and persistent fever that is not very responsive to normal doses of paracetamol (acetaminophen) or ibuprofen. The fever may persist steadily for up to two weeks and is normally accompanied by irritability. Affected children develop red eyes, red mucous membranes in the mouth, red cracked lips, a "strawberry tongue", iritis, keratic precipitates (detectable by an ophthalmologist but usually too small to be seen by the unaided eye), and swollen lymph nodes. Skin rashes occur early in the disease, and peeling of the skin in the genital area, hands, and feet (especially around the nails and on the palms and soles) may occur in later phases. Some of these symptoms may come and go during the course of the illness. If left untreated, the symptoms will eventually relent, but coronary artery aneurysms will not improve, resulting in a significant risk of death or disability due to myocardial infarction (heart attack). If treated in a timely fashion, this risk can be mostly avoided and the course of illness cut short.

- High-grade fever (greater than 39 °C or 102 °F; often as high as 40 °C or 104 °F) that normally lasts for more than a week if left untreated.
- Red eyes (conjunctivitis) without pus or drainage, also known as "conjunctival injection"
- Bright red, chapped, or cracked lips
- Red mucous membranes in the mouth
- Strawberry tongue, white coating on the tongue or prominent red bumps (papillae) on the back of the tongue
- Red palms of the hands and the soles of the feet.
- Swollen hands and feet
- Rash which may take many forms, but not vesicular (blister-like), on the trunk

- Swollen lymph nodes (frequently only one lymph node is swollen), particularly in the neck area
  Joint pain (arthralgia) and swelling, frequently symmetrical Irritability· Tachycardia (rapid heart beat)
- Peeling (desquamation) palms and soles (later in the illness); peeling may begin around the nails
  Beaus lines (transverse grooves on nails)

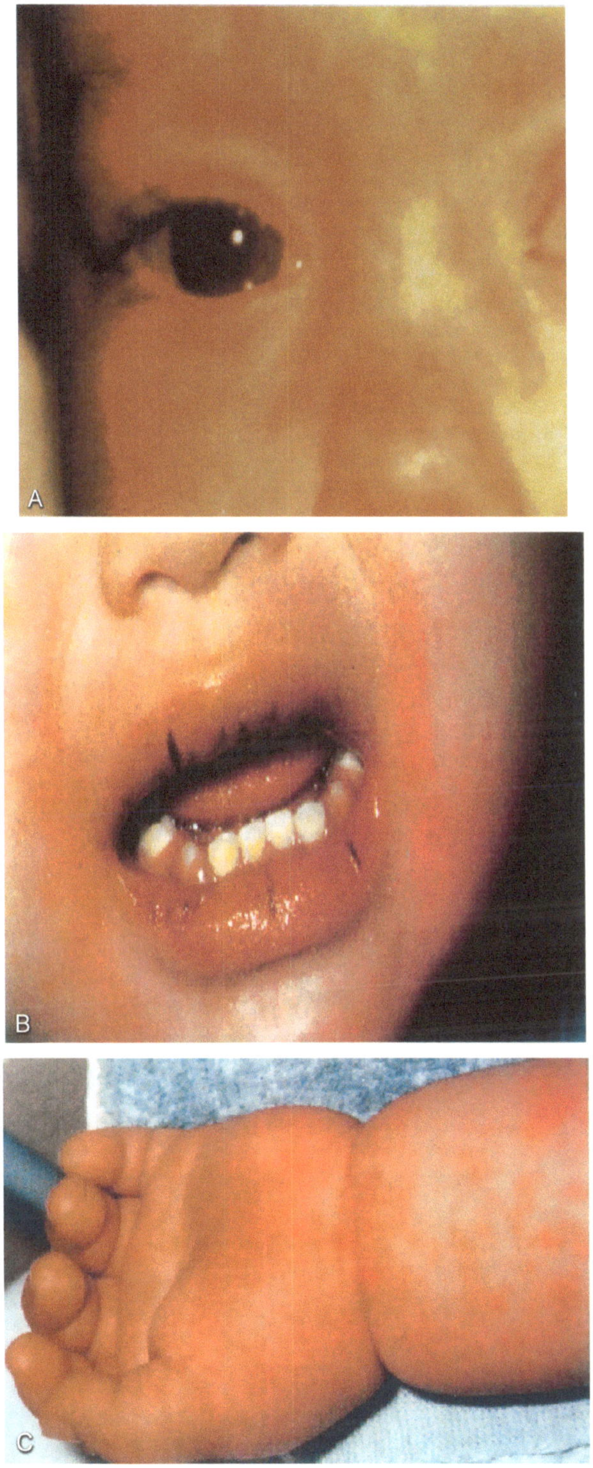

Fig. 40.87(A to C): *Showing different manifestations of Kawasaki's disease. (Upper) redness of conjuntiva with facial rash. (middle) red fissured lips and strawberry tongue (lower) redness of the palm and edema of the hand with induration*

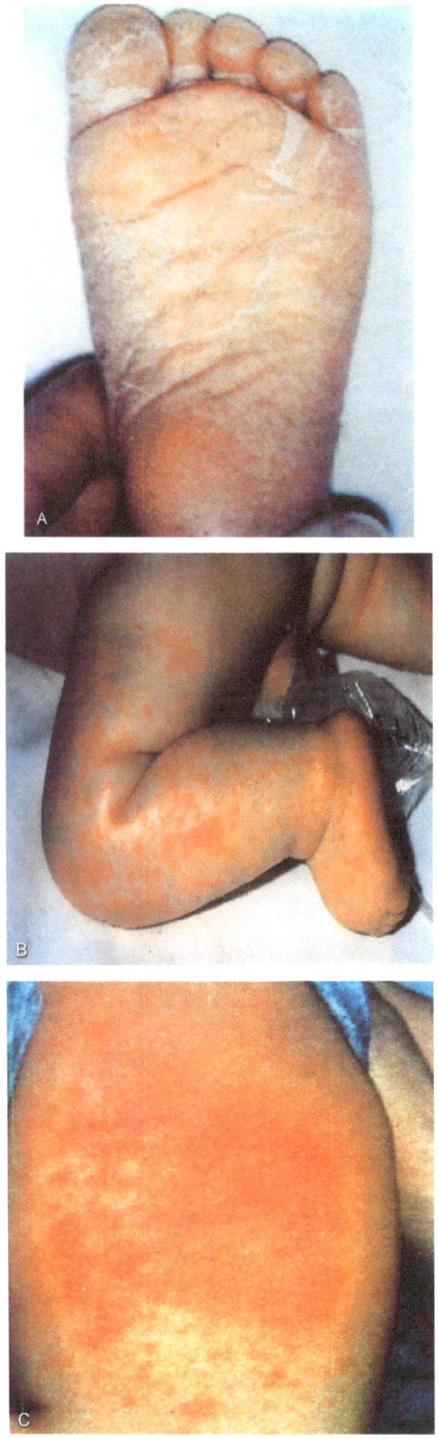

Fig. 40.88(A to C): *Showing different manifestations of Kawasaki's disease(Upper) desquammation of the foot in the subacute phase (middle) Skin rash with edema and redness of the foot (lower) erythema and induration around a BCG vaccination site*

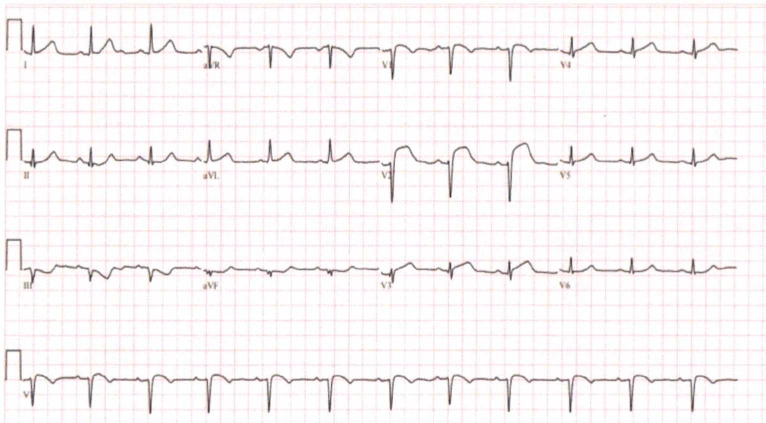

Fig. 40.89: *12-lead ECG from 12 -months old girl with Kawasaki disease. The ECG showing ST elevation in leadss 11,111,aVF and V4-V6 as acute coronary syndrome*

Blood Tests

Complete blood count (CBC) may reveal normocytic anemia and eventually thrombocytosis

- **Erythrocyte sedimentation rate (ESR)** will be elevated
- **C-reactive protein (CRP)** will be elevated
- **Liver function tests** may show evidence of hepatic inflammation and low serum albumi

Other tests (may or may not be performed)

Electrocardiogram may show evedence of ventricular dysfunction or, occasionally, arrhythmia due to myocarditis

Echocardiogram may show subtle coronary artery changes or, later, true aneurysms.

Ultrasound or computerized tomography may show hydrops (enlargement) of the gallbladder

- Urinalysis may show white blood cells and protein in the urine (pyuria and proteinuria) without evidence of bacterial growth Lumbar puncture may show evidence of aseptic meningitis.

Angiography was historically used to detect coronary artery aneurysms and remains the gold standard for their detection, but is rarely used today unless coronary artery aneurysms have already been detected by echocardiography. If not treated in time it can cause many heart problems

Diagnosis

Kawasaki disease can only be diagnosed clinically (by medical signs and symptoms), as there exists no specific laboratory test that can tell if someone has it. It is normally difficult to establish the diagnosis, especially early in the

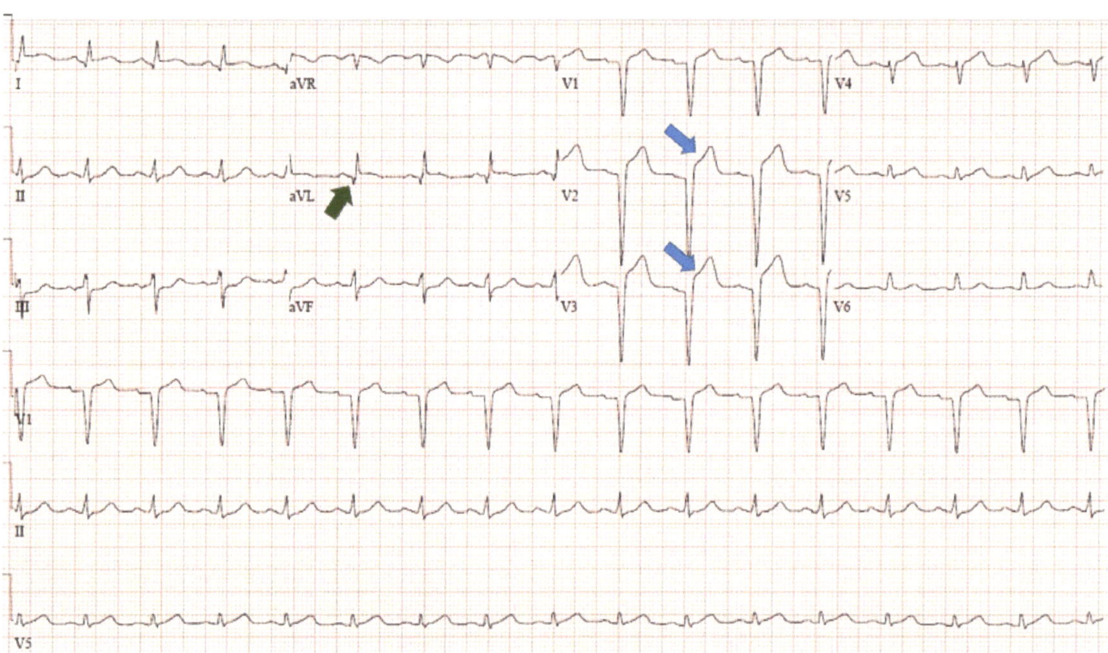

Fig. 47.90: *12-lead ECG Acute ST elevation infarction with delayed presentation (ST Elevation and Q waves present in a patient with Kawasaki disease*

course of illness, and frequently children are not diagnosed until they have seen their doctor several times, or visited a number of different health care providers. Many other serious illnesses can cause similar symptoms, and must be considered in the differential diagnosis, including scarlet fever, toxic shock syndrome, and juvenile idiopathic arthritis.

Classically, five days of fever plus four of five diagnostic criteria must be met in order to establish the diagnosis. The criteria are:

1. Erythema of the lips or oral cavity or cracking of the lips;
2. Rash on the trunk;
3. Swelling or erythema of the hands or feet;
4. Red eyes (conjunctival injection)
5. Swollen lymph node in the neck of at least 15 millimeters.

Many children, especially infants, eventually diagnosed with Kawasaki disease do not exhibit all of the above criteria. In fact, many experts now recommend treating for Kawasaki disease even if only three days of fever have passed and at least three diagnostic criteria are present, especially if other tests reveal abnormalities consistent with Kawasaki disease. In addition, the diagnosis can be made purely by the detection of coronary artery aneurysms in the proper clinical setting.

Treatment

Children with Kawasaki disease should be hospitalized and cared for by a physician who has experience with this disease. When in an academic medical center, care is often shared between pediatric cardiology and pediatric infectious disease specialists, although no infectious agent has been demonstrated. It is imperative that treatment be started as soon as the diagnosis is made to prevent damage to the coronary arteries. Intravenous immunoglobulin (IVIG) is the standard treatment for Kawasaki disease and is administered in high doses with marked improvement usually noted within 24 hours. If the fever does not respond, an additional dose may have to be considered. IVIG by itself is most useful within the first 7 days of onset of fever, in terms of preventing coronary artery aneurysm.

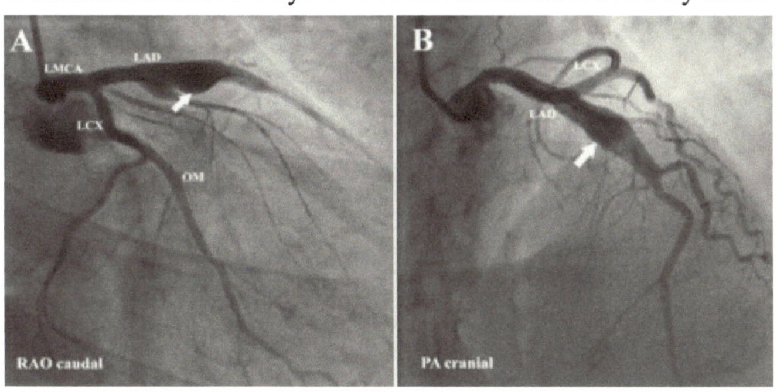

Fig. 40.91: *A&B:Coronary angiogram (after aspiration) showing fusiform aneurysm (10 mm×6 mm) of mid-left anterior descending coronary artery with TIMI 3 flow in distally (arrow). No thrombus seen. RAO-right anterior oblique view, PA- posterior anterior view, LMCA-left main coronary artery, LAD-left anterior descending coronary artery, LCX-left circumflex coronary artery, OM-obtuse marginal branch.in a young patient with Kawasaki disease*

Salicylate therapy, particularly aspirin, remains an important part of the treatment (though questioned by some) but salicylates alone are not as effective as Intravenous immunoglobulin. Aspirin therapy is started at high doses until the fever subsides, and then is continued at a low dose when the patient returns home, usually for 2 months to prevent blood clots from forming. Except for Kawasaki disease and a few other indications, aspirin is otherwise normally not recommended for children due to its association with Reye's syndrome.

Corticosteroids have also been used, especially when other treatments fail or symptoms recur, but in a randomized controlled trial, the addition of corticosteroid to immune globulin and aspirin did not improve outcome.There are also treatments for iritis and other eye symptoms.

Prognosis

With early treatment, rapid recovery from the acute symptoms can be expected and the risk of coronary artery aneurysms greatly reduced. Untreated, the acute symptoms of Kawasaki disease are self-limited (i.e. the patient will recover eventually), but the risk of coronary artery involvement is much greater. Overall, about 2% of patients die from complications of coronary vasculitis. Patients who have had Kawasaki disease should have an echocardiogram initially every few weeks, and then every 1–2 years to screen for progression of cardiac involvement. It is also not uncommon that a relapse of symptoms may occur soon after initial treatment with IVIG. This usually requires re-hospitalization and retreatment. Treatment with IVIG can cause allergic and non-allergic acute reactions, aseptic meningitis, fluid overload and, rarely, other serious reactions. Aspirin may increase the risk of bleeding from other causes and may be associated with Reye's syndrome. Overall, life-threatening complications resulting from therapy for Kawasaki disease are exceedingly rare, especially compared with the risk of non-treatment.

TYPHOID FEVER

Typhoid fever, also known as enteric fever, is a systemic infection by *Salmonella typhi* or by the related but less virulent *Salmonella paratyphi*. Since ancient times, these bacteria have thrived during wartime and during the breakdown of basic sanitation. Archeologists have found *S typhi* in Athenian mass graves from the era of the Peloponnesian Wars, implicating it as the cause of the Great Plague of Athens. *S typhi* persists mostly in developing nations where sanitation is generally poor. Although sporadic outbreaks occur in developed nations, most individuals with typhoid fever in such areas have recently returned from travel to an endemic region.

Of all *Salmonella* serotypes, only *S typhi* and *S paratyphi* are pathogenic exclusively in humans. Typhoid fever is a severe multisystemic illness characterized by the classic prolonged fever, sustained bacteremia without endothelial or endocardial involvement, agative, enteric, rond bacterial invasion of and multiplication within the mononuclear phagocytic cells of the liver, spleen, lymph nodes, and Peyer patches. Typhoid fever is potentially fatal if untreated. People are typically infected with *S typhi* and *S paratyphi* through food and beverages contaminated by a chronic stool carrier. Less commonly, carriers may shed the bacteria in urine. Individuals may also be infected by drinking sewage-contaminated water or by eating contaminated shellfish or faultily canned meat.

Salmonella is a genus in the family Enterobacteriaceae that has more than 2300 serotypes previously described in the Kauffman-White schema. Salmonellae are gram-negative, flagellate, nonsporulating, facultative anaerobic bacilli that ferment glucose, reduce nitrate to nitrite, and synthesize peritrichous flagella when motile. All but *S typhi* produce gas upon sugar fermentation.

Salmonellae are grouped based on the somatic O antigen and further divided into serotypes based on flagellar H and surface virulence (Vi) antigens. In particular, *S typhi,* the cause of typhoid fever, has O and H antigens, an envelope (K) antigen, and a lipopolysaccharide macromolecular complex called endotoxin that forms the outer portion of the cell wall. *S typhi, S paratyphi C,* and *Salmonella Dublin*are the only *Salmonella* serotypes that carry Vi antigen. Based on DNA studies, all salmonellae are now considered one of two species: *Salmonella enterica* (formerly called *Salmonella choleraesuis*) and *Salmonella* bongori. *S enterica* has 6 subspecies (I, II, IIIa, IIIb, IV, VI); *S bongori* has one (V). *S typhi* and *S paratyphi* are *S enterica* I subspecies, serotypes *typhi* and *paratyphi.*

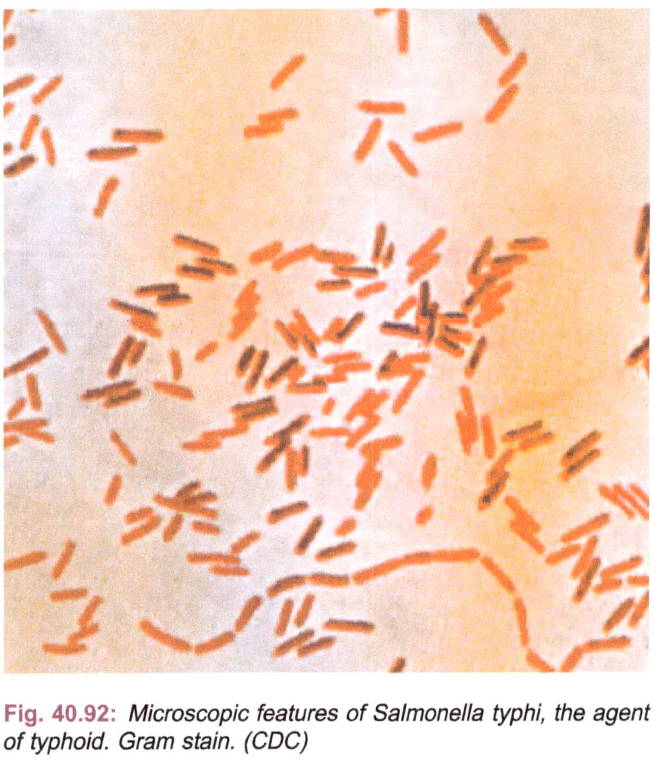

Fig. 40.92: *Microscopic features of Salmonella typhi, the agent of typhoid. Gram stain. (CDC)*

Pathophysiology: After ingestion by the host, *S typhi* invades through the gut and multiplies within the mononuclear phagocytic cells in the liver, spleen, lymph nodes, and Peyer patches of the ileum.

In studies of healthy, previously unvaccinated men, ingestion of 10^7 *S typhi* bacilli caused disease in 50% of volunteers. Investigations of outbreaks seem to indicate that an inoculum of as few as 200 organisms may lead to the disease. Perhaps such a discrepancy exists because many who ingest *S typhi* are not healthy men and have any one of a number of risk factors (*see* below). As the number of organisms increases, the incubation period decreases. The number of bacilli ingested does not change the subsequent clinical syndrome.

After successfully passing through the stomach, any *Salmonella* subspecies may be phagocytized by the gut's intraluminal dendritic cells, causing inflammation that leads to diarrhea. Only the subspecies *S enterica* causes severe disease in the rest of the body. Its specialized fimbriae adhere to the epithelium that overlies Peyer patches. Peyer patches are grossly visible aggregates of 5–100 lymphoid follicles in the small bowel submucosa; these patches are larger and more numerous distally. They are the primary mechanism for sampling antigens in the gut and initiating response. *S enterica* enters them via 1 of 3 pathways.

Intraluminal dendritic cells may infiltrate through the gut epithelium while carrying the bacterium. M cells may transport it as well. Immobile and interspersed among regular enterocytes in Peyer patches, M cells are epithelial cells that mature into professional phagocytes. They phagocytize bacteria such as *S enterica* and present them to macrophages and T cells in the lamina propria. Most interestingly, *S enterica* may convert normally nonphagocytic epithelial cells into bacterially-mediated endocytosis (BME).

In BME, *Salmonella* uses a type III secretion system—macromolecular channels that gram-negative bacteria such as *Salmonella* insert into eukaryotic cells and intracellular membranes to inject virulence proteins—to inject proteins SipA and SipC into the epithelial cell. These disrupt the normal brush border and force the cell to form membrane ruffles. The ruffles engulf the bacilli and create vesicles that carry them across the epithelial cell cytoplasm and the basolateral membrane. *Salmonella* pathogenicity island 1 (SPI-1) in the genome encodes the elements of BME.

In the submucosa, *Salmonella* enters macrophages via bacteria-triggered pinocytosis or via macrophage receptor–mediated phagocytosis. The intravacuolar environment activates the PhoP/PhoQ regulon, leading to modification of protein and lipopolysaccharide elements of the bacterial inner and outer membranes. Thus, *Salmonella* resists lysis and decreases host proinflammatory signaling. The bacterium also produces homocysteine to inactivate nitric oxide and enzymes against other microbicides. Finally, with the Vi antigen, a polysaccharide capsule, *S typhi* and *S paratyphi* further protect themselves from lysis within the macrophage and from neutrophils and complement

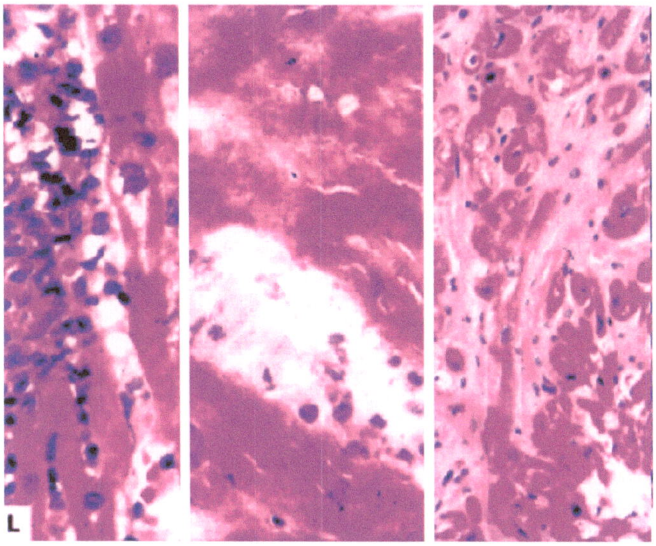

Fig. 40.93: *Serial biopsy samples taken from the patient with toxic typhoid myocarditis showing from left to right: acute myocarditis, healing myocarditis, All sections have the same magnification with haematoxylin and eosin stain*

without. The newly described *Salmonella* pathogenicity island 2 (SPI-2) encodes a type III secretion system that carries bacterial proteins across the vacuole membrane and into the cytosol. Other virulence factors from SPI-2 prevent or alter fusion of the *Salmonella*-containing vacuole with other intracellular compartments, rearrange the actin cytoskeleton around the vacuole, and may prevent the implantation of nicotinamide adenine dinucleotide phosphate (NADPH) oxidase and nitric oxide synthase into the vacuole membrane.

The infected macrophage provides *Salmonella* a vehicle safe from other elements of the immune system and in which it can multiply and travel. It passes through the mesenteric lymph nodes into the thoracic duct and the lymphatics beyond to seed the reticuloendothelial tissues—liver, spleen, bone marrow, and lymph nodes. In these havens, it multiplies until some critical density is reached. It causes the apoptosis in the macrophages and enters the bloodstream to attack the rest of the body. At this stage, the Vi antigen comes into play. It forms a capsule to protect the bacterium from complement and from phagocytic immune cells.

From blood or from the liver via bile ducts, it infects the gallbladder and reenters the gastrointestinal tract in the bile, spreading to other hosts via stool. In addition, it occasionally invades the urinary tract and spreads via urine. After primary intestinal infection, further seeding of the Peyer patches occurs through infected bile. They may become hyperplastic and necrotic with infiltration of mononuclear cells and neutrophils, forming ulcers that may hemorrhage through eroded blood vessels or perforate the bowel wall, causing peritonitis.

The host recognizes the invader with toll-like receptors 2, 4, and 5. These induce cytokines such as interferon alpha, interleukin (IL)–12, and tumor necrosis factor-alpha, which recruit macrophages and cause the high fevers of the disease. Macrophages and neutrophils suppress the active infection. Later, humoral and CD4 T-cell–mediated immunity clears it.

Physical: The classic signs of enteric fever include fever, toxemia, delirium, abdominal pain, constipation, and hepatosplenomegaly.

Fever occurs in 75–85% of patients in the first week and is often initially remittent but becomes steady. The individual's temperature often rises to as high as 103–104°F (39–40°C) by the beginning of week 2. Constipation often develops early and is likely due to obstruction at the ileocecal valve by swollen Peyer patches. It may last for the entire duration of illness.

At approximately the end of the first week of illness, about a third of patients develop bacterial emboli to the skin known as rose spots. These are considered a classic symptom in typhoid fever, but they occasionally appear in shigellosis and nontyphoidal salmonellosis. Rose spots constitute a subtle, extremely sparse (often ≤5 spots), salmon-colored, blanching, truncal, maculopapular rash with 1- to 4-cm lesions that generally resolve within 2–5 days. Relative bradycardia and a dicrotic pulse are also common during this stage of illness.

During the second week of illness, the patient is toxic-appearing and apathetic with sustained fever. The abdomen is slightly distended, and soft splenomegaly is common.

In the third week, the patient grows more toxic and anorexic with significant weight loss. The patient may have a thready pulse, tachypnea, conjunctivitis, and crackles over the lung bases. Pyrexia persists. The patient may enter into a typhoid state of apathy, confusion, and even psychosis. Patients may develop polyneuropathy. Abnormal cerebrospinal fluid should prompt a search for a different cause. Meanwhile, the patient commonly has pronounced abdominal distension. Some individuals may produce liquid, foul, green-yellow diarrhea (pea soup diarrhea). At this stage, the patient may die from overwhelming toxemia, myocarditis, intestinal hemorrhage, or perforation due to necrotic Peyer patches. Rare complications of enteric fever include pancreatitis, meningitis, orchitis, and osteomyelitis. During the fourth week, the fever, mental state, and abdominal distension slowly improve over a few days, but intestinal complications may still occur in surviving untreated individuals. Weight loss and debilitating weakness last months. Relapses occur in 10% of patients, mostly during the first 2–3 weeks of convalescence.

Chronic Carrier State

One to four percent of untreated patients become chronic carriers, defined as individuals who excrete *Salmonella* for more than 1 year. Some individuals may continue to excrete the bacterium for decades. Bladder infection with *Schistosoma haematobium* predisposes to urinary carriage. The parasite itself becomes a carrier. Stool carriage is more frequent in people with preexisting biliary abnormalities, perhaps because S *enterica* survives in gallstones, and these people have a greater incidence of cholecystitis. Chronic

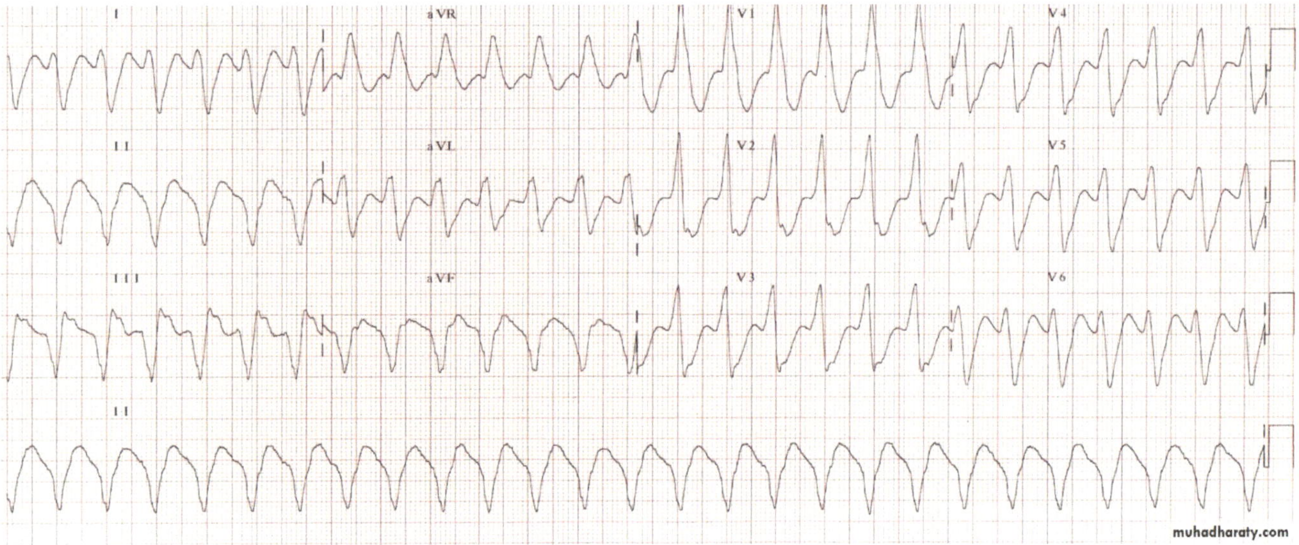

Fig. 40.94: *ECG showing regular broad complex tachycardia. as a part of typhoid toxic myocarditis*

carriers have a greater risk for carcinoma of the gallbladder and other gastrointestinal malignancies; chronic carriers had a 6-fold increase in the risk of death due to hepatobiliary cancer. This may be due to chronic inflammation caused by the bacterium.

Causes: *S typhi* and *S paratyphi* cause typhoid fever.

Lab Studies

- Typhoid fever causes various abnormalities in standard laboratory tests. Serological tests and cultures are the mainstay of diagnosis. DNA probes are used by researchers and are available to patients in well-funded facilities. The diagnosis is suggested by assays that identify *Salmonella* antibodies and antigens and is then confirmed by isolation of the organism.
- ***Standard laboratory tests:*** Most patients are moderately anemic, have an elevated erythrocyte sedimentation rate, thrombocytopenia, and relative lymphopenia. Most also have a slightly elevated prothrombin time (PT) and activated partial thromboplastin time, decreased fibrinogen levels, and levels of circulating fibrin degradation products that commonly rise to subclinical disseminated intravascular coagulation levels. Liver transaminase values and serum bilirubin levels are usually elevated to twice the reference range. Mild hyponatremia and hypokalemia are common.
- **Specific serological tests**
- Assays that identify *Salmonella* antibodies or antigens support the diagnosis but should be confirmed with cultures or DNA evidence.
- **The widal test** is more than a century old and was the standard serologic test for typhoid fever diagnosis for decades. Now, it is mostly of historical interest. It produces false-negative results in a significant proportion of patients who do not mount a detectable antibody response. It is highly nonspecific, especially in endemic areas where cross-reacting antigens from similar organisms are common. ***The Widal test measures agglutinating antibodies against H and O antigens of S typhi.***
- In acute infection, O antibody appears first, rising progressively, later falling, and often disappearing within a few months. H antibody appears slightly later but persists longer and can be used to distinguish between various types of enteric fever.
- Indirect hemagglutination, indirect fluorescent Vi antibody, and indirect enzyme-linked immunosorbent assay for immunoglobulin M (IgM) and IgG antibodies to *S typhi* polysaccharide are available. Monoclonal antibodies against *S typhi* flagellin are promising developments.
- **Culture**

  Definitive diagnosis of typhoid fever generally requires isolation of the organism from blood, bone marrow, vomitus, fresh stool, or urine. A bone marrow aspirate (BMA) culture is the most sensitive method of isolating *S typhi*. The sensitivity is 90% at any point in the disease course for as long as 5 days after the initiation of antibiotics. The test is extremely painful. Clinicians should try to establish the diagnosis with less traumatic means.

  If patients present within the first week of the disease, blood, intestinal secretions, and stool culture results are usually positive in approximately 85–90% of patients with typhoid fever. They decline to 20–30% later in the course of the disease. In particular, stool culture results may be positive for several days after *S typhi* ingestion. This is because of inflammation from the intraluminal dendritic cells. Later in the illness, bacteria shed through the gallbladder again cause positive stool culture results. Multiple positive blood culture results are 73–97%

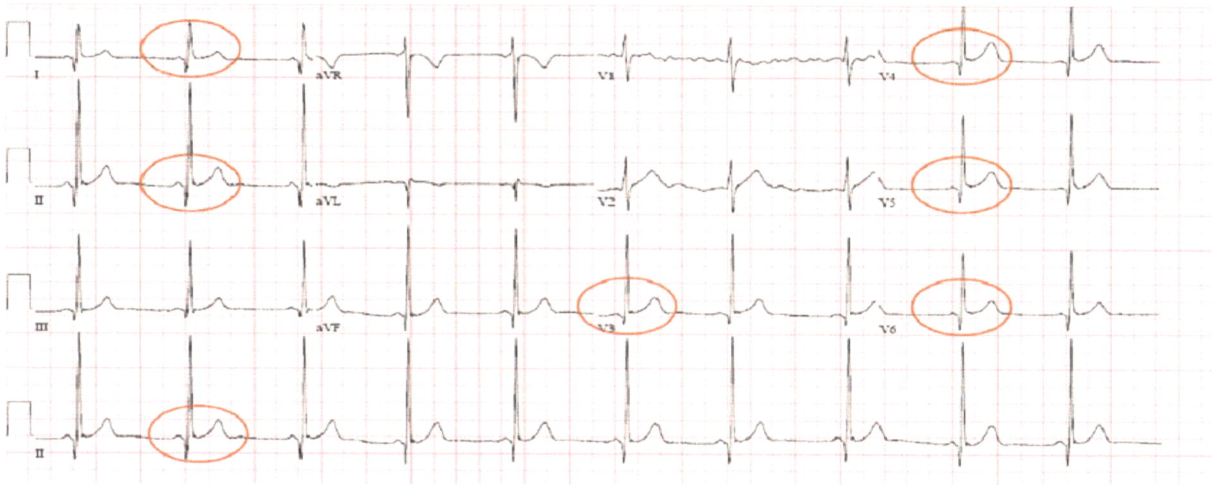

Fig. 40.95: *ECG showing diffuse ST elevations (circled), with an RSR' in V1 and V2. in acute myocarditis*

specific for typhoid fever. Large-volume blood culture and clot culture after serum removal increase sensitivity. Stool culture alone is less than 50% sensitive, and urine even less so. Cultures of punch biopsy samples of rose spots reportedly have a sensitivity of 63% and may show positive results even after antibiotics. A single rectal swab culture at hospital admission can be expected to detect *S typhi* in 30–40% of patients. *S typhi* has also been isolated from the cerebrospinal fluid, peritoneal fluid, mesenteric lymph nodes, resected intestine, pharynx, tonsils, abscess, bone, and urine, among others. After disease resolution, 3 stool cultures one month apart should be taken to rule out carrier state.
BMA and blood are cultured in a selective medium, such as 10% aqueous oxgall, or a nutritious medium, such as tryptic soy broth, and are incubated at 37°C for at least 7 days. Subcultures are made daily to one selective medium, such as MacConkey agar, and one inhibitory medium, such as *Salmonella-Shigella* agar. These conventional culture techniques usually take 48–72 hours from acquisition until the organism is identified.

- ***DNA testing:*** Polymerase chain reaction assays for identifying *S typhi* are available in some areas. However, this is used mostly for research since the test is generally too expensive for patients in developing countries.

Imaging Studies

Radiography of the kidneys, ureters, and bladder (KUB) are useful if the clinician suspects bowel perforation. CT scanning or MRI may be warranted to investigate abscesses that may occur in, among other sites, the liver or bones.

Procedures

The most sensitive method of isolating *S typhi* is obtaining a BMA culture

Histologic findings: The hallmark histologic finding in typhoid fever is infiltration of tissues by macrophages (typhoid cells) that contain bacteria, erythrocytes, and degenerated lymphocytes. Aggregates of these macrophages are called typhoid nodules, which are found most commonly in the intestine, mesenteric lymph nodes, spleen, liver, and bone marrow but may be found in the kidneys, testes, and parotid glands. In the intestines, 4 classic pathologic stages occur in the course of infection: (1) hyperplastic changes, (2) necrosis of the intestinal mucosa, (3) sloughing of the mucosa, and (4) the development of ulcers. The ulcers may perforate into the peritoneal cavity.

In the mesenteric lymph nodes, the sinusoids are enlarged and distended by large collections of macrophages and reticuloendothelial cells. The spleen is enlarged, red, soft, and congested; its serosal surface may have a fibrinous exudate. Microscopically, the red pulp is congested and contains typhoid nodules. The gallbladder is hyperemic and may show evidence of cholecystitis. A liver biopsy specimen from a person with typhoid often shows cloudy swelling, balloon degeneration with vacuolation of hepatocytes, moderate fatty change, and focal typhoid nodules. Intact typhoid bacilli can be observed at these sites.

Complications

- ***Intestinal manifestations***
  The 2 most common complications of enteric fever are intestinal hemorrhage (12% in one British series) and perforation (3-4.6% of hospitalized patients).
  From 1884–1909 (i.e. preantibiotic era), the mortality rate in patients with intestinal perforation in typhoid fever was 66–90% but now is significantly lower. Approximately 75% of patients have guarding, rebound tenderness, and rigidity, particularly in the right lower quadrant.
  Diagnosis is particularly difficult in the approximately 25% of patients with perforation and peritonitis who do not have the classic physical findings. Often, the discovery of free intra-abdominal fluid may be the only sign of perforation.
- ***Hepatobiliary manifestations***
  Mild elevation of transaminases without symptoms is common in persons with typhoid fever.
  Jaundice may occur in persons with enteric fever and may be due to hepatitis, cholangitis, cholecystitis, or hemolysis.
  Pancreatitis and simultaneous acute renal failure and hepatitis with hepatomegaly have been reported.

Cardiopulmonary

Nonspecific electrocardiographic changes occur in 10–15% of patients with typhoid. Toxic myocarditis occurs in 1–5% of persons with typhoid and is a significant cause of death in disease-endemic countries.

Toxic myocarditis occurs in patients who are severely ill and toxemic and is characterized by tachycardia, weak pulse and heart sounds, hypotension, and **electrocardiographic abnormalities** (Figs 47.94 and 47.95).

- Pericarditis rarely occurs, but peripheral vascular collapse without other cardiac findings is increasingly described. Pulmonary manifestations have also been reported in patients with typhoid fever.
- **Neuropsychiatric manifestations**
  In the past 2 decades, reports from the disease-endemic areas have documented a wide spectrum of neuropsychiatric manifestations of typhoid fever.
  A toxic confusional state, characterized by disorientation, delirium, and restlessness, is characteristic of late-stage typhoid. Occasionally, these and other neuropsychiatric features may dominate the clinical picture at an early stage.
  Facial twitching or convulsions may be the presenting feature; sometimes, paranoid psychosis or catatonia may develop during convalescence. Meningismus is not uncommon, but frank meningitis is rare. Encephalomyelitis may develop, and the underlying pathology may be that of demyelinating leukoencephalopathy. Rarely, transverse myelitis, polyneuropathy, or cranial mononeuropathy may develop.
  Other less commonly reported events are spastic paraplegia, peripheral or cranial neuritis, Guillain-Barré syndrome, schizophrenialike illness, mania, and depression.
- ***Hematologic manifestations***
  Subclinical disseminated intravascular coagulation occurs commonly in persons with typhoid fever.
  Hemolytic-uremic syndrome is rare.
  Hemolysis may also be associated with glucose-6-phosphate dehydrogenase deficiency.
- ***Genitourinary manifestations***
  Approximately 25% of patients excrete *S typhi* in their urine at some point during their illness.
  Immune complex glomerulitis and proteinuria have been reported, and IgM, C3 antigen, and *S typhi* antigen can be demonstrated in the glomerular capillary wall.
  Nephritic syndrome may complicate chronic *S typhi* bacteremia associated with urinary schistosomiasis.
- ***Musculoskeletal manifestations***
  Skeletal muscle characteristically shows Zenker degeneration, particularly affecting the abdominal wall and thigh muscles.

Clinically evident polymyositis may occur.

CNS Manifestations

Focal intracranial infections are uncommon.
Recently, multiple brain abscesses have been reported.

Prognosis

The prognosis depends on the geographical area and its demographics. Generally, the mortality rate in untreated disease is 10–20%. In properly treated disease, it is less than 1%.

Between 10% and 20% of patients treated with antibiotics have a relapse after initial recovery. A relapse typically occurs approximately 1 week after therapy is discontinued, but relapse after 70 days has been reported. The blood culture results are again positive, and high serum levels of H, O, and Vi antibodies and rose spots may reappear. A relapse generally is milder and shorter than the initial illness. Rarely, second or even third relapses may occur. Notably, the relapse rate is much lower following treatment with the new quinolone drugs, which have effective intracellular penetration

Medical care: Health care workers caring for patients with typhoid fever should pay strict attention to adequate hand washing and safe disposal of feces and urine. Antibiotic therapy is essential and should begin empirically if the clinical evidence is strong. Patients must receive adequate fluids, electrolytes, and nutrition. Antimicrobials shorten the course, reduce the rate of complications if begun early, and drastically reduce the case-fatality rate.

Surgical care: Surgery is usually indicated in cases of intestinal perforation. Most surgeons prefer simple closure of the perforation with drainage of the peritoneum. Small bowel resection is indicated for patients with multiple perforations.

If antibiotic treatment fails to eradicate the hepatobiliary carriage, the gallbladder should be resected. Cholecystectomy is not always successful in eradicating the carrier state because of persisting hepatic infection.

Physicians should consult an infectious disease specialist: Consultation with a surgeon is indicated upon suspected gastrointestinal perforation, serious gastrointestinal hemorrhage, cholecystitis, or extraintestinal complications (arteritis, endocarditis, organ abscesses).

Antibiotics should be started empirically while the results of confirmatory tests are pending. The literature describes varying medication recommendations. The regional sensitivity profiles in the antibiotic sensitivity of typhoid vary; thus, the authors' opinion is that these should be taken into account in the initial choice of treatment. Final sensitivity results should be used to determine the definitive treatment.

In absolute numbers, most patients in the United States with typhoid fever were infected in Latin America. However, the greatest risk of infection is travel to India and Pakistan. Because *S typhi* and *S paratyphi* rarely develop antibiotic resistance during treatment, patients who relapse may be given the same drug. However, relapse should dictate a search for anatomical, pathological, or genetic predispositions.

Drug therapy—Chloramphenicol was introduced in 1948 and was once the mainstay of treatment. By the 1970s, widespread resistance to the drug developed. Ampicillin and co-trimoxazole became treatments of choice. However, in the late 1980s, some *S typhi* strains developed simultaneous plasmid-mediated resistance to all 3 drugs. Fluoroquinolones and third-generation cephalosporins have filled the breach, but some resistance exists to both.

Resistance to ciprofloxacin is increasing. Up to 50% of the isolates from Finns with typhoid fever returning from Southeast Asia had reduced susceptibility to ciprofloxacin, with a minimum inhibitory concentration (MIC) of 0.125-0.250—a 9-fold increase. For therapeutic purposes, intermediate susceptibility should be regarded as full resistance. Ciprofloxacin is no longer a good first-line treatment for *S typhi* infection that arises in Southeast Asia. When last evaluated, the rate of intermediate sensitivity in strains was 3.7% in the Americas ($P = 0.132$), 4.7% ($P = 0.144$) in Sub-Saharan Africa, and 10.8% ($P = 0.706$) in the Middle East.

Uncomplicated typhoid fever from the western hemisphere should be treated empirically with ciprofloxacin for 7 days. The treatment for cases from Southeast Asia is controversial. Some authorities recommend high-dose ciprofloxacin in patients from areas with typhoid fever that is resistant to nalidixic acid. (Nalidixic acid is not used clinically but as an in vitro stand-in for measuring fluoroquinolone resistance.) The authors consider this inadequate, as reports of treatment failure under those conditions have increased. The authors recommend empiric first-line therapy with trimethoprim/sulfamethoxazole and second-line therapy with ampicillin or chloramphenicol. Resistance to these agents in Southeast Asia has declined to 5–10%.

Resistance to ceftriaxone is only sporadic in Southeast Asia and elsewhere. Ceftriaxone should be the first-line empiric treatment for severe typhoid fever, and the cours should last 10–14 days.

Clinicians should consider a 48-hour course of dexamethasone if the patient has shock or altered mental status. This may reduce the mortality risk from 56% to 10%. Corticosteroids are reserved for the only the most ill patients because they may increase the risk of relapse.

THYROID HORMONAL DISORDERS AFFECTING

Cardiovascular System

Increased or reduced action of thyroid hormone on certain molecular pathways in the heart and vasculature causes relevant cardiovascular derangements. It is well established that overt hyperthyroidism induces a hyperdynamic cardiovascular state (high cardiac output with low systemic vascular resistance), which is associated with a faster heart rate, enhanced left ventricular (LV) systolic and diastolic function, and increased prevalence of supraventricular tachyarrhythmias — namely, atrial fibrillation — whereas overt hypothyroidism is characterized by the opposite changes. However, whether changes in cardiac performance associated with overt thyroid dysfunction are due mainly to alterations of myocardial contractility or to loading conditions remains unclear. Extensive evidence indicates that the cardiovascular system responds to the minimal but persistent changes in circulating thyroid hormone levels, which are typical of individuals with subclinical thyroid dysfunction.

Subclinical hyperthyroidism is associated with increased heart rate, atrial arrhythmias, increased LV mass, impaired ventricular relaxation, reduced exercise performance, and increased risk of cardiovascular mortality. Subclinical hypothyroidism is associated with impaired LV diastolic function and subtle systolic dysfunction and an enhanced risk for atherosclerosis and myocardial infarction. Because all cardiovascular abnormalities are reversed by restoration of euthyroidism ("subclinical hypothyroidism") or blunted by β-blockade and L-thyroxine (L-T4) dose tailoring ("subclinical hyperthyroidism"), timely treatment is advisable in an attempt to avoid adverse cardiovascular effects. Interestingly, some data indicate that patients with acute and chronic cardiovascular disorders and those undergoing cardiac surgery may have altered peripheral thyroid hormone metabolism that, in turn, may contribute to altered cardiac function. Preliminary clinical investigations suggest that administration of thyroid hormone or its analogue 3,5-diiodothyropropionic acid greatly benefits these patients, highlighting the potential role of thyroid hormone treatment in patients with acute and chronic cardiovascular disease.

Thyroid hormone has relevant effects on the cardiovascular system (Klein and Ojamaa, 2001). Many symptoms and

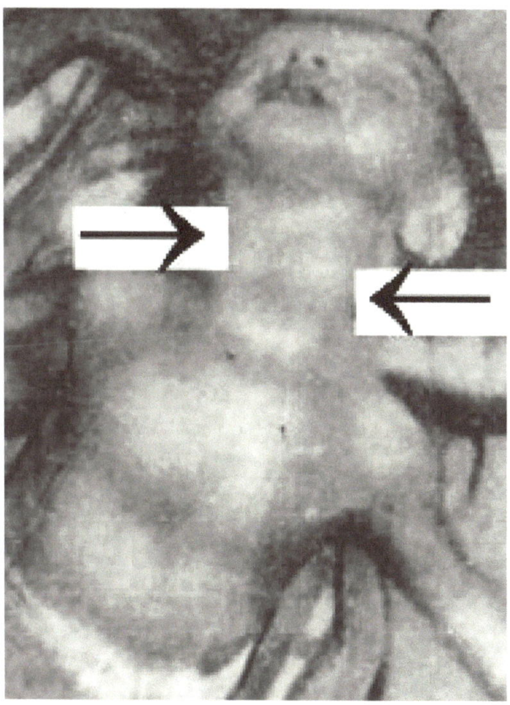

Fig. 40.96: *Photograph of a 12 hours newborn baby with goitrous hypothyroidim with the a history of mother consuming 0.8 g of pottassium iodide for many years in asthma mixture which she was prescribed by the physician. The baby had significant goitre (arrows),marked dyspnoea and huge cardiomegaly and signs of biventricular failure. The baby expired 12 hrs after birth before further measures could be initiated . This case was later published by Dr K.C.Verma and Girja Dhar in journal of the Indian Medical Asoociation. Feb 16,1977*

Table 40.3: *Normal range of TSH, T4 and T3 in infancy and childhood*

	TSH mIU/mL	*T4 g/dL*	*T3 ng/dL*
Cord blood	3–12	8–13	0–70
Newborn	3–18	11–24	75–260
1–5 yrs	2–10	7–15	100–260
5–10 yrs	2–10	6–13	90–240
10–16 yrs	2–10	5–12	80–110
Thereafter	2–10	5–12	115–190

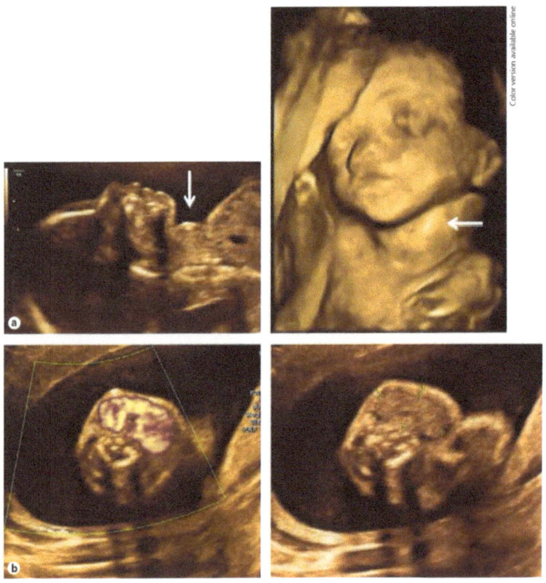

Fig 40.97.a Sagittal (left) and 3D views of the neck at GW 22, showing a large goiter (arrow). b Transverse view with and without power Doppler of the neck at GW 22, hypervascularity in the large goiter is apparent (left)

signs recognized in patients with overt hyperthyroidism and hypothyroidism are due to the increased or reduced action of thyroid hormone on the heart and the vascular system, respectively, and the related hemodynamic derangements. In recent decades, it has emerged that subclinical thyroid dysfunction may affect the cardiovascular system, which may increase cardiovascular risk. It is becoming increasingly apparent that acute and chronic cardiovascular disease may alter thyroid hormone metabolism and contribute to cardiovascular impairment. This chapter will provide an overview of the basic mechanisms underlying the effects of thyroid hormone on the cardiovascular system and their clinical correlates, then address the potential benefit of thyroid hormone treatment in patients with cardiovascular disorders

Most of the molecular and cellular mechanisms responsible for the cardiovascular effects of thyroid hormone have been clarified. Thyroid hormone may exert both genomic and nongenomic effects on cardiac myocytes. The genomic effects of thyroid hormone are mediated by the transcriptional activation or repression of specific target genes that encode both structural and functional proteins (Dillmann, 1990). This process begins with the entry of triiodothyronine (T3), the biologically active thyroid hormone, into the cardiomyocyte through specific transport proteins located within the cell membrane (Everts et al., 1996). To date, there is no clear evidence of a biologically relevant conversion of thyroxine (T4) to T3 in cardiomyocytes (Everts et al., 1996). Once in the cardiomyocyte, T3 enters the nucleus and interacts with specific transcriptional activators (nuclear receptor {alpha}1) or repressors (nuclear receptor {alpha}2). Occupancy of these receptors by T3, in combination with recruited cofactors, allows the thyroid hormone-receptor complex to bind (nuclear receptor {alpha}-1) or release (nuclear receptor {alpha}-2) specific sequences of DNA (thyroid-responsive elements) that, in turn, by acting as cis- or trans-regulators, modify the rate of transcription of specific target genes (Brent, Among various proteins whose expression is modulated at transcriptional level the most-extensively characterized are myosin heavy chains (Morkin, 1993; Ojamaa et al., 1996b) and the sarcoplasmic reticulum protein involved in the regulation of intracellular calcium handling, namely, calcium-activated ATPase and its inhibitory cofactor, phospholamban (Dillmann, 1990; Kiss et al., 1994). Many studies in vitro and in experimental rats incontrovertibly show that thyroid hormone upregulates the expression of the {alpha}-isoform of the myosin heavy chain in cardiomyocytes, while it downregulates the β-isoform (Morkin, 1993; Ojamaa et al. 1996b). There is some evidence that this regulation also occurs in humans (Ladenson et al., 1992). However, the magnitude of this phenomenon is certainly less pronounced than in rodents — a finding that fuels uncertainties about the functional correlate of this molecular effect. In humans, the β-isoform of the myosin heavy chain is more prevalent than the {alpha}-isoform (Magner et al., 1988; Ladenson et al., 1992)

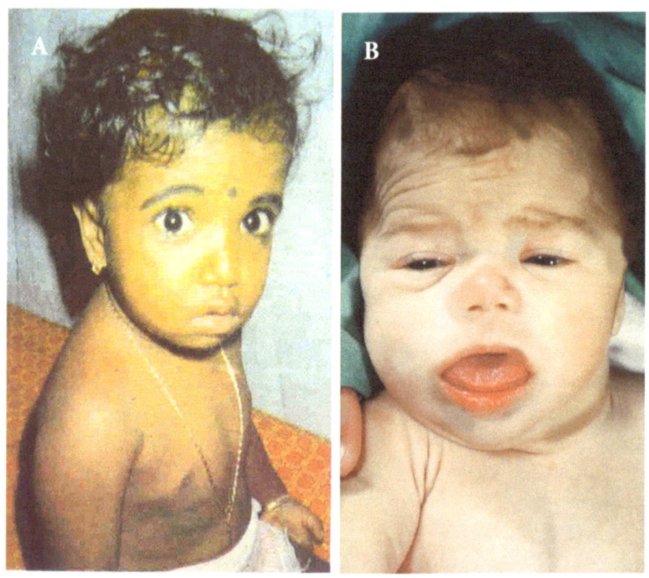

Fig.40.98 Photographs of two children (A) of 3 yrs old girl showing rough, dry skin,and facial puffiness. (B) facilal paillor, protruded tongue in a 2 yrs old child with congenital hypothyroidism

and the ratio is only marginally modified by thyroid hormone (Ladenson et al., 1992).

In contrast, several lines of evidence suggest that some abnormalities of cardiac function in patients with thyroid dysfunction directly reflect the effects of thyroid hormone on calcium-activated ATPase and phospholamban, which are involved primarily in the regulation of systodiastolic calcium concentrations in cardiomyocytes (Dillmann, 1990; Kiss et al., 1994). Sarcoplasmic reticulum calcium-activated ATPase is responsible for the rate of calcium reuptake into the lumen of the sarcoplasmic reticulum during diastole that, in turn, is a major determinant of the velocity of myocardial relaxation after contraction (Dillmann, 1990; Kiss et al., 1994). However, the performance of sarcoplasmic reticulum calcium-activated ATPase is influenced by the level of expression of phospholamban: the higher the phospholamban expression, the lower the sarcoplasmic reticulum calcium-activated ATPase activity (Kiss et al., 1994). In this regard, it has been extensively demonstrated that thyroid hormone upregulates expression of the sarcoplasmic reticulum calcium-activated ATPase and downregulates expression of phospholamban, thereby enhancing myocardial relaxation (Dillmann, 1990; Kiss et al., 1994). Indeed, the improved calcium reuptake during diastole may favorably affect myocardial contractility. In fact, the greater reduction in cytoplasmatic concentration of calcium at end-diastole increases the magnitude of the systolic transient of calcium that, in turn, augments its availability for activation of tropo-myosin units. In fact, in phospholamban-deficient mice, cardiac contractility was found to be increased, with no further increase after thyroid hormone treatment (Kiss et al., 1998). This finding strongly supports the key role of sarcoplasmic reticulum proteins and their effects on intracellular calcium handling in thyroid hormone-mediated changes in systo-diastolic cardiac function in patients with thyroid dysfunction. In this context, it is important to recognize that thyroid hormone also modifies the expression of other ion channels, such as Na+/K+-activated ATPase, Na+/Ca++ exchanger, and some voltage-gated K+ channels (Kv1.5, Kv4.2, Kv4.3), thereby coordinating the electrochemical and mechanical responses of the myocardium (Gick et al., 1990; Ojamaa et al., 1999).

In addition to these genomic effects, thyroid hormone produces changes in cardiac inotropism and chronotropism more rapidly than would be expected from regulation of gene expression, which usually take minutes to hours to be phenotypically and functionally appreciable. This calls into question the involvement of nongenomic mechanisms (Davis and Davis, 1993; Walker et al., 1994). Some evidence indicates that thyroid hormone promotes the acute phosphorylation of phospholamban and that this action attenuates the inhibitory effect of phospholamban on sarcoplasmic reticulum calcium-activated ATPase (Ojamaa et al., 2002). Interestingly, the fact that this process is mediated at least in part by the activation of intracellular kinase pathways involved in signal transduction of the adrenergic stimulus (Ojamaa et al., 2002) may help to explain functional analogies between the cardiovascular effects of thyroid hormone and those promoted by the adrenergic system (Levey and Klein, 1990). Indeed, although most of the cardiovascular manifestations associated with hyperthyroidism and hypothyroidism mimic a condition of increased and reduced adrenergic activity, respectively, the sensitivity of the cardiovascular system to adrenergic stimulation does not seem to be substantially altered in these conditions (Hoit et al., 1997; Ojamaa et al., 2000).

Thyroid hormone also exerts an important effect on the vascular system. It acutely reduces peripheral vascular resistance by promoting relaxation in vascular smooth-muscle cells (Klemperer et al., 1995; Ojamaa et al., 1996a; Park et al., 1997). A single study has reported that chronic thyroid hormone excess exerts profound effects on vascular reactivity by improving both endothelium-dependent and -independent mechanisms (Napoli et al., 2001).

Overt Hyperthyroidism

Palpitation is one of the most-common symptoms associated with overt hyperthyroidism (Nordyke et al., 1988). Continuous, ambulatory, 24-hour electrocardiogram (ECG) monitoring characteristically demonstrates that heart rate is constantly increased during the day and exaggerated in response to exercise, although its circadian rhythm usually is preserved (von Olshausen et al., 1989; Cacciatori et al., 1996). Analysis of heart rate variability reveals sympatho-vagal unbalancing with a relative increase in sympathetic tone (Cacciatori et al., 1996). In this respect, although ß-adrenergic blockade usually attenuates tachycardia in patients with overt hyperthyroidism, heart rates remain slightly higher, in comparison with euthyroid controls. This supports the notion that thyroid hormone is able to directly affect sinus node firing (Sun et al., 2001). About 5–10% of overt hyperthyroid patients have atrial fibrillation, which may be the presenting problem (Sawin et al., 1994; Auer et al., 2001). Atrial fibrillation usually reverts to sinus rhythm with achievement of euthyroidism (Nakazawa et al., 1982), the reversion rate decreasing with

Table 40.4: *Severity of hypothyroidism in relation to thyroid hormone deficiency*

Iodine deficiency	*None*	*Mild*	*Moderate*	*Severe*
Median urine iodine, mcg/L	>100	50-99	20-49	<20
Goiter prevalence	<5%	5-20%	20-30%	>30%
Neonatal thyroid stimulating hormone (TSH), >5 IU/mL whole blood	<3%	3-20%	20-40%	>40%
Cretinism	0	0	+	+

Table 40.4: *Severity of hypothyroidism in relation to thyroid hormone deficiency*

Symptoms palpitations
Exertional dyspnoea
Angina exercise intolerance
Cold intolerance
Physical signs systolic hypertension
Peripheral oedema
Arrhythmia low-volume pulse
Narrow pulse pressure
Peripheral oedema
ECG sinus tachycardia (most common)
Atrial flutter/fibrillation
Left ventricular hypertrophy bradycardia
Prolonged PR/QT intervals
Second/third degree heart block
T wave abnormalitues
Low-voltage ECG (pericardial effusion) blood tests increased serum cholesterol
Increased CRP

age and duration of arrhythmia (Nakazawa et al., 1982; Nordyke et al., 1988). Therefore, achievement of the euthyroid state should be the primary treatment strategy of atrial fibrillation associated with overt hyperthyroidism. β-adrenergic blockade may be used effectively to control the ventricular rate. In all instances, electrical or pharmacological cardioversion should be an option only after achievement of euthyroidism. In this context, it remains controversial whether overt hyperthyroid patients with atrial fibrillation should receive anticoagulant therapy. In general, the risk of bleeding with anticoagulant therapy always should be weighed against the risk of systemic embolization (Gilligan et al., 1996) and the decision made on a case-by-case basis. In general, it would be appropriate to administer anticoagulant agents to older patients with known or suspected heart disease or with atrial fibrillation of longer duration (Petersen and Hansen, 1988; Gilligan et al., 1996)

Systolic arterial pressure is almost invariably increased and diastolic arterial pressure decreased in subjects with overt hyperthyroidism, so that pulse pressure is characteristically wider and mean arterial pressure is only marginally decreased (Graettinger et al., 1959; Theilen and Wilson, 1967; DeGroot and Leonard, 1970). These hemodynamic changes are associated with a remarkable increase in cardiac output and a notable reduction in peripheral vascular resistance, thereby resulting in the classic hyperdynamic cardiovascular state (Graettinger et al., 1959; Theilen and Wilson, 1967; DeGroot and Leonard, 1970).

The main determinants of increased at-rest left ventricular (LV) performance in patients with overt hyperthyroidism have not been definitively established (Biondi et al., 2002a). The high cardiac output state results from a remarkably faster heart rate and a slightly augmented stroke volume that, in turn, is associated with normal or marginally enlarged LV end-diastolic size and normal or marginally decreased LV end-systolic size

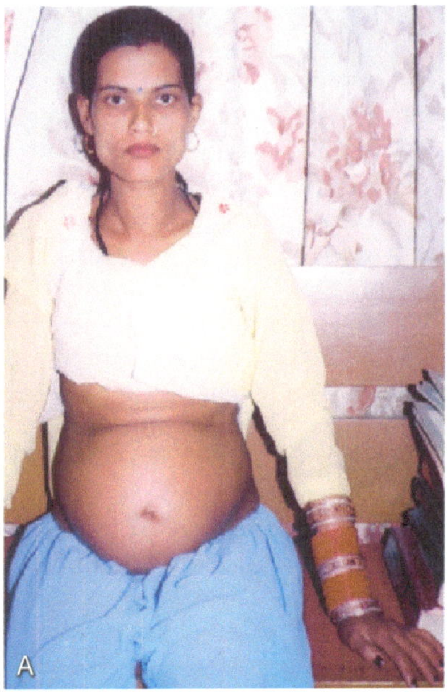
A

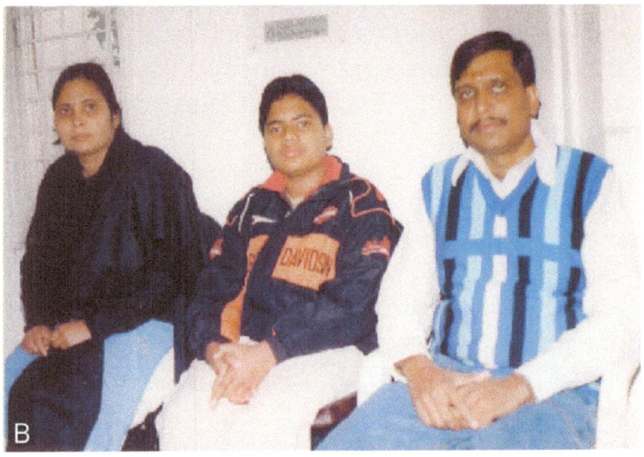
B

Fig. 40.99: *(Upper) showing pregnant young lady with hyperthyroidism under treatment (Lower) a family of hypothyroidism (husband, wife and their child)*

(Biondi et al., 2002a). As a result, LV ejection fraction, an index of overall systolic chamber function, characteristically is increased in overt hyperthyroid subjects (Biondi et al., 2002a). Whether this process is sustained mainly by a true enhancement of myocardial contractility or by the interaction of hemodynamic factors is unclear (Biondi et al., 2002a). Studies by Merillon and colleagues (1981) and by Feldman and coworkers (1986) are emblematic of the controversy surrounding this argument.

Merillon and coworkers (1981) assessed LV function in seven overt thyrotoxic subjects by cardiac catheterization, compared with 11 euthyroid controls atrially paced at a near-identical heart rate. They found no differences between the two groups in such parameters of contractile performance as LV ejection fraction, rate of rise of LV pressure as a proportion of the total pressure, velocity of circumferential fiber shortening, and ratio of LV end-systolic pressure to end-systolic volume. Conversely, it was noted that atrial pacing, but not hyperthyroidism, was accompanied by a marked reduction in both end-diastolic volume and pressure and by a significant increase in

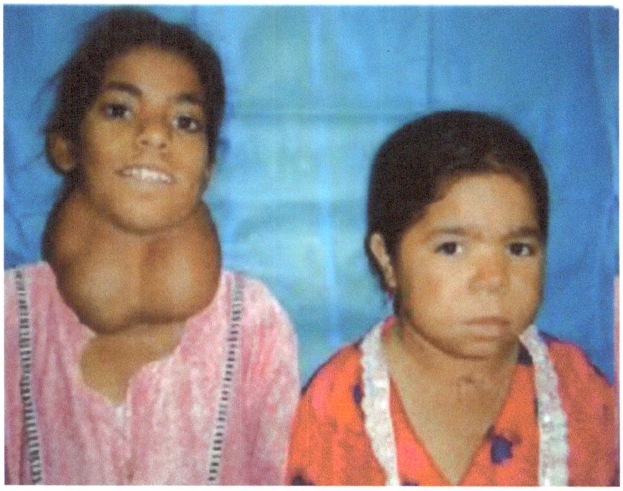

Fig. 40.100: *Photographs of two children showing multinodular thyroid goitor(left) and hypothyroidism without goitor (right)*

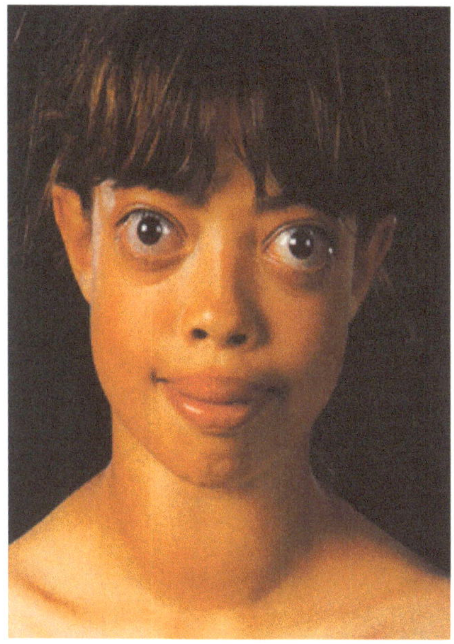

Fig.40.101: *Photograph showing enlargement of thyroid gland ,exophthalmos ,thin physique in 18 yrs old male suffering from hyperthyroidism who clinically presented with atrial fibrrilation and cardiomegaly*

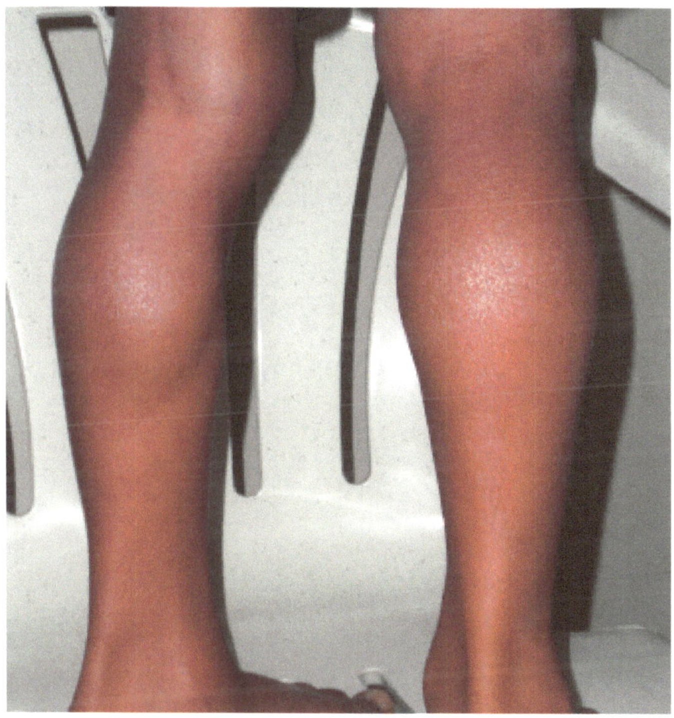

Pseudohypertrophy of calf muscles.

Fig.40.102: *Photographs of a 10 yrs old boy showing calf muscle hypertrophy with hypothyroidism (Kocker -Debrie-semilangene syndrome)*

systemic vascular resistance and mean aortic pressure. As expected, cardiac performance was not increased in atrially paced subjects. Although atrial pacing and hyperthyroidism are not strictly comparable (acute vs. chronic condition), the authors concluded that there was no realistic increase in the true level of myocardial contractility independent of changes in heart rate and preload in human hyperthyroidism.

Feldman and colleagues (1986) studied LV function in 11 hyperthyroid patients by means of echocardiography and in 11 age-matched normal subjects. They found no differences between the two groups in LV end-diastolic diameter or in end-systolic meridional wall stress. Differently, the rate-corrected mean velocity of circumferential fiber shortening (a measure of LV function claimed to be independent of preload and heart rate) was much higher in hyperthyroid patients. As a result, when LV end-systolic wall stress was related to the rate-corrected velocity of fiber shortening, the values of hyperthyroid patients were above the mean regression line for normal subjects, reflecting the presence of an increased contractile state. The authors, however, did not consider that the normal end-diastolic dimension, despite the augmented heart rate in their patients, corresponded to an effective increase in preload, given the inverse relationship between the two variables. Furthermore, the noninvasive method of assessing myocardial contractility by relating the rate-corrected circumferential fiber-shortening velocity to meridional LV end-systolic wall stress may overestimate myocardial performance in pathophysiological states characterized by simultaneous increases in preload and heart rate.

Based on these remarks, it may be assumed that the notably faster heart rate in hyperthyroid patients masks the actual increase in cardiac preload, leading to an underestimation of the extent to which the Frank-Starling mechanism contributes to improving cardiac performance (Biondi et al., 2002a). Indeed, there is evidence that cardiac preload is increased in overt hyperthyroidism. Some studies have demonstrated clearly that blood volume is enlarged in patients with overt hyperthyroidism (Gibson and Harris, 1939; Anthonisen et al., 1960). Other studies

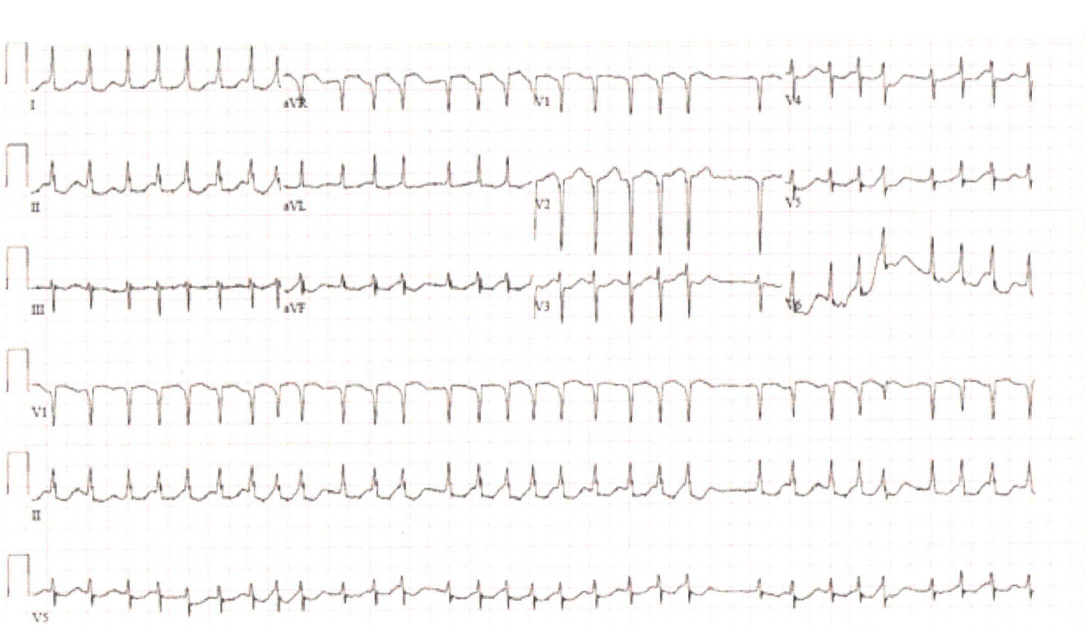

Fig. 40.103: *Electrocardiogram showing atrial fibrillation. P waves are absent and replaced by irregular electrical activity. The ventricular rate is irregular and chaoticin a patient with hyperthyroidism*

showed that the renin-angiotensin-aldosterone system is activated in hyperthyroid patients (Resnick and Laragh, 1982). In addition, thyroid hormone has been shown to upregulate erythropoietin secretion and, in turn, red blood cell mass, which may also contribute to the increase in total blood volume (Gibson and Harris, 1939; Graettinger et al., 1959; Klein and Levey, 1984). Moreover, the analysis of LV diastolic function in different investigations has almost invariably revealed an increase in indices of early LV filling and a faster LV relaxation independent of the effect of heart rate (Lewis et al., 1979; Friedman et al., 1982; Mintz et al., 1991; Kahaly et al., 1999). This pattern of diastolic function is consistent with a greater venous return and enhanced ventricular suction, suggesting that the improvement in diastolic function would allow the increased venous return to be accommodated without relevant changes in filling pressure. This interpretation is supported by the observation of comparable values of LV end-diastolic volume and pressure in hyperthyroid patients and normal subjects (Merillon et al., 1981).

It is, therefore, conceivable that the hyperthyroid heart increases its performance through the advantageous modulation of hemodynamic loads, rather than through recourse to its inotropic reserve (Biondi et al., 2002a). In this regard, it is important to underline that the mechanisms that utilize myocardial contractility involve an ever and necessarily greater myocardial metabolic demand. On the contrary, recourse to the hemodynamic loads to improve cardiac performance is an energetically favorable mechanism. Indeed, recourse to the latter mechanism optimizes the cardiac mechanic-energetic utilization in a condition such as hyperthyroidism, in which a clear increase of myocardial energetic consumption is already present (Bengel et al., 2000).

The complicated and delicate interaction between the different factors determining cardiac function in the patient with overt hyperthyroidism may explain, at least in part, two clinical observations. The first, and more frequent, is reduced exercise tolerance (Kahaly et al., 1998,1999); the second–less-frequently encountered than in the past — is development of congestive heart failure (CHF) (Magner et al., 1988). On the one hand, reduced exercise tolerance of hyperthyroid patients may result from their reduced cardiovascular reserve (Kahaly et al., 1998,1999). In fact, the mechanisms used by the cardiovascular system during exercise are almost largely used at rest. On the other hand, CHF may be precipitated by the occurrence of atrial fibrillation. The loss of atrial contribution to ventricular filling and the reduced diastolic time may severely compromise diastolic dynamics, increasing end-diastolic pressure and promoting systemic congestion. Occasionally, CHF may develop as a result of the so-called "rate-related cardiomyopathy" (Magner et al., 1988).

Subclinical Hyperthyroidism

Subclinical hyperthyroidism is characterized by subnormal or suppressed thyrotropin (TSH) serum levels in the presence of circulating thyroid hormones in the normal range for the general population (Biondi et al., 2002c). It may be due to an intrinsic pathology of the thyroid gland (endogenous subclinical hyperthyroidism) but, more often, is the consequence of suppressive or replacement L-thyroxine (L-T4) therapy (exogenous subclinical hyperthyroidism) (Biondi et al., 2002c). Exogenous subclinical hyperthyroidism is the condition more-frequently seen in clinical practice (Biondi et al., 2002c).

Over past decades, a number of studies have investigated the effects of subclinical hyperthyroidism on the heart,

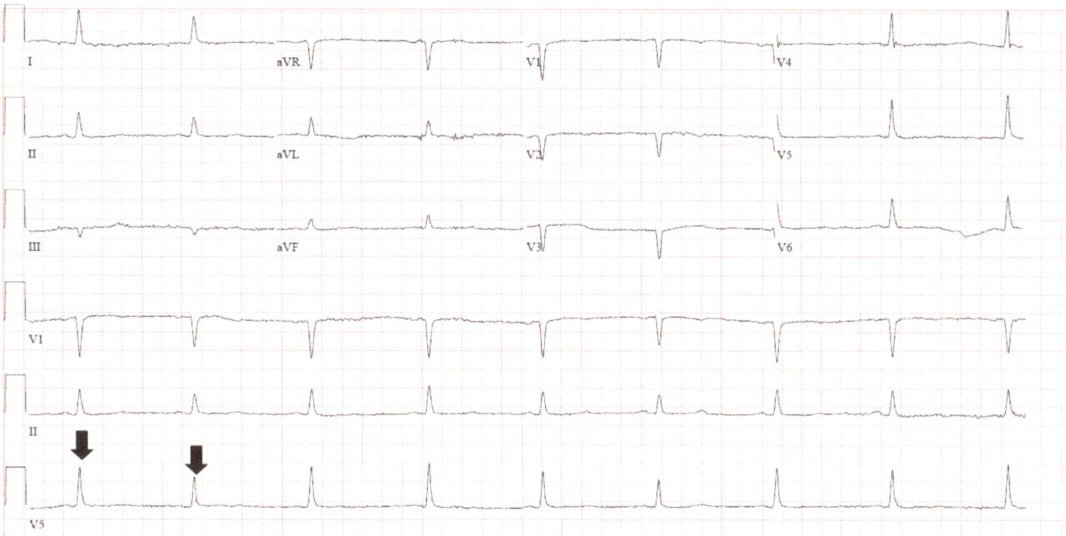

Fig.40.104: *The patient's ECG on arrival to the ED showing low-voltage QRS complexes, electrical alternans (arrows), bradycardia (52 beats/min), and a prolonged QT interval.typical of severe myxoedema.*

showing that this condition may be associated with important abnormalities of cardiac structure and function (Biondi et al., 2002c). The more-consistent abnormalities found in patients with subclinical hyperthyroidism are increased heart rate and prevalence of supraventricular arrhythmias and enhanced LV mass (Biondi et al., 1993, 1994, 1996, 1999b, 2000; Fazio et al., 1995; Ching et al., 1996; Shapiro et al., 1997; Mercuro et al., 2000). The latter feature often is associated with slightly enhanced systolic function and almost always with impaired diastolic function due to slowed myocardial relaxation (Biondi et al., 1993, 1994, 1996, 1999b, 2000; Fazio et al., 1995; Ching et al., 1996; Shapiro et al., 1997; Mercuro et al., 2000). The increase in LV mass is due to increased wall thickness without changes of cavity dimension ("concentric remodeling"). It rarely corresponds to an actual LV hypertrophy and is related to the duration of subclinical hyperthyroidism rather than to circulating thyroid hormone levels. The mechanism responsible for the increase in LV mass has not been completely clarified. In general, it is assumed to develop in response to a chronic hemodynamic overload due to the mild hyperkinetic cardiovascular state (Klein, 1988; Fazio et al., 1995). In fact, as happens with classic models of overload-induced cardiac hypertrophy, the increase of LV mass observed in patients with subclinical hyperthyroidism is associated with slowed myocardial relaxation and impaired ventricular filling. It has been suggested that this diastolic dysfunction results from altered intracellular calcium handling due to reduced expression of sarcoplasmic reticulum calcium ATPase and/or increased expression of phospholamban, with the consequent delayed sarcoplasmic reuptake of calcium. However, this view would contrast with the well-known effects of thyroid hormone on such genes (Dillmann, 1990; Kiss et al., 1994). Therefore, it may be hypothesized that, in the long-term, the effects of chronically increased cardiac workload on calcium metabolism would prevail on those promoted by thyroid hormone. Be that as it may, abnormalities of LV morphology and function promptly normalize with achievement of euthyroidism and are effectively attenuated by β-blocking drugs (Biondi et al., 1994, 1995, 1999b, 2000). This supports the concept that cardiac involvement in subclinical hyperthyroidism is reversible and mostly determined by functional mechanisms.

Importantly, compelling evidence exists that subclinical hyperthyroidism is associated with increased cardiovascular mortality (Parle et al., 2001). Although the mechanism responsible for this association remains obscure, several factors may contribute to this phenomenon (Biondi et al., 2002b). There are indications that patients with subclinical hyperthyroidism, particularly the elderly, have an increased risk of atrial fibrillation (Sawin et al., 1994; Auer et al., 2001), which may enhance the incidence of thromboembolic events (Petersen and Hansen, 1988; Ladenson, 1993). It has been shown that the increase of LV mass per se, even in the absence of a clear LV hypertrophy, and of heart rate are associated with an increased risk of sudden death (Haider et al., 1998; Greenland et al., 1999). Moreover, it is well-recognized that diastolic dysfunction may precede development of more-severe LV dysfunction. Indeed, especially in the elderly, it may precipitate cardiac decompensation and CHF. Therefore, the current opinion is to avoid or correct subclinical hyperthyroidism in all patients affected with benign thyroid disease (Biondi et al., 2002c). On the contrary, when subclinical hyperthyroidism is a therapeutic indication (e.g. in patients with differentiated thyroid cancer), L-T4 should be administered at the lowest dose sufficient to achieve a stable TSH suppression, eventually associated with chronic ß-blockade (Biondi et al., 2002c). Contextually, subclinical hyperthyroidism should be suspected in all subjects with a history of atrial fibrillation, especially in the elderly and in those with underlying cardiac disease who complain of worsening of angina pectoris or cardiac decompensation.

Overt Hypothyroidism

The cardiovascular effects of thyroid hormone deficiency are opposite to those caused by thyroid hormone excess. However, the clinical presentation of overt hypothyroidism is not obvious and most patients have few symptoms and signs (Klein and Ojamaa, 2000). Bradycardia and systemic hypertension, with narrow pulse pressure and slightly increased mean arterial pressure, and some degree of exercise impairment are the most-common findings in patients with overt hypothyroidism (McAllister et al., 1995; Klein and Ojamaa, 2000).

Many patients with overt hypothyroidism have abnormal standard ECG, including QT interval lengthening and flattening or inversion of the T wave (Fredlund and Olsson, 1983; Klein and Ojamaa, 2000), which reflects the prolonged cardiac action potential (Ojamaa et al., 1999). In addition, overt hypothyroid patients are more prone to ventricular arrhythmias, particularly in the presence of an underlying ischemic heart disease, due to increased electrical dispersion in the myocardium (Fredlund and Olsson, 1983; Klein and Ojamaa, 2000).

The prevalence of systemic hypertension is nearly three-fold higher in patients with overt hyperthyroidism than in euthyroid subjects. In addition, in patients with systemic hypertension, overt hypothyroidism is associated with higher blood pressure (Endo et al., 1979; Saito et al., 1983; Streeten et al., 1988; Klein, 1989; Fletcher and Weetman, 1998; Fommei and Iervasi, 2002). Two factors contribute to systemic hypertension in overt hypothyroidism. The first, and certainly the most-widely recognized, is the remarkable increase in peripheral vascular resistance (Klein and Ojamaa, 2000). The second, and more-recently documented, is the increase in arterial stiffness, which likely results from myxedema of the arterial wall (Dernellis and Panaretou, 2002; Obuobie et al., 2002). In general, systemic hypertension associated with overt hypothyroidism is poorly controlled by conventional treatments, whereas it promptly improves with achievement of euthyroidism (Dernellis and Panaretou, 2002). This finding would encourage the routine assessment of thyroid function in all patients with preexisting systemic hypertension that becomes resistant to pharmacological treatment.

The most-consistent cardiac abnormality recognized in patients with overt hypothyroidism is impairment of LV diastolic function, which is characterized by slowed myocardial relaxation and impaired early ventricular filling (Crowley et al., 1977; Wieshammer et al., 1989). LV systolic function usually is only marginally subnormal, as demonstrated by slightly reduced values of ejection fraction and stroke volume (Crowley et al., 1977; Wieshammer et al., 1989). On the one hand, the reduced cardiac preload, in combination with bradycardia and slightly depressed myocardial contractility, accounts for a subnormal cardiac output in overt hypothyroidism (Crowley et al., 1977; Wieshammer et al., 1989). On the other hand, the lower cardiac performance and the abnormalities in peripheral and proximal vascular function may contribute to the poor exercise tolerance in overt hypothyroidism (McAllister et al., 1995).

Occasionally, cardiac function may be further compromised by the development of pericardial effusion, which occurs with severe, long-standing overt hypothyroidism (Ladenson et al., 1992). In addition, overt hypothyroidism may be associated with some increase in LV mass. However, as shown by necropsy and ultrasound investigations, the increase in LV mass does not correspond to myocardial hypertrophy sensu strictu but rather to interstitial myxedema (Aber, 1964). By increasing wall stiffness, cardiac myxedema may further compromise LV mechanics, contributing to reduced cardiac output.

In this context, it is important to recall that although overt hypothyroidism is associated with a lower myocardial oxygen demand, myocardial mechanical work efficiency is worse than in euthyroid controls and improves with achievement of euthyroidism (Bengel et al., 2000). The increase in peripheral vascular resistance and arterial stiffness in overt hypothyroidism contributes to increased cardiac afterload, one of the major factors determining myocardial oxygen consumption (Bengel et al., 2000). The disproportionate increase in myocardial oxygen uptake with respect to the level of cardiac performance may, therefore, explain at least in part why overt hypothyroidism may precipitate or worsen angina in patients with suspected or known ischemic heart disease (Keating et al., 1960) and why some of these patients have an improvement in anginal symptoms after thyroid hormone replacement is initiated.

Overt hypothyroidism may be particularly hazardous in the elderly, independent of the presence of underlying cardiovascular disease. Aging is accompanied by the development of cardiac hypertrophy and interstitial fibrosis, which may be responsible per se for diastolic dysfunction and reduced cardiovascular performance. Therefore, the onset of overt hypothyroidism in this vulnerable population occasionally may precipitate cardiac decompensation and CHF. In a single study, it was estimated that approximately 30–50% of elderly subjects with heart failure have normal values of ejection fraction (diastolic heart failure) (McDermott et al., 1995). Noteworthy, diastolic heart failure was strongly associated with hypothyroidism and was more prevalent in women (McDermott et al., 1995). Therefore, thyroid function should be routinely assessed in older patients with newly diagnosed or worsening heart failure.

Subclinical Hypothyroidism

Subclinical hypothyroidism (SH), defined by elevated serum TSH level in the presence of normal levels of free thyroid hormones, is common in the adult population, especially among women above 60 years of age (Tunbridge et al., 1977; Canaris et al., 2000). Up to two thirds of patients have serum TSH between 5–10 mU/L and thyroid autoantibodies (Tunbridge et al., 1977; Canaris et al., 2000). Almost half of these individuals may progress to overt thyroid failure (Vanderpump et al., 1995; Huber et al., 2002). Striking evidence indicates that elevated TSH levels in SH patients do not reflect pituitary compensation to maintain euthyroidism but mild tissue hypothyroidism sensu strictu (Andersen et al., 2002). Several changes in metabolic and organ function indexes have been reported in most clinical investigations of patients with persistent SH (Biondi et al., 2002c). Deviation from normality progressively increases with serum TSH level ("dosage effect" phenomenon) (Lekakis et al., 1997; Bindels et al., 1999; Faber et al., 2002). In general, resting heart rate and blood pressure are normal in SH subjects (Biondi et al., 1999a; Monzani et al., 2001; Di Bello et al., 2002; Vitale et al., 2002). However, significant hypofunctional abnormalities in the parasympathetic nervous system and an increased prevalence of systemic hypertension have been reported in patients with SH (Kahaly, 2000; Luboshitzky et al., 2002).

The most-consistent cardiac abnormality recognized in SH patients is LV diastolic dysfunction, characterized by slowed myocardial relaxation and impaired early ventricular filling, both at rest and with exercise (Biondi et al., 1999a; Monzani et al., 2001; Di Bello et al., 2002; Vitale et al., 2002; Brenta et al., 2003). Often, this is associated with a variable impairment in LV systolic function at rest (Biondi et al., 1999a; Monzani et al., 2001; Di Bello et al., 2002; Vitale et al., 2002), which becomes more consistent on exercise (Foldes et al., 1987; Kahaly, 2000; Brenta et al., 2003). In a comprehensive study of exercise capacity, it was reported that SH is associated with impairment of several exercise-related cardiopulmonary responses, resulting in some degree of exercise impairment (Kahaly, 2000).

Recently, a strong association between SH and atherosclerotic cardiovascular disease, independent of the traditional risk factors (i.e. hypercholesterolemia, hypertension, smoking, diabetes mellitus), was noted in a large cross-sectional survey of postmenopausal women (the Rotterdam Study) (Hak et al., 2000). Although the mechanism responsible for this association remains to be clarified, compelling evidence indicates that SH is associated with an atherogenic lipid profile, characterized by increased circulating levels of total and low-density cholesterol and increased levels of oxidized low-density lipoproteins (Duntas, 2002; Duntas et al., 2002). It has been reported that SH may affect the hemostatic profile, thereby promoting a hypercoagulable state (Müller et al., 2001). Moreover, a reduced endothelium-dependent, flow-mediated vasodilation, which is an early marker of atherosclerosis, has been reported in patients with SH (Lekakis et al., 1997).

Importantly, when SH patients are treated with L-T4, most metabolic and cardiovascular abnormalities improve or even normalize (Danese et al., 2000; Biondi et al., 2002c). However, whether patients with SH should be treated remains the subject of disagreement (Chu and Crapo, 2001; McDermott and Ridgway, 2001).

Amiodarone and Thyroid Disease

Amiodarone, a class III antiarrhythmic agent, is widely used in atrial and ventricular rhythm disturbances. The high iodine content of amiodarone (3mg iodine per 100mg amiodarone) can result in hypothyroidism (5–25 per cent of treated patients) or hyperthyroidism (2–10 per cent).[5]

The baseline serum TSH, free T4 and T3, and antithyroid antibodies should be measured before starting amiodarone and monitored every six months.

Amiodarone-induced hyperthyroidism is described as type-1 in patients with existing thyroid disease or goitre and type-2 in euthyroid patients. Hypothyroidism should be treated with thyroxine replacement.

Treatment of both types of amiodarone-induced hyperthyroidism is more difficult. It is relatively resistant to the thio-ureas owing to high intrathy-roid iodine content, and the effect of radioactive iodine is poor because iodine uptake by the thyroid is reduced.

A pragmatic approach is to treat patients with high-dose carbimazole. Resistance to carbimazole should raise the possibility of type-2 disease.

Treatment with potassium perchlorate, with or without oral prednisolone 30–40mg per day, should be considered. Refractory cases may need thyroidectomy.

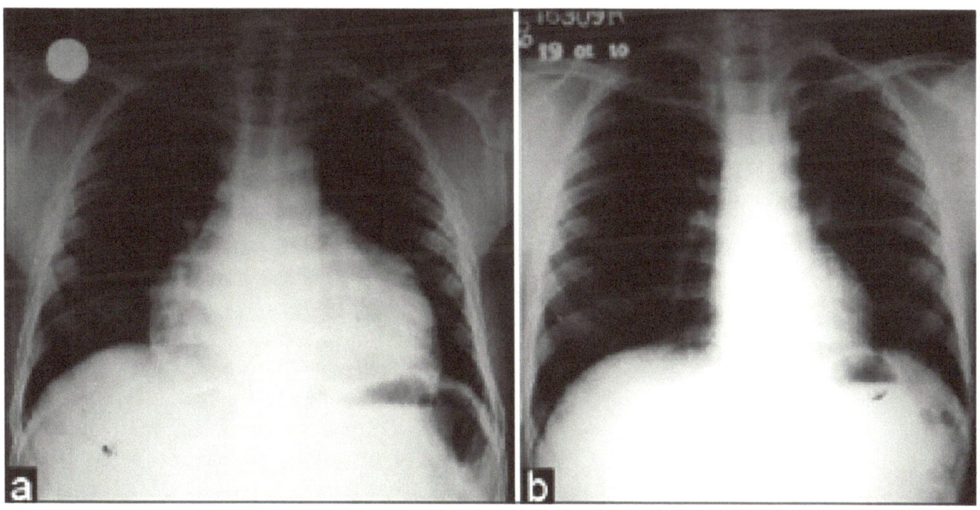

Fig. 40.105: *(a) Chest X-ray PA view showing cardiomegaly before treatment. (b) Chest X-ray PA view showing resolution of cardiac enlargement after thyroxine supplementation at follow-up (8 months)*

Conclusion

Thyroid dysfunction causes remarkable cardiovascular derangements. Because signs and symptoms referable to the cardiovascular system may be the only manifestations of overt thyroid dysfunction and because persistent subclinical thyroid dysfunction may notably increase the cardiovascular risk, thyroid status should be systematically investigated in all patients with newly diagnosed or worsening cardiovascular disease, especially the elderly. In addition, patients with acute or chronic cardiovascular disorders have abnormalities in peripheral thyroid hormone metabolism that may alter cardiac function. The finding that administration of thyroid hormone or its analog 3,5-diiodothyropropionic acid may greatly benefit these patients should foster further investigation in this area.

THALASSEMIAS AND HEART DISEASE

Thalassemia (British spelling, "thalassaemia") is an inherited autosomal recessive blood disease. In thalassemia, the genetic defect results in reduced rate of synthesis of one of the globin chains that make up hemoglobin. Reduced synthesis of one of the globin chains can cause the formation of abnormal haemoglobin molecules, and this in turn causes the anemia which is the characteristic presenting symptom of the thalassemias.

Thalassemia is a quantitative problem of too few globins synthesized, whereas sickle-cell disease (a haemoglobinopathy) is a qualitative problem of synthesis of an incorrectly functioning globin (Figs 47.106–108).

Thalassemias usually result in under production of normal globin proteins, often through mutations in regulatory genes. Hemoglobinopathies imply structural abnormalities in the globin proteins themselves [1]. The two conditions may overlap, however, since some conditions which cause abnormalities in globin proteins (hemoglobinopathy) also affect their production (thalassemia). Thus, some thalassemias are hemoglobinopathies, but most are not. Either or both of these conditions may cause anemia. The disease is particularly prevalent among Mediterranean peoples, and this geographical association was response between ble for its naming: Thalassa (èÜëáóóá) is Greek for the sea, Haema (áßìá) is Greek for blood. In Europe, the highest concentrations of the disease are found in Greece, including the Greek islands; in parts of Italy, in particular, the lower Po valley; in southern Italy; and in the Italian islands. Sicily, Sardinia (Italian islands), Corsica (French island) and Cyprus and Crete (Greek islands) are heavily affected in particular; the higher incidence in these islands likely is because of the higher inbreeding that occurs in isolated populations. But Asia now has even greater prevalence, with the highest concentration of carriers (18% of the population) in the Maldives.

Prevalence

Generally, thalassemias are prevalent in populations that evolved in humid climates where malaria was endemic, but affects all races. Thalassemias are particularly associated with Arabs, people of Mediterranean origin, and Asians.[2] The Maldives has the highest incidence of Thalassemia in the world with a carrier rate of 18% of the population. The estimated prevalence is 16% in people from Cyprus, 3–14% in Thailand, and 3–8% in populations from Bangladesh, China, India, Malaysia and Pakistan. There are also prevalences in descendants of people from Latin America, and Mediterranean countries (e.g. Greece, Italy, Portugal, Spain, and others). A very low prevalence has been reported from people in northern Europe (0.1%) and Africa (0.9%), with those in northern Africa having the highest prevalence.[4] Ancient Egyptians suffered from Thalassemia and it was particularly common in populations of indigenous ethnic minorities such as the Beja, Hadendoa, Saiddi and Siwans.

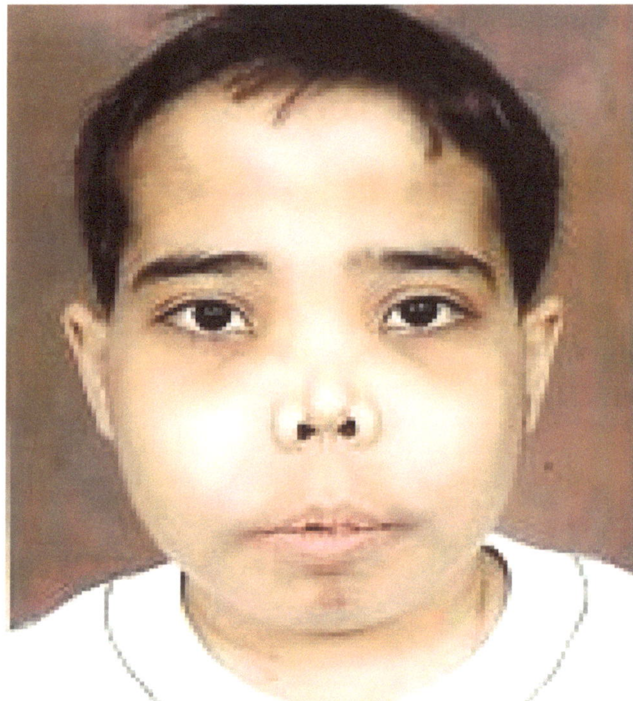

Fig. 40.106: *Photograph showing prominence of frontal, parietal, and maxillary bones due to bone marrow hypertrophy ,depressed bridge of nose and typical pallor giving an impression of 'mongoloid facies' in a young patient with thalassemia major*

Pathophysiology

The thalassemias are classified according to which chain of the hemoglobin molecule is affected (*see* hemoglobin for a description of the chains). In α thalassemias, production of the α globin chain is affected, while in α thalassemia production of the α globin chain is affected.

Thalassemia produces a deficiency of β or α globin, unlike sickle-cell disease which produces a specific mutant form of α globin. α globin chains are encoded by a single gene on chromosome 11; α globin chains are encoded by two closely linked genes on chromosome 16. Thus in a normal person with two copies of each chromosome, there are two loci encoding the β chain, and four loci encoding the β chain.[3]

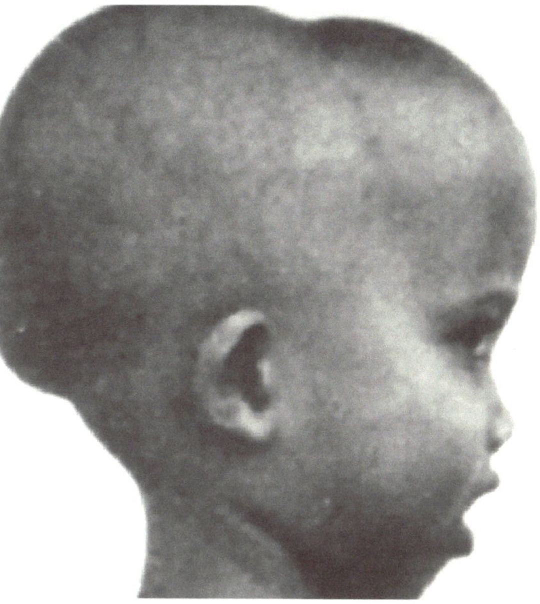

Fig. 40.107: *Showing enlargement of skull bones in a child with longstanding beta -thalassemia*

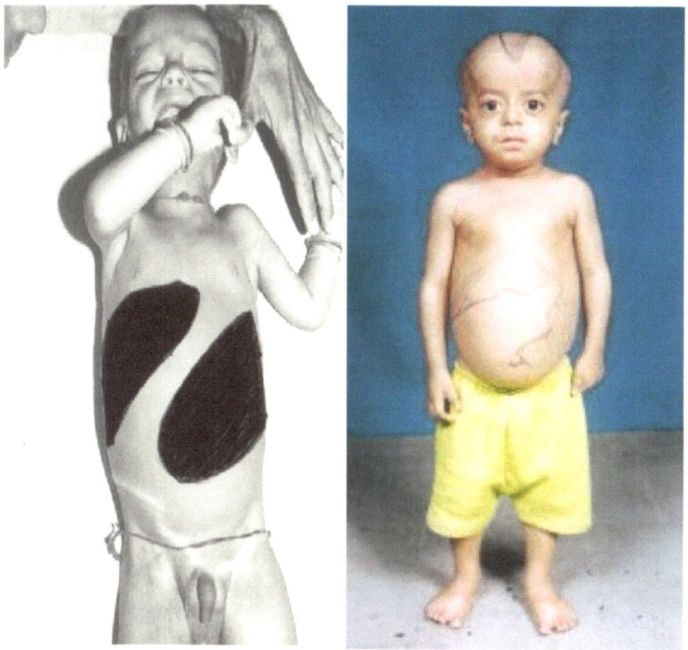

Fig. 40.108: *Photographs showing splenohepatomegaly in two young children with thalassemia major*

Deletion of one of the α loci has a high prevalence in people of African-American or Asian descent, making them more likely to develop α thalassemias. α thalassemias are common in African-Americans, but also in Greeks and Italians.

Alpha (α) thalassemias: The α thalassemias involve the genes HBA1 (Online 'Mendelian Inheritance in Man' (OMIM) 141800) and HBA2 (Online 'Mendelian Inheritance in Man' (OMIM) 141850), inherited in a Mendelian recessive fashion. It is also connected to the deletion of the 16p chromosome. α thalassemias result in decreased alpha-globin production, therefore fewer alpha-globin chains are produced, resulting in an excess of β chains in adults and excess β chains in newborns. The excess β chains form unstable tetramers (called Hemoglobin H or HbH of 4 beta chains) which have abnormal oxygen dissociation curves. There are four genetic loci for α globin, two of which are maternal in origin and two of which are paternal in origin. The severity of the á thalassemias is correlated with the number of affected á globin loci: the greater the number of affected loci, the more severe will be the manifestations of the disease.

- If one of the four á loci is affected, there is minimal effect. Three α-globin loci are enough to permit normal hemoglobin production, and there are no clinical symptoms. They have been called silent carriers. They may have a slightly reduced mean corpuscular volume and mean corpuscular hemoglobin.

If two of the four á loci are affected, the condition is called alpha thalassemia trait. Two á loci permit nearly normal erythropoiesis, but there is a mild microcytic hypochromic anemia. The disease in this form can be mistaken for iron deficiency anemia and treated inappropriately with iron. Alpha thalassemia trait can exist in two forms: one form, associated with Asians, involves cis deletion of two alpha loci on the same chromosome; the other, associated with Blacks, involves trans deletion of alpha loci on different (homologous) chromosomes.

- If three loci are affected, the condition is called Hemoglobin H disease. Two unstable hemoglobins are present in the blood: Hemoglobin Barts (tetrameric γ chains) and Hemoglobin H (tetrameric β chains). Both of these unstable hemoglobins have a higher affinity for oxygen than normal hemoglobin, resulting in poor oxygen delivery to tissues. There is a microcytic hypochromic anemia with target cells and Heinz bodies (precipitated HbH) on the peripheral blood smear, as well as splenomegaly. The disease may first be noticed in

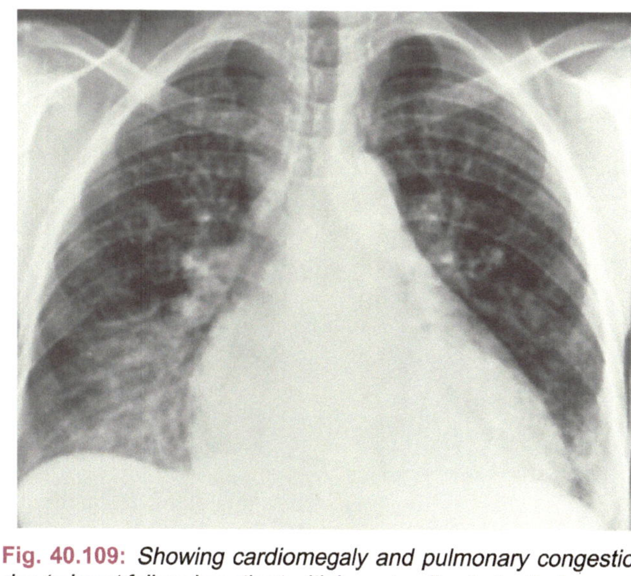

Fig. 40.109: *Showing cardiomegaly and pulmonary congestion due to heart failure in patient with longstanding beta -thalassemia*

childhood or in early adult life, when the anemia and splenomegaly are noted.

- If all *four* loci are affected, the fetus cannot live once outside the uterus and may not survive gestation: most such infants are dead at birth with *hydrops fetalis*, and those who are born alive die shortly after birth. They are edematous and have little circulating hemoglobin, and the hemoglobin that is present is all tetrameric ã chains (hemoglobin Barts)

Beta (β) thalassemias

Beta thalassemias are due to mutations in the HBB gene on chromosome 11 (Online 'Mendelian Inheritance in Man' (OMIM) 141900), also inherited in an autosomal-recessive fashion. The severity of the disease depends on the nature of the mutation. Mutations are characterized as (β^o) if they prevent any formation of β chains; they are characterized as (β^+) if they allow some β chain formation to occur. In either case there is a relative excess of β chains, but these do not form tetramers: rather, they bind to the red blood cell membranes, producing membrane damage, and at high concentrations they form toxic aggregates. Any given individual has two α globin alleles.

- If only *one* α globin allele bears a mutation, the disease is called **α thalassemia minor** (or sometimes called **β thalassemia trait**). This is a mild microcytic anemia. In most cases β thalassemia minor is asymptomatic, and many affected people are unaware of the disorder. Detection usually involves measuring the mean corpuscular volume (size of red blood cells) and noticing a slightly decreased mean volume than normal. The patient will have an increased fraction of Hemoglobin A2 (>2.5%) and a decreased fraction of Hemoglobin A (<97.5%).

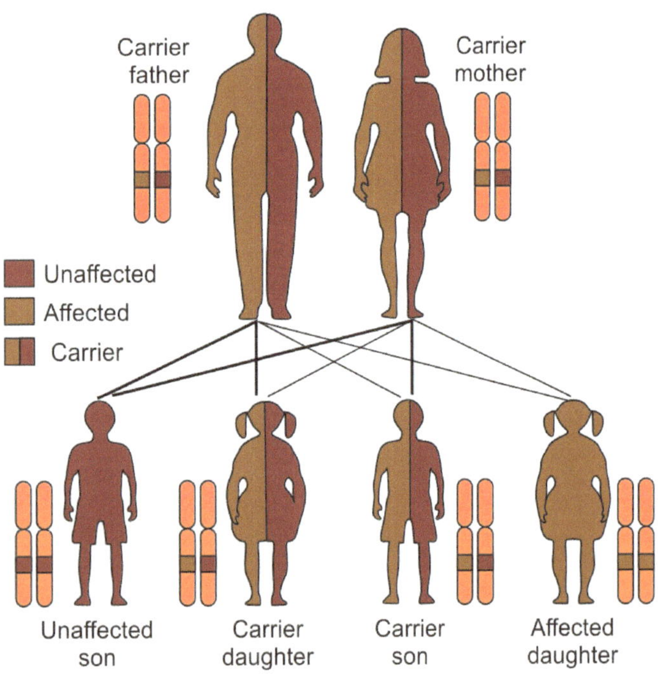

Fig. 47.110: *Diagram showing genetic transmission of beta - thalassemia*

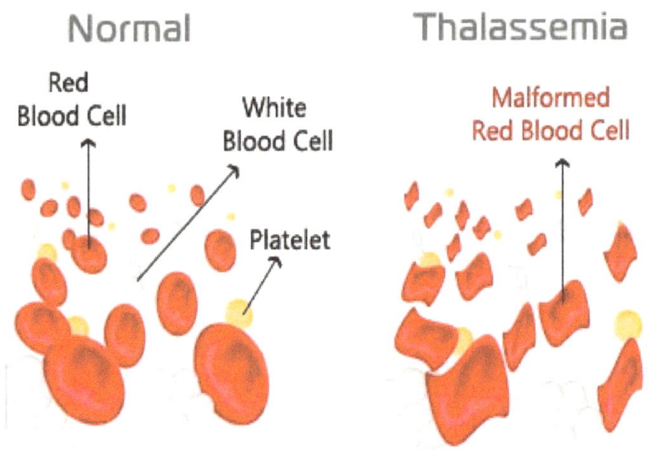

Fig.40.111: *Blood films comparing normal with that of thalassemic patient. Thalassemiais an inherited blood disorder characterised by abnormal formation of hemoglobin (absent or decreased) and red blood cells in the body.*

If *both* alleles have thalassemia mutations, the disease is called **β thalassemia major** or **Cooley's anemia**. This is a severe microcytic, hypochromic anemia. Untreated, this progresses to death before age twenty. Treatment consists of periodic blood transfusion; splenectomy if splenomegaly is present, and treatment of transfusion-caused iron overload. Cure is possible by bone marrow transplantation.

Thalassemia intermedia is a condition intermediate between the major and minor forms. Affected individuals can often manage a normal life but may need occasional transfusions, e.g. at times of illness or pregnancy, depending on the severity of their anemia.

The genetic mutations present in â thalassemias are very diverse, and a number of different mutations can cause reduced or absent β globin synthesis. Two major groups of mutations can be distinguished:

Nondeletion forms: These defects generally involve a single base substitution or small deletion or inserts near or upstream of the â globin gene. Most commonly, mutations occur in the promoter regions preceding the beta-globin genes. Less often, abnormal splice variants are believed to contribute to the disease.

Deletion forms: Deletions of different sizes involving the a globin gene produce different syndromes such as (b^o) or hereditary persistence of fetal hemoglobin syndromes.

Delta (δ) thalassemia

As well as alpha and beta chains being present in hemoglobin about 3% of adult hemoglobin is made of alpha and delta chains. Just as with beta thalassemia, mutations can occur which affect the ability of this gene to produce delta chains. A mutation that prevents formation of any delta chains is termed a $delta^0$ mutation, whereas one that decreases but does not eliminate production of delta chain is termed a $delta^+$ mutation. When one inherits two $delta^0$

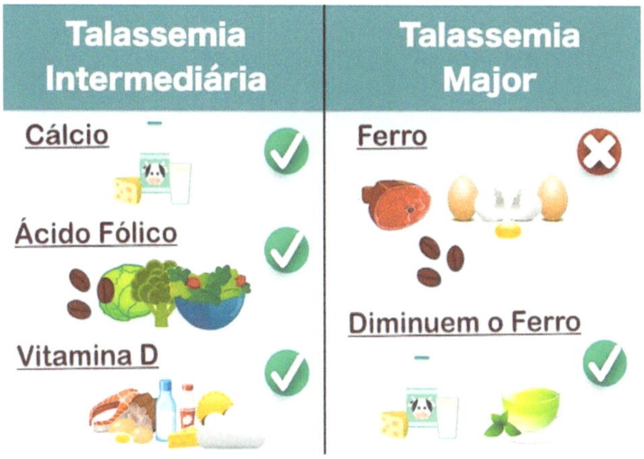

Fig.40.112 Diet In thalassemia intermedia, the patient has moderate anemia and may not need a blood transfusion, it is necessary to increase the levels of calcium, vitamin D and folic acid to improve quality of life. Thalassemia major is the most severe form of the disease, in which the patient needs to receive blood transfusions frequently. Due to transfusions, there is an accumulation of iron in the body that can be harmful to organs such as the heart and liver. Thus, excess iron-rich foods such as liver, red meat, seafood, egg yolks and beans should be avoided

mutations, no hemoglobin A2 (alpha2, delta2) can be formed. Hematologically, however, this is innocuous because only 2–3% of normal adult hemoglobin is hemoglobin A2. The individual will have normal hematological parameters (erythrocyte count, total hemoglobin, mean corpuscular volume, red cell distribution width). Individuals who inherit only one delta thalassemia mutation gene will have a decreased hemoglobin A2, but also no hematological consequences. The importance of recognizing the existence of delta thalassemia is seen best in cases where it may mask the diagnosis of beta thalassemia trait. In beta thalassemia, there is an increase in hemoglobin A2, typically in the range of 4–6% (normal is 2-3%). However, the co-existence of a delta thalassemia mutation will decrease the value of the hemoglobin A2 into the normal range, thereby obscuring the diagnosis of beta thalassemia trait. This can be important in genetic counseling, because a child who is the product of parents each of whom has beta^0 thalassemia trait has a one in four chance of having beta thalassemia major.
In combination with other hemoglobinopathies

Thalassemia can co-exist with other hemoglobinopathies. The most common of these are:

- Hemoglobin E/thalassemia: common in Cambodia, Thailand, and parts of India; clinically similar to â thalassemia major or thalassemia intermedia. hemoglobin S/thalassemia, common in African and Mediterranean populations; clinically similar to sickle cell anemia, with the additional feature of splenomegaly
- Hemoglobin C/thalassemia: common in Mediterranean and African populations, hemoglobin C/â^o thalassemia causes a moderately severe hemolytic anemia with splenomegaly; hemoglobin C/â$^+$ thalassemia produces a milder disease.

Treatment and Complications

Anyone with thalassemia should consult a properly qualified hematologist. Thalassemias may co-exist with other deficiencies such as folic acid (or folate, a B-complex vitamin) and iron deficiency (only in Thalassemia Minor).

Thalassemia Major and Intermedia

Thalassemia Major patients receive frequent blood transfusions that lead to iron overload. Iron chelation treatment is necessary to prevent iron overload damage to the internal organs in patients with Thalassemia Major. Because of recent advances in iron chelation treatments, patients with Thalassemia Major can live long lives if they have access to proper treatment. Popular chelators include deferoxamine and deferiprone. Of the two, deferoxamine is preferred; it is more effective and is associated with fewer side-effects.

The most common complaint by patients receiving deferoxamine is that it is difficult to comply with the intravenous chelation treatments because they are painful and inconvenient. The oral chelator deferasirox (marketed as Exjade by Novartis) was approved for use in 2005 in some countries. It offers some hope with compliance but is very expensive, and has been associated with deaths from toxicity.

Untreated thalassemia Major eventually leads to death usually by heart failure, therefore birth screening is very important. In recent years, bone marrow transplant has shown promise with some patients of thalassemia major. Successful transplant can eliminate the patients dependencies in transfusions.

All Thalassemia patients are susceptible to health complications that involve the spleen (which is often enlarged and frequently removed) and gall stones. These complications are mostly prevalent to thalassemia Major and Intermedia patients. Thalassemia Intermedia patients vary a lot in their treatment needs depending on the severity of their anemia.

Thalassemia Minor

Contrary to popular belief, Thalassemia Minor patients should not avoid iron-rich foods by default. A serum ferritin test can determine what their iron levels are and guide them to further treatment if necessary. Thalassemia Minor, although not life threatening on its own, can affect quality of life due to the effects of a mild to moderate anemia. Studies have shown that Thalassemia Minor often coexists with other diseases such as asthma, and mood disorders.

Complications

- Iron overload
- Traditionally, ferritin level assessment has been the most commonly used test for indirect evaluation of body iron stores, even though it reflects only 1% of the total iron storage pool. The test is not perfect or accurate, as various conditions complicate the interpretation of its values. For this reason, reliance on serum ferritin assessment alone

can lead to an inaccurate assessment of body iron stores in patients with iron overload who have been transfused heavily and who have levels in excess of the upper limit for the physiologic ferritin synthesis (400 mcg/L). At high levels, the test loses its clinical relevance since ferritin can be released from damaged cells in certain pathologic conditions.

Furthermore, certain drugs and clinical conditions such as ascorbate deficiency, fever, acute and chronic infections, and hemolysis may influence the ferritin level, producing misleading values. Despite its deficiencies, and for lack of a better practical, noninvasive test, ferritin assessment continues to be the most commonly used tool to diagnose and to monitor iron overload.

MRI or CT scanning is used to assess liver iron levels as a measure of total body iron load.

Liver biopsy may be performed to assess liver iron concentration, which is considered the most sensitive method to assess body iron burden. Again, this procedure is an invasive one and not without complications. Furthermore, because iron distribution in the thalassemic liver is uneven and could be affected by fibrosis, one can expect conflicting and inaccurate results in some patients. Grading of stainable iron or measuring parenchymal iron by atomic absorption spectroscopy has been helpful in measuring tissue iron levels, with good correlation to calculated body iron burden.

Cardiac Complications

- Most deaths in patients with thalassemia are due to cardiac involvement. These complications range from constrictive pericarditis to heart failure and arrhythmias.
- Transfusional hemosiderosis has been classified into 3 stages based on the number of blood units given. The higher the number of PRBC units given, the more advanced the stage. Advanced stage is associated with more severe clinical symptoms and more abnormal findings on cardiac function studies.
- Cardiac hemosiderosis does not occur without significant accumulation of iron in other tissues.
- Chelation therapy has shown promising results in patients with cardiac symptoms due to iron overload.
- Ventricular myocardium is the first site of cardiac iron deposition, while the conduction system is usually the last to be affected. The value of endomyocardial biopsy, which has been used to evaluate iron deposits in the heart, has been questioned. Iron has been reported as absent from the right ventricular subendocardium in some patients with cardiac iron overload.

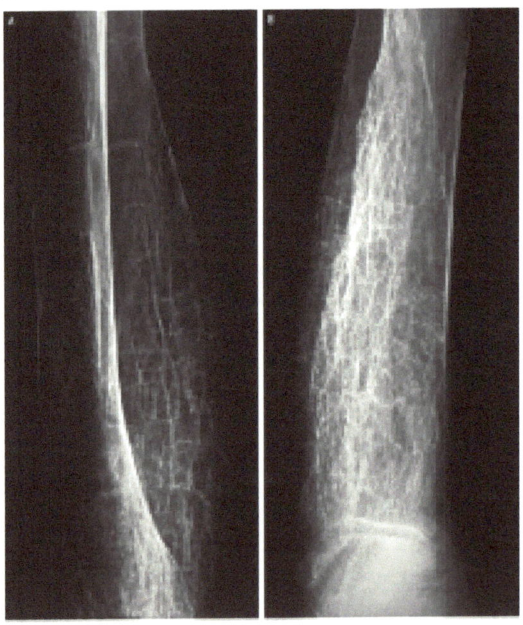

Fig. 40.113: *Showing a cobwebbing trabecular pattern of long bones in patient with longstanding beta -thalassemia*

Echocardiography,radionuclide cineangiogrphy, **and 24-hour ECG** are to be used to monitor these patients

Hepatic Complications

Patients who have received regular blood transfusions for some time develop liver enlargement due to swelling of the phagocytic and parenchymal cells from the deposition of hemosiderin.

- Liver enzyme levels are not typically elevated unless hemosiderin deposition is associated with hepatitis.
- Chelation therapy may prevent or delay progressive liver disease, which may end in cirrhosis.

Long-term Therapy Complications

Because of improved medical care, patients with thalassemia are surviving their disease longer and reaching old age. With this longer survival comes new issues related to complications that need to be addressed.

HCV has emerged as the paramount risk in patients who have been receiving blood transfusions all their lives. HCV screening was initiated in 1990. Since then, according to the Registry of the TCRN, the incidence rate of HCV has dropped significantly. The current prevalence of HCV in patients with thalassemia older than 25 years is 70%, as opposed to only 5% in those with thalassemia aged 15 years or younger.

Unfortunately, a high incidence rate of HCV continues in developing countries, leading to an increased incidence of fibrosis, cirrhosis, and hepatocellular carcinoma (HCC), especially in the presence of a second risk factor such as iron overload. For this reason, many centers advocate screening patients with HCV every 6 months by obtaining a fetoprotein (AFP) and an ultrasound of the liver. According to the TCRN, approximately 33% of patients with thalassemia major who are also HCV positive develop a spontaneous clearance of the HCV. Two-thirds of patients with b thalassemia major have multiple calcified bilirubin stones by age 15 years.

Hematologic Complications

Recently, thrombosis was encountered in relatively significant numbers of patients with thalassemia. In a study of 83 patients with thalassemia intermedia, a 26% incidence

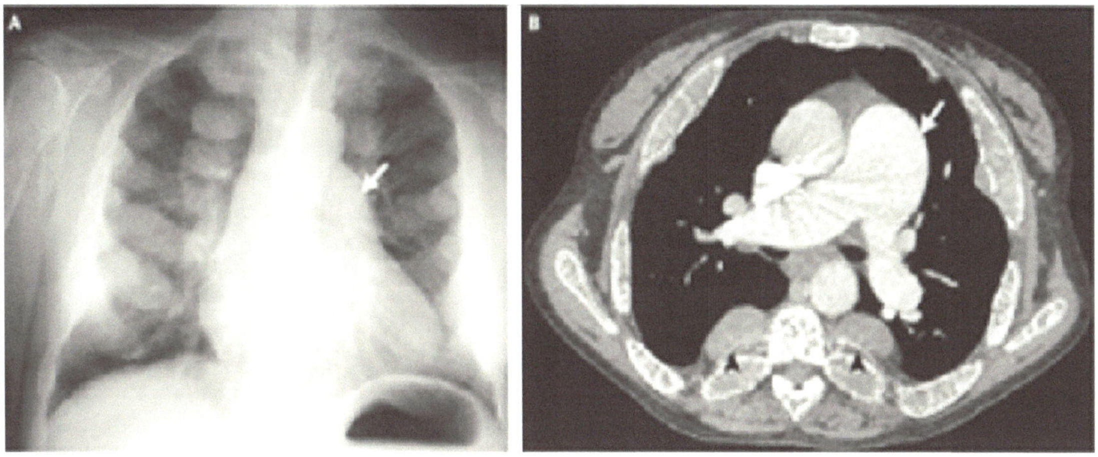

Fig. 40.114: *Chest radiography (Panel A, arrow) and computed tomography (Panel B, arrow) show enlarged central pulmonary arteries owing to pulmonary arterial hypertension. In patients with thalassemia, such enlargement is thought to arise from chronic anemia, hemolysis, and an increased tendency for microscopic thrombi to form within the pulmonary vasculature. Bilateral paravertebral soft-tissue masses (Panel B, arrowheads), as well as marked medullary expansion of the bony structures (with the ribs showing the most pronounced involvement), were also present, findings that are associated with compensatory extramedullary hematopoiesis*

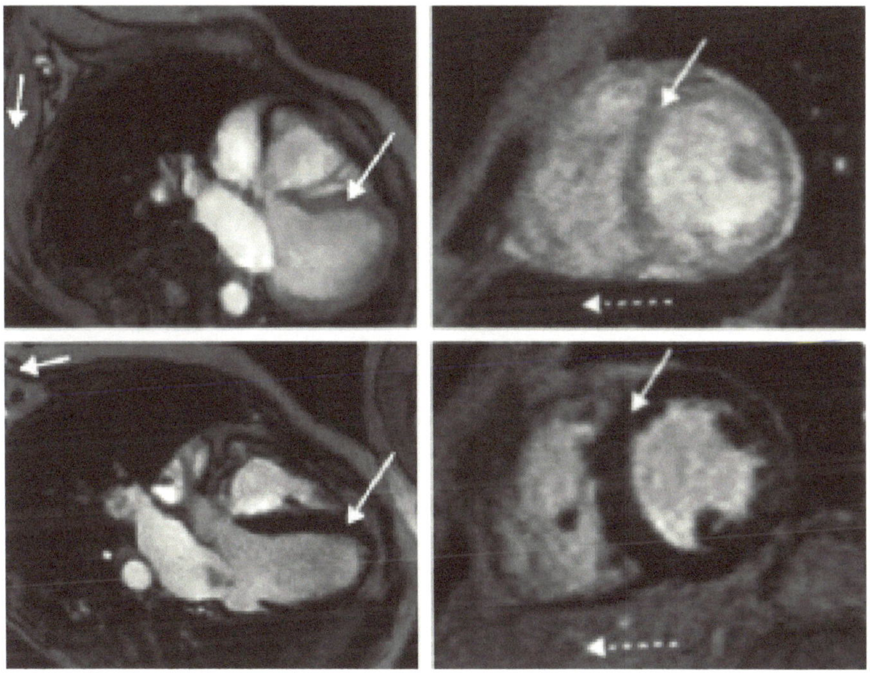

Fig. 40.115: *Magnetic resonance scans in patients with thalassemia major.Left scans are horizontal long axis, the right ones mid-short axis. (A) Low myocardial iron deposition. The left ventricular volumes are normal, and myocardial signal intensity (long arrow) is similar to that arising from skeletal muscle (short arrow). Left ventricular ejection fraction was 70%. In this case, the liver is very dark (dotted arrow), indicating heavy hepatic iron deposition despite the normal myocardial appearances. (B) Severe myocardial iron overload. The myocardial signal intensity is dark (long arrow) compared with skeletal muscle (short arrow). The ventricle is dilated and thickened. Cine imaging showed greatly reduced systolic function (left ventricular ejection fraction 39%) with a restrictive filling pattern. Liver signal in this case is well preserved (dotted arrow)*

rate of VTEs was encountered, while only 2% of 65 patients with thalassemia major developed VTE.

- One study determined that most of the patients with thalassemia intermedia who developed VTE had been splenectomized. Based on this fact, several centers recommend some type of prophylactic therapy to prevent thrombosis in such patients. Short-term antithrombotic therapy, both perioperatively and in the presence of thrombotic risk factors, is recommended. Patients who have undergone splenectomy and have a platelet count in excess of 600,000/µL receive low-dose daily aspirin. Development of pulmonary hypertension in such patients as a result of small pulmonary thrombi represents a significant indication of the increased risk for clotting. Based on the observation of hypercoagulable state in patients with thalassemia, exaggerated by splenectomy, the role of such a procedure in patients with thalassemia needs to be reconsidered.

Endocrine Complications

People with thalassemia major frequently exhibit features of diabetes mellitus; 50% or more exhibit clinical or subclinical diabetes. This is believed to be due to defective pancreatic production of insulin, but insulin resistance also has been implicated.

Glucose intolerance encountered in these patients usually correlates with the numbers of transfusions received and the patient's age and genetic background.

A recent study compared the incidence of endocrinopathy in patients with thalassemia with the incidence in patients with sickle cell disease and a similar iron overload due to transfusion. The study also compared patients with sickle cell disease who received transfusion with those who did not receive transfusion. The study showed that patients with thalassemia are far more prone to develop various endocrinopathies than patients with sickle cell disease. Furthermore, the incidence did not differ between patients with sickle cell disease who received transfusion and those who did not. However, the duration of transfusion was found to be a significant predictor. Thus, the underlying disease may modulate iron-related endocrine injury.

Growth Retardation

Growth retardation is frequently severe in patients with thalassemia. This retardation is caused, in part, by the diversion of caloric resources for erythropoiesis, as well as by the chronic anemia, since hypertransfusion usually restores normal growth. Unless chelation therapy is initiated early in life, patients rarely grow normally. Excessive chelation with DFO may also cause growth retardation.

The direct cause of growth retardation in these patients is thought to be an impaired growth hormone production or deficiency in production of somatomedin by the hemosiderotic liver. Involvement of the adrenal glands or the thyroid gland may also contribute to growth failure.

Fertility and Pregnancy Complications

Adult patients with thalassemia major are known to have low fertility; this is attributed to the commonly encountered hypogonadotrophic hypogonadism.

Both primary and secondary sexual characteristics are usually delayed in both males and females.

Females are frequently oligomenorrheic or amenorrheic. Pregnancy complications are also seen frequently and are likely due to endocrinologic and cardiac complications. Case reports demonstrated, however, that successful pregnancy and delivery of healthy babies is possible in women with thalassemia major.

Early intervention with hormonal therapy and aggressive chelation to prevent permanent damage may help to preserve fertility.

Transfusion complications: The most common complications of blood transfusion

Chelation Therapy Complications

These complications and the specific adverse effects of DFO

Viral hepatitis: Viral hepatitis has been reported in nontransfused patients with iron overload, suggesting that iron overload predisposes patients to viral hepatitis, as was stated above.

Prognosis

The prognosis depends on the type and severity of thalassemia. As stated above, the clinical course of thalassemia varies greatly from mild or even asymptomatic to severe and life threatening.

Prevention

Screening and Prevention

In persons with b thalassemia trait, confirming the diagnosis is usually easy. In such situations, genetic counseling is necessary, and, if both parents are carriers, a detailed discussion with the couple should include all possible outcomes. These include the 1 in 4 chance of having a severely affected or completely healthy child and a 1 in 2 chance of having a child with heterozygous thalassemia.

For a thalassemia carriers, confirmation is not that simple. Hb electrophoresis is usually not informative. For this reason, more sophisticated studies are warranted if confirmation is critical. Genetic counseling should be provided for patients with b thalassemia if a sibling or a family member is known to be affected.

Prenatal DNA testing has been available for several years. The decision to perform prenatal diagnosis in parents known to be at risk for having a child with thalassemia is complex and is usually influenced by several factors, such as religion, culture, education, and the number of children in the family. Genetic counseling by professionals that addresses the details of both the genetic risks and the testing risks involved is expected to help the parents make an informed and intelligent decision concerning the procedure. Unfortunately, such tests are not available in certain areas of the world where they are needed most. Extensive screening programs and prenatal diagnosis has resulted in a significant decline in the incidence of b thalassemia in some of the high-risk Mediterranean countries.

Successful prevention programs in different parts of the world have resulted in an impressive decline in the number of patients with severe forms of thalassemia. Ferrara, Cyprus, Sardinia, Greece, and the United Kingdom were among the first to report a significant decline in the birth rate of children with thalassemia major. Many other regions with more limited resources are following their steps with remarkable success. In addition to the effective prenatal diagnosis adopted in the countries mentioned, other measures such as premarital screening programs, genetic counseling, and restrictions on issuing marriage certificates and licenses also proved to be effective. Because many of the countries where thalassemia prevails are poor and cannot afford sophisticated preventive programs, more practical approaches are clearly needed.

Screening of children, pregnant women, and individuals visiting public health facilities is effective in identifying individuals at risk who require further testing. A simple CBC count, with emphasis on the RBC counts and indices, including the MCV, MCH, and RDW, is the main component of such screening processes. Persons suspected to be positive for thalassemia are checked for elevated levels of Hb A_2, Hb F, or both for confirmation. In some situations, this simple method is not adequate, and further testing, including analyses of globin chain synthesis, must be performed to reach a final diagnosis.

Prenatal Diagnosis

Globin chain synthesis, which was once used in postnatal diagnosis, was also used on fetal cells obtained by fetoscopy to screen the fetus. This test reveals imbalanced production of certain globin chains that are diagnostic of thalassemia.

Since polymerase chain reaction (PCR) techniques have become available, several new methods are now in use to identify affected babies or carrier individuals accurately and quickly. The DNA material is obtained by chorionic villus sampling (CVS), and mutations that change restriction enzyme cutting sites can be identified. Because many of the mutations that cause a and b thalassemia have become known in recent years, identifying such mutations on the amplified b-globin gene region is now possible with specific labeled oligonucleotide probes. Some of the new techniques can give accurate results in less than 3 hours.

IDIOPATHIC DILATED CARDIOMYOPATHY (DCM)

Idiopathic dilated cardiomyopathy (DCM) refers to congestive cardiac failure secondary to dilatation and systolic dysfunction (with or without diastolic dysfunction) of the ventricles (predominantly left) in the absence of congenital, valvular, or coronary artery disease or any systemic disease known to cause myocardial dysfunction. DCM is the most common type of heart muscle disease in children.

All 4 cardiac chambers are dilated and are sometimes hypertrophied. Dilation is more pronounced than hypertrophy, and the left ventricle is affected more often than the right ventricle. The cardiac valves are intrinsically normal, although the mitral and tricuspid valve rings are dilated, and the valve leaflets do not appose each other in systole, giving rise to varying degrees of mitral regurgitation, tricuspid regurgitation, or both. Persistent mitral regurgitation leads to thickening of the mitral valve leaflets, and, at times, distinguishing this thickening from other causes of mitral regurgitation is difficult. Thrombus formation (secondary to the low-flow cardiac output state) is often seen in the left ventricular apex and, at times, is seen in the atria. Occasionally, the right ventricle is preferentially involved in the cardiomyopathic process; this often indicates a familial basis.

Pathophysiology

Injury to the myocardial cell is the initiating factor that leads to cell death. If considerable cell loss occurs, the myocardium fails to generate enough contractile force to produce adequate cardiac output. This results in the activation of compensatory mechanisms, including the renin-angiotensin-aldosterone system, sympathetic stimulation, antidiuretic hormone production, release of atrial natriuretic peptide, tumor necrosis factor (TNF)-a, and mechanical factors, such as increased end-diastolic stretch on the ventricle.

These compensatory mechanisms help to maintain cardiac output in the initial phase; however, as myocardial damage progresses, persistent and excessive activation can be detrimental to cardiac function, leading to overt congestive heart failure. Over-stretching of the ventricles causes myocardial thinning, cavity dilation, secondary valvular regurgitation, and compromised myocardial

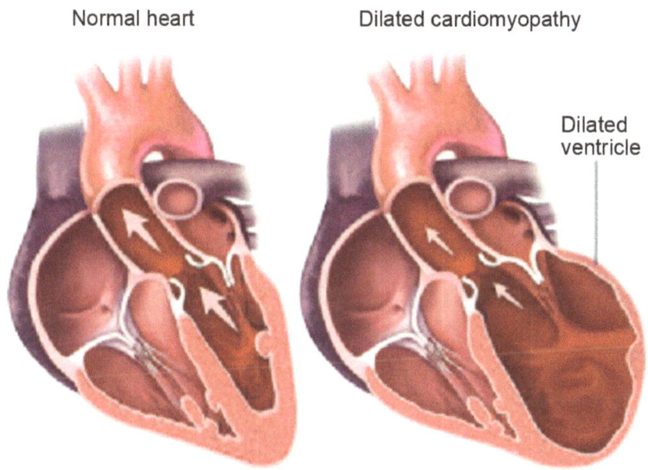

Fig. 40.116: *A comparison in the cross-section between a normal heart and a heart affected by DCM*

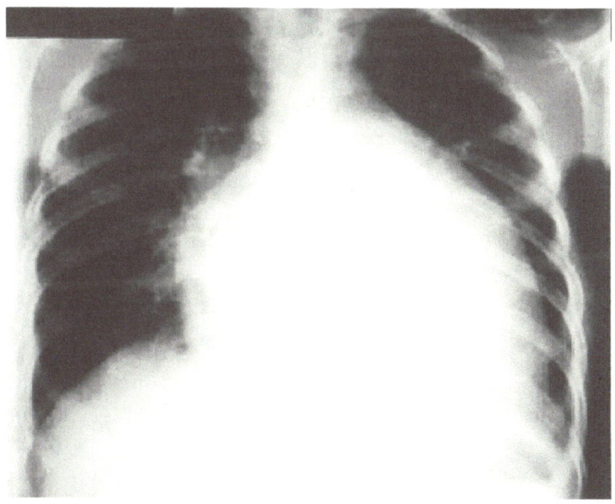

Fig. 40.117: *X-ray chest PA view showing massive cardiomegaly involving almost all chambers of the heart in Idiopathic dilated cardiomyopathy*

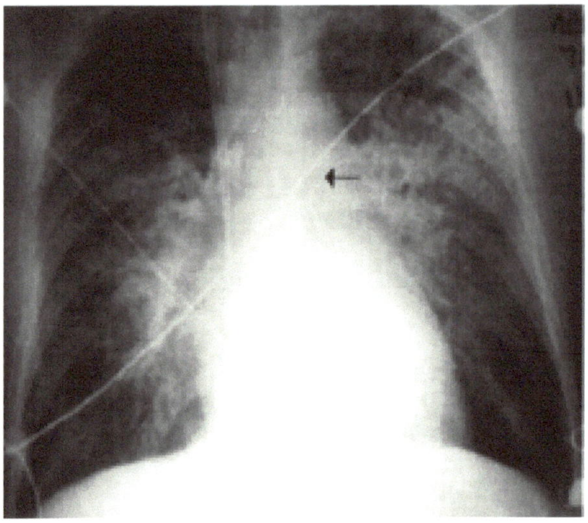

Fig. 40.118: *Cardiogenic alveolar oedema. Symmetrical air space opacity with perihilar predominance is one characteristic pattern produced by cardiogenic patient with dilated cardiomyopathy*

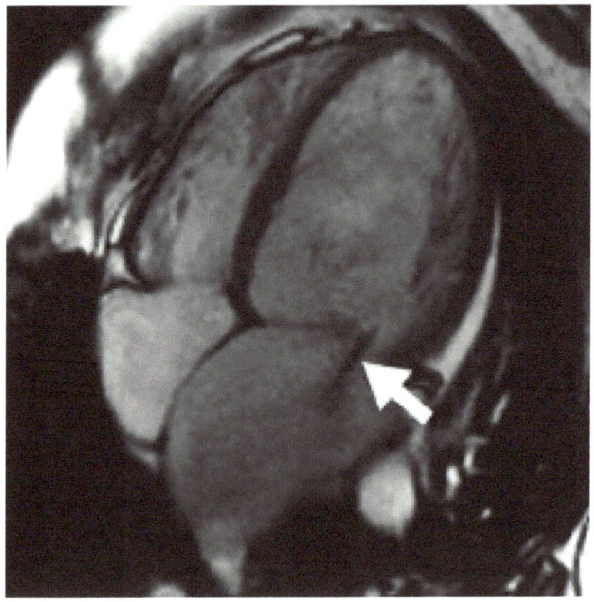

Fig. 40.119: *Idiopathic dilated cardiomyopathy in a 18-year-old girl with shortness of breath. Four-chamber steady-state free-precession MR image shows marked dilation of LV , which measures 68 mm. Note black jet (arrow) from mitral regurgitation, a common finding in dilated cardiomyopathy*

perfusion. The resulting subendocardial ischemia perpetuates myocyte damage. Myocardial remodeling is an important contributor to worsening heart failure. Lost myocyte cells are replaced with fibrous tissue, thereby decreasing the compliance of one or more ventricles and adversely affecting performance. Aldosterone, angiotensin II, catecholamines, endothelins, and mechanical factors, such as excessive myocardial stretch and ischemia, have been identified as mediators of remodeling. Apoptosis is a process of programmed cell death and is now believed to play a role in the continuing loss of myocardial cells in chronic heart failure. Overloading of myocytes possibly triggers apoptosis without fibrosis.

Heightened peripheral vasoconstriction, abnormal and excessive remodeling of the peripheral vasculature, and abnormalities in endothelium-dependent vasodilation contribute to the progression of heart failure. Abnormal responses to muscarinic stimulation along with a defect in the endothelial nitric oxide pathway have been suggested as the potential underlying mechanisms.

Altered gene expressions resulting in calcium-handling abnormalities, down regulation of myosin or conversion to the less-active beta isoform, and abnormal beta-receptor signal transduction have all been identified at the molecular level in the chronically failing heart.

Incidence

The reported incidence rate is 0.57 cases per 100,000 children. The incidence rate in Finland is 2.6 cases per 100,000 children. No reliable figures are available for the rest of the world.

- Genetic causes account for more than 30% of DCM.

Mortality/Morbidity

Mortality and morbidity have greatly decreased because of advances in medical management. Studies from 1975-1990 reported 70% survival at 2 years and 52% survival at 11.5 years of follow-up. Studies from 1992-1997 document more than 85% survival at 5 years. In general, approximately one third of patients die from the disease, one third of patients continue to have chronic heart failure requiring therapy, and one third of patients experience improvement in their condition.

Causes of death include heart failure, ventricular arrhythmias, and transplantation-related complications (less common).

Gender Distribution

DCM is reportedly more common in boys than in girls, and some forms are clearly X-linked.[1]

Age Distribution

All age groups are affected. However, studies suggest that DCM is more common in infancy (age [1] Fetal presentation is uncommon.

History

- Onset is usually insidious but may be acute in as many as 25% of patients, especially if exacerbated by a complicating lower respiratory infection.
- Cough, poor feeding, irritability, and shortness of breath are usually the initial presenting symptoms.
- Pallor, sweating, easy fatigability, failure to gain weight, and decreased urine output may be observed.
- Wheezing may be an important clinical sign, suggesting congestive heart failure manifestation in infants.
- Chest pain, palpitations, orthopnea, hemoptysis, frothy sputum, sudden death, abdominal pain, syncope, and

neurologic deficit are other symptoms at presentation (20%).

- Cardiomegaly that is incidentally detected on a chest radiograph or an arrhythmia that is incidentally detected on an ECG may be the basis for initial cardiac referral.
- Approximately 50% of patients with dilated cardiomyopathy (DCM) have a history of preceding viral illness. A detailed family history for familial cardiomyopathy is revealing in as many as 25% of cases.

Physical Examination

In a patient with established disease, features of congestive heart failure are dominant.

The infant or young child with the disease is often tachypneic, tachycardic with weak peripheral pulses, and has cool extremities and hepatomegaly. Blood pressure is low with a decreased pulse pressure. In extreme cases, patients may present in shock.

Older children may show dependent edema, elevated jugular venous pulses, and fine basal crepitations in the lungs.

Major cardiac findings include cardiomegaly, quiet precordium, tachycardia, gallop rhythm (S_3 and/or S_4), accentuated P-2, and murmurs of mitral and tricuspid regurgitation. Murmurs may be inconspicuous initially if the patient presents with acute heart failure.

Infants often present with predominantly respiratory signs and, in the absence of a precordial heave or prominent murmur, the underlying cardiac disease may remain undiagnosed until cardiomegaly is detected on a chest radiograph.

Causes

Various factors have been identified as causes of myocardial damage. However, in the vast majority of patients, no specific etiology is demonstrable (idiopathic). Systemic carnitine deficiency and anthracycline-induced cardiomyopathy are notable exceptions.

Three major factors have been implicated in the pathogenesis of myocardial damage in DCM: preceding viral myocarditis, autoimmunity, and underlying genetic predisposition.

Viral Myocarditis

Currently, no methods can be used to distinguish cardiovirulent strains of enteroviruses from those that are not virulent. Furthermore, the presence of a virus a patient with DCM does not necessarily establish a causal relationship. Demonstration of viral DNA or RNA by polymerase chain reaction (PCR) is a more reliable method for revealing viral myocarditis. Unfortunately, obtaining myocardial tissue is invasive. The exact mechanism of myocardial damage (rapid destruction or a long-term slowing of cardiomyocyte function) also remains unclear.

Autoimmunity

Animal studies have shown that DCM is an autoimmune disease in genetically predisposed strains of mice. Approximately 30–40% of adult patients with DCM have organ-specific and disease-specific autoantibodies. The absence of these antibodies in the remaining patients may be related to the stage of disease progression. The notion that an insult such as viral myocarditis initiates an autoimmune process with superantigen-triggered immune responses, resulting in massive T-lymphocyte activation and myocardial damage, has been postulated.

Genetic Predisposition

Genetic causes account for 25–50% of DCM cases.

The role of genetic factors is exemplified by the studies on familial DCM.

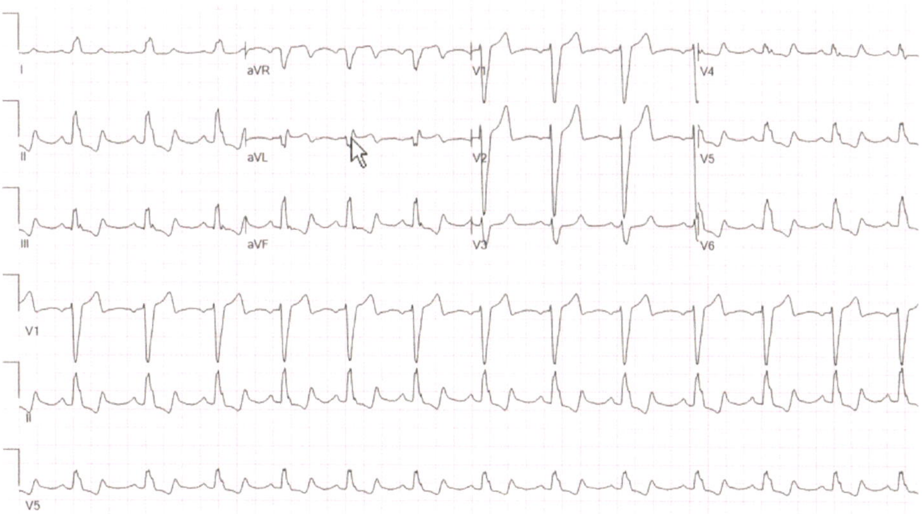

Fig. 40.120: *Idiopathic dilated cardiomyopathy: An ECG of a patient with nonischemic dilated cardiomyopathy showing LBBB. There is discordant ST depression > 1 mm in leads V4-V5. The QRS amplitude in these leads is less than 6 mm. Therefore, the BARCELONA criteria for OMI are met and are thus falsely positive, whereas the Sgarbossa and Smith criteria are not met and are true negatives*

Patients with familial DCM have an increased frequency of human leukocyte antigen (HLA)-DR4. The frequency of HLA-DQA1 0501 alleles has been reported to be significantly higher in patients with idiopathic DCM.

Autosomal dominant and recessive inheritance, X-linked transmission, and polygenic and mitochondrial inheritance have all been documented.

Mutation analysis: Mutation screening of the exons that code for actin, α myosin heavy chain (*MYH7* gene), cardiac troponin T (*TNNT2* gene), phospholamban (*PLN* gene), titin, αβ-crystallin, and the cardio-specific exon of metavinculin (*VCL* gene) could be helpful in detecting some forms of familial DCM.

- **Anthracyclines and cardiomyopathy:** Anthracyclines, which are widely used in the management of childhood malignancies, account for as many as 30% of cases of DCM in the United States and a lesser percentage in other countries. Besides DCM, the other manifestations of anthracycline cardiotoxicity include restrictive cardiomyopathy (symptomatic and asymptomatic), asymptomatic left ventricular enlargement, and more subtle changes of cardiac function. ·Early diagnosis requires periodic Doppler echocardiography studies during therapy and for several years after cessation of treatment. It also requires more widespread use of load-independent measurements of cardiac contractility (like stress velocity index), which incorporate measurements of contractility, afterload, and preload.

Cardiotoxicity has 2 types: early onset and late onset. The early onset type may be acute nonprogressive orchronically progressive.

Acute-onset type is defined as left ventricular dysfunction during or immediately following infusion of anthracycline and is attenuated by discontinuation of therapy. With use of low-dose regimens, this type is becoming rare. ECG changes include nonspecific ST segment and T wave changes, decreased QRS voltage, prolonged QT interval, and sinus tachycardia. Less commonly, ventricular, junctional, or supraventricular tachycardia or atrioventricular and bundle branch blocks. Blood levels of cardiac troponin T (cTnT) are a specific marker of this type of injury.

Early onset chronically progressive toxicity presents within one year of completion of therapy and persists or progresses even after discontinuation of therapy. Clinical features are similar to any other type of cardiomyopathy and include ECG changes, left ventricular dysfunction, arrhythmias, reduced exercise-stress capacity, and even overt signs of heart failure. Blood levels of cTnT are elevated. Presence of early onset cardiotoxicity is believed to be a harbinger of poor patient outcome.

Late-onset toxicity clinically manifests after a latent period of one or more years following completion of therapy. This type of manifestation is presumably due to diminished left ventricular contractility and an inappropriately thin left ventricular wall, resulting in elevated wall stress and progressive left ventricular dysfunction. Myocyte loss underlies all these sequelae, and alteration of myocellular protein transcription by anthracyclines may contribute. Thus, the latent period is not latent at all, and more sensitive markers may be abe to detect the changes earlier. Late-onset asymptomatic toxicity has also been reported, but more detailed questioning often reveals easy fatigability or dyspnea in many of these patients.

Risk factors contributing to the development of cardiotoxicity include the following: (1) the total cumulative dose of the drug received (20% mortality with cumulative dose >550 mg/m^2, 65% frequency of subtle Echo changes with dose >400 mg/m^2, and histologic evidence of toxicity with >240 mg/m^2), (2) female sex (higher cellular concentrations because of higher body fat percentage), (3) young children, (4) rate of drug administration (maximum risk with doses >50 mg/m^2/dose), (5) concomitant cardiac radiation exposure or use of amsacrine, (6) black race, and (7) trisomy 21.

Lab Studies

Full blood counts, erythrocyte sedimentation rate, and C-reactive proteins may show evidence of acute inflammation in the presence of active myocarditis.

Similarly, creatine kinase–myocardial fraction may be elevated.

Rising titers of specific viral-neutralizing antibodies in the serum and positive viral cultures from nasopharyngeal or stool swabs may suggest a viral etiology; however, this does not necessarily mean a cause-and-effect relationship. Serum carnitine levels (total and free) are low when the disease is due to systemic carnitine deficiency.

Arterial blood gas (ABG) analysis reveals early stages of mild respiratory alkalosis and, later, mild hypoxemia secondary to pulmonary edema. In advanced disease, mixed acid-base disturbances with metabolic acidosis indicate the need for intravenous inotropes and ventilatory assistance.

Imaging Studies

Chest radiography: Chest radiography reveals cardiomegaly with a prominent left ventricular apex and prominent pulmonary artery segment. Elevation of left main bronchus reflects dilation of the left atrium. This can result in compression of the left lower lobe bronchus when combined with a dilated pulmonary artery, leading to collapse of the left lower lobe of the lung

Pulmonary venous congestion and frank pulmonary edema are often evident. When present, pleural effusion is better appreciated in the erect and lateral decubitus films. Massive cardiomegaly resembling pericardial effusion is the hallmark of established disease.

Rarely, in fulminant cases, cardiomegaly may not be prominent because the ventricle has not had time to dilate despite the presence of features of pulmonary edema.

Echocardiography and Doppler studies: These form the basis for the diagnosis of dilated cardiomyopathy (DCM) in most patients. Marked dilation of the left ventricle with

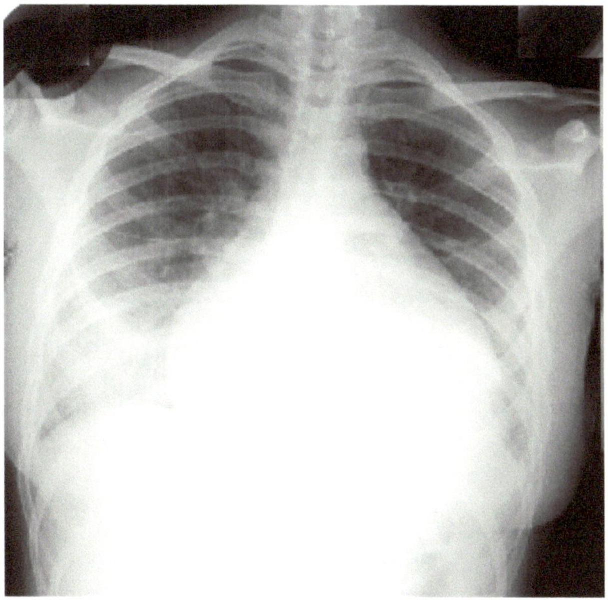

Fig. 40.121: *X- ray chest PA view demonstrates cardiomegaly, pulmonary edema and pleural effusions. as a result of Congestive Heart Failure due to Viral Myocarditis*

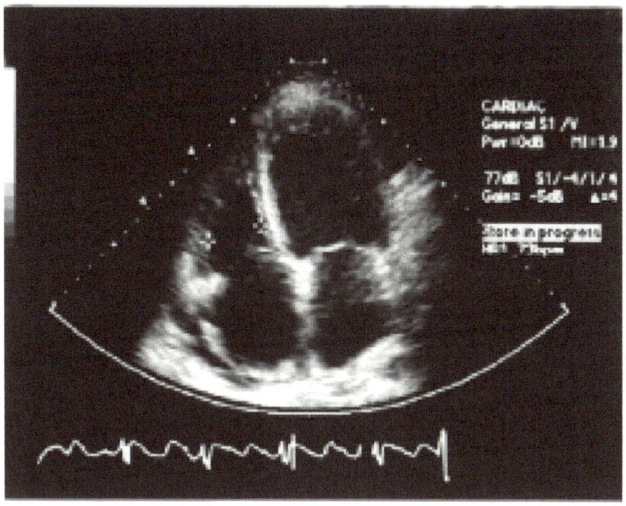

Fig. 40.122: *2D echo-cardiogram. Four-chamber view shows atrial and ventricular dilatation in viral myocarditis*

global hypokinesia is the hallmark of the disease. Left ventricular fractional shortening is usually less than 25% (ejection fraction Doppler studies show varying degrees of mitral regurgitation secondary to left ventricular dilation and possible papillary muscle dysfunction. Mitral regurgitation is more prominent in follow-up studies after commencing therapy when the cardiac output has improved. Left ventricular ejection parameters show decrease in peak velocity and peak acceleration, prolongation of the pre-ejection period, and decrease in ejection time. These flow measurements are dependent on loading conditions. The dilatation of the mitral valve ring and the altered shape of the left ventricle cavity, which leads to change in the direction of the papillary muscles, are used to explain the secondary mitral regurgitation seen in a large proportion of children with DCM. Tissue Doppler studies have recently been reported in children with DCM .

Parameters of diastolic dysfunction are not reliable in the presence of established systolic dysfunction and mitral regurgitation; however, they may be useful in the early stages of the disease. Diastolic dysfunction is not as typical or as pronounced as it is in hypertrophic cardiomyopathy. Long-standing cases show evidence of pulmonary hypertension in the form of right ventricular dilation and hypertrophy and tricuspid regurgitation. Tricuspid regurgitation and pulmonary regurgitation velocities give an estimate of the pulmonary artery systolic and diastolic pressures respectively. In severe cases, swirling echodensity (smoke or spontaneous echocardiographic contrast) can be observed along the outer ventricular wall, moving from the mitral valve towards the aortic valve. Occasionally, thrombi can be visualized in the left ventricular apex and in the left atrium. Pericardial effusion also may be present. Echocardiography can exclude other heart diseases, both congenital and acquired. Cardiomyopathy secondary to severe aortic stenosis, coarctation of aorta or congenital mitral valve dysplasia, and anomalous left coronary artery arising from pulmonary artery (ALCAPA) are the major differential diagnoses. At times, identifying cardiomyopathy secondary to congenital mitral regurgitation (dysplastic mitral valve without stenosis) is difficult, but the abnormal anatomy of the mitral valve leaflets should help. The echo-dense papillary muscles and the dilated proximal right coronary artery and continuous retrograde flow of blood into the origin of pulmonary artery all direct the attention of the cardiologist to ALCAPA, a potentially treatable that mimics DCM.

Radionuclide imaging: First-pass test and multiple gated acquisition (MUGA) scans help to measure the left and right ventricular stroke volumes and cardiac outputs. They are also helpful in documenting dyskinetic segments in the ventricular walls. Although theoretically superior to echocardiographic measurements, their practical application is limited because of a lack of standardization and because of nonreproducibility, especially in children. Thallium studies can identify areas of decreased myocardial perfusion, although this is seldom required.

Gallium citrate Ga 67 scintigraphy and indium In-111 altumomab pentetate antimyosin antibody cardiac imaging have been suggested to help identify ongoing inflammation noninvasively. They may be used to identify patients who might benefit from myocardial biopsy

Other Tests

Electrocardiography

ECG changes are usually nonspecific. Some patients have sinus tachycardia, downward frontal plane QRS axis, left atrial enlargement, left ventricular hypertrophy, deep Q waves with ST segment depression, and tall T waves in leads I, aVL, V_5, V_6 (the latter reflect left ventricular volume overload). In more advanced disease, right axis deviation, right atrial enlargement, and right ventricular hypertrophy are seen (because of pulmonary hypertension).

The main role of ECG is to detect evidence of myocardial ischemia (pathologic Q waves with ST elevation and T-wave inversion in leads I, aVL, V_5, V_6) that might point to anomalous coronary artery as the etiology of the cardiomyopathy. A segmental myocarditis may result in ECG features of myocardial infarction.

Cardiac arrhythmias, such as supraventricular/ventricular ectopy or tachycardia, may be revealed. These might indicate an underlying myocarditis or cardiomyopathy; wever, if sustained, the arrhythmia may be the cause of the cardiomyopathy rather than the result (i.e. tachycardia-mediated cardiomyopathy).

Procedures

Cardiac catheterization and angiography: Children with DCM are at a particular risk for complications during cardiac catheter studies and angiography. Should be performed by experienced pediatric cardiologists and only when absolutely essential.

At present, preparation for cardiac transplant and need for myocardial biopsy are the main indications for performing the procedure.

Patients should be under optimum medical therapy and kept hemodynamically stable before and after catheterization. Careful observation is required during the procedure for ventricular arrhythmias and hemodynamic deterioration.

Echocardiography should be considered after catheterization to identify any pericardial effusion secondary to subclinical perforation of the myocardium, especially if a biopsy has also been performed.

Aortography may be performed to identify a coronary artery anatomy, and left ventricular angiography may be performed to assess mitral valve function. The number of biopsy specimens collected should be limited to the minimum required (usually 4–8). Usual findings include elevated filling pressures in all the cardiac chambers (especially the left ventricle), pulmonary wedge pressure, and reduced cardiac output and stroke volume. Mixed venous oxygen saturation and reduced arterial saturation reflect low cardiac output and pulmonary edema. Pulmonary and systemic vascular resistances are elevated. With end-stage disease, the peak systolic left ventricular and aortic pressures drop.

Myocardial Biopsy

At present, preparation for cardiac transplant and post-transplant follow-up monitoring for rejection are the main indications for biopsy. If facilities are available, molecular or metabolic studies can be additional indications for academic and research purposes. Rarely, suspected metabolic diseases (isolated myocardial carnitine deficiency, rare forms of glycogen storage disease, fatty acid oxidation defects) or persistent myocarditis might require biopsy for confirmation Specimens should be subjected to both light and electron microscopy. PCR and metabolic studies should be performed when indicated. The most important aspect is the availability of a sufficient level of expertise for interpretation of the findings. PCR has been used to aid the detection of viral antigens in myocardial tissue in patients with DCM. Studies have revealed an association between viral antigens and DCM. However, a proportion of the studies gave negative results. A recently published meta-analysis of the studies on DCM gave an odds ratio of 3.8 to the association between presence of viral antigens in DCM. The results are influenced by factors like contamination from the reference strain used in the laboratory and choice of the controls. It also is not clear whether these positive cases among DCM actually represented acute myocarditis rather than DCM.

Medical care: Perform general supportive measures during acute-stage management, including endotracheal intubation and mechanical ventilation, vasoactive infusions, and fluid/acid-base management. Treat chest infections appropriately. Treat anemia appropriately.

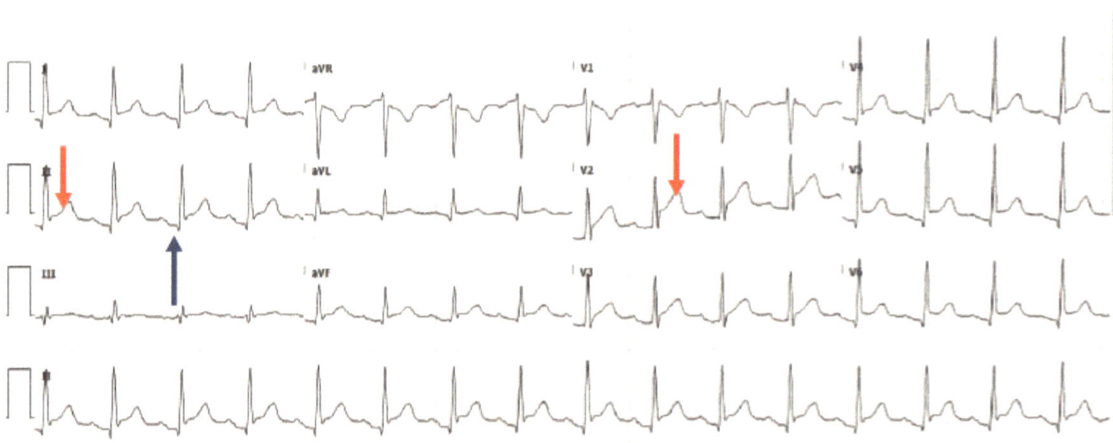

Fig. 40.123: *Electrocardiography shows sinus rhythm with diffuse ST elevation (red arrow) in most leads, except in aVR with PR depression (black arrow) when the patient was referred to the local hospital emergency department. suggesting a diffuse myocarditis*

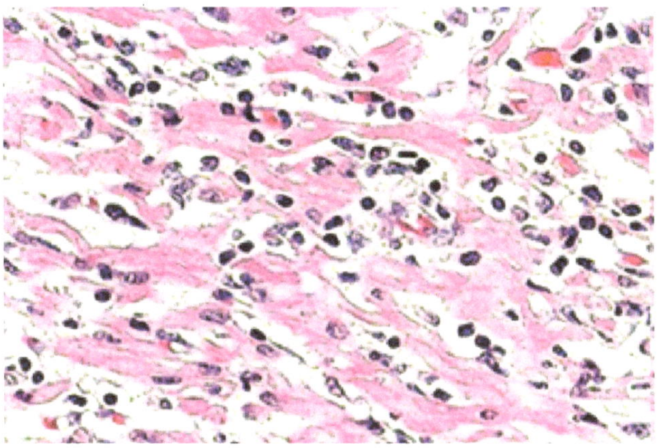

Fig.40.124: *There is myocyte necrosis along with inflammation consisting of mononuclear cells, typical for a viral myocarditis.*

- Oxygen inhalation is of benefit only in the presence of hypoxia (as with pneumonia or pulmonary edema).
- Carnitine supplements (100 mg/kg IV infusion over 30 min, followed by 100 mg/kg/d as continuous infusion for 24–72 h; 25–50 mg/kg/dose PO bid/tid, not to exceed 200 mg/kg/d) reverse the myocardial dysfunction in most patients affected by systemic carnitine deficiency.
- Coenzyme Q10 has also been used in children with dilated cardiomyopathy (DCM), with variable results.

Decreased serum levels of growth hormone (GH), which acts on cardiac myocytes primarily through insulinlike growth factor (IGF)-1, are associated with impaired myocardial growth and function, which can be improved with the restoration of GH/IGF-1 homeostasis. Based on this hypothesis and on observation of benefits in animal models, GH therapy has been used in children with DCM, but the results have not been conclusive.

Surgical Care

Cardiac transplantation is currently the optimal treatment for DCM-induced resistant chronic congestive heart failure in children.

- Limiting factors include availability of a suitable donor, complications of rejection, and lifelong immunosuppression. Survival rates of as much as 92% at 5 years have been reported.
- Palliative surgical measures are associated with significant mortality and morbidity rates despite advances. Resection of a large segment of the hypertrophied ventricular muscle **(Batista procedure)** and repair or replacement of mitral valve to minimize volume overload of left ventricle have been used as palliative measures. Cardiomyoplasty is the transposition of electrically transformed skeletal muscle to provide systolic and diastolic augmentation to the native heart.
- **Implantable mechanical support devices,** modified for used in infants and children, have been introduced to support the failing heart until a suitable donor is available for transplantation (bridge to transplant). Major limitations include infection, thromboembolism, disturbance from noise, and the need to recharge batteries frequently.
- **Cardiac resynchronization therapy** using a biventricular pacemaker has been shown to be effective in adults with DCM. In addition, these devices are available with

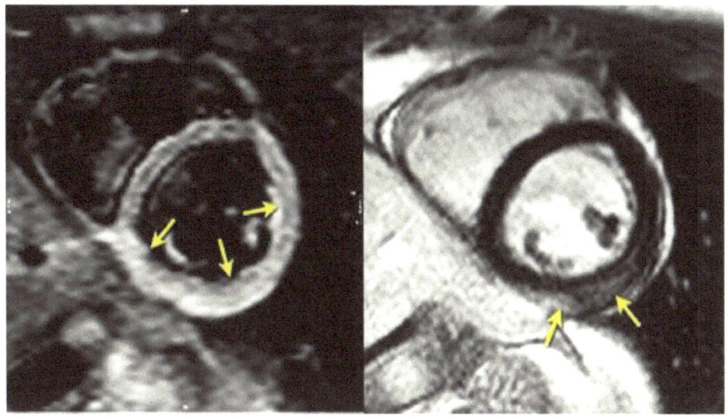

Fig.40.125: Reversible myocardial injury in a patient with clinically acute myocarditis. Upper, short-axis view before (left) and early after (right) injection of gadolinium showing myocardial hyperemia with regionally more pronounced uptake in the anteroseptal segment (arrows). Lower, myocardial edema (arrows; left); late gadolinium enhancement image without apparent high–signal intensity areas indicating the absence of necrosis in the edematous regions (right). The quantitative evaluation (early gadolinium enhancement ratio) indicated a globally increased early gadolinium uptake

Diet

Foods to eat:	Foods to avoid:
Foods which contain healthy fats such as walnuts, salmon, soybean oils Plenty of fruits such as melon, kiwi fruit Plenty of vegetables such as spinach, broccoli, kale	Fatty Foods such as fried chicken, fried potatoes Salty Foods Sugary Foods such as sodas, chocolate

defibrillator backup for patients at risk for ventricular arrhythmias. They are being used in children with DCM, with early favorable results.

- Prolonged support of left ventricular function with these devices has shown restoration of the native cardiac function, enabling removal of the device in a few cases. This raises the possibility that mechanical intervention at an earlier stage in viral myocarditis and DCM might prevent the deterioration of cardiac function. Recent adult studies have documented myocardial recovery and successful explantation of the left ventricular assist system, even after they were on the device for a year. A lesser degree of fibrotic changes in the left ventricle could predict better chances of recovery.

Activity

- Enforced bed rest is impractical and probably unnecessary.
- Often, restriction of physical activity is self-enforced.
- Infants might need intravenous alimentation for relief from feeding activity.
- Apart from the above, activity to the limit of tolerance should be allowed and encouraged.
- In patients with chronic illness, regular graded exercise has been shown to improve effort tolerance and quality of life.
- All feasible support should be provided for peer interaction and participation in normal life activities. Restricted life activities, frequent diagnostic and therapeutic interventions, and an uncertain prognosis make these children prone to psychological problems that may significantly influence prognosis and outcome.

Among the described abnormalities are inhibition of emotions, marked anxiety, depressive reaction with loneliness, low self-esteem, feelings of inadequacy, emotional lability, impulsiveness, and weakness of self-identity.

Medical therapy is largely directed at the symptoms and is aimed at the underlying heart failure. Diuretics, angiotensin-converting enzyme (ACE) inhibitors, and beta-blockers form the initial therapy. Diuretics may provide an improvement in symptoms, whereas ACE inhibitors appear to prolong survival. Beta-blockers also have a long-term positive effect on outcome. Intravenous infusions of vasoactive agents may be required in patients with resistant heart failure. Recently, the use of beta-blockers has become more extensive in childhood dilated cardiomyopathy (DCM) drug therapy.

Antibiotics for endocarditis prophylaxis are administered to patients with certain cardiac conditions, such as DCM, before performing procedures that may cause bacteremia.

Complications

Congestive heart failure

- Pneumonia
- Cardiac arrhythmias (supraventricular and ventricular)
- Infective endocarditis
- Thromboembolism
- Venous thrombosis
- Cardiac cirrhosis
- Post-transplant complications
- Sudden, unexplained death

Prognosis

- If a treatable cause is discovered, prognosis is better.
- Prognosis is worst for cardiomyopathy secondary to storage diseases that do not have effective therapy.
- History of viral illness in the 3 months before onset may suggest a better prognosis.
- In DCM with no obvious detectable etiology, outcome depends on severity of myocardial dysfunction, improvement during the first year after onset, compliance to therapy, and availability of timely transplant.
- Degree of depression of fractional shortening or ejection fraction at time of initial echocardiography, elevation of left ventricular end diastolic pressure, and cardiothoracic ratio have all been applied as predictors of outcome, although they are not often predictive. Other possible prognostic factors include age at onset (better for infants), presence of symptomatic arrhythmias, and thromboembolic episodes.
- Arrhythmic death can occur even after the left ventricular ejection fraction has returned to normal.
- Following cardiac transplant, survival rates of as much as 77% at 1 year and as much as 65% at 5 years have been reported in children.
- Schoolteachers should be informed of the child's condition. Teachers and other caregivers should be adequately trained for first aid and cardiopulmonary resuscitation (CPR).
- Family members should be screened with ECG and echocardiography to detect asymptomatic cases.
- Pregnancy imposes special demands on the cardiac reserve, and the decision to have children has to be individualized, depending mainly on the degree of exercise tolerance and the severity of ventricular dysfunction and cardiomyopathy

Acute and Chronic Pericarditis

Pericarditis is inflammation of the pericardium, often with fluid accumulation. Pericarditis may be caused by many disorders (e.g. infection, MI, trauma, tumors, metabolic disorders) but is often idiopathic. Symptoms include chest pain or tightness, often worsened by deep breathing. Cardiac output may be greatly reduced. Diagnosis is based on symptoms, a friction rub, ECG changes, and evidence of pericardial fluid accumulation on x-ray or echocardiogram. Finding the cause requires further evaluation. Treatment depends on the cause, but general measures include analgesics, anti-inflammatory drugs, and sometimes surgery. Pericarditis is the most common pericardial disorder. Congenital pericardial disorders are rare.

Anatomy and Pathophysiology

The pericardium has 2 layers. The visceral pericardium is a single layer of mesothelial cells that is attached to the myocardium, folds back (reflects) on itself over the origin of the great vessels, and joins with a tough, fibrous layer to envelop the heart as the parietal pericardium. The sac created by these layers contains a small amount of fluid (< 25 to 50 mL), composed mostly of an ultrafiltrate of plasma. The pericardium limits distention of the cardiac chambers and increases the heart's efficiency. The pericardium is richly innervated with sympathetic and somatic afferents. Stretch-sensitive mechanoreceptors sense changes in cardiac volume and tension and may be responsible for transmitting pericardial pain. The phrenic nerves are embedded in the parietal pericardium and are vulnerable to injury during surgery on the pericardium. Pericarditis may be acute or chronic. Acute pericarditis develops quickly, producing an inflammatory reaction. Chronic pericarditis (defined as persisting > 6 mo) develops more slowly; its prominent feature is effusion. Acute disease may become chronic. Adverse hemodynamic effects and rhythm disturbance are rare, although cardiac tamponade is possible. Occasionally, pericarditis produces a marked thickening and stiffening of the pericardium (constrictive pericarditis). Pericarditis can lead to inflammation of the epicardial myocardium.

Pericardial effusion is accumulation of fluid in the pericardium. The fluid may be serous fluid (sometimes with fibrin strands), serosanguineous fluid, blood, pus, or chyle.

Cardiac tamponade occurs when a large pericardial effusion impairs cardiac filling, leading to low cardiac output and sometimes shock and death. If fluid (usually blood) accumulates rapidly, even small amounts (e.g. 150 mL) may produce tamponade because the pericardium cannot stretch quickly enough to accommodate it. Slow

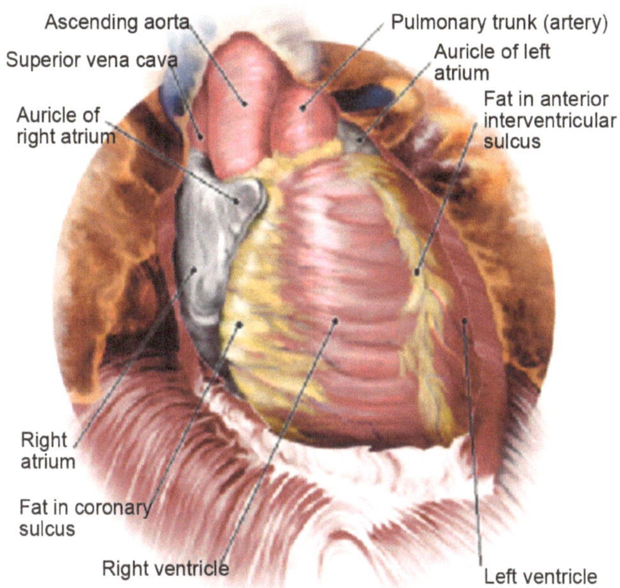

Fig. 40.126: *Showing anatomy of sac after exposing two layers ofpericardium*

Table 40.3: *Causes of acute pericarditis*

Causes
Idiopathic
Viral infections (echovirus, influenza virus, coxsackie B virus, HIV*)
Bacterial infections† (streptococci; staphylococci; gram-negative bacilli; in children, *Haemophilus influenzae*)
Fungal infections (histoplasmosis, coccidioidomycosis, candidiasis, blastomycosis)
Parasitic infections (toxoplasmosis, amebiasis, echinococcosis)
Autoimmune disorders (RA, SLE, scleroderma)
Inflammatory disorders (amyloidosis, inflammatory bowel disease, sarcoidosis)
Uremia
Trauma
MI
Post-MI (Dressler's) syndrome
Post pericardiotomy
Drugs (eg, hydralazine, isoniazid, methysergide, phenytoin, procainamide)

* If patients with AIDS develop lymphoma, Kaposi's sarcoma, or certain infections (ie, *Mycobacterium avium*, *M. tuberculosis*, *Nocardia*, other fungal or viral infections), pericarditis may follow.

† Tuberculous pericarditis accounts for < 5% of cases of acute or subacute pericarditis in the US but the majority of cases in some areas of India and Africa.

accumulation of up to 1500 mL may not produce tamponade. Loculated effusion may produce localized tamponade on the right or left side of the heart.

Constrictive pericarditis, which is uncommon, results from marked inflammatory, fibrotic thickening of the pericardium. Sometimes the visceral and parietal layers adhere to each other or to the myocardium. The fibrotic tissue often contains Ca deposits. The stiff, thickened pericardium markedly impairs ventricular filling, decreasing stroke volume and cardiac output. Significant pericardial fluid accumulation is rare. Rhythm disturbance is common. The diastolic pressures in the ventricles, atria, and venous beds become virtually the same. Systemic venous congestion occurs, causing considerable transudation of fluid from systemic capillaries, with dependent edema and, later, ascites. Chronic elevation of systemic venous and hepatic venous pressure may lead to cardiac cirrhosis. Constriction of the left atrium, the left ventricle, or both may elevate pulmonary venous pressure Etiology.

Acute pericarditis may result from infection, autoimmune and inflammatory disorders, uremia, trauma, MI, or certain drugs.

Pericarditis

Causes of Acute Pericarditis

Infectious pericarditis is most often viral. Purulent bacterial pericarditis is uncommon but may follow infective endocarditis, pneumonia, septicemia, penetrating trauma, or cardiac surgery. Often, the cause cannot be identified (called nonspecific or idiopathic pericarditis), but many of these cases are probably viral. Overall, the most common causes are viral and idiopathic. Acute MI causes 10 to 15% of cases of acute pericarditis. Post-MI syndrome (Dressler's syndrome) is a less common cause now, occurring mainly when reperfusion with percutaneous transluminal coronary angioplasty (PTCA) or thrombolytic drugs is ineffective in patients with transmural infarction. Pericarditis occurs after pericardiotomy (called postpericardiotomy syndrome) in 5 to 30% of cardiac operations.

Myocardial Infarction

Post-MI (Dressler's) syndrome

Post pericardiotomy

Drugs (e.g. hydralazine, isoniazid, methysergide, phenytoin, procainamide)

***If patients with AIDS develop lymphoma, Kaposi's sarcoma, or certain infections** (i.e. Mycobacterium avium, M. tuberculosis, Nocardia, other fungal or viral infections), may follow.

Tuberculous pericarditis accounts for < 5% of cases of acute or subacute pericarditis in the US but the majority of cases in some areas of India and Africa. Chronic pericardial effusion or constrictive pericarditis may follow almost any disorder that causes acute pericarditis, as well as TB, tumor, irradiation, rheumatoid disease, and cardiac surgery. Sometimes no cause of chronic pericarditis is identified. Pericarditis with large effusion (serous, serosanguineous, or bloody) is most commonly caused by metastatic tumors, most often by lung or breast carcinoma, sarcoma (especially melanoma), leukemia, or lymphoma. Fibrosis of the pericardium may follow purulent pericarditis or myocardial infection (myocarditis—a common cause in young people) or accompany a connective tissue disorder.

In elderly patients, common causes are malignant tumors, MI, and TB. Hemopericardium (accumulation of blood within the pericardium) may lead to pericarditis or pericardial fibrosis; common causes include chest trauma, iatrogenic injury (e.g. from cardiac catheterization, pacemaker insertion, or central venous line placement), and rupture of a thoracic aortic aneurysm (Fig. 47.128).

Symptoms, Signs and Diagnosis

Some patients present with symptoms and signs of inflammation (acute pericarditis); others present with those of fluid accumulation (pericardial effusion). Symptoms and signs vary depending on the severity of inflammation and the amount and rate of fluid accumulation. Even a large amount of pericardial fluid may be asymptomatic if it develops slowly (e.g. over months).

Acute Pericarditis

Acute pericarditis tends to cause chest pain and a pericardial rub, sometimes with dyspnea. The first evidence can be tamponade, with hypotension, shock, or pulmonary edema. Because the innervation of the pericardium and myocardium is the same, the chest pain of pericarditis is sometimes similar to that of myocardial inflammation or ischemia: Dull or sharp precordial or substernal pain may radiate to the neck, trapezius ridge (especially the left), or shoulders. Pain ranges from mildespecially the left), or shoulders. Pain ranges from mild to severe. Unlike ischemic chest pain, pain due to pericarditis is usually aggravated by thoracic motion, cough, breathing, or swallowing food; it may be relieved by sitting up and leaning forward. Tachypnea and nonproductive cough may be present; fever, chills, and weakness are common. In 15 to 25% of patients with idiopathic pericarditis, symptoms recur intermittently for months or years. The most important physical finding is a triphasic or a systolic and diastolic precordial friction rub. However, the rub is often intermittent and evanescent; it may be present only during systole or, less frequently, only during diastole. If no rub is heard with the patient seated and leaning forward, auscultation may be attempted with the patient on all fours and listening with the diaphragm of the stethoscope. Sometimes, a pleural component to the rub is noted during breathing, which is due to inflammation of the pleura adjacent to the pericardium. Considerable amounts of pericardial fluid may muffle heart sounds, increase the area of cardiac dullness, and change the size and shape of the cardiac silhouette. If acute pericarditis is suspected, hospitalization is sometimes required for initial evaluation. ECG and chest X-ray are done. If symptoms or signs of elevated right-sided pressure, tamponade, or an enlarged cardiac silhouette are present, echocardiography to check for effusion and cardiac filling abnormalities is also done. Blood tests may detect leukocytosis and an elevated ESR, but these findings are nonspecific. The diagnosis is based on the presence of typical clinical findings and

ECG abnormalities: Serial ECGs may be needed to show abnormalities. The ECG in acute pericarditis may show abnormalities confined to ST segments and T waves, usually in most leads Peri carditis: Acute pericarditis: Stage

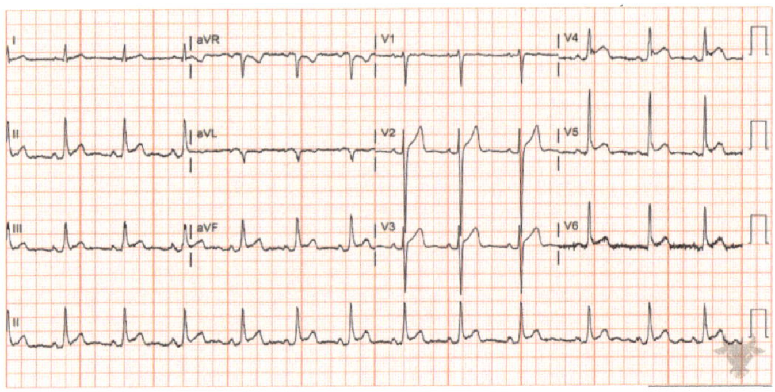

Fig. 40.127: *ECG in acute pericarditis showing wide spread concave ST elevation and depression of PR segment*

1 ECG.). The ST segments in 2 or 3 of the standard leads become elevated but subsequently return to baseline. Unlike MI, acute pericarditis does not cause reciprocal depression in ST segments (except in leads aVR and V_1), and there are no pathologic Q waves. The PR segment may be depressed. After several days or longer, T waves may become flattened and then inverted throughout the ECG, except in lead aVR; T-wave inversion occurs after the ST segment has returned to baseline and thus differs from the pattern of acute ischemia or MI .

Acute Pericarditis

ECG

J points, except aVR and V_1, are elevated. T waves are essentially normal. PR segments, except aVR and V_1, are depressed. PR deviations are commonly absent in one limb

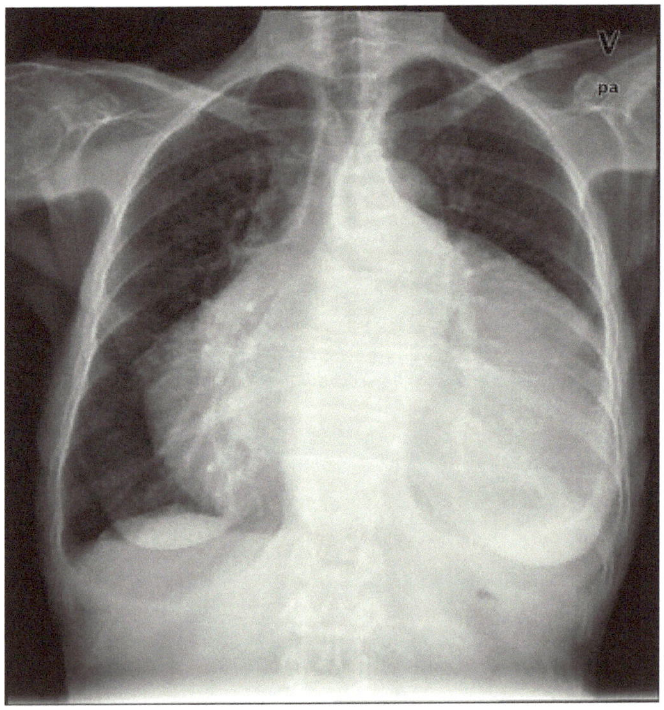

Fig. 40.128: *Photograph of X-ray chest showing money bag apprearance of cardiac silhoute in patient with moderate pericardial effusion*

lead (here, aVL). Because the pain of pericarditis may resemble that of acute MI or pulmonary infarction, additional tests (e.g. serum cardiac marker measurement, lung scan) may be required if the history and ECG findings are atypical for pericarditis. Troponin is almost always elevated in acute pericarditis due to epicardial inflammation so it cannot discriminate between acute infarction and pulmonary embolism. The CPK level is usually normal in acute pericarditis unless myocarditis is also present. Postpericardiotomy and post-MI syndromes may be difficult to identify and must be distinguished from recent MI, pulmonary embolism, and pericardial infection after surgery. Pain, friction rub, and fever appearing 2 wk to several months after surgery and a rapid response to aspirin, NSAIDs, or corticosteroids aid diagnosis.

Tuberculoma of Left Ventricle

it may be seen as a part of wide spread systemic tuberculosis or rarely as an independant pathology

Pericardial effusion: Pericardial effusion is often painless, but when it occurs with acute pericarditis, pain may be present. Typically, heart sounds are muffled. A pericardial rub may be heard. With large effusions, compression of the base of the left lung can decrease breath sounds (heard near the left scapula) and produce crackles (rales). Arterial pulse, jugular venous pulse, and BP are normal unless intrapericardial pressure increases substantially, causing tamponade. In the post-MI syndrome, pericardial effusion can occur with fever, friction rub, pleurisy, pleural effusions, and joint pain. This syndrome usually occurs within 10 days to 2 mo after MI. It is usually mild but may be severe. Occasionally, the heart ruptures post-MI, causing hemopericardium and tamponade, usually 1 to 10 days post-MI and more commonly in women. Diagnosis is suggested by clinical findings but often is suspected only after finding an enlarged cardiac silhouette on chest x-ray. On ECG, QRS voltage is often decreased, and sinus rhythm remains in about 90% of patients. With large, chronic effusions, the ECG may show electrical alternans (i.e. P, QRS, or T wave amplitude increases and decreases on alternate beats). Electrical alternans is associated with variation in cardiac position (swinging heart). Echocardiography has a high degree of sensitivity and specificity for detecting pericardial fluid. Patients with a normal ECG, small (< 0.5 L) effusion, and no suspicious findings from the history and examination may be observed with serial examination and echocardiography. Other patients must be evaluated further to determine etiology. Cardiac tamponade the clinical findings are similar to those of cardiogenic shock: decreased cardiac output, low systemic arterial pressure, tachycardia, and dyspnea. Neck veins are markedly dilated. Severe cardiac tamponade is nearly always accompanied by a fall of > 10 mm Hg in systolic BP during inspiration (pulsus paradoxus—*see* Approach to the Cardiac Patient: Pulsus paradoxus). In advanced cases, pulse may disappear during inspiration. (However, pulsus paradoxus can also occur in COPD, bronchial asthma, pulmonary embolism, right ventricular infarction, and

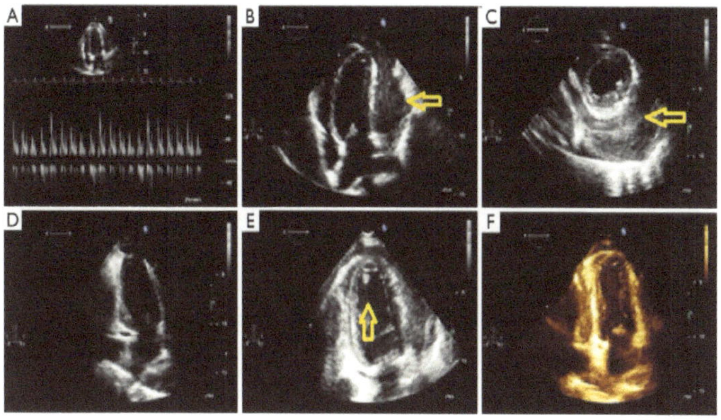

Fig.40.129 TTE images of the patient before, in the middle and after treatment. (A) (Inspiratory view), (B) (four chamber view) and (C) (two chamber view) show the pericardial thickness (yellow arrow); (D) shows four chamber view before cardiac tuberculoma appears; (E) displays the tuberculoma at the apex of LV (yellow arrow) and (F) shows disappearance of the tuberculoma after treatment. TTE, transthoracic echocardiography; LV, left ventricular.

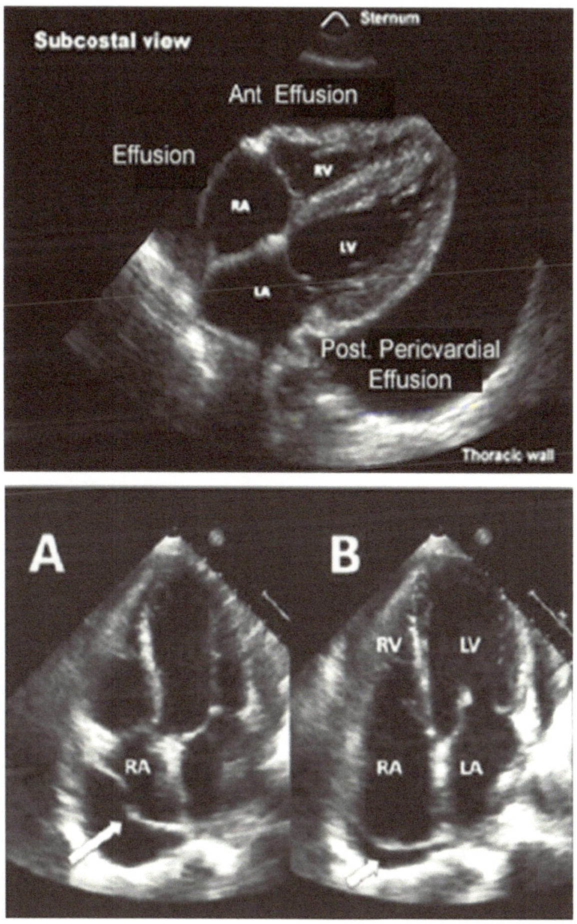

Fig. 40.130: *(Upper) Echocardiogram showing anterior and posterior pericardial effusion in the pericardial sac surrounding the heart (Bottom) A. (left) Apical 4C View showing pericardial effusion (arrow) with collapse of right atrium during diastole. B (Right) circumferential small effusion surrounding the right atrium (arrow)*

noncardiogenic shock.) Heart sounds are muffled unless the effusion is small. Low voltage and electrical alternans on the ECG suggest cardiac tamponade, but these findings lack sensitivity and specificity. When tamponade is suspected, echocardiography is done unless even a brief delay might be life threatening. Then pericardiocentesis is done immediately for diagnosis and treatment. On an echocardiogram, respiratory variation of transvalvular and venous flows and compression or collapse of right cardiac chambers in the presence of a pericardial effusion support the diagnosis. If tamponade is suspected, right heart (Swan-Ganz) catheterization may be done. In cardiac tamponade, there is no early diastolic dip in the ventricular pressure record.In the atrial pressure curve, x descent is preserved and y descent is lost. In contrast, in severe congestive states due to dilated cardiomyopathy, pulmonary artery occlusion or left ventricular diastolic pressure usually exceeds right atrial mean pressure and right ventricular diastolic pressure by ≥ 4 mm Hg. Constrictive pericarditis Fibrosis or calcification rarely produces symptoms unless constrictive pericarditis develops. The only early abnormalities may be elevated ventricular diastolic, atrial, pulmonary, and systemic venous pressures. Symptoms and signs of peripheral venous congestion (e.g. peripheral edema, neck vein distention, hepatomegaly) may appear with an early diastolic sound (pericardial knock), often best heard during inspiration. This sound is due to abrupt slowing of diastolic ventricular filling by the rigid pericardium. Ventricular systolic function (based on ejection fraction) is usually preserved. Prolonged elevation of pulmonary venous pressure results in dyspnea (particularly during exertion) and orthopnea. Fatigue may be severe. Distention of neck veins with a rise in venous pressure during inspiration (Kussmaul's sign) is present; it is absent in tamponade. Pulsus paradoxus is rare and is usually less severe than in tamponade. Lungs are not congested unless severe left ventricular constriction develops. Diagnosis may be suspected based on ECG, chest X-ray, and Doppler echocardiography findings, but cardiac catheterization and CT (or MRI) are usually required. Because ventricular filling is restricted,ventricular pressure tracings show a sudden dip followed by a plateau (resembling a square root sign) in early diastole. Rarely, right heart biopsy is needed to exclude restrictive cardiomyopathy.ECG changes are nonspecific. QRS voltage is usually low. T waves are usually nonspecifically abnormal. Atrial fibrillation occurs in about 1D 3 of patients; atrial flutter is less common. Lateral chest X-rays often show pericardial calcification best, but the finding is nonspecific. The changes on echocardiogram are also nonspecific. When the right and left ventricular filling pressures are equally elevated, Doppler echocardiography helps distinguish constrictive pericarditis from restrictive cardiomyopathy. During inspiration, mitral diastolic flow velocity usually falls > 25%in constrictive pericarditis but < 15% in restrictive cardiomyopathy. In constrictive pericarditis, inspiratory tricuspid flow velocity increases more than it normally does, but it does not do so in restrictive cardiomyopathy. Determining tissue velocities at the mitral annulus may be helpful when excessively high left atrial pressure blunts respiratory variation in transvalvular velocities. If clinical and echocardiographic findings suggest constrictive pericarditis, right heart cardiac catheterization is done. It helps confirm and quantify the abnormal hemodynamics that define constrictive pericarditis: Mean pulmonary artery occlusion pressure (pulmonary capillary wedge pressure), pulmonary artery diastolic pressure, right ventricular end-diastolic pressure, and mean right atrial pressure are all at about 10 to 30 mm Hg. The pulmonary artery and right ventricular systolic pressures are normal or modestly elevated, so that pulse pressures are small. In the atrial pressure curve, x and y descents are typically accentuated; in the ventricular pressure curve, a diastolic dip occurs at the time of rapid ventricular filling. These changes almost always occur with significant constrictive pericarditis. Right ventricular systolic pressure of > 50 mm Hg often occurs

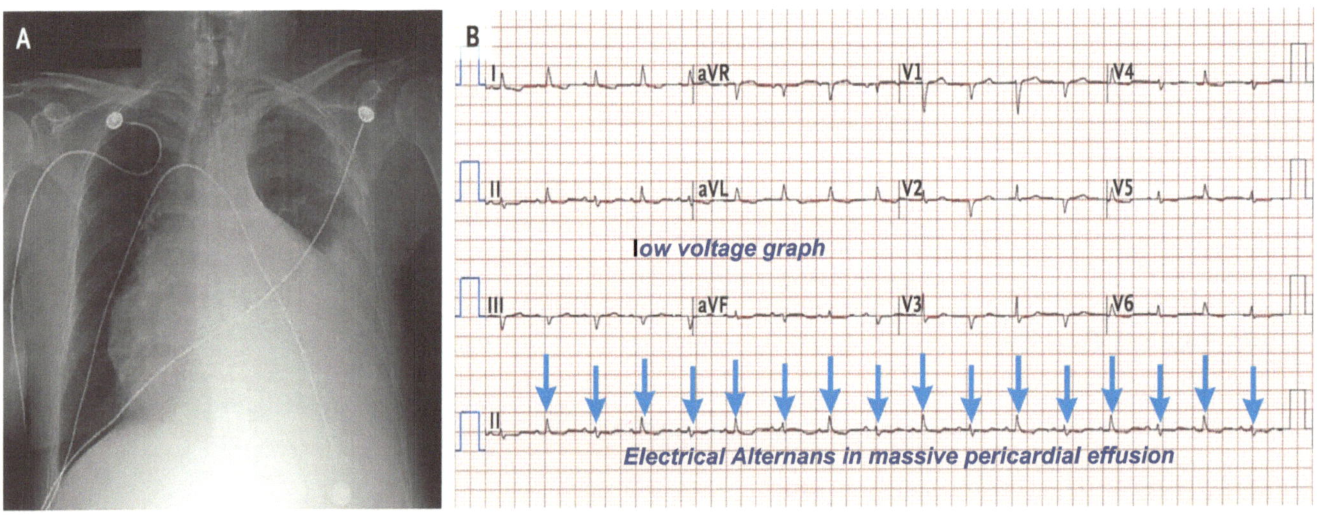

Fig. 40.131: (A)**Chest x-ray showed larged pericardial effusion** (B) *ECG showing low voltage graph with electrical alternans (Blue arrows) in massive Pericardial Effusion:(cardiac tamponade)*

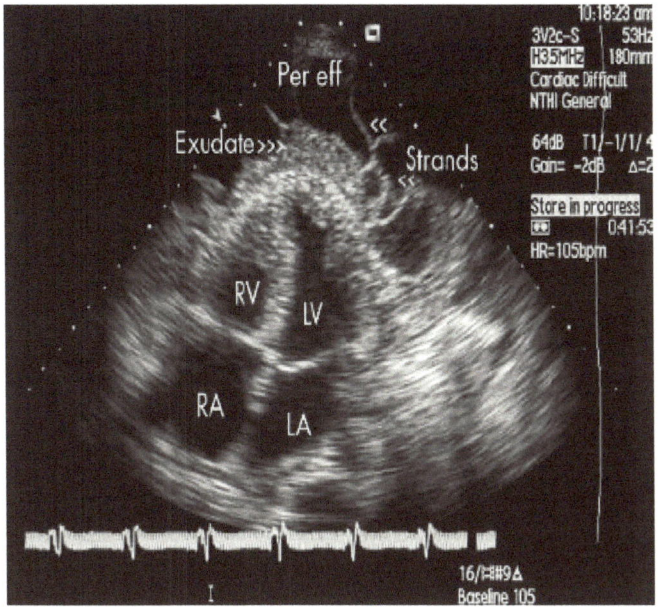

Fig.40.132:Apical four chamber view of a two dimensional echocardiogram of a patient with tuberculous pericardial effusion showing multiple fibrin strands as linear or band like structures crossing the pericardial space or protruding from the epicardium or parietal pericardium and exudates. LA, left atrium; LV, left ventricle; Per eff, pericardial effusion; RA, right atrium; RV, right ventricle.

in restrictive cardiomyopathy but less often in constrictive pericarditis. When the pulmonary artery occlusion pressure equals the right atrial mean pressure and an early diastolic dip in the ventricular pressure curve occurs with large X and y waves in the right atrial curve, either disorder may be present. CT or MRI can identify pericardial thickening

> 5 mm. Such thickening with typical hemodynamic changes can confirm a diagnosis of constrictive pericarditis. When no pericardial thickening or fluid is seen, the diagnosis of restrictive cardiomyopathy is favored but not proved; a normal pericardial thickness does not exclude the diagnosis of constrictive pericarditis. Diagnosis of cause After pericarditis is diagnosed, tests to determine etiology and the effect on cardiac function are done. In a young, previously healthy adult who presents with a viral infection and pericarditis, an extensive evaluation is usually unnecessary. Differentiating viral from idiopathic pericarditis is difficult, expensive, and generally of little practical importance. A biopsy of pericardial tissue or aspiration of pericardial fluid may be needed to establish a diagnosis. Acid-fast stains and cultures of pericardial fluid help identify infectious causes. Samples are examined for malignant cells. However, complete drainage of a newly identified pericardial effusion is usually unnecessary for diagnosis. Persistent (usually > 3 mo) or progressive effusion, particularly when the etiology is uncertain, also warrants pericardiocentesis. The choice between needle pericardiocentesis and surgical drainage depends on institutional resources and physician experience, the etiology of the effusion, the need for diagnostic tissue samples, and the prognosis of the patient. Needle pericardiocentesis is often best when the etiology is known or the presence of tamponade is in question. Surgical drainage is best when the presence of tamponade is certain but the etiology is unclear. Laboratory tests of pericardial fluid other than culture and cytology are usually nonspecific. But specific diagnoses are sometimes possible using newer visual, cytologic, and immunologic analysis of fluid obtained via pericardioscopic-guided biopsy. Cardiac catheterization is useful for evaluating pericarditis and identifying the cause of reduced cardiac function. CT or MRI can help identify metastases, although echocardiography is usually sufficient. Other tests include CBC, acute-phase reactants, routine chemistries, cultures, autoimmune tests, and, when appropriate, tests for HIV, histoplasmosis complement fixation (in endemic areas), streptozyme, and neutralizing antibodies for coxsackievirus, influenza virus, and echovirus. Anti-DNA and anti-RNA antibody tests may be useful. A PPD skin test is done. Treatment Hospitalization to watch for complications is usually advisable. Possible causative drugs (e.g. anticoagulants, procainamide, phenytoin) are stopped. For cardiac tamponade, immediate pericardiocentesis is done.

Echocardiography may be used to guide the needle as agitated saline is injected through it. Once in place, the needle should be clamped next to the skin to prevent it from entering further than necessary and possibly puncturing the heart or injuring a coronary vessel.

ECG monitoring is essential for detecting arrhythmias produced when the myocardium is touched or punctured. As a rule, right atrial pressure and pulmonary artery occlusion pressure (pulmonary capillary wedge pressure) are monitored. Fluid is withdrawn until intrapericardial pressure falls below right atrial pressure, usually to subatmospheric levels. If continued drainage is needed, a plastic catheter may be passed through the needle into the pericardium and the needle withdrawn. The catheter may be left in place for 2 to 4 days. Pain can usually be controlled with aspirin 325 to 650 mg po q 4 to 6 h or other NSAIDs (e.g. ibuprofen 600 to 800 mg po q 6 to 8 h) for 1 to 4 days; duration of therapy varies, and patients should be treated until an effusion, if present, has resolved. Colchicine 1 mg/day, added to NSAIDs or given alone, is effective for the initial episode of pericarditis and helps prevent recurrences. The intensity of therapy is dictated by the patient's distress. Severe pain may require opioids and corticosteroids (e.g. prednisone 60 to 80 mg po once/day for 1 wk, followed by rapid tapering of the dose). Corticosteroids are particularly useful in acute pericarditis due to uremia or a connective tissue disorder, but tuberculous and pyogenic pericarditis should be excluded before corticosteroid therapy is initiated. Intrapericardial instillation of triamcinolone(300 mg/m2) avoids systemic adverse effects and is highly effective. Anticoagulants are usually contraindicated in acute pericarditis because they may cause intrapericardial bleeding and even fatal tamponade; however, they can be given in early pericarditis complicating acute MI. Uncommonly, pericardial resection is required. Infections are treated with specific antimicrobial drugs. Complete drainage is often necessary. In postpericardiotomy syndrome, post-MI syndrome, or idiopathic pericarditis, antibiotics are not indicated. An NSAID at full doses may control pain and effusion. When required to control pain, fever, and effusion, prednisone 20 to 60 mg po once/day may be given for 3 to 4 days. If the response is satisfactory, the dose is gradually reduced, and the drug may be stopped in 7 to 14 days. But sometimes many months of treatment are needed. For pericarditis due to rheumatic fever, another connective tissue disorder, or tumor, therapy is directed at the underlying process. For pericardial effusion due to trauma, surgery is sometimes required to repair the injury and evacuate blood from the pericardium. Pericarditis due to uremia may respond to increased frequency of hemodialysis, aspiration, or systemic or intrapericardial adrenal corticosteroids. Intrapericardial triamcinolone may be useful. Chronic effusions are best treated by treating the cause, if known. Recurrent or persistent symptomatic effusions may be treated with balloon pericardiotomy, a surgical pericardial window, or sclerosing drugs (e.g. tetracycline). Recurrent effusion due to malignant tumor invasion may be treated with sclerosing drugs. Asymptomatic effusions of unknown cause may require only observation. Congestion in chronic constrictive pericarditis may be alleviated with bed rest, salt restriction, and diuretics. Digoxin is indicated only if atrial arrhythmias or ventricular systolic dysfunction is present. Symptomatic constrictive pericarditis usually requires pericardial resection. However, patients with mild symptoms, heavy calcification, or extensive myocardial damage may be poor surgical candidates. The mortality rate for pericardial resection may approach 40% in New York Heart Association (NYHA) functional class IV patients. Patients who have constrictive pericarditis due to irradiation or a connective tissue disorder are especially likely to have severe myocardial damage and may not benefit from pericardial resection.

Complications

Most cases of acute idiopathic pericarditis resolve without complications or recurrence. Complications may include:

Pericardial effusion

- Constrictive pericarditis
- Cardiac tamponade
- Fibrinous pericarditis

Fibrinous pericarditis is an exudative inflammation.

The pericardium is infiltrated by the fibrinous exudate. This consists of fibrin strands and leukocytes. Fibrin describes an amorphous, eosinophilic (pink) network. Leukocytes (mainly neutrophils) are found within the fibrin deposits and intrapericardic. Vascular congestion is also present. The myocardium has no changes. Sometimes referred to as having "Bread and Butter Appearance"

Pericarditis Due to Tuberculosis

Pericarditis caused by tuberculosis is difficult to diagnose, because definitive diagnosis requires culturing *Mycobacterium tuberculosis* from aspirated pericardial fluid or pericardial biopsy, which requires high technical skill and is often not diagnostic (the yield from culture is low even with optimum specimens). The Tygerberg scoring system helps the clinician to decide whether pericarditis is due to tuberculosis or whether it is due to another cause: night sweats (1 point), weight loss (1 point), fever (2 point), serum globulin > 40g/l (3 points), blood total leucocyte

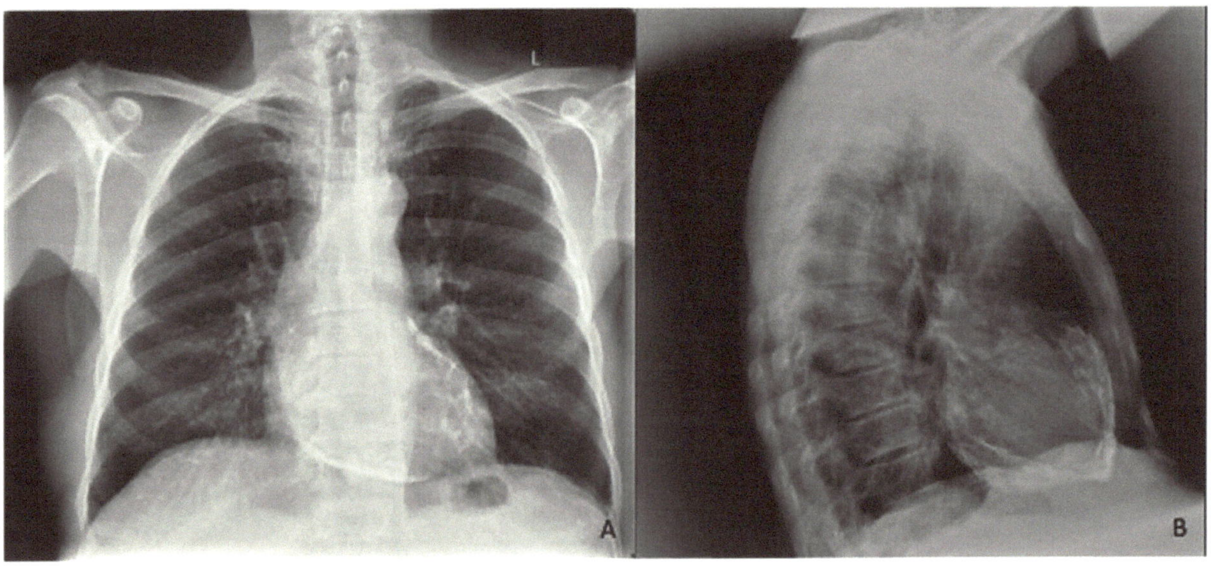

Fig. 40133: *Chest X-ray (PA and Lateral views) obtained on initial presentation showing dense circumferential calcification of pericardium in patient with chronic pericarditis*

count <10 × 10^9/l (3 points); a total score of 6 or more is highly suggestive of tuberculous pericarditis. Pericardial fluid with an interferon- level greater than 50pg/ml is highly specific for tuberculous pericarditis.

Treatment

The treatment in viral or idiopathic pericarditis is with non-steroidal anti-inflammatory drugs. Severe cases may require: pericardiocentesis

- Antibiotics
- Steroids
- Colchicine
- Surgery

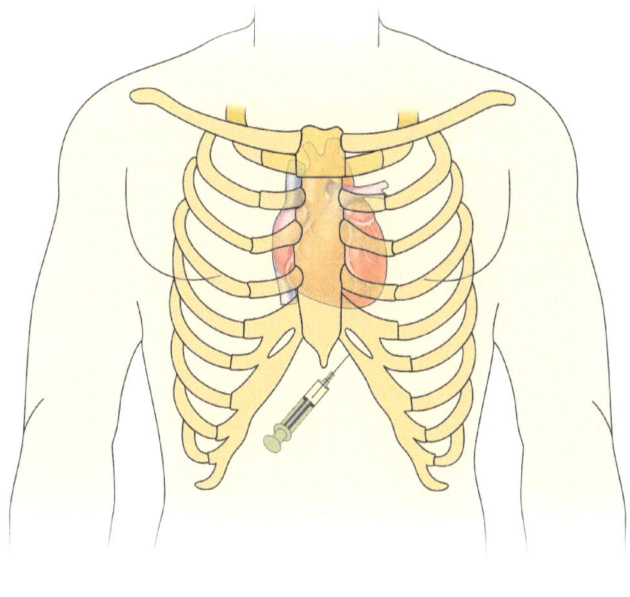

Fig. 40.134: *Placement and angle at which the fluid aspirating needle should be directed in the procedure of pericardiocentesis*

Pericardiocentesis

Except in emergencies (e.g. cardiac tamponade), pericardiocentesis, a potentially lethal procedure, should be done using echocardiographic guidance in a cardiac catheterization laboratory and should be supervised by a cardiologist or thoracic surgeon if possible. Resuscitation equipment must be at hand. IV sedation (e.g. morphine 0.1 mg/kg or meperidine 1 mg/kg plus midazolam 3 to 5 mg) is desirable. The patient should be recumbent, with the head elevated 30° from the horizontal. Under aseptic conditions, the skin and subcutaneous tissues are infiltrated with lidocaine. A 75 mm short-beveled, 16-gauge needle is attached via a 3-way stopcock to a 30 or 50 mL syringe. The pericardium may be entered via the right or left xiphocostal angle or from the tip of the xiphoid process with the needle directed inward, upward, and close to the chest wall. The needle is advanced with constant suction applied to the syringe.

BIBLIOGRAPHY AND ACKNOWLEDGMENTS

1. Abd-Alla, M. D., T. F. Jackson, V. Gathiram, A. M. el-Hawey, and J. I. Ravdin. 1993. Differentiation of pathogenic Entamoeba histolytica infections from nonpathogenic infections by detection of galactose-inhibitable adherence protein antigen in sera and feces. J. Clin. Microbiol. 31:2845-2850.
2. Acquatella, H. 2007. Echocardiography in Chagas heart disease. Circulation 115:1124-1131.
3. Adair, O. V., N. Randive, and N. Krasnow. 1989. Isolated toxoplasma myocarditis in acquired immune deficiency syndrome. Am. Heart J. 118:856-857.
4. Adams, J. H., L. Haller, F. Y. Boa, F. Doua, A. Dago, and K. Konian. 1986. Human African trypanosomiasis (T. b. gambiense): a study of 16 fatal cases of sleeping sickness with some observations on acute reactive arsenical encephalopathy. Neuropathol. Appl. Neurobiol. 12:81-94.
5. Adams, J. L. 1962. Acute toxoplasmosis with involvement of the heart. N. Z. Med. J. 61:20. [PubMed]
6. Adkins, R. B., Jr., and A. H. Dao. 1984. Pulmonary dirofilariasis: a diagnostic challenge. South. Med. J. 77:372-374.
7. Aerts, D., P. Truc, L. Penchenier, Y. Claes, and D. Le Ray. 1992. A kit for in vitro isolation of trypanosomes in the field: first trial with sleeping sickness patients in the Congo Republic. Trans. R. Soc. Trop. Med. Hyg. 86:394-395.
8. Aikat, B. K., S. R. Bhusnurmath, A. K. Pal, P. N. Chhuttani, and D. V. Datta. 1978. Amoebic liver abscess—a clinicopathological study. Indian J. Med. Res. 67:381-391.
9. Ammann, R. W., and J. Eckert. 1996. Cestodes. Echinococcus. Gastroenterol. Clin. North Am. 25:655-689.
10. Amorim, D. S., and J. A. Marin Neto. 1995. Functional alterations in the autonomic nervous system in Chagas' heart disease. Sao Paulo Med. J. 113:772-784.
11. Ancelle, T., A. De Bruyne, D. Poisson, and J. Dupouy-Camet. 2005. Outbreak of trichinellosis due to consumption of bear meat from Canada, France, September 2005. Euro Surveill. 10:E051013.3.
12. Anderson, S. E., and J. S. Remington. 1975. The diagnosis of toxoplasmosis. South. Med. J. 68:1433-1443.
13. Andrade, L. O., and N. W. Andrews. 2005. The Trypanosoma cruzi-host-cell interplay: location, invasion, retention. Nat. Rev. Microbiol. 3:819-823.
14. Andrade, Z. A. 1999. Immunopathology of Chagas disease. Mem. Inst. Oswaldo Cruz 94(Suppl. 1):71-80.
15. Andy, J. J., J. P. O'Connell, R. C. Daddario, and W. C. Roberts. 1977. Trichinosis causing extensive ventricular mural endocarditis with superimposed thrombosis. Evidence that severe eosinophilia damages endocardium. Am. J. Med. 63:824-829.
16. Angel, S. O., M. Matrajt, J. Margarit, M. Nigro, E. Illescas, V. Pszenny, M. R. Amendoeira, E. Guarnera, and J. C. Garberi. 1997. Screening for active toxoplasmosis in patients by DNA hybridization with the ABGTg7 probe in blood samples. J. Clin. Microbiol. 35:591-595.
17. Arness, M. K., J. D. Brown, J. P. Dubey, R. C. Neafie, and D. E. Granstrom. 1999. An outbreak of acute eosinophilic myositis attributed to human Sarcocystis parasitism. Am. J. Trop. Med. Hyg. 61:548-553.

18. Bailey, J. W., and D. H. Smith. 1994. The quantitative buffy coat for the diagnosis of trypanosomes. Trop. Doct. 24:54-56.

19. Balasegaram, M., H. Young, F. Chappuis, G. Priotto, M. E. Raguenaud, and F. Checchi. 2009. Effectiveness of melarsoprol and eflornithine as first-line regimens for gambiense sleeping sickness in nine Medecins Sans Frontieres programmes. Trans. R. Soc. Trop. Med. Hyg. 103:280-290.

20. Barnard, P. M., L. A. MacGregor, and H. F. Weich. 1989. Primary echinococcus cyst of the heart. A case report. S. Afr. Med. J. 76:275-277.

21. Barry, J. D. 1997. The relative significance of mechanisms of antigenic variation in African trypanosomes. Parasitol. Today 13:212-218.

22. Barsoum, R. S. 2004. Parasitic infections in organ transplantation. Exp. Clin. Transplant. 2:258-267.

23. Bastien, P. 2002. Molecular diagnosis of toxoplasmosis. Trans. R. Soc. Trop. Med. Hyg. 96(Suppl. 1):S205-S215.

24. Beaver, P., R. Jung, and E. Cupp. 1984. Clinical parasitology. Lea and Febiger, Philadelphia, PA.

25. Berensztein, C. S., D. Pineiro, M. Marcotegui, R. Brunoldi, M. V. Blanco, and J. Lerman. 2000. Usefulness of echocardiography and Doppler echocardiography in endomyocardial fibrosis. J. Am. Soc. Echocardiogr. 13:385-392.

26. Berger, P. B., J. Duffy, G. S. Reeder, B. L. Karon, and W. D. Edwards. 1994. Restrictive cardiomyopathy associated with the eosinophilia-myalgia syndrome. Mayo Clin. Proc. 69:162-165.

27. Bern, C., and S. P. Montgomery. 2009. An estimate of the burden of Chagas disease in the United States. Clin. Infect. Dis. 49:e52-e54.

28. Bern, C., S. P. Montgomery, B. L. Herwaldt, A. Rassi, Jr., J. A. Marin-Neto, R. O. Dantas, J. H. Maguire, H. Acquatella, C. Morillo, L. V. Kirchhoff, R. H. Gilman, P. A. Reyes, R. Salvatella, and A. C. Moore. 2007. Evaluation and treatment of Chagas disease in the United States: a systematic review. JAMA 298:2171-2181.

29. Bern, C., S. P. Montgomery, L. Katz, S. Caglioti, and S. L. Stramer. 2008. Chagas disease and the US blood supply. Curr. Opin. Infect. Dis. 21:476-482.

30. Bertrand, E., F. Serie, I. Kone, J. Rive, P. Campaore, L. Sentilhes, and J. Philippe. 1973. Symptomatologie generale de la trypanosomiase humaine Africaine au moment du depistage. Med. d'Afrique Noire 20:303-314.

31. Bertrand, E., F. Serie, J. Rive, and I. Kone. 1973. La symptomatologie cardio-vasculaire dans la trypanosomiase humaine Africaine a Trypanosoma gambiense. Med. d'Afrique Noire 20:327-339.

32. Bhalla, A., A. Sood, and A. Sachdev. 2008. Heart involvement in disseminated cysticercosis—a case report and review of literature. Indian Heart J. 60:260-262.

33. Bhatia, G. 1997. Echinococcus. Semin. Respir. Infect. 12:171-186.

34. Biava, M. F., A. Dao, and B. Fortier. 2001. Laboratory diagnosis of cystic hydatic disease. World J. Surg. 25:10-14.

35. Bisser, S., V. Lejon, P. M. Preux, B. Bouteille, A. Stanghellini, M. O. Jauberteau, P. Buscher, and M. Dumas. 2002. Blood-cerebrospinal fluid barrier and intrathecal immunoglobulins compared to field diagnosis of central nervous system involvement in sleeping sickness. J. Neurol. Sci. 193:127-135.

36. Bittencourt, A. L. 1976. Congenital Chagas disease. Am. J. Dis. Child. 130:97-103.

37. Blessmann, J., H. Buss, P. A. Nu, B. T. Dinh, Q. T. Ngo, A. L. Van, M. D. Alla, T. F. Jackson, J. I. Ravdin, and E. Tannich. 2002. Real-time PCR for detection and differentiation of Entamoeba histolytica and Entamoeba dispar in fecal samples. J. Clin. Microbiol. 40:4413-4417.

38. Blum, J., C. Schmid, and C. Burri. 2006. Clinical aspects of 2541 patients with second stage human African trypanosomiasis. Acta Trop. 97:55-64. [PubMed]

39. Blum, J. A., C. Burri, C. Hatz, L. Kazumba, P. Mangoni, and M. J. Zellweger. 2007. Sleeping hearts: the role of the heart in sleeping sickness (human African trypanosomiasis). Trop. Med. Int. Health 12:1422-1432.

40. Bobic, B., D. Sibalic, and O. Djurkovic-Djakovic. 1991. High levels of IgM antibodies specific for Toxoplasma gondii in pregnancy 12 years after primary toxoplasma infection. Case report. Gynecol. Obstet. Invest. 31:182-184.

41. Bocchi, E. A., and A. Fiorelli. 2001. The paradox of survival results after heart transplantation for cardiomyopathy caused by Trypanosoma cruzi. First Guidelines Group for Heart Transplantation of the Brazilian Society of Cardiology. Ann. Thorac. Surg. 71:1833-1838.

42. Boggild, A. K., J. S. Keystone, and K. C. Kain. 2004. Tropical pulmonary eosinophilia: a case series in a setting of nonendemicity. Clin. Infect. Dis. 39:1123-1128.

43. Bohne, W., J. Heesemann, and U. Gross. 1994. Reduced replication of Toxoplasma gondii is necessary for induction of bradyzoite-specific antigens: a possible role for nitric oxide in triggering stage conversion. Infect. Immun. 62:1761-1767.

44. Borst, P., and S. Ulbert. 2001. Control of VSG gene expression sites. Mol. Biochem. Parasitol. 114:17-27.

45. Boschetti, A., and J. Kasznica. 1995. Visceral larva migrans induced eosinophilic cardiac pseudotumor: a cause of sudden death in a child. J. Forensic Sci. 40:1097-1099.

46. Botero, D., H. B. Tanowitz, L. M. Weiss, and M. Wittner. 1993. Taeniasis and cysticercosis. Infect. Dis. Clin. North Am. 7:683-697.

47. Bouraoui, H., B. Trimeche, A. Mahdhaoui, A. Majdoub, J. Zaaraoui, S. H. Ernez, J. Gouider, and H. Ammar. 2005. Echinococcosis of the heart: clinical and echocardiographic features in 12 patients. Acta Cardiol. 60:39-41.

48. Bracha, R., L. S. Diamond, J. P. Ackers, G. D. Burchard, and D. Mirelman. 1990. Differentiation of clinical isolates of Entamoeba histolytica by using specific DNA probes. J. Clin. Microbiol. 28:680-684.

49. Britto, C. C. 2009. Usefulness of PCR-based assays to assess drug efficacy in Chagas disease chemotherapy: value and limitations. Mem. Inst. Oswaldo Cruz 104(Suppl. 1):122-135.

50. Brown, C. R., and R. McLeod. 1990. Class I MHC genes and CD8+ T cells determine cyst number in Toxoplasma gondii infection. J. Immunol. 145:3438-3441.

51. Brown, R. L. 1991. Successful treatment of primary amebic meningoencephalitis. Arch. Intern. Med. 151:1201-1202.

52. Bustamante, J. M., H. W. Rivarola, A. R. Fernandez, J. E. Enders, R. Fretes, J. A. Palma, and P. A. Paglini-Oliva. 2003. Indeterminate Chagas' disease: Trypanosoma cruzi strain and re-infection are factors involved in the progression of cardiopathy. Clin. Sci. (Lond.) 104:415-420.

53. Cameron, E. W. 1978. The treatment of pleuropulmonary amebiasis with metronidazole. Chest 73:647-650. [PubMed]
54. Campbell, D., and K. Chadee. 1997. Survival strategies of Entamoeba histolytica: modulation of cell-mediated immune responses. Parasitol. Today 13:184-190. [PubMed]
55. Candolfi, E., R. Pastor, R. Huber, D. Filisetti, and O. Villard. 2007. IgG avidity assay firms up the diagnosis of acute toxoplasmosis on the first serum sample in immunocompetent pregnant women. Diagn. Microbiol. Infect. Dis. 58:83-88.
56. Carod-Artal, F. J., A. P. Vargas, T. A. Horan, and L. G. Nunes. 2005. Chagasic cardiomyopathy is independently associated with ischemic stroke in Chagas disease. Stroke 36:965-970.
57. Carrasco, H. A., J. S. Barboza, G. Inglessis, A. Fuenmayor, and C. Molina. 1982. Left ventricular cineangiography in Chagas' disease: detection of early myocardial damage. Am. Heart J. 104:595-602.
58. Carrasco, H. A., H. Parada, L. Guerrero, M. Duque, D. Duran, and C. Molina. 1994. Prognostic implications of clinical, electrocardiographic and hemodynamic findings in chronic Chagas' disease. Int. J. Cardiol. 43:27-38.
59. Carter, R. F. 1972. Primary amoebic meningo-encephalitis. An appraisal of present knowledge. Trans. R. Soc. Trop. Med. Hyg. 66:193-213.
60. Castro, A. M., A. O. Luquetti, A. Rassi, G. G. Rassi, E. Chiari, and L. M. Galvao. 2002. Blood culture and polymerase chain reaction for the diagnosis of the chronic phase of human infection with Trypanosoma cruzi. Parasitol. Res. 88:894-900.
61. Castro, J. A., M. M. de Mecca, and L. C. Bartel. 2006. Toxic side effects of drugs used to treat Chagas' disease (American trypanosomiasis). Hum. Exp. Toxicol. 25:471-479.
62. CDC. 2004. Trichinellosis associated with bear meat—New York and Tennessee, 2003. MMWR Morb. Mortal. Wkly. Rep. 53:606-610.
63. Chappuis, F., L. Loutan, P. Simarro, V. Lejon, and P. Buscher. 2005. Options for field diagnosis of human African trypanosomiasis. Clin. Microbiol. Rev. 18:133-146.
64. Chappuis, F., N. Udayraj, K. Stictenroth, A. Meussen, and P. A. Bovier. 2005. Eflornithine is safer than melarsoprol for the treatment of second-stage Trypanosoma brucei gambiense human African trypanosomiasis. Clin. Infect. Dis. 41:748-751.
65. Checchi, F., J. A. Filipe, M. P. Barrett, and D. Chandramohan. 2008. The natural progression of gambiense sleeping sickness: what is the evidence? PLoS Negl. Trop. Dis. 2:e303.
66. Cheever, A. W., I. A. Kamel, A. M. Elwi, J. E. Mosimann, R. Danner, and J. E. Sippel. 1978. Schistosoma mansoni and S. haematobium infections in Egypt. III. Extrahepatic pathology. Am. J. Trop. Med. Hyg. 27:55-75.
67. Chen, Y., Y. Zhang, B. Yang, T. Qi, H. Lu, X. Cheng, and H. Tachibana. 2007. Seroprevalence of Entamoeba histolytica infection in HIV-infected patients in China. Am. J. Trop. Med. Hyg. 77:825-828.
68. Cheung, Y. Y., S. Steinbaum, W. T. Yuh, and L. Chiu. 1987. MR findings in extracranial cysticercosis. J. Comput. Assist. Tomogr. 11:179-181.
69. Clumeck, N. 1991. Some aspects of the epidemiology of toxoplasmosis and pneumocystosis in AIDS in Europe. Eur. J. Clin. Microbiol. Infect. Dis. 10:177-178.
70. Collomb, H., and D. Bartoli. 1967. The heart in human African trypanosomiasis caused by Trypanosoma gambiense. Bull. Soc. Pathol. Exot. Filiales 60:142-156.
71. Compton, S. J., C. L. Celum, C. Lee, D. Thompson, S. M. Sumi, T. R. Fritsche, and R. W. Coombs. 1993. Trichinosis with ventilatory failure and persistent myocarditis. Clin. Infect. Dis. 16:500-504.
72. Conter, R. L., H. A. Pitt, R. K. Tompkins, and W. P. Longmire, Jr. 1986. Differentiation of pyogenic from amebic hepatic abscesses. Surg. Gynecol. Obstet. 162:114-120.
73. Cordon-Obras, C., P. Berzosa, N. Ndong-Mabale, L. Bobuakasi, J. N. Buatiche, P. Ndongo-Asumu, A. Benito, and J. Cano. 2009. Trypanosoma brucei gambiense in domestic livestock of Kogo and Mbini foci (Equatorial Guinea). Trop. Med. Int. Health 14:535-541.
74. Cunha-Neto, E., A. M. Bilate, K. V. Hyland, S. G. Fonseca, J. Kalil, and D. M. Engman. 2006. Induction of cardiac autoimmunity in Chagas heart disease: a case for molecular mimicry. Autoimmunity 39:41-54.
75. Cunha-Neto, E., V. Coelho, L. Guilherme, A. Fiorelli, N. Stolf, and J. Kalil. 1996. Autoimmunity in Chagas' disease. Identification of cardiac myosin-B13 Trypanosoma cruzi protein crossreactive T cell clones in heart lesions of a chronic Chagas' cardiomyopathy patient. J. Clin. Invest. 98:1709-1712.
76. Cunha-Neto, E., M. Duranti, A. Gruber, B. Zingales, I. De Messias, N. Stolf, G. Bellotti, M. E. Patarroyo, F. Pilleggi, and J. Kalil. 1995. Autoimmunity in Chagas disease cardiopathy: biological relevance of a cardiac myosin-specific epitope crossreactive to an immunodominant Trypanosoma cruzi antigen. Proc. Natl. Acad. Sci. U. S. A. 92:3541-3545.
77. Dannemann, B. R., D. M. Israelski, G. S. Leoung, T. McGraw, J. Mills, and J. S. Remington. 1991. Toxoplasma serology, parasitemia and antigenemia in patients at risk for toxoplasmic encephalitis. AIDS 5:1363-1365.
78. Dao, A. H., and R. Virmani. 1986. Visceral larva migrans involving the myocardium: report of two cases and review of literature. Pediatr. Pathol. 6:449-456.
79. de Carvalho, V. B., E. F. Sousa, J. H. Vila, J. P. da Silva, M. R. Caiado, S. R. Araujo, R. Macruz, and E. J. Zerbini. 1996. Heart transplantation in Chagas' disease. 10 years after the initial experience. Circulation 94:1815-1817.
80. de Cleva, R., P. Herman, V. Pugliese, B. Zilberstein, W. A. Saad, J. J. Rodrigues, and A. A. Laudanna. 2003. Prevalence of pulmonary hypertension in patients with hepatosplenic Mansonic schistosomiasis—prospective study. Hepatogastroenterology 50:2028-2030.
81. De Cock, C., J. Lemaitre, and F. E. Deuvaert. 1998. Loeffler endomyocarditis: a clinical presentation as right ventricular tumor. J. Heart Valve Dis. 7:668-671.
82. deGhetaldi, L. D., R. M. Norman, and A. W. Douville, Jr. 1983. Cerebral cysticercosis treated biphasically with dexamethasone and praziquantel. Ann. Intern. Med. 99:179-181.
83. Dempsey, W. L., and J. M. Mansfield. 1983. Lymphocyte function in experimental African trypanosomiasis. V. Role of antibody and the mononuclear phagocyte system in variant-specific immunity. J. Immunol. 130:405-411.

84. Denie, C., F. Vachiery, A. Elman, T. Soupison, A. Gadano, R. Moreau, and D. Lebrec. 1996. Systemic and splanchnic hemodynamic changes in patients with hepatic schistosomiasis. Liver 16:309-312.

85. de Raadt, P., and J. W. Koten. 1968. Myocarditis in rhodesiense trypanosomiasis. East Afr. Med. J. 45:128-132.

86. Derouin, F., and H. Pelloux. 2008. Prevention of toxoplasmosis in transplant patients. Clin. Microbiol. Infect. 14:1089-1101.

87. Derrick, E. H. 1948. A fatal case of generalized amoebiasis due to a protozoan closely resembling, if not identical with Iodamoeba butschlii. Trans. R. Soc. Trop. Med. Hyg. 42:191-198.

88. Despommier, D. D. 1998. How does Trichinella spiralis make itself at home? Parasitol. Today 14:318-323.

89. Dubey, J. P., H. R. Gamble, D. Hill, C. Sreekumar, S. Romand, and P. Thuilliez. 2002. High prevalence of viable Toxoplasma gondii infection in market weight pigs from a farm in Massachusetts. J. Parasitol. 88:1234-1238.

90. Dubey, J. P., D. S. Lindsay, and C. A. Speer. 1998. Structures of Toxoplasma gondii tachyzoites, bradyzoites, and sporozoites and biology and development of tissue cysts. Clin. Microbiol. Rev. 11:267-299.

91. Duma, R. J., H. W. Ferrell, E. C. Nelson, and M. M. Jones. 1969. Primary amebic meningoencephalitis. N. Engl. J. Med. 281:1315-1323.

92. Dupouy-Camet, J. 2008. Presidential address of ICT12 Conference: "Trichinella and trichinellosis—a never ending story." Vet. Parasitol. 159:194-196.

93. Dupouy-Camet, J., S. L. de Souza, C. Maslo, A. Paugam, A. G. Saimot, R. Benarous, C. Tourte-Schaefer, and F. Derouin. 1993. Detection of Toxoplasma gondii in venous blood from AIDS patients by polymerase chain reaction. J. Clin. Microbiol. 31:1866-1869.

94. Dursun, M., E. Terzibasioglu, R. Yilmaz, B. Cekrezi, S. Olgar, K. Nisli, and A. Tunaci. 2008. Cardiac hydatid disease: CT and MRI findings. Am. J. Roentgenol. 190:226-232.

95. Eberly, M. D., E. K. Soh, S. P. Bannister, H. Tavaf-Motamen, and J. S. Scott. 2008. Isolated cardiac cysticercosis in an adolescent. Pediatr. Infect. Dis. J. 27:369-371.

96. Eckert, J., and P. Deplazes. 2004. Biological, epidemiological, and clinical aspects of echinococcosis, a zoonosis of increasing concern. Clin. Microbiol. Rev. 17:107-135.

97. Enanga, B., R. J. Burchmore, M. L. Stewart, and M. P. Barrett. 2002. Sleeping sickness and the brain. Cell. Mol. Life Sci. 59:845-858.

98. Engman, D. M., and J. S. Leon. 2002. Pathogenesis of Chagas heart disease: role of autoimmunity. Acta Trop. 81:123-132.

99. Erentug, V., N. Bozbuga, K. Kirali, I. Mataraci, C. Kaymaz, M. Balkanay, E. Akinci, G. Ipek, and C. Yakut. 2004. Cardiac hydatid cysts: surgical treatment and results. J. Card. Surg. 19:358-360.

100. Hotez. 2009. The unfinished public health agenda of Chagas disease in the era of globalization. PLoS Negl. Trop. Dis. 3:e470.

41 Heart Transplant in Children and Adolescents

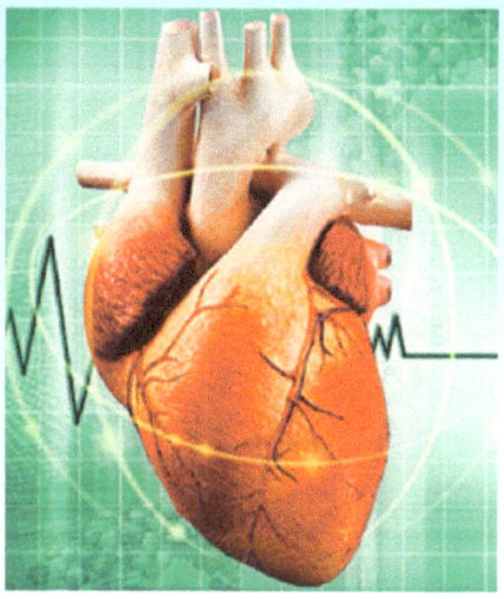

Heart transplantation, has been recently accepted as treatment of choice for children and adolescents with end stage heart disease. Selection of patients, follow up and management of post transplant patients as well as the surgical procedure and the immediate postoperative management are very important factors in their survival. Results from recent studies of long term survival following pediatric heart transplantation is now excellent but limited long term follow-up data is available as this operation has only been performed for about two decades. One year survival is now over 90% and five year survival is estimated to be close to 70% in major transplant centers around the world. Post transplant coronary artery disease is mainly responsible for the decreased long term survival. Complications of immunosuppression such as infections, lymphoprolifrative disorders and depressed renal function are still common but usually not life threatening. Non-compliance with medication was observed amongst teenage recipients and can have lethal consequences. Despite this, it has been shown that heart transplantation can provide good quality of life and prolong survival in pediatric patients with end-stage heart disease.

A heart transplant is surgery done to remove a heart that is not working properly, in order to replace it with a healthy donor heart. A successful heart transplant in a child will extend the child's life and help him grow and develop more normally.

The first human heart transplant was done in 1967. At the Hospital for Sick Children, the first heart transplant was performed in 1990. The hospital now performs about 15 heart transplants each year, about 80% of Canada's paediatric heart transplants. At HSC, the survival for standard and moderate risk cases is 86% and 75% overall.

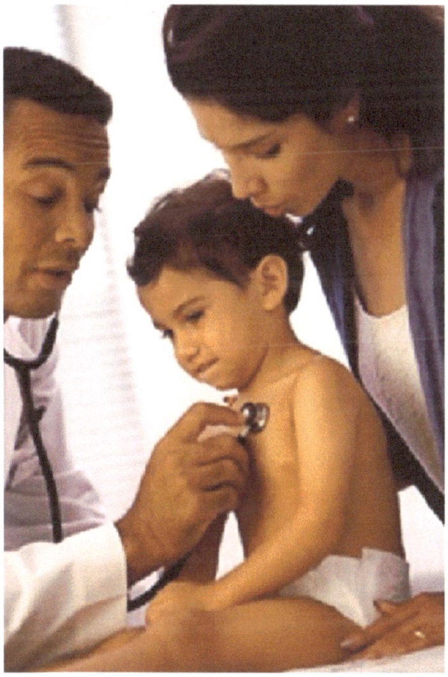

Fig. 41.1: *A young child being examined by a cardiac surgeon preoperatively for his medical fitness*

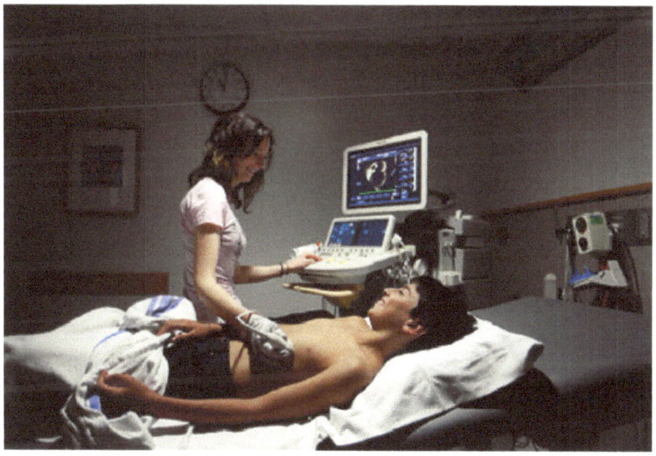

Fig. 41.2: *Teenager is being examined preoperatively with echoardiography for the degree of heart failure*

Table 41.1: *Description fo status levels in the united network of organ sharing list*

Status	*Description*
IA	Must be an inpatient Life expectancy < 7 days VAD related infection (including the pocket and the driveline) Extracorporeal membrane oxygenation (ECMO) Intraaortic balloon pump with inotropic criteria Continuous invasive hemodynamic monitoring with inotropic criteria Life-threatening arrhythmias Mechanical ventilation 30 Days following medical stabilization after VAD implantation
IB	Inotrope dependent VAD not meeting criteria for IA status
II	Not inotrope dependent
VII	Inactive on list because of improved clinical status or short term contraindications to cardiac transplantation (e.g. active infection)

Inotrope Criteria for Status IA

1. Two or more inotropes, regardless of dose
2. Intravenous milrinone, at least 0.5 μg/kg/min by continuous infusion
3. Intravenous dobtuamine, at least 7.5 μg/kg/min by continuous infusion

Heart transplantation is not a cure. It is a very complex process that includes lots of medications, tests, procedures, and an intensive follow-up. As a parent, it can seem overwhelming. Just remember that you will have the ongoing support of the transplant team from start to finish. Team members will teach you what you need to know to help your child. The application of heart transplantation to infants and children has come of age. While many programs were outgrowths of adult heart transplant programs, most pediatric heart transplant programs have separate teams devoted to the care of infants and children. Most programs now have 5-year survival rates in excess of 70%. But, while an additional 5 years of life is important for all, the goal of pediatric heart transplantation is to provide as much of a normal life span for these children as possible. This chapter describes the unique aspects of heart transplantation as applied to infants and children (Figs 51.9, 51.10 and 51.14).

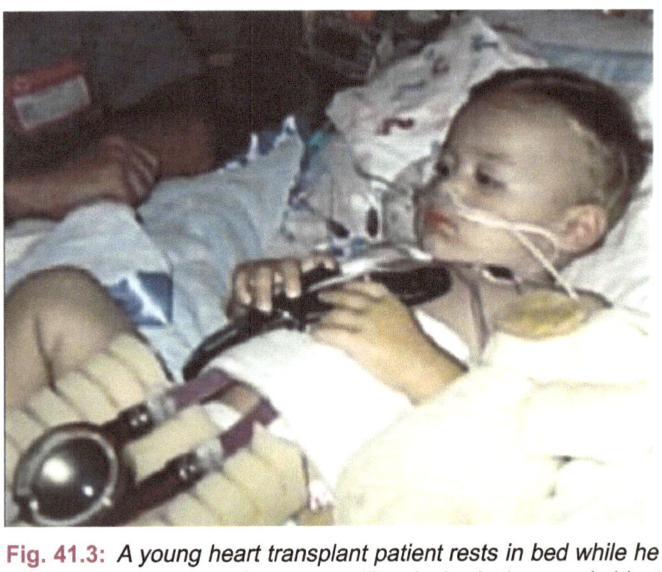

Fig. 41.3: *A young heart transplant patient rests in bed while he is kept alive with an artificial heart. The device is the round object in the lower part of the abdomen between two lower limbs*

Medical history: The first pediatric heart transplant was performed in 1968 when the heart of an anencephalic infant was transplanted into an 18-day-old infant with Ebstein anomaly. This neonate died 5 hours after the procedure. Older children occasionally underwent transplants during the 1970s and early 1980s. Routine successful cardiac transplantation began after the introduction of cyclosporine and with the pioneering efforts of Bailey and his team at Loma Linda University Children's Hospital in 1985.

Incidence: An estimated 10% of congenital heart disease cases have been deemed uncorrectable. One of the most common indications for infant heart transplantation is hypoplastic left heart syndrome (HLHS). This occurs in about 1 in 6,000 live births. Congenital cardiomyopathy occurs in approximately 1 in 10,000 live births.

Global burden: Worldwide, approximately 300–350 pediatric heart transplant procedures are performed each year, representing about 10% of the total number of heart transplants performed.

Etiology: The 4 etiologies leading to conditions that might require heart transplantation are errors in the formation of the heart, cardiac tumors, infections, and toxins (either endogenous or exogenous) leading to damage to the myocardium. Many of the congenital anomalies, including congenital cardiomyopathy, now are known to have specific chromosomal abnormalities associated with them. A good example is the "Catch-22" syndrome, a 22q11 band deletion associated with DiGeorge syndrome and interrupted aortic arch.

Box40.1 *Staff Members of the transplant*

Transplant cardiologists
Cardiovascular surgeons
Clinicalnursespecialists/nurse practitionerstransplant nurses
Social workers
Psychiatrists
Clinical dieticians
Occupational therapists
Physiotherapists
Pharmacists
Adolescent medicine physicians
Discharge planners
Information coordinators
Cardiology, transplant, and cardiovascular surgery fellows (physicians in training)
The donor heart

Box 40.2: *Indications for heart transplant surgery*

Conditions considered for pediatric heart transplantation include the following:

1. Cardiomyopathy (dilated, hypertrophic, restrictive)
2. Anatomically uncorrectable congenital heart disease (hypoplastic left heart syndrome, pulmonary atresia with intact ventricular septum plus sinusoids, congenitally corrected transposition of the great arteries with single ventricle and heart block, severely unbalanced atrio-ventricular septal defects)
3. Congenital heart disease at high risk for repair (severe Shone complex, interrupted aortic arch and severe subaortic stenosis, critical aortic stenosis with severe endocardial fibroelastosis, Ebstein anomaly in a symptomatic newborn)
4. Refractory heart failure after previous cardiac surgery
5. Unresectable symptomatic cardiac neoplasms

Age Factor

It is usually considered to suitable patients from infancy through to 18 years of age. In some cases heart transplantation is an option prior to a baby being delivered if the heart disease is diagnosed before birth and there are no other problems with the baby.

Pathophysiology: The pathophysiology of conditions requiring heart transplantation is obviously as varied as the conditions themselves. Inherent in each condition, however, is the underlying principle of the inability of the pump to supply adequate perfusion for end-organ health and well being. Details of the pathophysiology of each condition should be obtained from the section in this text dedicated to that condition.

Care of your Child while Waiting for a Donor Heart

You child's cardiologist will still be the main doctor caring for your child's heart problem while you wait for a donor heart. Your cardiac clinic nurse will know that your child is waiting for a heart transplant. While your child waits for a heart, you will see your transplant nurse from time to time. If your child's condition is more serious and she can't be cared for at home, she will be looked after in the hospital.

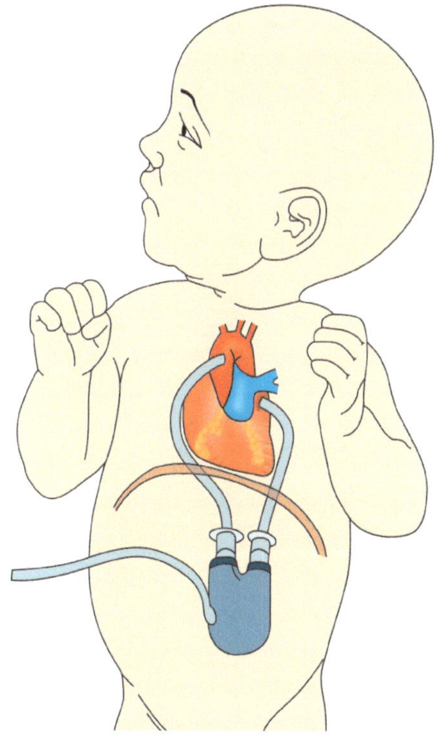

Fig. 41.4: *Diagrammatic representation ofAn artificial heart which has been fitted into the child just before heart transplantation*

There is no way of knowing how long your child may have to wait for a donor heart. Your child will be put on a waiting list and will get a donor heart when an appropriate one becomes available. The wait for a heart could be anywhere from days to months, depending on your child's size and blood type, and how sick your child is. This will all be explained to you in detail if your child gets listed for a heart transplant. Unfortunately not many transplant organs are available. In Canada, about one in 4 people die while waiting for an organ transplant. There are only 1four donors for every one million people in Canada.

You and your family may find the time you spend waiting for a donor heart very frightening and difficult. This is particularly true if your child's condition gets worse. Your social worker will help you to plan for this stressful time (Box 51.2).

Depending on the severity of the condition, your child may need to stay in hospital while he waits for a heart. The transplant team will also help you make sure your child is in the best possible health at all times in case a heart becomes available. You will be alerted immediately when a suitable heart is available.

Keeping your child as healthy as possible before the heart transplant is very important. In particular, you need to make sure your child eats healthy foods and stays active. Your child's clinical dietician will help you choose the right foods to keep your child as healthy as possible before the heart transplant. Your child needs physical activity and exercise to keep the joints moving and the muscles strong. Your physiotherapist will help your child stay as active as possible before the transplant.

Emergency During Waiting for Transplant

If you are worried about your child's condition during the wait for a donor heart, call your cardiac clinic nurse. She will contact your child's cardiologist to confirm next steps. If you don't live near the hospital that will perform the transplant, you may need to move closer to the hospital. You will have to move near the hospital while you wait for a donor heart. The transplant team assesses each patient individually and makes recommendations about the need for family relocation. If this is necessary, there are multiple resources available to help you with this.

When a donor heart becomes available The hospital will call you or page you. If your child is not in the hospital, you will need to come to the hospital as soon as you can so that the staff can prepare your child for surgery. Different members of the medical team will help get your child ready for surgery.

Once at the hospital, your child will get an IV, have his blood tested (along with possibly other tests), have a bath or shower, and not be able to eat or drink anything.

The surgeon, transplant cardiologist, anesthesiologist, and nurses will see your child. Sometimes, after you've been called to the hospital, the doctors decide that the donor heart is not suitable. This can be very disappointing, however it is more important that the donor heart be suitable. This is best for your child's health. If this should happen, your child's name will stay on the waiting list and the search for a suitable donor will continue.

The systems in place to match appropriate organs with appropriate recipients are very reliable. In extremely rare cases, there are reports in the media of patients who receive organs that aren't suitable for them. Safeguards are continually implemented and expanded to ensure this doesn't happen. Isolated incidents such as these should not cast doubt on the very dependable systems that are in place.

Evaluation of the Donor Heart Before Transplant?

A number of things are important in determining the suitability of a donor for your child including weight and the results of the heart tests on the organ donor. It doesn't matter if the donor is the same sex or ethnic background as the recipient. A team of surgeons at the donor hospital assesses the donor heart and surgically removes it for transfer back to the hospital. At the donor hospital — where the donor's heart was removed — the heart (also called the "graft") will be stopped with a fluid in a process called cardioplegia. It's then put in salt water and transported, in an ice cooler, to the hospital where the transplant patient is waiting (Fig. 51.1).

Clinical considerations in heart transplant patients: Infants with serious congenital heart disease generally present in the newborn period with varying degrees of cyanosis, tachypnea, tachycardia, dysrhythmias, poor perfusion, feeding intolerance, and other symptoms of heart failure. Symptoms of heart failure, either of rapid or slow onset, are associated with the cardiomyopathies. Children with tumors may present with congestive heart failure (CHF) or with syncope or cardiac arrest from arrhythmias. Specific presentations for each of the diagnoses can be found in the appropriate sections of this text. An increasing number of congenital lesions are diagnosable by fetal ultrasound. In the author's experience, almost half of all infants with hypoplastic left heart syndrome are diagnosed in utero.

High risk children for corrective operation: Patients with potentially correctable congenital heart disease but at greatly increased operative risk also should be considered for transplantation. This decision is somewhat dependent on the surgical results at specific institutions. Lesions that should be considered include complex truncus arteriosus (with severe truncal valve insufficiency, interrupted aortic arch, or coronary artery anomalies), some severe forms of Shone complex, and complex interrupted aortic arch.

Contraindications in cardiac transplant surgery: Some anatomic considerations specifically referable to transplantation exist. The major anatomic contraindication is small pulmonary arteries that cannot be satisfactorily enlarged surgically. Other features that could preclude safe heart transplantation include subsets of anomalous pulmonary venous connection without a suitable pulmonary venous confluence for direct anastomosis to the donor left atrium. Few absolute contraindications to pediatric heart transplantation exist. Many children who are quite ill can make a remarkable recovery once a new heart restores adequate perfusion. The following, however, are considered incompatible with successful transplantation:

- Irreversible elevated pulmonary vascular resistance (> or = 5 Wood units M^2) (Table 41.2)

Table 41.2: *Modified recipient containdictions to heart transplantation*

Absolute contraindications
Severe irreversible pulmonary hypertension (>6 wood units)
Active systemic infection
Active systemic disease with poor prognosis
Active gastrointestinal bleeding
Probable contraindications
Irreversible renal and/or hepatic dysfunction
Hepatitis B positive serology
HIV positive serology
Active alcohol or drug abuse
Recent pulmonary infarction
Peripheral vascular or cerebrobascular disease
Psychosocial instability and lack of compliance
Potential contraindications
Hepatitis C positive serology
Chronic obstructive pulmonary disease
Renal insufficiency
Hepatic insufficiency
Peptic ulcer disease
Diverticular bowel disease
Active or recent malignancy
Diabetes mellitus
Excessive obesity

- Diffuse hypoplasia of right and left pulmonary arteries
- Total anomalous pulmonary venous connection without pulmonary venous confluence
- Ectopia cordis
- Active systemic infection
- Infection with HIV or chronic active hepatitis B or C
- Malignancy without cure or of recent onset
- Severe primary renal or hepatic dysfunction
- Multiorgan system failure
- Major central nervous system abnormality
- Severe dysmorphism
- Marked prematurity (<36 wk)
- Low birth weight (<2 kg)
- Positive drug screen
- Lack of family support

Lab Studies

- ***Blood type:*** To be used to list for an appropriate organ
- ***Infection screening:*** CBC with differential, urine and blood cultures, cytomegalovirus (CMV) titer, hepatitis B surface antigen (HBsAg), HIV test, rapid plasma reagin (RPR) test, endotracheal tube (ETT) aspirate (if applicable)
- ***Assess renal and liver function:*** Electrolytes, BUN, creatinine, and liver profile
- Assess pretransplant sensitization - Panel reactive antibody

Imaging studies: Head ultrasound, CT scan, MRI, EEG as appropriate to assess neurological status
- Chest X-ray (Fig. 51.6)
- Renal ultrasound

Diagnostic Tests

1. Echocardiogram to assess anatomy and function (Fig. 51.2)
2. Cardiac catheterization

May be needed to assess anatomy, rule out pulmonary venous drainage abnormalities, assess pulmonary artery adequacy, and assess pulmonary vascular resistance Recipients with elevated pulmonary vascular resistance (PVR) are at increased risk for acute right heart failure in the early posttransplant period (Fig. 51.8).

In the first few months of life, if the main and branch pulmonary arteries are of normal caliber and distribution, the elevated PVR of the newborn period usually rapidly normalizes shortly after transplantation. If there is pulmonary venous obstruction, pulmonary artery pressures may not normalize as quickly.

Estimation of pulmonary artery pressures may be possible by echocardiography but usually requires cardiac catheterization for a more formal analysis. Elevated PVR that is reactive (i.e. responds to vasodilator therapy) usually can be managed with oxygen and/or intravenous vasodilator therapy in the pretransplant period. This can lead to a decrease in the PVR, simplifying the posttransplant management. Elevated PVR that is fixed is an indicator of significant risk for acute graft failure.

Surgical intervention

Donor operation: Attention to detail during the procurement of the donor organ and gentle handling of the donor organ is as important as the implantation of the organ. The donor operation must be tailored to the anatomic needs of the recipient. Recipient anomalies of pulmonary venous connection often require complete resection of the donor left atrium, dividing each donor pulmonary vein separately. In the case of anomalies of systemic venous return, extended removal of the superior vena cava, left innominate vein, and inferior vena cava may be required.

The pediatric cardioplegia solution usually is either the University of Wisconsin solution or Roe solution.

Preoperative assessment in a transplant patient: Meticulous care of the child awaiting transplant is essential to ensure the best possible outcome. For patients with ductal dependent physiology, the lowest dose possible of

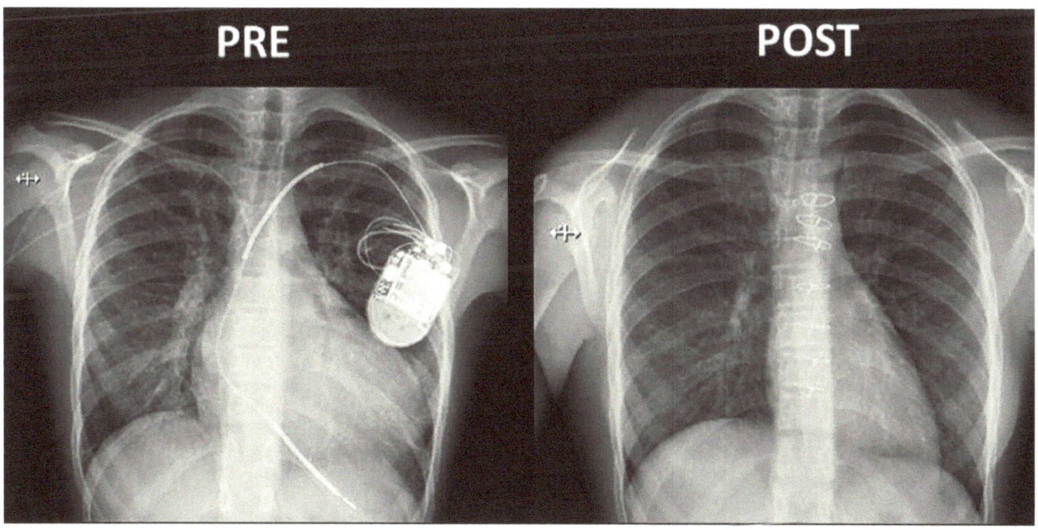

Fig. 41.5: *Chest radiographs before and after heart transplantation On the left, chest radiograph shows damage to the heart of an 11-year-old girl with severe dilated cardiomyopathy. An implantable cardioverter defibrillator and a peripherally inserted central catheter for delivering intravenous milrinone infusion are visible. On the right, radiography shows the same patient's chest after heart transplantation.*

prostaglandin (0.1–0.2 mcg/kg/min) should be used. The authors usually use a peripherally inserted central catheter (PICC) line, with a second heparin lock in place in the advent of sudden loss of the primary intravenous site. Oxygenation must be managed to balance the pulmonary and systemic blood flows. This may require adding nitrogen to the inspired gas mixture to render delivered oxygen at less than a fractional inspired oxygen (FiO_2) of 0.21. An important complication is a significantly restricted interatrial communication. Balloon atrial septostomy or surgical septectomy may be necessary. Among all children waiting for heart transplantation, the mortality prior to transplantation is approximately 15–20%. Mortality during the waiting period for infants with HLHS is significant when the infant has to wait longer than about 3 months, with infants only occasionally surviving until aged 6 months. In the group of less critically ill children (United Network for Organ Sharing [UNOS] status II), pretransplant mortality by 12 months is about 10%.

Intra-operative assessment: The operative method of transplantation in children with cardiomyopathy is the same as for adults. A median sternotomy is utilized to perform thymectomy and expose the recipient's native heart. If the donor heart is significantly larger than the native heart, the entire left pericardium anterior to the phrenic nerve is removed. Single venous and arterial cannulation generally is employed. A standard orthotopic technique utilizing biatrial or bicaval connection is used. Modifications for anatomy specific to congenital heart disease are as follows

- For the infant with hypoplastic left heart syndrome, the ductus arteriosus is isolated and cannulated for arterial perfusion through a stab wound in the distal main

a b

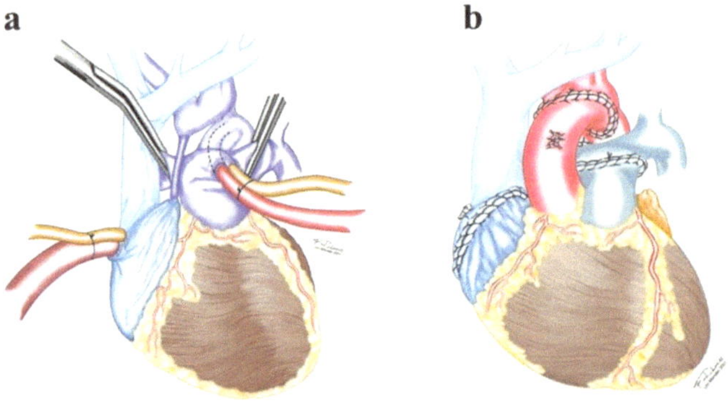

Fig.41.6: *Illustration (a) Heart-lung machine connection for HLHS; (b) Anastomosis in heart transplantation for HLHS.*

pulmonary artery. All aortic arch vessels are isolated with loose tourniquets during the initial cooling phase in preparation for reconstruction. Implantation of the allograft is accomplished with systemic hypothermia, performing the atrial anastomoses under low-flow perfusion, with the pulmonary artery clamped and systemic perfusion maintained by means of the arterial cannula positioned in the ductus arteriosus. The aortic arch is then reconstructed under circulatory arrest with the arch vessel tourniquets tightened. The excision of ductal tissue at its entrance into the distal arch is important in providing secure aortic tissue for the anastomosis and to minimize the likelihood of a posttransplant stenosis in this area. The pulmonary artery anastomosis is completed while rewarming the patient.

Other complex congenital heart anomalies, such as transposition of the great arteries, often can be managed by direct anastomosis if sufficient lengths of donor arterial and venous connections are procured.

Postoperative evaluation: Management of the child who has undergone heart transplantation is similar to management for any pediatric cardiac surgery. Those details specifically referable to heart transplantation include the following

- ***Prostaglandin therapy:*** For those patients on prostaglandin E (PGE) prior to transplantation, continuing for at least 1–2 days and then gradually weaning over 2–3 days to prevent rebound pulmonary hypertension is advisable.
- ***Pulmonary hypertension:*** The donor right ventricle is not tolerant of significant pulmonary hypertension and, for this reason, acute graft failure is one of the largest contributors to early mortality. Optimal therapy includes sedation, vasodilator therapy, alkalinization through hyperventilation, inotropic agents with minimal pulmonary vasoconstrictive effects, and inhaled nitric oxide when available.
- ***Pulmonary management:*** Many children receive donor organs that are larger than their native hearts. This leads to compression of lung parenchyma. Aggressive pulmonary toilet is indicated and close observation for respiratory compromise is required, especially after the initial extubation.

Perioperative immunosuppression: A number of protocols exist for immunosuppression in the perioperative and postoperative period. The following protocol is used at Loma Linda University Children's Hospital. Cyclosporine (CSA) is begun at 0.1 mg/kg/h IV when the donor is identified, stopped during surgery, and restarted after transplantation. This is switched to oral dosing when possible with a target trough CSA level of 250–300 ng/mL. Methylprednisolone is given IV at a dose of 20 mg/kg every 12 hours for 4 doses. Antithymocyte induction therapy (Thymoglobulin) is given for recipients older than 30 days at a dose of 1.5 mg/kg/d once daily for the first 5 days. Azathioprine is started at 3 mg/kg/d IV or PO given once daily and adjusted downward as necessary to maintain a white blood cell count.

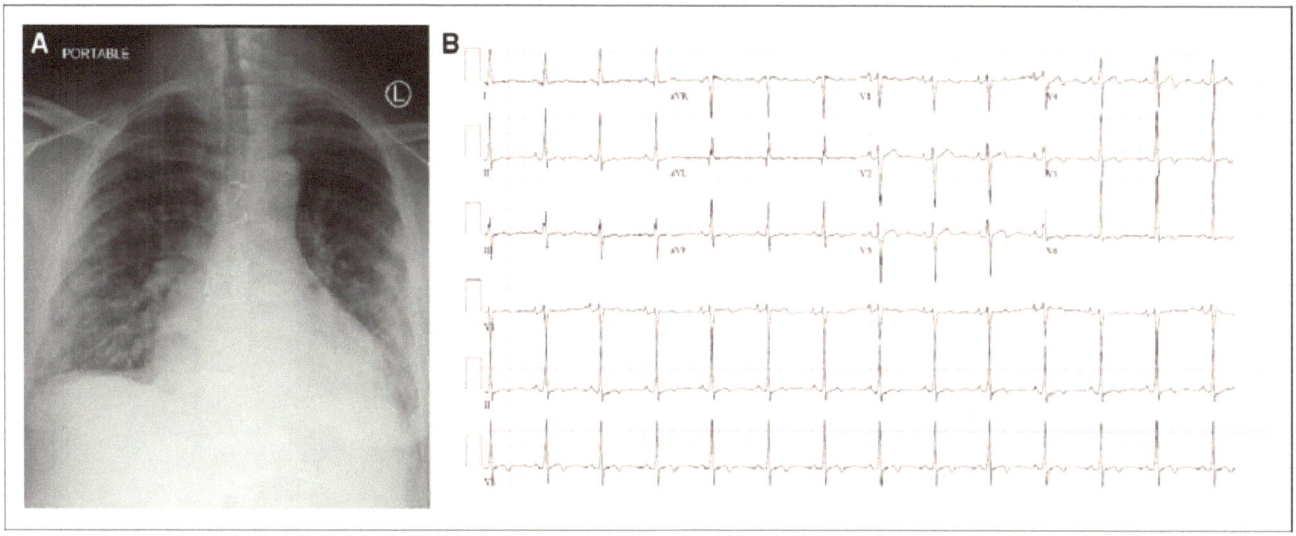

Fig.41.7 Heart transplant recipient. Chest radiography with multifocal bilateral patchy airspace opacities (A). ECG with normal sinus rhythm with new nonspecific ST changes and T wave inversions in inferior and lateral leads (B).

Adjunctive therapy includes intravenous immune globulin at a dose of 2 g/kg given over 24 hours beginning right after the transplant. Ranitidine is given while on methylprednisolone. Ganciclovir is given IV for 2 weeks for those recipients who are CMV positive or who receive a CMV positive donor. Aspirin at 3–5 mg/kg/d is given if the platelet count is chronically over 500 × 10/L.

Follow-up of transplant cases: Close outpatient follow-up is essential to ensure long-term success. The highest risk for complications occurs in the first few months after transplantation, and, for this reason, the child should remain near the transplant center for the initial follow-up. The outpatient-testing schedule at Loma Linda University Children's Hospital is as follows:

- Physician visits are twice weekly for 6 weeks, then less frequently as rejection free interval increases. Minimum visit frequency is monthly for the first year and every 3 months thereafter.
- **Echocardiogram/ECG** is obtained twice weekly for 4 weeks, then less often as the rejection free interval increases and should be performed at the same time as the routine physician visits thereafter. Full-study echocardiogram is obtained at 1 month, 3 months, and 12 months to evaluate the aortic arch in patients with arch reconstruction
  Chest X-ray is taken monthly for 3 months, at 6 and 12 months, then annually
- **Cyclosporine trough level** is assessed twice weekly for 2 weeks after discharge, weekly for 4 weeks, monthly for the first year, and then every 3 months thereafter. **Target CSA levels (with favorable rejection history)** are 250-300 ng/mL for 6 months, 200–250 ng/mL for 6–12 months, and then 125–150 ng/mL thereafter.
- **CBC with platelets** is obtained every 2 weeks for 2 months, then monthly for the first year and every 3 months thereafter.
- **Basic electrolytes** are obtained at the same time as the CBC for the first year with complete metabolic profile

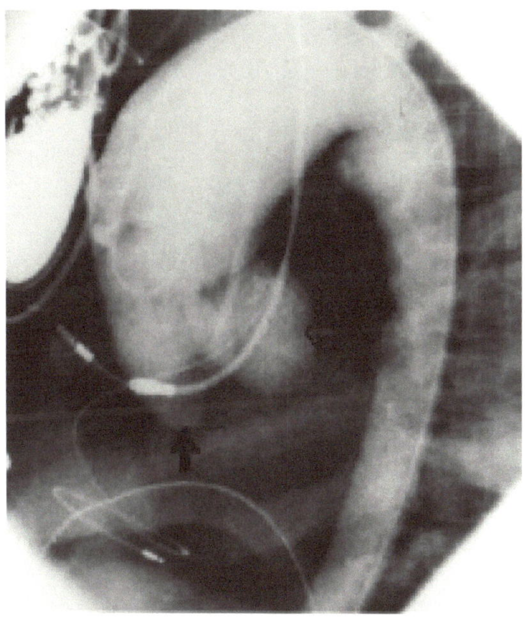

Fig. 41.8: Lateral aortogram confirming false aneurysm posteriorly (open arrow). Note large ascending aorta and absence of distal aortic rupture after heart transplantation (closed arrow = native aortic root)

Table 41.3: *Acute cardiac transplant rejection*

Acute cellular grade 2 or greater
Methylprednisolone 1000 mg IV q.d. × 3 days
Prednisone 0.6 mg/kg tapering to 0.2 mg/kg over 3 weeks
Cellular recurrent grade 2 or greater
Methylprednisolone 500–1000 mg IV q.d. × 3 days
Prednisone 0.6 mg/kg with 2 week taper
RATG or OKT3
Change Cyclosporine to Tacrolimus
Cellular, Intractable
Total lymphoid irradiation 800 cGy total dose twice weekly (mantel and inverted Y distributions)

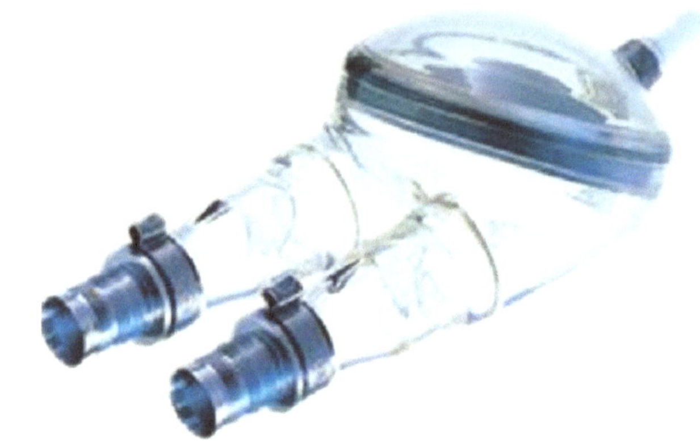

Fig. 41.9: *Showing EXCOR Pediatric blood pump 30ml forchildren up to 66 pounds device stabilizes pediatric patients waiting for heart transplants*

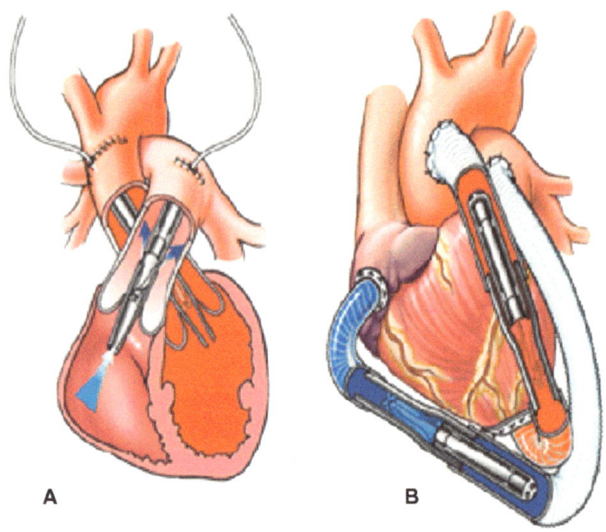

Fig. 41.10: *(A) Shows partial implantation of artificial (Pedipump) providing support to the ldamaged left ventricle. (B) Shows completion of implantation in a newborn patient with end stage cardiac failure*

Table 41.4: *Sample endomyocardial biopsy schedule*

Weeks after transplantation	*Biopsy frequency*
1–4	Weekly
5–12	Every 2 weeks
13–24	Monthly
25–52	Every 2 months
Year 2	Every 3–4 months
Years 3–4	Every 6 months
>4 years	Only if clinically indicated
After biopsy with	2 weeks after initial biopsy acute rejection

every 3 months.

- **CMV immunoglobulin G (IgG) titer and Epstein-Barr virus (EBV) titers** are assessed at 6 months, 12 months, and then annually until conversion. (Antigen load by PCR may replace/supplement these values.)
- **HIV and HBsAg tests are obtained at 6 months.**
- **Developmental assessment is conducted at age 4 months and 18 months for infant recipients.**
- **Speech and language evaluation is conducted at age 3 years for infant recipients.**
- **Standard psychometric testing is conducted at age 5 years for those transplanted during infancy.**

Isotopic glomerular filtration rate (GFR) is assessed at 3 months, 12 months, and every year thereafter for those transplanted during infancy. Isotopic GFR is assessed every 2 years for those transplanted after the first year and for those children who are older than 2 years and whose most recent GFR is more than 100 mL/min/1.73 m^2.

- **Renal ultrasound is performed at 3 months, 12 months, and then every other year.**
- Metabolic exercise stress testing is started at age 6 years for those transplanted while younger than 6 years; test annually for all children older than 6 years.
- **Endomyocardial biopsy** is obtained annually for those who are newborn to aged 2 years at transplant; at 1 month, 3 months, 12 months, and annually thereafter for children aged 2–8 years at transplant; and prior to discharge, at 1 month, 2 months, 3 months, 6 months, 12 months, and annually thereafter for patients aged 9 years or older at transplant.

Coronary angiography is performed annually, starting at the first anniversary of transplant. (Consider intravascular ultrasound for children aged 6 years or older.) All routine vaccinations, except live virus vaccines (e.g. oral polio, varicella vaccine, measles-mumps-rubella [MMR]) should be given, starting as early as 6 weeks after transplantation (Fig. 51.19).

Development of Coronary Atheresclerosis after Heart Transplant

Post-transplant coronary artery disease is another form of rejection also known as chronic vascular rejection or graft vasculopathy. The blood is supplied to the heart by little blood vessels called coronary arteries. After transplant, for reasons not fully understood, the coronary arteries can become narrow and thick. This is not the same kind of coronary artery disease you may have heard about in adult patients with heart disease or heart attacks. There are no good catheter lab or surgical options to treat post-transplant coronary artery disease. All patients after heart transplant undergo testing regularly to look for signs of coronary artery disease. Important things to help slow down or prevent coronary artery disease include a heart healthy diet, regular exercise, proper taking of all medications (for example, immunosuppression, blood pressure medications, cholesterol medications). Some children may require another heart transplant if the coronary artery disease becomes severe enough (Fig. 51.9).

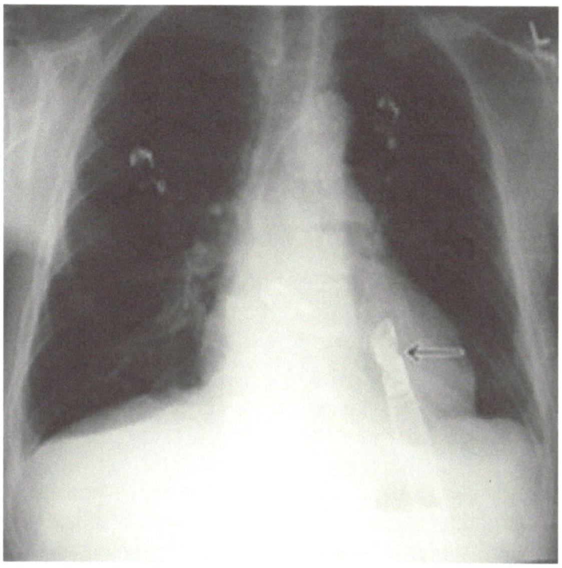

Fig. 41.11: *Frontal views of the chest show a Thoratec left VAD (arrow)*

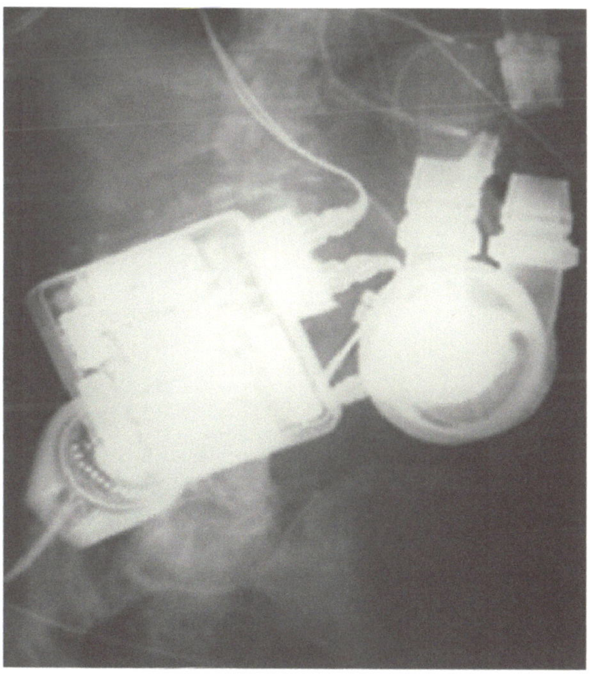

Fig. 41.12: *Abdominal image shows a heartmate VAD*

Risk of Infections after Transplant

Some parts of your child's immune system may be weaker because of the immunosuppressants she is taking for the new heart. Your child will get common illnesses, just like other children, that will not require any pecial treatment or precautions. However, certain infections may be more concerning in a patient who has had a transplant and require special monitoring or treatment including the chicken pox, and 2 specific viruses called cytomegalovirus (CMV) and Epstein-Barr virus (EBV). Information about this will be included in all of your post-transplant teaching and also provided to your family doctor or paediatrician after transplant (Table 51.6).

To prevent infection, you should keep your child away from crowded places for the first 3 months after the operation. This means that your child will not be able to school, the movies, restaurants, or swimming pools where there are large crowds. Your child will also need to stay away from other children or adults who have a cold, a cold sore, the flu, or diarrhea.

Lymphoproliferative Disease after Transplant

Post-transplant lymphoproliferative disorder (PTLD) is caused by an infection of the white blood cells in the body with Epstein Barr virus (EBV). This virus lives in your body once you have had it but, in most people, the immune system keeps it under control. Patients on immunosuppressant drugs may have a more difficult time controlling this virus in the body and it can cause the white blood cells to multiply out of control leading to varying stages of lymphoma, a type of cancer. Any post-heart transplant patient is susceptible to this, therefore, your child will be followed very regularly for the levels of EBV in the blood. She may require ultrasounds, X-rays, or other types of scans to look for tumours. If she does develop EBV, EBV disease, or any form of PTLD, she may require IV medications for many months to treat it. This can be administered at home. If the disease progresses, there may be a need for stronger forms of chemotherapy, but this is very rare.

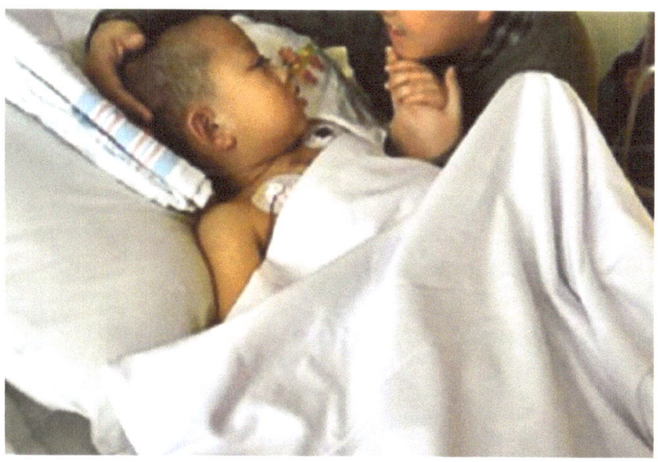

Fig. 41.13: *A 5year old child finally gets his permanent heart transplant after 7 months waiting with Pediatric blood pump (Pedipump)*

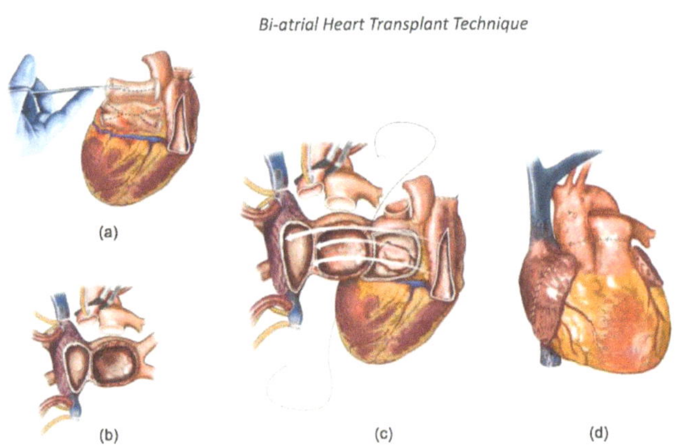

Fig.41.14 (A) Bi-atrial heart transplant technique. (a) Preparation of the donor heart at the back table. (b) Recipients atrial cuffs after cardiectomy. (c) Lines of anastomoses for left and right atriums. (d) Final sutures line as seen anteriorly after completion of aortic and PA anastomoses.

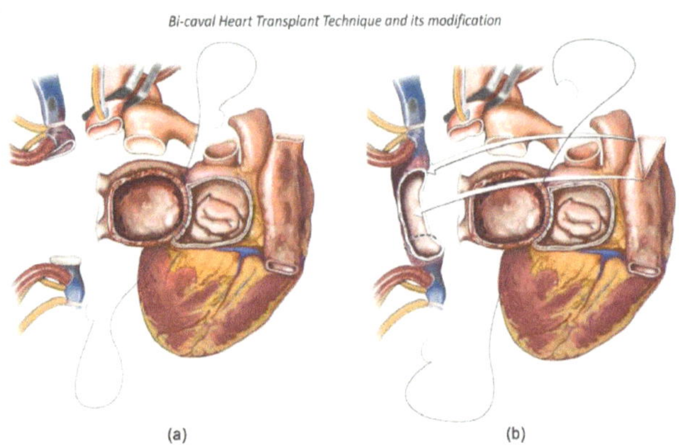

Fig.41.14 (B) Bicaval technique of heart transplant. (a) Standard bi-caval technique, which include complete excision of the right atrium and bicaval separation. (b) Modified bi-caval technique, include partial excision of the right atrium by keeping the posterior wall that connects the SVC and IVC.

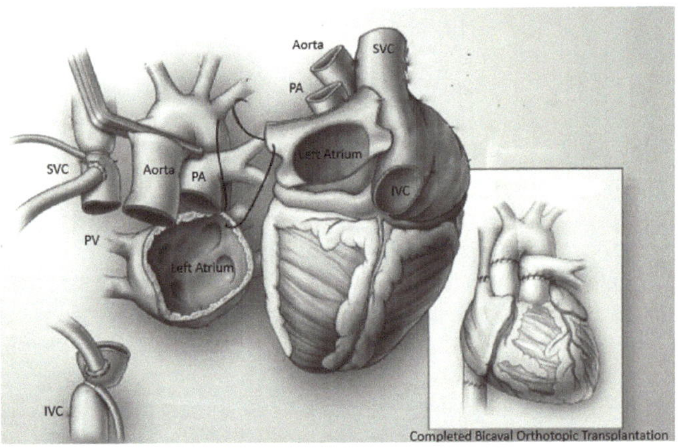

Fig.41.14 (C) An illustration of the recipient mediastinum and the donor heart with the first stitch at the level of the donor left atrial appendage and recipient left superior pulmonary vein. The illustration on the right showed the completion of a bicaval orthotopic heart transplantation. PA, pulmonary artery; PV, pulmonary vein; SVC, superior vena cava; IVC, inferior vena caca.

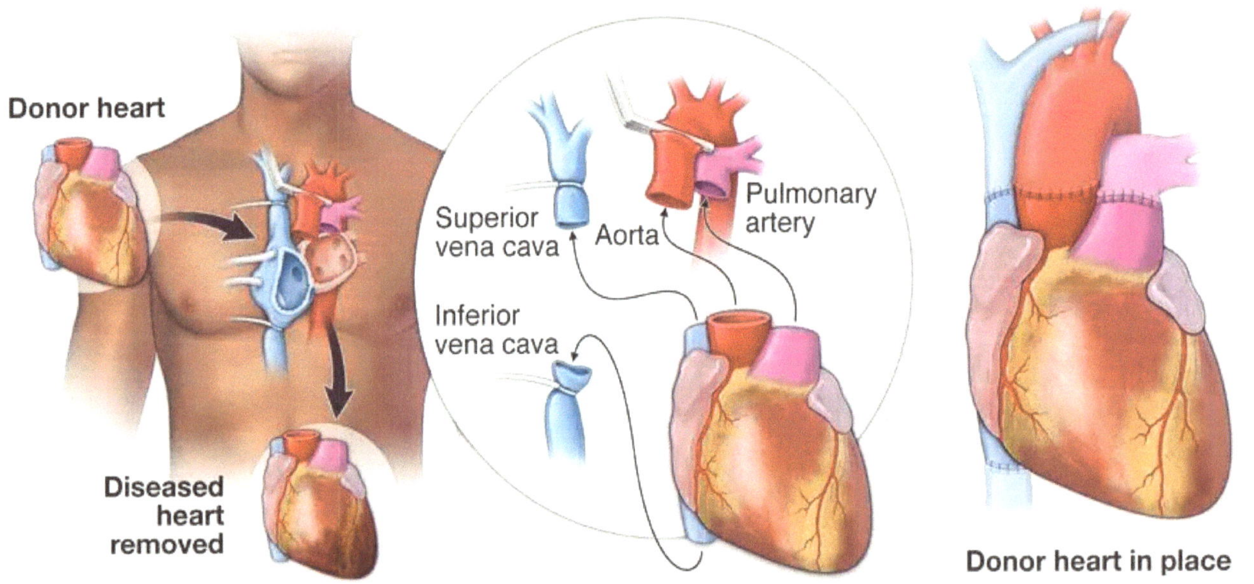

Fig. 41.15 During a heart transplant, your chest is opened (called sternotomy) and your failing heart is removed and replaced by a healthy heart from a deceased donor. you're placed on a heart-lung machine, which will take over for your heart to pump blood and to help you continue breathing during the surgery.

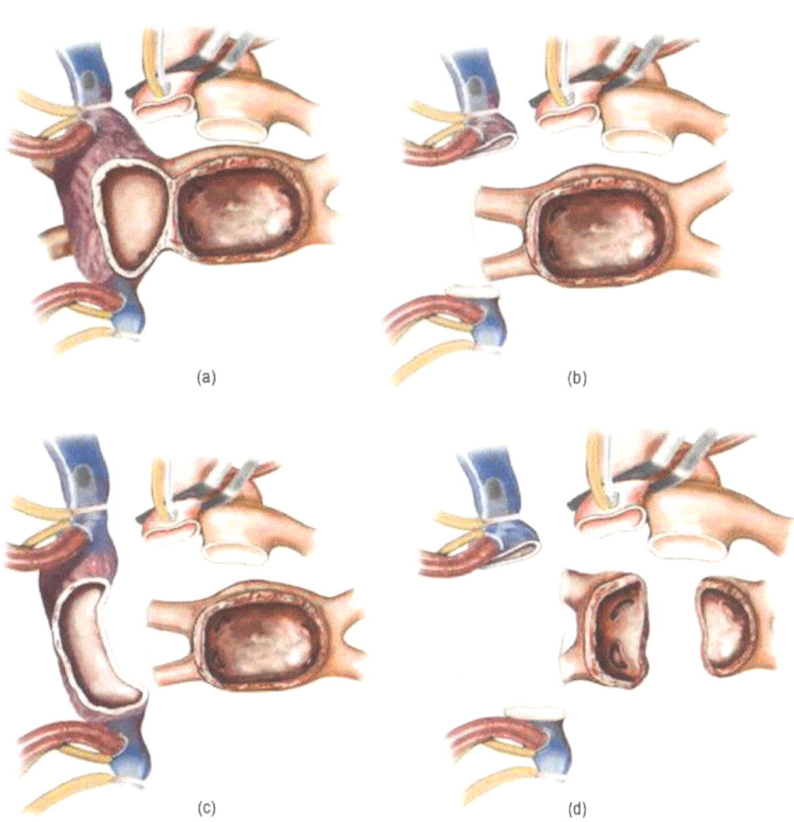

Fig. 41.16: *Summary of recipient's preparation for different heart transplant techniques. Preparations for bi-atrial (a), bi-caval (b), modified bi-caval (c), and total heart transplant (d) techniques.*

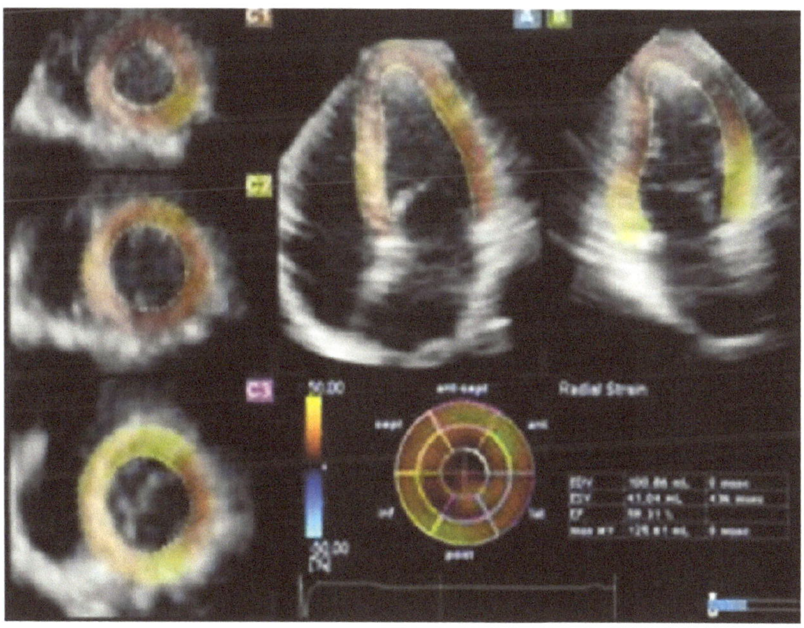

Fig. 41.17: *Analysis of myocardial deformation in heart transplant patients Echocardiography has become vitally important for cardiac assessment of patients following heart transplant (HTx). The present work will investigate whether the contractile behaviour of the transplanted heart differs in general from that of healthy subjects. Myocardial deformation will therefore be evaluated using three-dimensional speckle tracking technology. The transplant patients will undergo regular echocardiographic examinations as a part of outpatient follow-up examinations. The purpose of the study is to develop prognostic echocardiographic parameters in order to detect threatened rejection of the transplant earlier on*

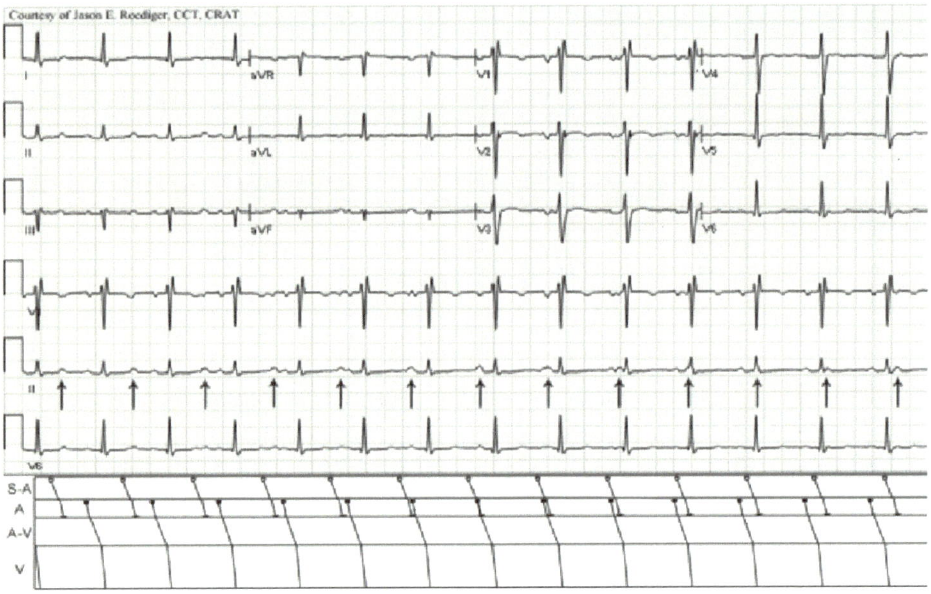

Fig. 41.18: *ECG shows Orthotopic heart transplant. Recipient P-waves (arrows)*

Table 41.5: *ECG alternations in heart transplant patients*

General specifications

1. The recipient retains the posterior walls of his own atria.
2. The recipient's atria are vascularized by bronchial collateral vessels.
3. The transplanted heart is denervated and lacks autonomic neural control.
4. The EKG changes in these patients are mainly due to the remnant activity of the recipients atria, injury to the donor heart during the transplant procedure, and increased PVR in the recipient.
5. Atrial arrhythmias and ventricular conduction defects are common.
6. Role of the ECG in acute rejection is controversial.
7. MI may occur as a result of accelerated atherogenesis

1. Two sets of P waves

The recipients native P waves are of a small amplitude donor P waves have normal amplitude and configuration

The suture line between the donor and the recipient atria blocks any interchange of the electrical impulses from the two sources. Atrial dissociation is present.

The donor P wave is conducted and stimulates the ventricles. The recipients atrial impulses are not conducted.

The rate of the denervated donor's heart is faster than that of the recipient's atrial remnant rate. in one series, two sets of P waves were identified in 86% of patients.

P waves of the recipient atrial remnants may not be seen because of their small amplitude or the presence of sinus node dysfunction or atrial fibrillation prior to the transplantation. May also lose the sinus node artery during surgery.

a. fib/flutter may be present in one set of atria while NSR is present in the other pair making interpretation difficult.

2. RBBB (complete or incomplete)

Occurs in 83% of patients in Chou's experience, in 45% in another series.

3. LAHB

Occurs in about 25% of patients

4. Bradyarrhythmias due to sinus node dysfunction

Cause not explained by rejection or ischemic time during transplant

Subsidiary pacemakers may be unreliable in providing an escape rhythm and sudden death may occur.

Permanent pacemaker may be required.

PACs, PSVTs, afib and aflutter are seen postoperatively. Some investigators have felt that these episodes are associated with rejection episodes.

Presence of complex VEA is associated with accelerated atherosclerosis and early death.

5. ST-segment and T-wave changes

Some patients may develop diffuse ST-segment elevation followed by evolutionary changes of the ST segment and T wave changes consistent with acute pericarditis in the early post-operative period. as a rule these changes are transient

6. ECG Evidence of rejection

Originally though that low voltage was indicative of rejection but this has been called into question

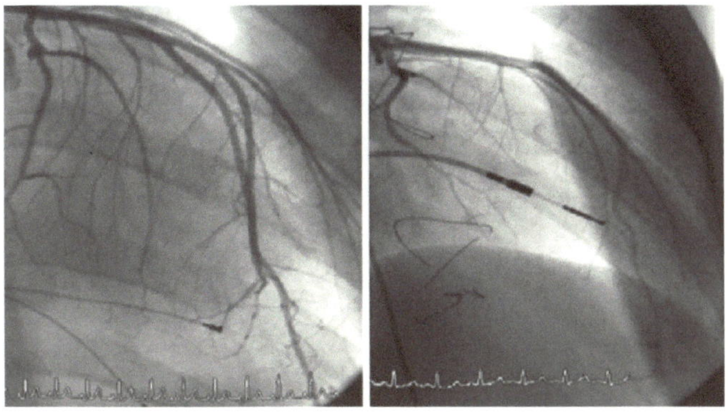

Fig. 41.19: *Angiographic studies from 2 patients. Left: a patient without signs of CAD right: signs of CAD with peripheral obliterations and B2 lesions with an intramyocardial pacemaker electrode (IMEG) in place*

Child's Diet After Heart Transplant

The immunosuppressant medicines may affect your child's appetite and weight after the operation, so a clinical dietician will help you and your child make sure that she eats healthy foods. Keeping a good weight will keep your child's new heart healthy.

It is important that your child eat foods that have little cholesterol and not too much salt. Foods with a lot of animal fat and cholesterol may make the chance of getting post-transplant coronary artery disease higher. Foods high in cholesterol can cause a thickening of the coronary arteries. Your child may also have high blood pressure after the transplant, so should not eat foods high in salt. The foods your child eats may change greatly after the operation. This is particularly true if, before the operation, your child had a restricted salt and fluid diet. After the transplant, your child should have lots of liquids to make sure that the medicines are well washed out through the kidneys.

Role of Exercise after Heart Transplant Surgery

After your child gets a new heart, she will be able to do lots of new things. A physiotherapist will work with you and your child so that she can get stronger and be able to exercise more. Your child will start doing exercises, called a physiotherapy program, in the hospital. Your child should continue to do this physiotherapy program after she goes home from the hospital (Fig. 51.20).

Appropriate time of Discharge from the Hospital

Your child can go home when you, your child, and the heart transplant team believe the time is right. Often transplant patients start off on day passes, and then night passes, before they are completely discharged from the hospital. If you live more than a few hours away from the hospital, you'll need to find a place to stay close to the hospital for the first few weeks, and then a few months in the city.

Often getting your child ready to go home is a time filled with excitement and worry. After all, you will now be the main person caring for your child. You will be giving your child new medicines. You will also be arranging for all his regular medical needs, such as blood tests, heart biopsies, echocardiograms, electrocardiograms, and visits to the clinic. You may find this scary and wonder if you can deal with all this at home. This is very normal (Fig. 51.13).

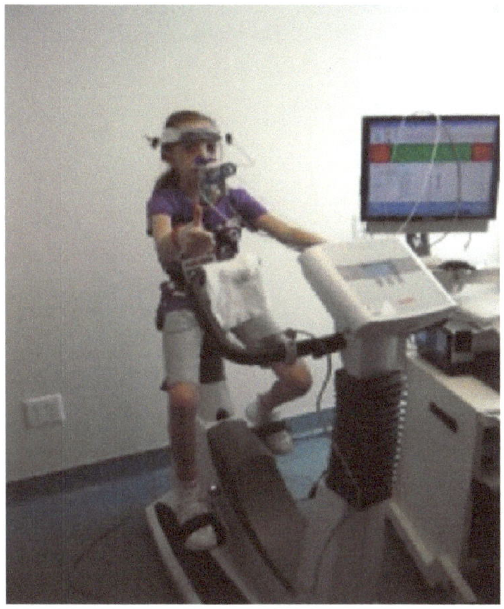

Fig. 41.20: *Young child with heart transplant is undergoing exercise stress test for knowing functional status of the heart*

To help with your child's care at home, the hospital may arrange for nurses to come to your home and check on your child. You'll also have help from a social worker and will come to clinic about twice a week for the first few weeks.

Prevention of Common Childhood Illnesses in a Trasplant Patient

Brothers and sisters may get the common childhood conditions like coughs and colds, vomiting and diarrhea. Try to make sure that all members of your family wash their hands a lot. This is particularly important when you and your family change diapers and before making all meals and snacks.

For the first 3 months after the operation, let your child have only 2 visitors at a time. Make sure your child's friends do not visit when they have a fever, runny nose, cold, cough, vomiting, diarrhea, or rash. It is a good idea to ask all your visitors to wash their hands when they come to visit.

Make sure that all your pets have regular check-ups and have no fleas. Do not let your child touch your cat's litter box. That way your child should not get the germ called toxoplasmosis that cats sometimes have. Also, try to make sure that you and your child wash your hands after playing with cats and kittens.

Return of transplant child to his/her school or day **care**

In general, your child can return to school or day care 3 months after the transplant. Parents often go to the school before the child returns to talk to the child's teachers about what the child has been through. Members of the transplant team will send the school general information about having a student with a transplant and will be available to answer

Table 41.6: *Antimicrobial prophylaxis regimen post cardiac transplantation*

	Donor CMV negative	*Donor CMV positive*
Recipient CMB negative	No treatment	DHPG prophylaxis 34 days/Cytovene/ Cytogam
Recipient CMB positive	DHPG prophylaxis 24 days	DHPG prophylaxis 24 days
DHPG (Gancivlovir IV) 24 day Regimen	5 mg/kg IV b.i.d. for 14 days	
	6 mg/kg IV q.d. for 10 days	
	5 mg/kg IV b.i.d. for 14 days	
	6 mg/kg IV b.i.d. for 20 days	
Cytovene (Ganciclovir PO		
1000 mg PO TID for 6 weeks		
Cytogam (IgG Gamma Globulin)		
Within 72 hours posttransplant:	150 mg/kg	
Weeks 2, 4, 6, 8 posttransplant:	100 mg/kg	
Weeks 12 and 16 posttransplant:	50 mg/kg	
Pneumocystic Carinii Pneumonia Prophylaxis		
Bactrim SS 1 table q.d. for life		
If bactrim allergic: Pentamidine 300 mg nebulized Q month		
Aspergillus prophylaxis		
Amphotericin B aerosolized: 20 mg b.i.d. while hospitalized		

any questions that the school might have. Immunosuppressant drugs

Complications in Heart Transplant Children

The most significant causes of death after transplantation include early graft failure (either primary graft failure or secondary to pulmonary hypertension), allograft rejection, infection, allograft vasculopathy, and malignancy.

Evaluation of an allograft rejection: The diagnosis of rejection is made based on clinical signs and symptoms, echocardiographic changes, and endomyocardial biopsy. Clinical clues to rejection include a decrease in the child's activity or feeding, low-grade fever, persistent resting tachycardia, ventricular ectopy, S_3 gallop, tachypnea/dyspnea, hepatic congestion, ileus, and other signs and/or symptoms of low cardiac output. Echocardiographic criteria for rejection are somewhat controversial, but include findings reflective of an increase in left ventricular mass, impairment of systolic and diastolic function, new pericardial effusion, and new mitral insufficiency. Endomyocardial biopsies are graded according to the criteria of the International Society for Heart and Lung Transplantation, with most centers only treating biopsies with a 3A (i.e. lymphocytic infiltration with myocyte degeneration) or greater histology.

Rejection is treated with bolus steroid therapy. The authors use methylprednisolone IV at a dose of 20 mg/kg/dose every 12 hours for 8 doses. For recurrent rejection or rejection accompanied by hemodynamic compromise, antithymocyte therapy is added. Various agents are available, such as Orthoclone OKT3 (monoclonal mouse derived), antithymocyte gamma globulin (ATGAM) (polyclonal equine derived), and Thymoglobulin (polyclonal rabbit derived). The authors use Thymoglobulin at a dose of 1.5 mg/kg/dose given over 6 hours daily for 10 days. The target T-cell count (CD3 by flow cytometry) is 150/mL or less

Many options for adjusting immunosuppression protocols exist, depending on rejection history. Several programs now use tacrolimus and/or mycophenolic acid as primary immunosuppression therapy. These can also be used as

Table 41.7: *Stanford immunosuppressive regimen for cardiac transplantation*

Induction Immunosupression	
Methylprednisolone	**500 mg IV coming off bypass**
Daclizumab	**1 mg/kg coming off bypass (q2weeks for a total of 5 weeks)**
Maintenance immunosuppression	
Sirolimus	2 mg per day 4 hours after Cyclosporine dose
Corticosteroids	Methylprednisolone 125 mg IV q8h for 3 doses post op
	Prednisone 1.0 mg/kg divided b.i.d. Days 1–14
	Prednisone Days 14 + tper to off as tolerated
Cyclosporine	25 mg p.o. b.i.d. postoperative day 1

"rescue" therapy for recalcitrant rejection. Total lymphoid irradiation also can be used for cases of rejection particularly difficult to treat.

- **Infection is an expected complication,** with a significant number of recipients experiencing one or more potentially serious infections in the first few months after transplantation. These infections in the early post-operative period usually are bacterial and include wound infections, pneumonia, bacteremia, and urinary tract infections. CMV is a significant complication. *Pneumocystis carinii* occurs but is less frequent. Other opportunistic infections should be anticipated and aggressively treated when present.

Malignancy usually posttransplant ***lymphoproliferative disease associated with EBV infection, occurs in 2–10% of children.***

When the histology is low-grade (polymorphous hyperplasia), it usually responds to short-term cessation of immunosuppression. Higher-grade lymphomas also may respond to this therapy, with chemotherapy reserved for rapidly progressive or persistent disease. A more recent development is the ability to use anti-CD20 monoclonal antibody (rituximab) to treat those tumors that express CD20.

- **Allograft vasculopathy** has emerged as the most important limiting factor for long-term survival. At 10 years after transplantation, as many as 20% of recipients will have developed significant allograft vasculopathy. Since the donor heart is denervated, children with graft vasculopathy rarely present with angina. They may have atypical angina such as shoulder or back pain, or, more frequently, abdominal pain. They also may present with syncope or sudden death. Significant vasculopathy that is diagnosed by coronary angiography probably is best treated with retransplantation (Figs 51.8 and 51.26).

Other modalities that have been useful in diagnosis are treadmill testing and dobutamine stress echocardiography. Data in adult heart transplantation suggest that calcium channel blockers and 3-hydroxy-3-methylglutaryl-coenzyme A reductase (HMG-CoA) inhibitors may help prevent allograft vasculopathy, but data in children are lacking. Some transplant centers treat all children with these agents while others use them only in high-risk patients.

- Nephrotoxicity is the most import nonlethal complication. Hypertension, metabolic acidosis, and other metabolic abnormalities may be observed with varying frequency. Adjusting the calcineurin inhibitor to the lowest level possible helps ameliorate these problems. Minimizing steroid dosing also helps significantly with hypertension and with issues relating to growth and bone density.

Prognosis after Transplant Surgical Intervention

In the current era in experienced centers, expected 1-year survival is 80–90%, 2-year survival is 80–85%, and 5-year survival is approximately 70–80%. Mortality while waiting for a donor organ is additive to these survival figures. A survival advantage appears to exist for infants transplanted in the first month of life compared to infants transplanted during the remainder of the first year of life. This likely is related to immunologic and nonimmunologic factors.

The condition of the children who have survived beyond 10 years after transplant is good. Two thirds of infant recipients who are older than 10 years are described as developmentally normal by their parents. More formal psychometric testing shows that infant heart transplant recipients score lower on IQ testing than normal controls, with about a 10-point decrement in standardized testing.

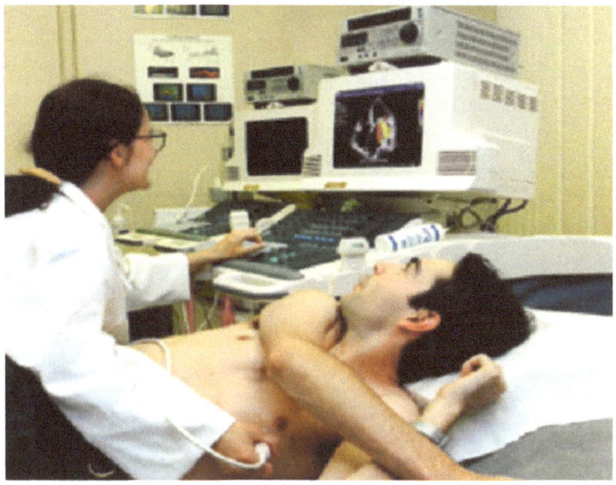

Fig. 41.21: *Teenager patient who received heart transplantation 6 months back is being investigated with Strain and strain rate images for focal stenoses of coronary arteries. These patient are more prone to premature atherosclerosis and coronary artery disease*

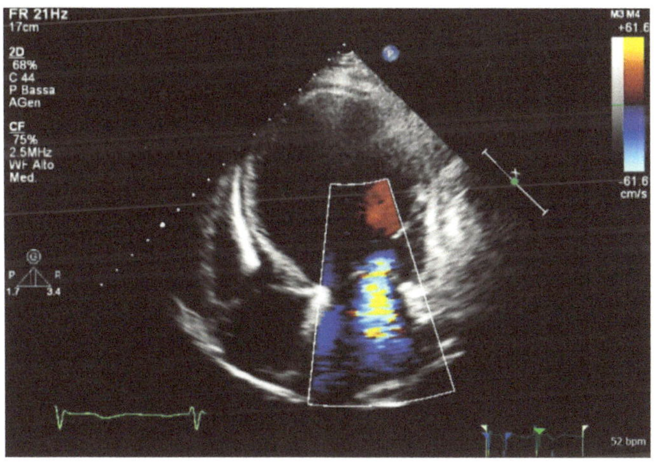

Fig. 41.22: *Two-dimensional transthoracic echocardiography of dilated cardiomyopathy, apical four-chamber view, color Doppler study. Presence of significant functional mitral regurgitation due to dilatation of the mitral valve annulus and tethering of mitral valve leaflets*

This is similar to infants undergoing other similar congenital heart surgery. In the absence of long-term higher-dose steroids, children grow appropriately after heart transplantation. Recent data indicate that they progress through puberty in a normal fashion. In the absence of repeated graft rejection or graft vasculopathy, cardiac function and exercise tolerance are normal.

Rejection of the heart transplant: Rejection is the body's way of responding to something it thinks does not belong in the body. Some rejection is expected after the transplant. Most rejection events are mild and your child may not have any signs of the rejection. Rejection of your child's new heart could happen at any time, but happens most often during the first year after the heart transplant operation. There are different kinds of rejection. The most common type is called acute cellular rejection. There are more rare types of rejection that some patients are at higher risk of experiencing. If this is the case for your child, it will be explained to you by the Transplant team.

Method of detection of rejection: A heart biopsy is one way to find out if your child's body is rejecting the new heart. It involves removing a small piece of heart muscle tissue for examination. Biopsies will be done regularly to check for rejection, though less often if your child is a newborn or infant.

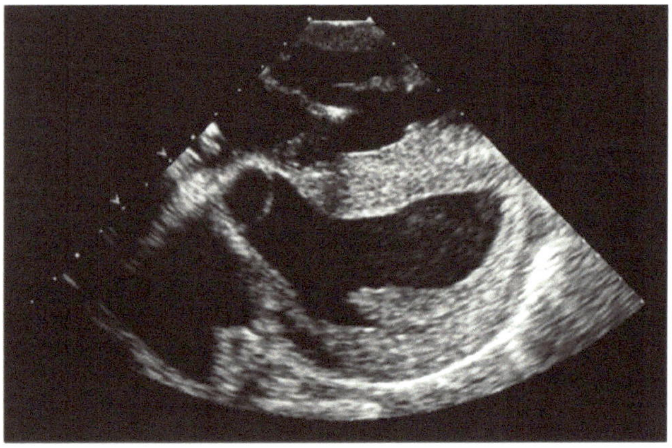

Fig. 51.23: *Epicardial echocardiogram performed on a young female with hyperacute rejection, taken 4 days after transplant. The patient had presented with immediate systolic and diastolic dysfunction on reperfusion at the time of transplant, with progressive thickening of the myocardium over the first few days despite intensive antirejection treatment and ECMO rescue. Note the diffuse, infiltrative appearance of the myocardium.*

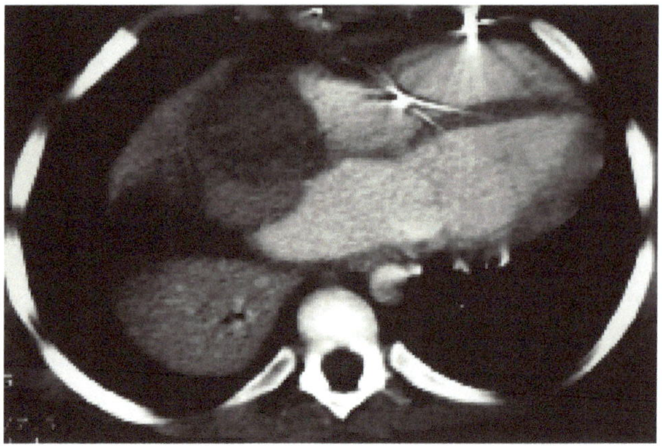

Fig. 51.24: *Axial CT scan with contrast through mid chest region showing right pleural effusion and circular shadow adjacent to right atrium.after heart transplantation*

Immunosuppressive therapy: Immunosuppressant medications are the medications given to stop your child's body from rejecting the new heart. They are started in the operating room and your child will need to continue taking them for the rest of her life. The health of your child's new heart will depend on her taking these medications exactly as they are prescribed every day. Although these are critical for the health of your child's heart, they do have side effects which may need other medications to treat. All of these things will be explained and taught to you while your child is in the hospital. This will continue in the outpatient clinic visits (Table 51.8).

Type of immunosuppressant drugs used in heart transplant patients

Your child will need to take immunosuppressants for the rest of his life. These drugs are used to prevent and treat rejection. There are 3 groups of immunosuppressants:

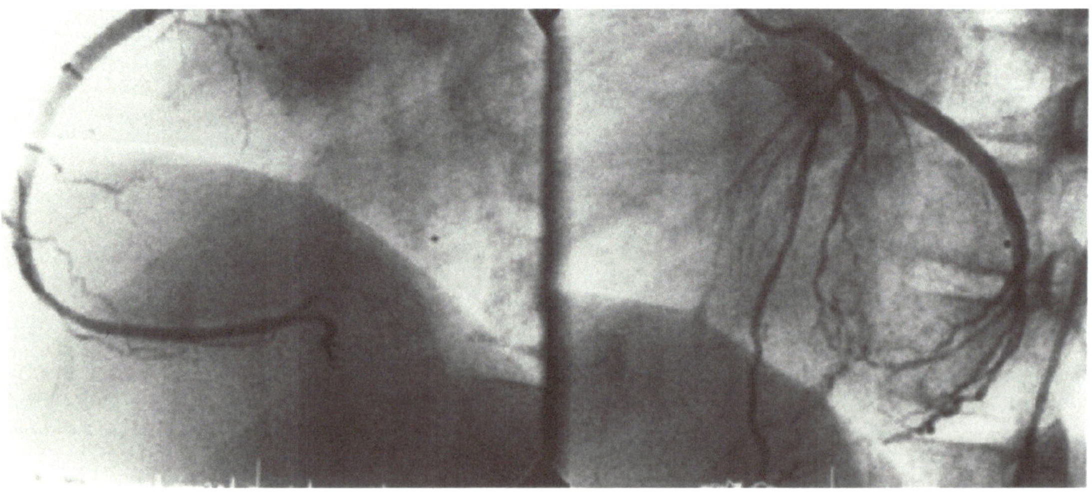

Fig. 51.25: *Selective right and left coronary angiograms showing graft dysfunction in a patient 5 years after transplant*

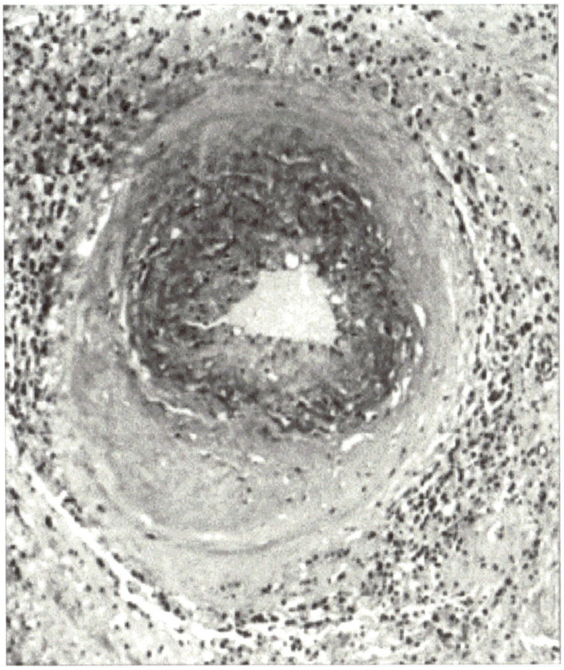

Fig. 41.26: *Postmortem histopathologic section of left anterior descending coronary artery from patient who died suddenly 8 years after heart transplantation. Note the extensive myointimal proliferation with obliteration of the coronary lumen. A mononuclear cell infiltrate is evident in the adventitia and a small number of lymphocytes infiltrate the vascular wall. Hematoxylin and Eosin, 20×*

cyclosporine or FK506 azathioprine or mycophenolate mofetil prednisone Cyclosporine (Table 51.8).

Cyclosporine

Cyclosporine helps prevent the body from rejecting the transplanted heart.

Cyclosporine is usually given twice a day, 12 hours apart at the same times each day. Blood levels of cyclosporine are checked to make sure your child is receiving the correct amount.

Food affects how the body absorbs cyclosporine. To maintain constant blood levels, your child must always take cyclosporine the same way — either always with food or always without food.

You may mix cyclosporine with water, juice or milk. Mixing improves the taste. Never use grapefruit juice or fruit juices containing grapefruit juice. It increases the amount of cyclosporine in the blood.

Do not use a Styrofoam cup to mix the cyclosporine as some of the medication will be absorbed by the Styrofoam. Cyclosporine will stick to rubber nipples. Do not put a soother or a bottle in an infant's mouth for at least 5 minutes after giving cyclosporine.

Cyclosporine is stored at room temperature. Do not store cyclosporine in direct sunlight or in the refrigerator. The shade of yellow of liquid cyclosporine may vary but it must be clear. Do not use if it is cloudy. Keep the foil on the cyclosporine capsules until just before you give them to your child.

If a cyclosporine dose is missed, give your child the missed dose soon as you remember. If it is almost time for the next dose, do not give the missed dose at all but give the regular dose as scheduled. Contact your clinical nurse specialist or transplant nurse if there has been more than 1 dose of cyclosporine missed or if your child is not taking her cyclosporine.

If your child throws up within 30 minutes of giving the cyclosporine dose, give your child the full dose again.

If your child throws up between 30 minutes and 1 hour of giving the cyclosporine dose, give your child half the dose.

If your child throws up more than 1 hour after giving the dose of cyclosporine, do not repeat the medication.

Most common side effects of cyclosporine increase in bodily and facial hair found mostly on eyebrows, arms and back bleeding, tender or overgrown gums high blood pressure shakiness in the hands and feet damage to the kidneys changes in the blood such as higher potassium levels and lower magnesium levels. If your child has diarrhea, this can affect the amount of cyclosporine absorbed. If your child has diarrhea or 6 watery bowel movements in 12 hours, contact your clinical nurse specialist or transplant nurse.

Several other medications may change the way cyclosporine works. Some raise the cyclosporine level in your child's blood and others lower the level. Always call your clinical nurse specialist or transplant nurse before using any new medications. If your child's paediatrician or family doctor orders a new medication for your child, you must ask the doctor to call us to make sure it is safe for your child to take that medication with cyclosporine.

If your child's paediatrician or family doctor orders a new medication or antibiotic for your child, you must ask the doctor to call the transplant clinic, or your child's clinical specialist nurse or transplant nurse, to make sure it is safe for your child to take that medication with cyclosporine. Your child should never take an antibiotic containing erythromycin while she is taking cyclosporine because the erythromycin causes the cyclosporine level to go very high.

FK506/Tacrolimus

FK506 helps prevent the body from rejecting the transplanted heart. If your child has had several rejection episodes while taking cyclosporine or has problems with the cyclosporine side effects, your child will be switched to FK506. Cyclosporine and FK506 are never used at the same time.

FK506 is given twice a day, 12 hours apart at the same times each day. Blood levels of FK506 are checked to make sure your child is receiving the correct amount.

Food affects how the body absorbs FK506. To maintain constant blood levels, your child should always take FK506 the same way — either always with food or always without food.

Table 41.8: *Clinically used immunosuppresive agents*

Agent	*Mechanism of action*	*Toxicities*
Induction immunosuppression		
Antilymphocyte/Antithymocyte	Deplete activated lymphocytes	Antibody response
Immunoglobulin	Deplete activated thymocytes	Allergic reaction
OKT3	Sequestration of $CD3^{+}$ T cells	Cytokine release syndrome
Interleukin-2	Inhibits T cell activation	None know
Receptor Blocker		
Maintenance Immunosuppression		
Glucocorticoids	Anti-inflammatory	Cushingoid habitus
		Glucose intolerance
		Osteoporosis
		Cataracts
		Hypertension
		Hyperlipidemia
		Poor wound healing
Cyclosporine	Calcineurin inhibitor	Nephrotoxicity
	Inhibits T cell proliferation	Neurotoxicity
		Hypertension
		Gingival hyperplasis
		Hyperlipidemia
Tacrolimus	Calcineurin inhibitor	Nephrotoxicity
	Inhibits T cell proliferation	Neurotoxicity
		Hypertension
		Gingival hyperplasis
		Diabetes
		Alopecia
Azathioprine	Purine analogue	Marrow toxicity
	Inhibits de novo and salvage purine synthesis pathways	Hepatotoxicity Hepatotoxicity
Mycophenolate	Inhibitis inosine mono-phosphate	Gastrointestinal distance
Mofetil	dehydrogenase: inhibits de novo purine synthesis	
Rapamycin	Inhibits T cell activation? unknown mechanism	Hyperlipidemia
		Myelosuppression

FK506 is stored at room temperature. Do not store FK506 in direct sunlight or in the refrigerator.

If a FK506 dose is missed, give your child the missed dose soon as you remember. If it is almost time for the next dose, do not give the missed dose at all but give the regular dose as scheduled. Contact your clinical nurse specialist or transplant Nurse if there has been more than 1 dose of FK506 missed or if your child is not taking his/her FK506. If your child throws up within 30 minutes of giving the FK506 dose, give your child the full dose again.If your child throws up between 30 minutes and 1 hour of giving the FK506 dose, give your child half the dose.

If your child throws up more than 1 hour after giving the dose of FK506 do not repeat the medication.

Side Effects of FK506? changes in the blood such as high blood sugar, high potassium levels and low magnesium levels shakiness in the hands and feet high blood pressure damage to the kidneys insomnia diarrhea or watery bowel movement.

If your child has diarrhea, this can affect the amount of FK506 absorbed. If your child has diarrhea or 6 watery bowel movements in 12 hours, contact your clinical nurse specialist or transplant nurse.

Several other medications may change the way FK506 works. Some raise the FK506 level in your child's blood and others lower the level. Always call your clinical nurse specialist or transplant nurse before using any new medications. If your child's paediatrician or family doctor orders a new medication or antibiotic for your child, you must ask the doctor to call the transplant clinic, or your child's clinical specialist nurse or transplant nurse, to make sure it is safe for your child to take that medication with

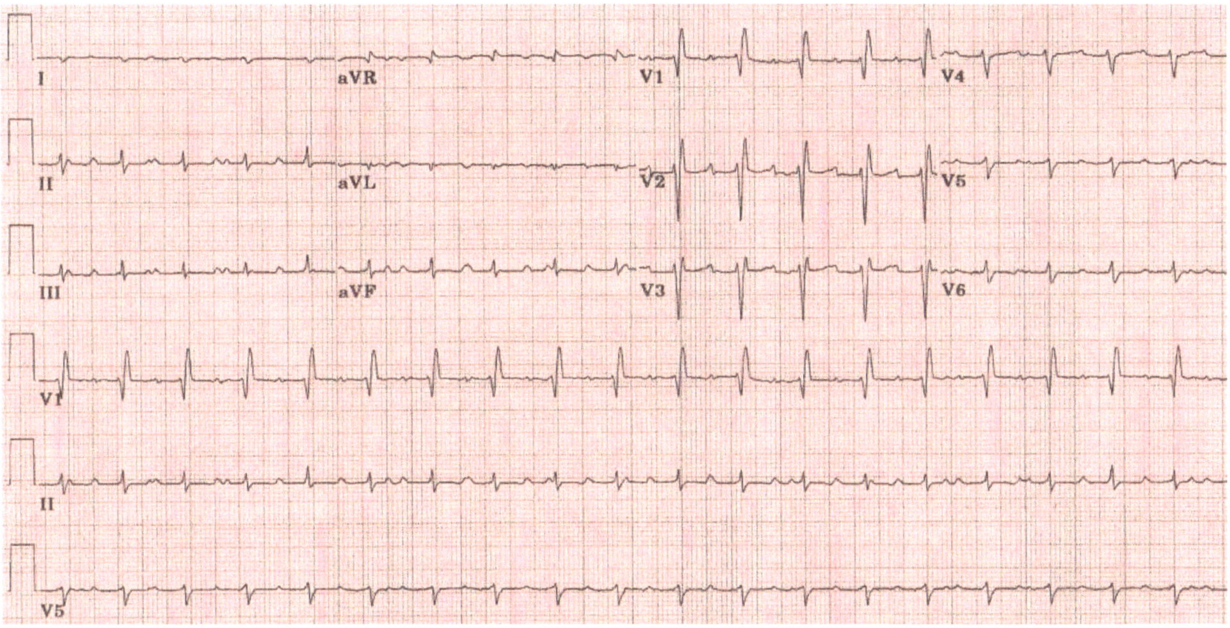

Fig. 51.27: *12 lead EKG shows accessory atrial activity (better seen in lead II at the end of the first complex in the middle between the second and third complex and after the third complex) due to some of the original sinus node still remains in addition to the donor sinus node after a cardiac transplant. Because of a suture line in the right atrium the ectopic atrial rhythm rarely conducts to the AV node. Right axis deviation and a rSR' which might suggest volume overload RVH also shown*

FK506. Your child should never take an antibiotic containing erythromycin while she is taking FK506 because the erythromycin causes the FK506 level to go very high.

Azathioprine

Azathioprine helps prevent the body from rejecting the transplanted heart.

Azathioprine is given once a day in the morning. Azathioprine should always be given with food. Azathioprine pills are stored at room temperature. Azathioprine liquid is stored in the refrigerator.

If an azathioprine dose is missed, give your child the missed dose soon as you remember. Contact your clinical nurse specialist or transplant nurse if there has been more than 1 dose of azathioprine missed or if your child is not taking her azathioprine.

If your child throws up within 30 minutes of giving the azathioprine dose, give your child the full dose again.

If your child throws up between 30 minutes and 1 hour of giving the azathioprine dose, give your child half the dose.

If your child throws up more than 1 hour after giving the dose of azathioprine, do not repeat the medication.

Side Effects of Azathioprine

Upset stomach
Bruising
Low white blood cell count in the blood

If your child has diarrhea, this can affect the amount of azathioprine absorbed. If your child has diarrhea or 6 watery bowel movements in 12 hours, contact your clinical nurse specialist or transplant nurse. Several other medications may change the way azathioprine works. Always call your clinical nurse specialist or transplant nurse before using any new medications.

Mycophenolate mofetil

Mycophenolate mofetil helps prevent the body from rejecting the transplanted heart. If your child has had several rejection episodes while taking azathioprine, your child will be switched to mycophenolate mofetil. Azathioprine and mycophenolate mofetil are never used at the same time.

Mycophenolate mofetil is usually given twice a day, 12 hours apart at the same times each day. Food affects how the body absorbs mycophenolate mofetil. The most important thing is that your child should always take mycophenolate mofetil the same way each day — either always with food or always without food.

If your child has an upset stomach, your transplant cardiologist may tell you to give the mycophenolate 3 to 4 times a day in a lower dose. Never change the times you give the mycophenolate mofetil or the dose on your own. Mycophenolate mofetil is stored at room temperature. Keep mycophenolate mofetil in its package until your child needs a dose.

If a mycophenolate mofetil dose is missed, give your child the missed dose soon as you remember. If it is almost time for the next dose, do not give the missed dose at all but give the regular dose as scheduled. Contact your clinical nurse specialist or transplant nurse if there has been more than 1 dose of mycophenolate mofetil missed or if your child is not taking her mycophenolate mofetil.

If your child throws up less than 30 minutes after giving the mycophenolate mofetil dose, give your child the full dose again.

If your child throws up more than 30 minutes after giving the dose of mycophenolate mofetil do not repeat the medication.

Side Effects of Mycophenolate Mofetil

Upset stomach
Diarrhea or watery bowel movement
Bruising

If your child has diarrhea, contact your clinical nurse specialist or transplant nurse. Your child's diarrhea may mean that your child's dose of mycophenolate mofetil or the number of times you give it during the day may need to be changed.

Several other medications may change the way mychophenolate mofetil works. Always call your clinical nurse specialist or transplant nurse before using any new medications.

Prednisone

When children have a heart transplant, prednisone does 2 things: Prednisone helps prevent the body from rejecting the transplanted heart (Box 51.3).

Prednisone is also used to treat rejection after biopsy. If your child has a rejection, the transplant cardiologist will increase the dose of prednisone. Sometimes, the pill or liquid prednisone isn't strong enough to treat the rejection. Your child may need to have an intravenous form of prednisone called methylprednisolone.

Prednisone is given once a day in the morning. When prednisone is used to treat a 3A rejection, your child may need to take it twice a day for 4 to 5 days. Your clinical nurse specialist or transplant nurse will tell you exactly what to do if your child's prednisone dose changes and your child needs to take it more than once a day. Prednisone should always be given with food. It should never be given when your child's stomach is empty.

Prednisone pills are stored at room temperature. Prednisone liquid is stored in the refrigerator.

If a prednisone dose is missed, give your child the missed dose soon as you remember. Contact your clinical nurse specialist or transplant nurse if there has been more than 1 dose of prednisone missed or if your child is not taking her prednisone.

Box 41.3 : *Side effects of prednisone*

Puffy cheeks
Weight gain
High blood pressure
Swelling of the hands and feet
Bbruise easily
Hungry
Upset stomach
Mood changes
Higher amounts of sugar in your child's blood
Eye problems called cataracts
Weak bones

If your child throws up within 1 hour after giving the prednisone dose, give your child the full dose again.

If your child throws up after 1 hour after giving the prednisone dose, do not repeat the prednisone.

What One should do if your Child has Diarrhea?

If your child has diarrhea, this can affect the amount of prednisone absorbed. If your child has diarrhea or 6 watery bowel movements in 12 hours, contact your clinical nurse specialist or transplant nurse.

Several other medications may change the way prednisone works. Always call your clinical nurse specialist or transplant nurse before using any new medications. Changes in the dose of prednisone must only be done by your transplant doctor. If your child's paediatrician or family doctor wants to change the prednisone dose, you must call the transplant clinic, or your child's clinical specialist nurse or transplant nurse, immediately.

Controversies in Childhood Heart Transplant and Future Challenges

The oldest newborn recipient of a heart transplant reached age 15 years in 2000. Longer-term prognosis is unknown. Significant numbers of children are now entering the second decade after their transplantation and are generally in good health. The biggest challenge in the long-term is preventing or treating graft vasculopathy. Retransplantation, at some point in time, probably is inevitable for most, if not all, children who have undergone heart transplantation. If the vasculopathy is diagnosed in a timely manner, these children tolerate the second transplant well, with better survival rates than for the primary transplant. The role of calcium channel blockers, HMG-CoA reductase inhibitors, and newer immunosuppressive agents (e.g. mycophenolate, sirolimus) in the prevention of vasculopathy remains to be determined.

The most appropriate initial immunosuppression protocol is not known. Probably, a different protocol exists for nearly each transplant center. Clear data are difficult to obtain because of the small number of transplants performed each year and the need for centers to standardize practice across institutions. In addition, while early rejection and survival are important therapeutic end points for research design, graft vasculopathy is the most important outcome measure. Vasculopathy does not become a significant issue for at least 5 years after transplantation. Much work remains to be done on this front.

Finally, donor supply is inadequate. Improved public and physician awareness of donor issues is the most important factor in increasing donor supply because many potential donors are not identified as such. Other more innovative and controversial sources of donors include resuscitation of asystolic donors and the use of xenografts.

BIBLIOGRAPHY AND ACKNOWLEDGMENT

1. Armitage JM, Fricker FJ, del Nido P, et al: A decade (1982 to 1992) of pediatric cardiac transplantation and the impact of FK 506 immunosuppression. J Thorac Cardiovasc Surg 1993 Mar; 105(3): 464–72; discussion 472–3.
2. Assaad A: Posttransplantation management of the newborn and the immunosuppressive role of prostaglandin E1. J Heart Lung Transplant 1993 Nov-Dec; 12(6 Pt 2): S191–4.
3. Bailey LL: Heart transplantation techniques in complex congenital heart disease. J Heart Lung Transplant 1993 Nov-Dec; 12(6 Pt 2): S168–75.
4. Bailey LL, Gundry SR, Razzouk AJ, et al: Bless the babies: one hundred fifteen late survivors of heart transplantation during the first year of life. The Loma Linda University Pediatric Heart Transplant Group. J Thorac Cardiovasc Surg 1993 May; 105(5): 805–14.
5. Bailey LL, Zuppan CW, Chinnock RE, et al: Graft vasculopathy among recipients of heart transplantation during the first 12 years of life. The Pediatric Heart Transplant Group. Transplant Proc 1995 Jun; 27(3): 1921–5.
6. Bauer J, Dapper F, Demirakca S, et al: Perioperative management of pulmonary hypertension after heart transplantation in childhood. J Heart Lung Transplant 1997 Dec; 16(12): 1238–47.
7. Baum D, Bernstein D, Starnes VA, et al: Pediatric heart transplantation at Stanford: results of a 15-year experience. Pediatrics 1991 Aug; 88(2): 203–14.
8. Baum M, Chinnock R, Ashwal S, et al: Growth and neurodevelopmental outcome of infants undergoing heart transplantation. J Heart Lung Transplant 1993 Nov-Dec; 12(6 Pt 2): S211–7.
9. Baum M, Freier MC, Freeman KR: Developmental outcomes and cognitive functioning in infant and child heart transplant recipients. Progress in Pediatric Cardiology 2000; 11: 159–163.
10. Berner M, Beghetti M, Spahr-Schopfer I, et al: Inhaled nitric oxide to test the vasodilator capacity of the pulmonary vascular bed in children with long-standing pulmonary hypertension and congenital heart disease. Am J Cardiol 1996 Mar 1; 77(7): 532–5.
11. Bork J, Chinnock R, Ogata K, Baum M: Infectious complications in infant heart transplantation. J Heart Lung Transplant 1993 Nov-Dec; 12(6 Pt 2): S199–202.
12. Boucek MM, Faro A, Novick RJ, et al: The Registry of the International Society of Heart and Lung Transplantation: Third Official Pediatric Report-1999. J Heart Lung Transplant 1999 Dec; 18(12): 1151–72.
13. Boucek MM, Mathis CM, Kanakriyeh MS, et al: Donor shortage: use of the dysfunctional donor heart. J Heart Lung Transplant 1993 Nov-Dec; 12(6 Pt 2): S186–90.
14. Boucek MM, Mathis CM, Boucek RJ Jr, et al: Prospective evaluation of echocardiography for primary rejection surveillance after infant heart transplantation: comparison with endomyocardial biopsy. J Heart Lung Transplant 1994 Jan-Feb; 13(1 Pt 1): 66–73.
15. Boucek RJ Jr, Naftel D, Boucek MM, et al: Induction immunotherapy in pediatric heart transplant recipients: a multicenter study. J Heart Lung Transplant 1999 May; 18(5): 460–9.
16. Burch M, Siddiqi SA, Celermajer DS, et al: Dilated cardiomyopathy in children: determinants of outcome. Br Heart J 1994 Sep; 72(3): 246–50.
17. Canter C, Naftel D, Caldwell R, et al: Survival and risk factors for death after cardiac transplantation in infants. A multi-institutional study. The Pediatric Heart Transplant Study. Circulation 1997 Jul 1; 96(1): 227–31.
18. Canter CE: Preoperative assessment and management of pediatric heart transplantation. Progress in Pediatric Cardiology 2000; 11: 91–97.
19. Cetta F, O'Leary PW, Seward JB, Driscoll DJ: Idiopathic restrictive cardiomyopathy in childhood: diagnostic features and clinical course. Mayo Clin Proc 1995 Jul; 70(7): 634–40.
20. Chartrand C, Guerin R, Kangah M, Stanley P: Pediatric heart transplantation: surgical considerations for congenital heart diseases. J Heart Transplant 1990 Nov-Dec; 9(6): 608–16; discussion 616–7.
21. Chen JM, Levin HR, Michler RE, et al: Reevaluating the significance of pulmonary hypertension before cardiac transplantation: determination of optimal thresholds and quantification of the effect of reversibility on perioperative mortality. J Thorac Cardiovasc Surg 1997 Oct; 114(4): 627–34.
22. Chiavarelli M, Gundry SR, Razzouk AJ, Bailey LL: Cardiac transplantation for infants with hypoplastic left-heart syndrome. JAMA 1993 Dec 22–29; 270(24): 2944–7.
23. Chinnock R, Baum M: Somatic growth in infant heart transplant recipients. Pediatr Transplant 1998 Feb; 2(1): 30–4.
24. Chinnock R, Emery J, Larsen R, et al: Methotrexate therapy for complex graft rejection in pediatric heart transplant recipients. The Pediatric Heart Transplant Team—Loma Linda. J Heart Lung Transplant 1995 Jul-Aug; 14(4): 726–33
25. Chinnock RE, Baum MF, Larsen R, Bailey L: Rejection management and long-term surveillance of the pediatric heart transplant recipient: the Loma Linda experience. J Heart Lung Transplant 1993 Nov-Dec; 12(6 Pt 2): S255–64.
26. Chinnock RE: Pediatric heart transplantation at Loma Linda: 1985 to 1996. Clin Transpl 1996; 145–51.
27. Chinnock RE, Torres VI, Jutzy RV, et al: Cardiac pacemakers in pediatric heart transplant recipients: incidence, indications, and associated factors. Pediatric Heart Transplant Group- Loma Linda. Pacing Clin Electrophysiol 1996 Jan; 19(1): 26–30.
28. Chinnock RE, Cutler D, Baum M: Clinical outcome 10 years after infant heart transplantation. Progress in Pediatric Cardiology 2000; 11: 165–169.
29. del Rio MJ: Transplantation in complex congenital heart disease. Progress in Pediatric Cardiology 2000; 11: 107–113.
30. Denfield SW, Rosenthal G, Gajarski RJ, et al: Restrictive cardiomyopathies in childhood. Etiologies and natural history. Tex Heart Inst J 1997; 24(1): 38–44.
31. Dent CL, Canter CE, Hirsch R, Balzer DT: Transplant coronary artery disease in pediatric heart transplant recipients. J Heart Lung Transplant 2000 Mar; 19(3): 240–8.
32. Fricker FJ, Addonizio L, Bernstein D, et al: Heart transplantation in children: indications. Report of the Ad Hoc Subcommittee of the Pediatric Committee of the American Society of Transplantation (AST). Pediatr Transplant 1999 Nov; 3(4): 333–42.

33. Fritzsche SD, McCabe JL, Chinnock RE: Rare combined heart and kidney transplant in a pediatric patient: a case study. J Transpl Coord 1999 Sep; 9(3): 145–8.
34. Fukushima N, Gundry SR, Razzouk AJ, Bailey LL: Risk factors for graft failure associated with pulmonary hypertension after pediatric heart transplantation. J Thorac Cardiovasc Surg 1994 Apr; 107(4): 985–9.
35. Gajarski RJ, Towbin JA, Bricker JT, et al: Intermediate follow-up of pediatric heart transplant recipients with elevated pulmonary vascular resistance index. J Am Coll Cardiol 1994 Jun; 23(7): 1682–7.
36. Hirsch R, Huddleston CB, Mendeloff EN, et al: Infant and donor organ growth after heart transplantation in neonates with hypoplastic left heart syndrome. J Heart Lung Transplant 1996 Nov; 15(11): 1093–100.
37. Hsu DT, Garofano RP, Douglas JM, et al: Exercise performance after pediatric heart transplantation. Circulation 1993 Nov; 88(5 Pt 2): II238–42.
38. Jacobs ML, Blackstone EH, Bailey LL: Intermediate survival in neonates with aortic atresia: a multi- institutional study. The Congenital Heart Surgeons Society. J Thorac Cardiovasc Surg 1998 Sep; 116(3): 417–31.
39. Jenkins PC, Flanagan MF, Jenkins KJ, et al: Survival analysis and risk factors for mortality in transplantation and staged surgery for hypoplastic left heart syndrome. J Am Coll Cardiol 2000 Oct; 36(4): 1178–85.
40. Kawauchi M, Gundry SR, de Begona JA, et al: Prolonged preservation of human pediatric hearts for transplantation: correlation of ischemic time and subsequent function. J Heart Lung Transplant 1993 Jan-Feb; 12(1 Pt 1): 55–8.
41. Kirklin JK: Pediatric cardiac transplantation. Ann Thorac Surg 2000 May; 69(5): 1627–8.
42. Kuhn MA, Jutzy KR, Deming DD, et al: The medium-term findings in coronary arteries by intravascular ultrasound in infants and children after heart transplantation. J Am Coll Cardiol 2000 Jul; 36(1): 250–4.
43. Larsen RL, Applegate PM, Dyar DA, et al: Dobutamine stress echocardiography for assessing coronary artery disease after transplantation in children. J Am Coll Cardiol 1998 Aug; 32(2): 515–20.
44. Loker J, Darragh R, Ensing G, Caldwell R: Echocardiographic analysis of rejection in the infant heart transplant recipient. J Heart Lung Transplant 1994 Nov-Dec; 13(6): 1014–8.
45. Lynch BJ, Glauser TA, Canter C, Spray T: Neurologic complications of pediatric heart transplantation. Arch Pediatr Adolesc Med 1994 Sep; 148(9): 973–9.
46. Moran AM, Lipshultz SE, Rifai N, et al: Non-invasive assessment of rejection in pediatric transplant patients: serologic and echocardiographic prediction of biopsy-proven myocardial rejection. J Heart Lung Transplant 2000 Aug; 19(8): 756–64.
47. Morrow WR, Naftel D, Chinnock R, et al: Outcome of listing for heart transplantation in infants younger than six months: predictors of death and interval to transplantation. The Pediatric Heart Transplantation Study Group. J Heart Lung Transplant 1997 Dec; 16(12): 1255–66.
48. Morrow WR, Frazier E, Naftel DC: Survival after listing for cardiac transplantation in children. Progress in Pediatric Cardiology 2000; 11: 99–105.
49. Pahl E, Crawford SE, Swenson JM, et al: Dobutamine stress echocardiography: experience in pediatric heart transplant recipients. J Heart Lung Transplant 1999 Jul; 18(7): 725–32.
50. Pahl E, Zales VR, Fricker FJ, Addonizio LJ: Posttransplant coronary artery disease in children. A multicenter national survey. Circulation 1994 Nov; 90(5 Pt 2): II56–60.
51. Pahl E: Transplant coronary artery diseasein children. Progress in Pediatric Cardiology 2000; 11: 137–143.
52. Pietra BA, Boucek MM: Immunosuppression for pediatric cardiac transplantation in the modern era. Progress in Pediatric Cardiology 2000; 11: 115–129.
53. Razzouk AJ, Chinnock RE, Dearani JA, et al: Cardiac retransplantation for graft vasculopathy in children: should we continue to do it? Arch Surg 1998 Aug; 133(8): 881–5.

42 Tele-Medicine in Pediatric Cardiology

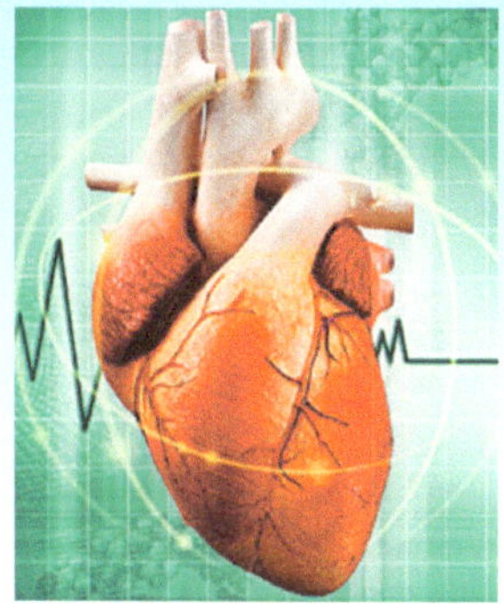

The newly developing field of telemedicine has the potential to benefit pediatric care by in creasing access to pediatric specialists and services. This report explores the current uses and limitations of telemedicine in pediatrics.

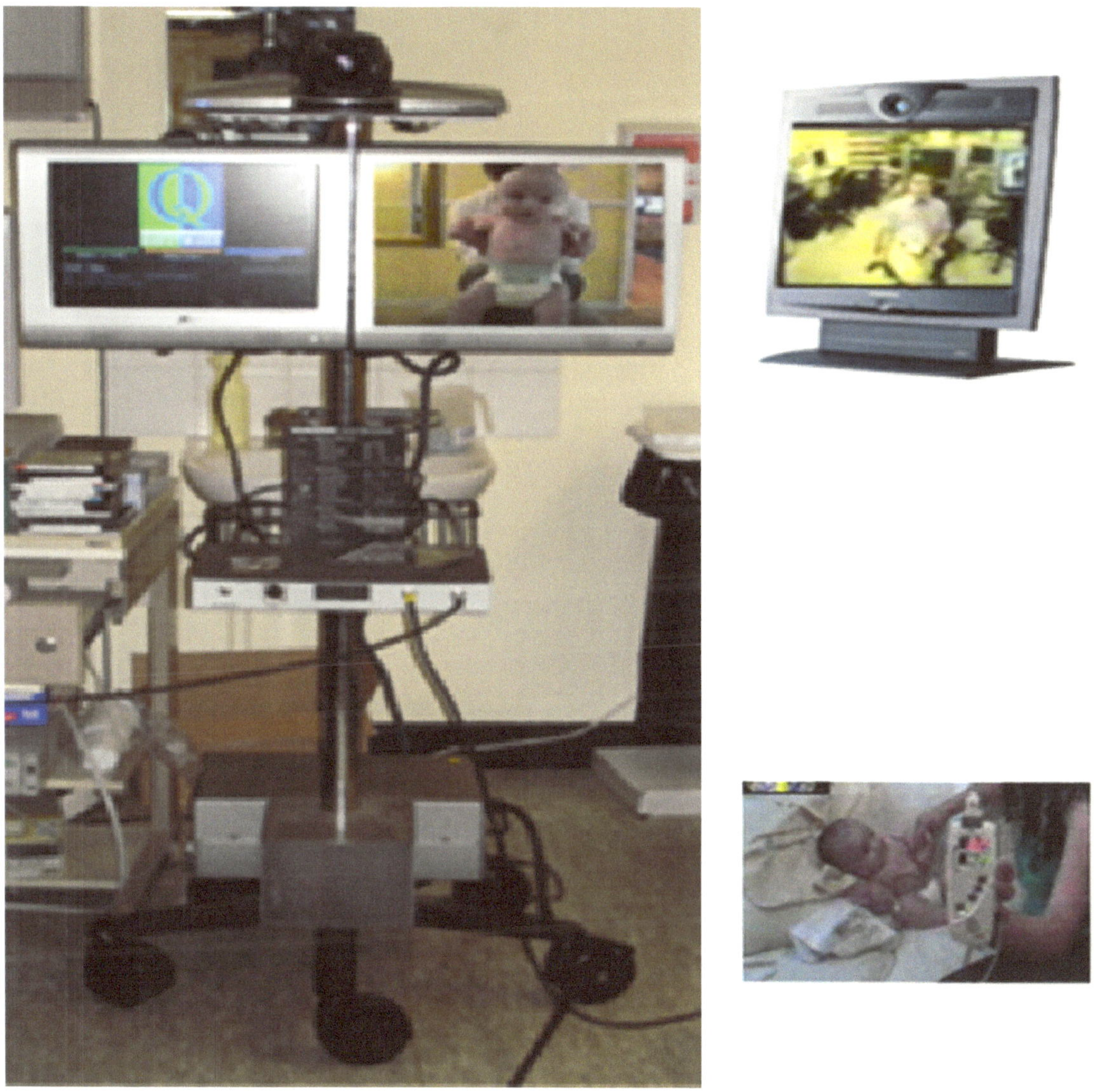

Fig. 42.1: *Telemedicine hardware needed for hospital-home videoconferencing. What the doctor sees and what the family sees*

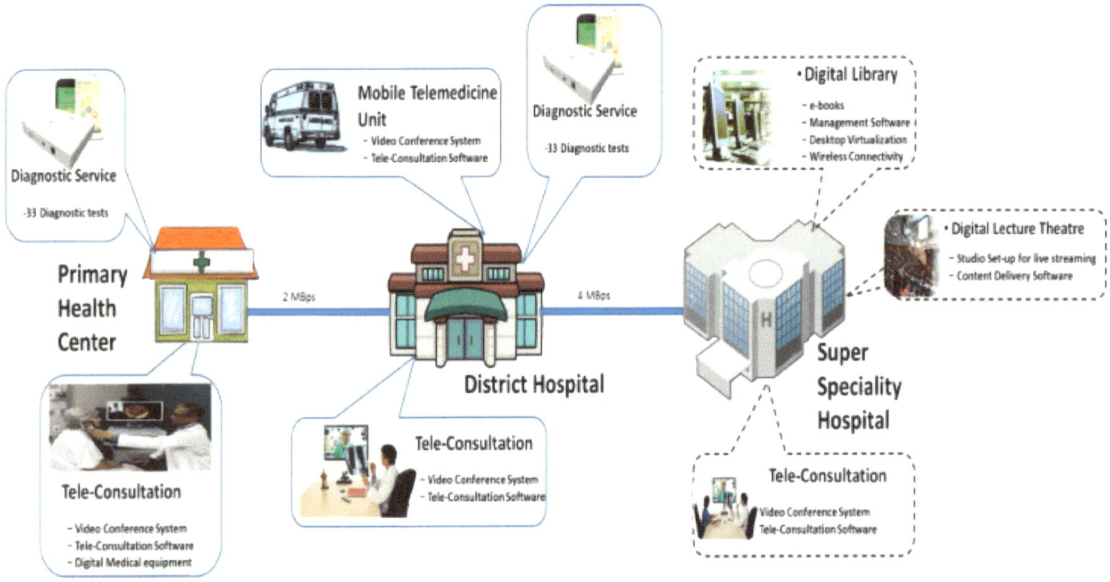

Fig 42.2 National Telemedicine Network (NTN)" has been envisaged to provide Telemedicine Services to the remote areas by upgrading existing Government Healthcare Facilities (MC, DH, SDH, PHC, and CHC) in States. Telemedicine nodes across India are being created inter connecting SDH/PHC/CHC, District Hospital and Medical College in every State for providing Citizen-centric services. This TM Network will start in Synchronous with the roll out of NOFN across country

Table 42.1 How congenital heart disease presents and the potential for telemedicine to support district general hospitals within a clinical network.

	Presentation	Urgency	Potential for telemedicine
Antenatal	Suspected CHD on routine anomaly scan Risk factor for CHD	Non-urgent	Support sonographers Streamline antenatal screening
Neonate	Cyanosis Murmur Clinical shock Abnormal femoral pulses Risk factor for CHD	Usually an emergency	Immediate diagnosis or exclusion of CHD Institute potentially life-saving therapy Decide upon need for transfer
Infant & Child	Murmur Tachypnoea Hepatomegaly Abnormal femoral pulses Failure to Thrive	Usually less urgent	Virtual clinics could help reconfigure workload for paediatric cardiologists

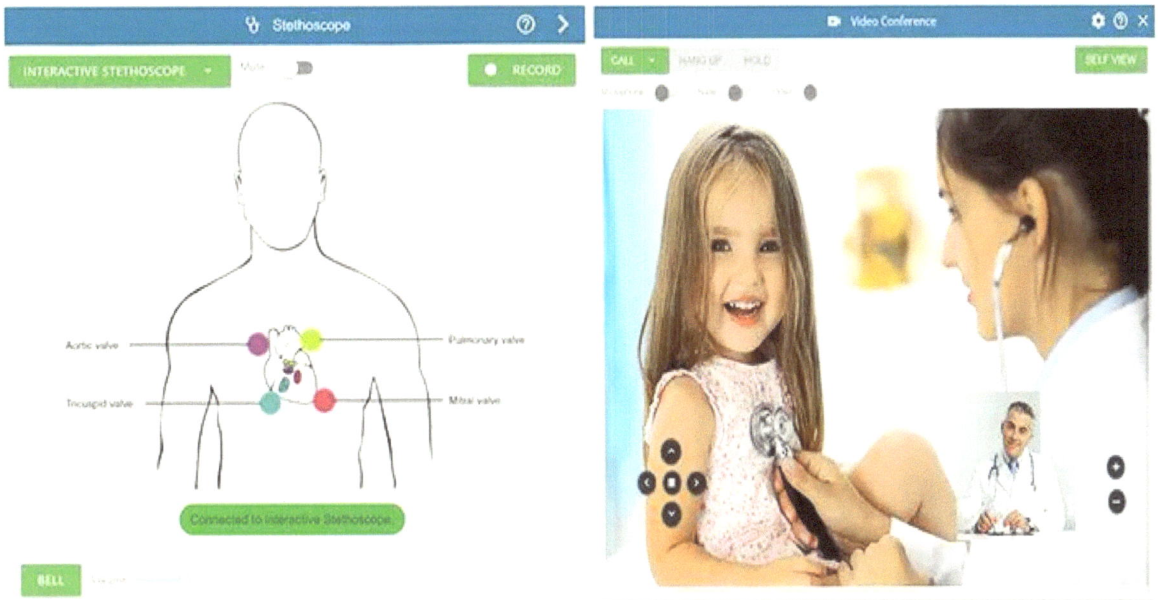

Fig 42.3 showing application of interactive digital stethoscope in a child with clinically diagnosed heart murmur

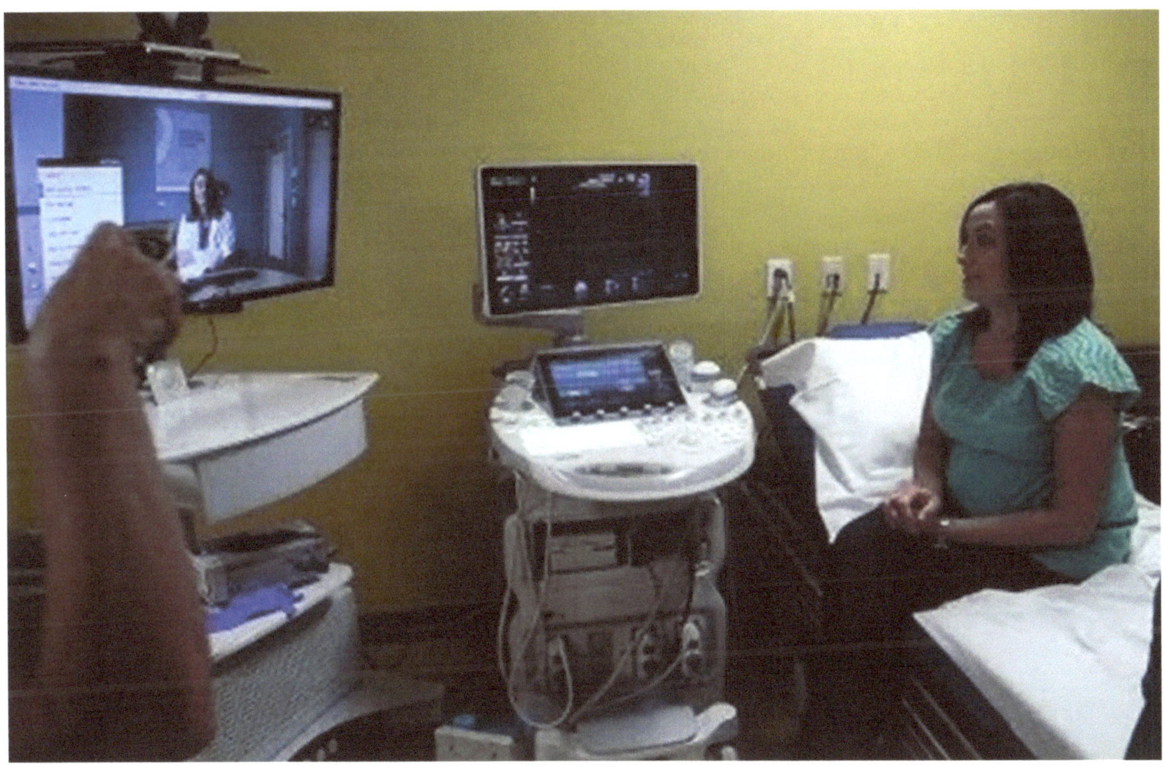

Fig 42.4 Through telemedicine ,pediatric cardiologist is explaining to the mother the type of cardiac defect her baby is having and what type of action is likely to taken in future.

Tele-echocardiography has the potential to bring real-time diagnoses to neonatal facilities without in-house pediatric cardiologists. Many neonates in rural areas, smaller cities, and community hospitals do not have immediate access to pediatric sonographers or echocardiogram interpretation by pediatric cardiologists. This can result in suboptimal echocardiogram quality, delay in initiation of medical intervention, unnecessary patient transport, and increased medical expenditures. Telemedicine has been used with increased frequency to improve efficiency of pediatric cardiology care in hospitals that are not served by pediatric cardiologists. Initial reports suggest that telecardiology is accurate, improves patient care, is cost-effective, enhances echocardiogram quality, and prevents unnecessary transports of neonates in locations that are not served by pediatric cardiologists (Fig. 53.1).

Echocardiography is often used to diagnose and exclude important cardiac diagnoses in children. Evolving telemedicine technology has the potential to improve access to echocardiography diagnoses in the intensive care unit, emergency room, and newborn nursery. The two primary modes of telemedicine practice are "store and forward" and "real-time" videoconferencing. A digital echocardiogram (often several one cardiac cycle loops) can be stored at one site and forwarded across a telemedicine network to a receiving station for review at a later time. Pediatric cardiologists often favor "real-time" telemedicine because of the ability to guide sonographers with limited experience in congenital heart disease. A complete telemedicine system requires a modified computer, a low- or high-speed connection, and telemedicine inputs. Several adult and pediatric clinical studies have shown telemedicine to be accurate, improve patient care, be cost-effective, enhance echocardiogram quality and sonographer proficiency, and promote practice expansion. Obstacles to widespread implementation of telemedicine include lack of standardization of telemedicine components, confusing legal issues and licensure requirements, and poor reimbursement.

Congenital Heart Diseases

Several telemedicine applications have become well established in paediatric cardiology but there is potential for improvement in and expansion of existing programmes and opportunities for new applications. This chapter shall discuss why telemedicine has an important role to play in paediatric cardiology, examine current applications from fetus to adult, including the evidence base and suggest what future steps may be taken to promote the use of telemedicine in paediatric cardiology. We shall also

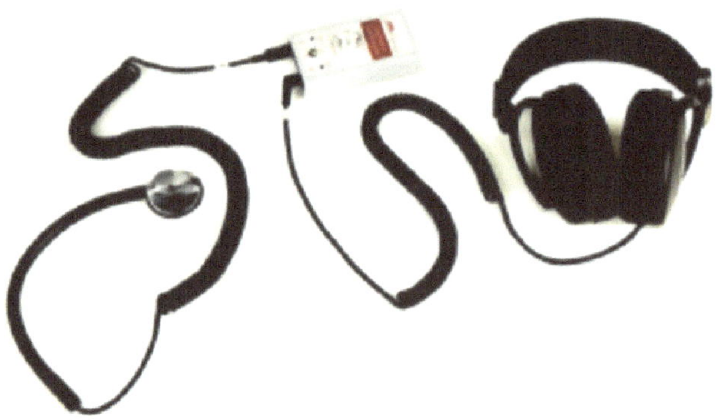

Fig.42.6 *AMD-3700 telephonic stethoscope The AMD-3700 features low data bandwidth and high performance. Each module can operate on either transmit or receive mode auscultation bandwidth: 20Hz to 1,400Hz at low data communications bandwidth (19,2 kbps). Plugging chest piece automatically switches unit from send to receive mode*

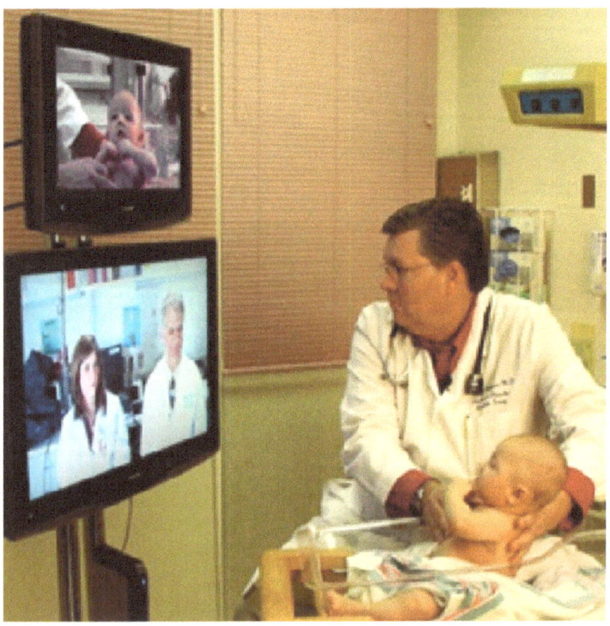

Fig. 42.5 *A telemedicine consultation for an infant with heart problem (top) and experts are advising accordingly (bottom)*

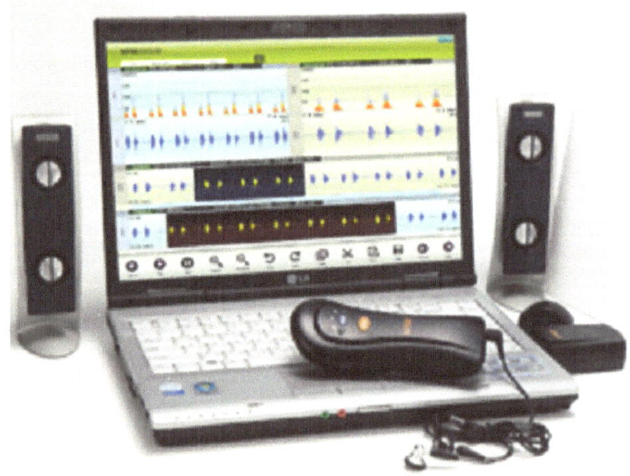

Fig. 42.7: *AMD-3130 E-scope stethoscope. The AMD-3130 E-scope stethoscope utilizes state of the art electronic technology to amplify heart, breath and Korotkoff sounds so they become much easier to hear. The sound is pure and clean. Compared to acoustic stethoscopes, murmurs and faint lows are much more distinguishable*

consider what equipment and personnel are necessary for successful telecardiology. However, before examining the role of telemedicine in paediatric cardiology, it is first important to understand what congenital heart disease is and how it presents to clinicians.

Why is Paediatric Cardiology Suited to Telemedicine

The single biggest reason why paediatric cardiology is suited to telemedicine is that it is a highly specialized field of medicine with a small cadre of professionals. Care is concentrated in a few regional centres. Therefore, large distances separate the patient and nonspecialist from expert advice. However CHD presents, it is unlikely that a nonspecialist will be confident in making a definitive diagnosis, counselling parents or instituting specific treatment without verification from a paediatric cardiologist. Fortunately, all forms of CHD can be diagnosed by a specialist using a combination of clinical examination including stethoscopy, ECG, chest X-ray and echocardigraphic images, i.e. on the analysis of data. These data are suitable for digitisation and electronic transmission and so used in telemedicine (Dowie et al., 2009). Babies with significant CHD may present to a hospital with on-site paediatric cardiology but considering only 13 hospitals in England and Wales have this facility compared with the 184 DGHs providing acute paediatric care, most will present to postnatal wards, neonatal units and emergency departments without on-site paediatric cardiology expertise (Workforce Review Team, 2009) .

Telemedicine can potentially support paediatricians faced with the predicament of a sick, cyanosed newborn baby with a suspected duct dependent CHD. Duct dependent lesions are a subgroup of severe CHD in which the circulation to either the lungs or body is dependent upon patency of the ductus arteriosus. This usually closes within the first 72 hours of life. In babies with duct dependent CHD, closure of the ductus arterious heralds the onset of severe symptoms. If not treated urgently duct dependent CHD is invariably fatal. The main differential diagnosis in this life-threatening scenario is persistent pulmonary hypertension of the newborn. The treatment of the two conditions is very different. Tele echocardiography interpreted by a paediatric cardiologist can offer timely diagnosis, institution of appropriate therapy and expedite or avoid transfer to a paediatric cardiology centre (Finley et al. 1997; Casey, 1999; Mulholland et al. 1999). Antenatal diagnosis of CHD is chiefly reliant upon an abnormality being suspected by a sonographer at a DGH, with very limited experience and knowledge of CHD during routine anomaly scanning.

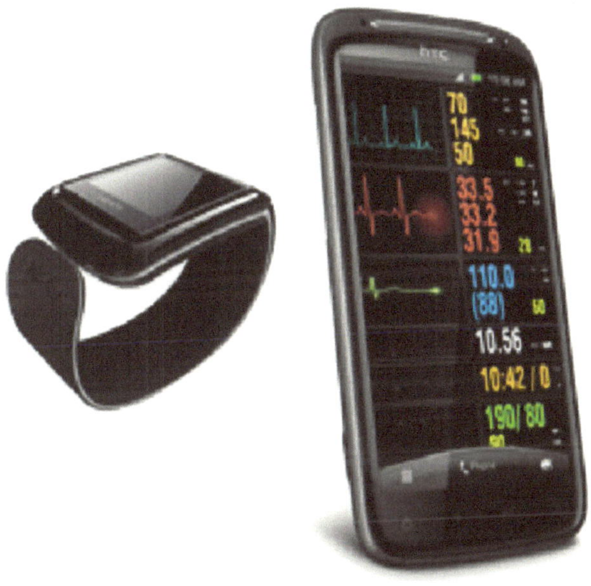

Fig.42.8: Wearable ECG monitor (wrist, wireless) CardioDefender is the first system to deliver mobile, real-time, beat-by-beat, and quantitative heart monitoring and automated reporting by combining patented analytical smartphone software with a Bluetooth device and electrodes

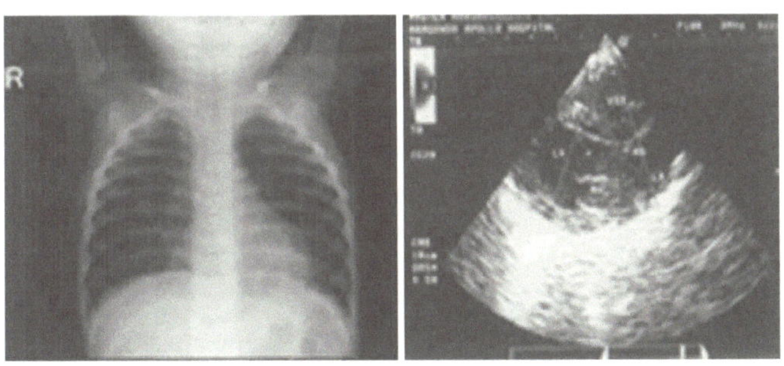

Fig.42.9: Chest X-ray and echocardiography as transmitted by internet

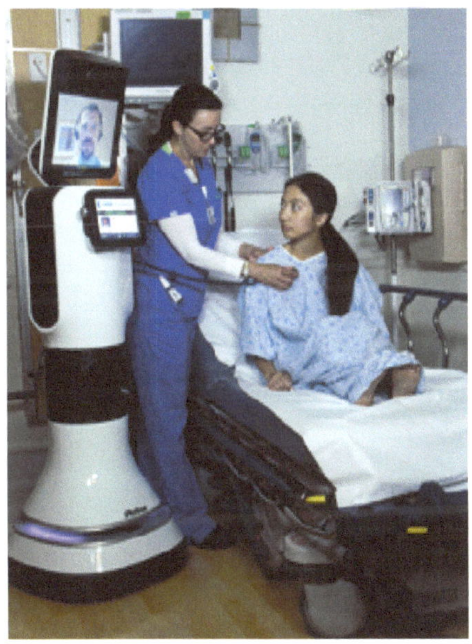

Fig. 42.10: In touch health's specialty is remote-controlled robots for critical care, enabling people to be seen by doctors soonerthan if they had to be in the same physical space as the physician. Getting a stroke victim, for example, to a specialist within 3 hours for diagnosis and treatment can make a huge difference to theatient. Similarly, specialists can provide care in intensive care units without having to physically be present which should lower health care costs and improve care

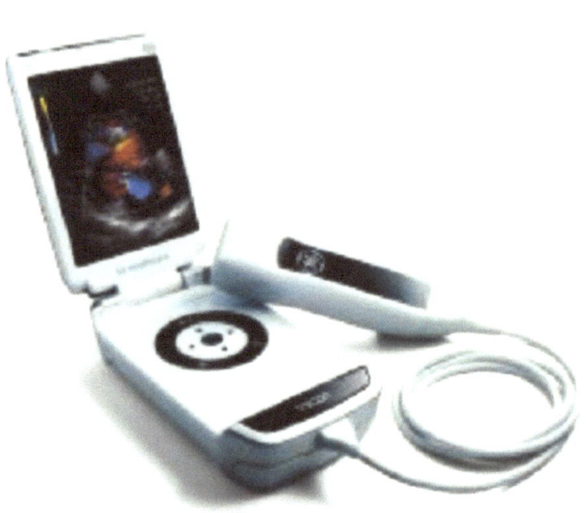

Fig.42.11: *Echocardiography is a natural application for telemedicine, as handheld ultrasound devices and cloud-based transmission solutions make it possible to perform a test at a remote location and have consultation, in real-time, by an expert thousands of miles away. Telemedicine can eliminate the need for travel, reduce wait time for test results, and is cost effective*

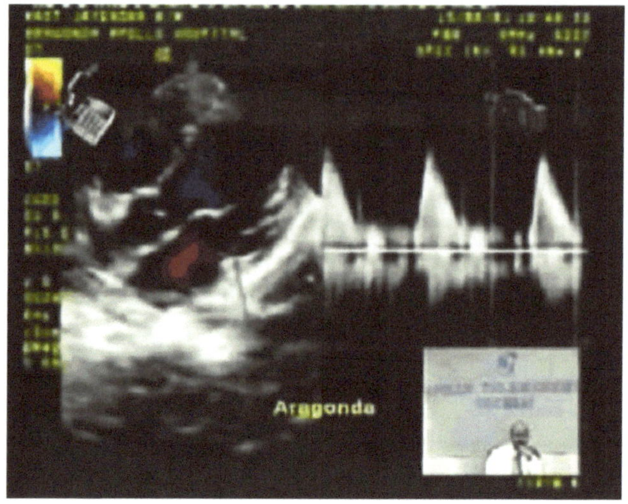

Fig.42.12: *Specialist viewing transmitted live echocardiography from a remote centre*

Telemedicine may offer support to these radiographers. Telemedicine may also facilitate a rationalization of paediatric cardiology outreach clinics. Paediatric cardiologists hold outreach clinics at a number of DGHs within their region, travelling on a half day or full day once a month or once every 2 or 3 months. Lower thresholds for referring asymptomatic children with clear cut innocent murmurs for "a second opinion" have swollen outreach clinics (Dowie et al. 2009); (Dowie et al. 2009). Further pressures have been placed on service provision because of the need to comply with guidelines recommending screening of babies with various syndromes and family screening of certain inheritable conditions. Thus, the paediatric cardiologist may be away from the tertiary unit on average at least once a week. Whilst an excellent service is provided at the outreach clinic, it does not seem to be efficient from the tertiary unit's perspective (Qureshi, 2008). It is understood that most patient's first port of call will be their DGH. Therefore, it is important to foster confidence and competence in managing children with CHD. On the other hand, patients with a clinical problem requiring a paediatric cardiology opinion that cannot wait for the next out reach clinic, need transferred to the tertiary centre for a specialist opinion. A recent innovation has been the curriculum for paediatricians with special expertise in cardiology. Several posts have been appointed in DGHs throughout the UK (Royal College of Paediatrics and Child Health, 2009). The role of the paediatrician with special expertise in cardiology is to unload some of the outpatient work currently being done by the tertiary centres (e.g. evaluation of children with asymptomatic murmurs or chest pain), to be the link person for children with CHD followed up at that DGH and to be competent at performing 2D echocardiography. These paediatricians will need to be supported by the relevant tertiary centre. One of the key methods of providing this support could be via telemedicine links. Congenital cardiac surgery for children for England is currently provided across 11 centres. Each tertiary centre serves several DGHs staffed by paediatricians. A tertiary congenital cardiology service is provided by cardiac surgeons, specializing in congenital cardiac surgery, and paediatric cardiologists. The role of telemedicine in diagnosing and excluding CHD has been recognized at a national level in the UK. Various models of care have been debated leading to a number of recommendations including the establishment of telemedicine links between DGHs and the tertiary unit in order to have echocardiograms interpreted by paediatric cardiologists at all hours, all the year round (Qureshi, 2008). A proposed restructuring of paediatric cardiology services in the UK would reduce the number of paediatric cardiology surgical centres from 11 to 6 (National Health Service, Specialized Services, 2011). Several tertiary care

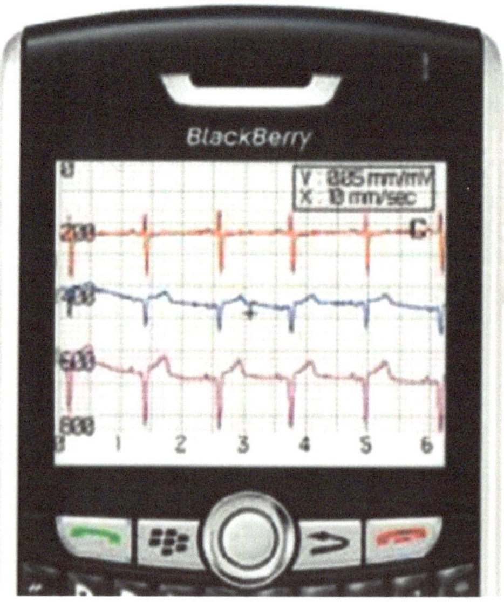

Fig. 42.13: *ECG record transmitted through mobile phone*

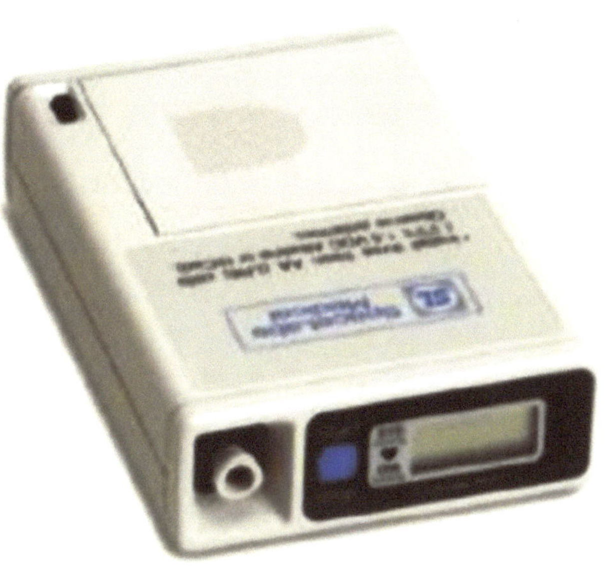

Fig. 42.14: *The features of ambulatory blood pressure monitoring recorder*

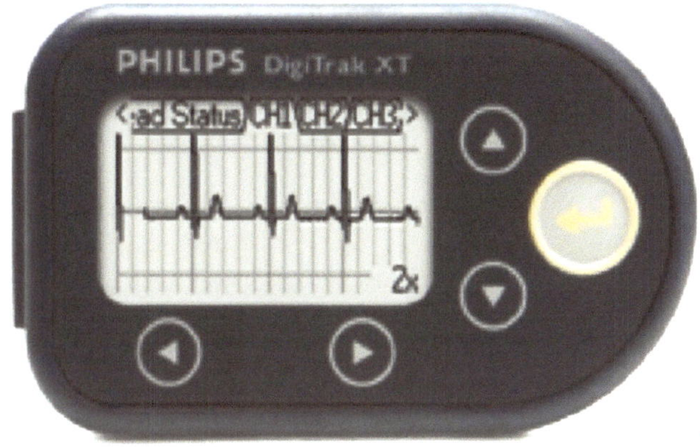

Fig. 42.15: *The features of cardiac event monitoring recorder*

centres will therefore need to significantly reorganize their working practices and become part of a large network of hospitals across a wide area. This development, which is likely to be adopted in other countries, is proposed in order to further centralise expertise and hopefully improve outcomes for patients. However, this may disadvantage paediatric cardiologists working in noncardiac centres and further isolate paediatricians in DGHs. The shared care of patients with CHD, between tertiary nonsurgical cardiac centres and the quaternary surgical centres, will necessitate excellent communication and case conferences. CHD case conferences are based around imaging data. It is easy to see that reliable telemedicine links between the various hospitals within this network will be essential.

In summary, congenital heart disease is potentially lethal. Its diagnosis is reliant upon interpretation of audio and visual data by a small number of experts, concentrated in a few tertiary units. Telemedicine seems to be the ideal tool to provide support to the nonspecialist thereby promoting access to specialist advice and improving patient care.

Common Diagnostic Difficulties for the Neonatologist

In terms of life or death of the patient, the defects that must be diagnosed are those causing cyanotic heart disease, major obstructive lesions of the left or right heart, and total anomalous pulmonary venous drainage (TAPVD). Cyanotic lesions such as transposition of the great arteries, pulmonary or tricuspid atresia, and other complex lesions with univentricular hearts do not usually present diagnostic difficulty if standard views can be obtained during the transmitted echocardiography. The diagnosis of TAPVD is the one likely to provide the most difficulty and is obviously a crucial one to make, particularly in babies where the differential diagnosis is persistent pulmonary hypertension. In our series, to date there has been only one patient with TAPVD. The correct diagnosis of supracardiac TAPVD was made with the transmitted scan, on which the pulmonary venous confluence and the ascending vein could be seen. The exclusion of a diagnosis of TAPVD requires a combination of imaging the pulmonary veins entering the left atrium and the demonstration of normal Doppler flow from them into left atrium. In the cases to date where a diagnosis of persistent pulmonary hypertension was being considered we have been able to satisfy ourselves that pulmonary venous drainage was normal.

For those with limited experience in echocardiography, obtaining good aortic arch views is one of the areas that causes most difficulty. The diagnosis of coarctation of aorta is essentially a clinical one, and if the femoral pulses are weak or absent in association with an arm-leg blood pressure gradient, the patient will require transfer to the regional centre for a definitive diagnosis.

The other common diagnostic dilemma for the neonatologist is in deciding whether the premature infant has a PDA, and, if there is one, how much is it contributing to the clinical condition of the patient? It is not practical to use a telemedicine link to confirm or exclude a PDA in all premature infants with this clinical problem. There is a case, however, for transmitting scans on ventilator dependent babies with chronic lung disease to determine whether a significant shunt through a PDA is exacerbating the problem. It is very useful in this situation to be able to answer the question by remote echocardiography and avoid transferring the ventilated patient.

Overview of Evidence Available in Paediatric Telecardiology

There is a substantial body of research to support the feasibility of many applications of telecardiology in both paediatric and adult populations. There is much less good quality evidence demonstrating its clinical utility and cost-effectiveness. Most of the evidence is from small or uncontrolled studies. This is particularly difficult in paediatric cardiology because the numbers of patients involved are necessarily smaller than adult studies. However, there are larger scale randomized control trials in tele-homecare. There is now robust evidence advocating

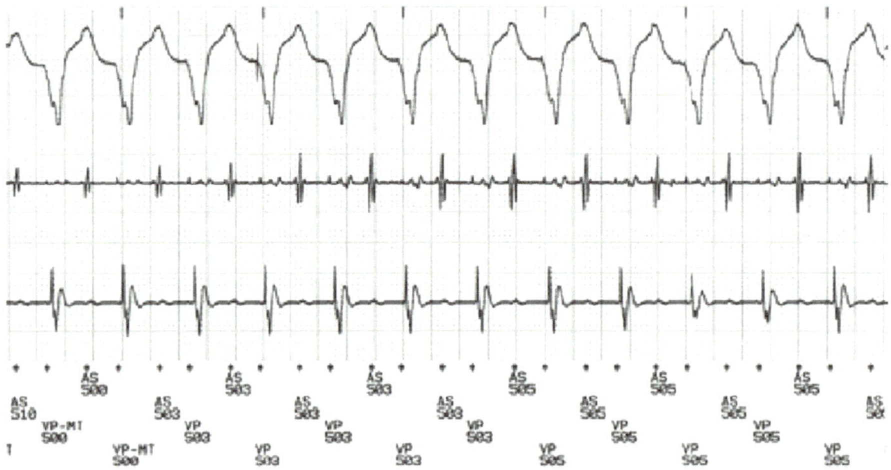

Fig. 42.16: *Telemetered ECG tracing with surface lead II (top) and intracardiac electrograms [atrial electrogram (center) and ventricular electrogram (lower)] and marker channel (bottom) showing pacemaker-mediated tachycardia (PMT). The intracardiac markers indicate that the retrograde P waves, labeled AS for atrial-sensed event, occur 280 milliseconds after the ventricular-paced beats, labeled VP*

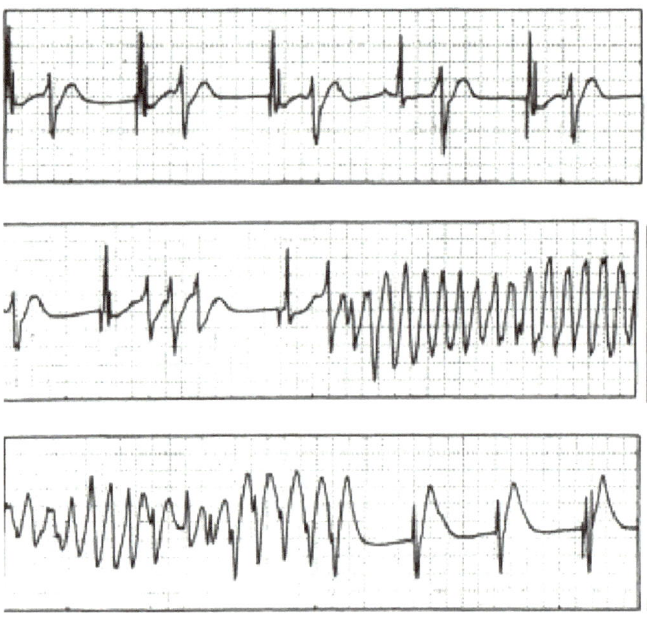

Fig.42.17: *Continuous telemetry strip showing episode of TdP in a patient with a dual chamber pacemaker. The patient with sinus node dysfunction was started on quinidine and diltiazem in the hospital. The normally functioning pacemaker was programmed to the DDD mode with a lower rate of 50 beats per minute. She developed a junctional escape rhythm at around 50 bpm. Late-coupled ventricular bigeminy is followed by a three-beat run of ventricular tachycardia and then a 6-second run of TdP. The apparent ventricular undersensing is the result of "safety pacing" after sensing the ventricular electrogram in the nonphysiologic AV delay period after the atrial artifact. Torsades de pointes was suppressed by increasing the pacing rate*

a role for telemonitoring and structured telephone support for patients with chronic heart failure.

There is also evidence suggesting that remote monitoring of pacemakers and implantable cardiac defibrillators is reliable, safe, that it may improve patient satisfaction and reduce costs. Large randomizes control trials are ongoing which should hopefully clarify the role of remote monitoring in this patient group (Burri and Senouf, 2009).

Telemedicine Applied to Specific Cardiology Situations

Telemedicine in fetal cardiology, there are a number of features of fetal cardiology that appear to make telemedicine an attractive proposition:

The clinical imperative

1. Fetal cardiology is a highly centralized subspeciality with even fewer specialists than paediatric cardiology.
2. Patients often travel large distances (up to 160 km in Northern Ireland) to attend a fetal cardiology clinic. The distance between home and the specialist centre is even greater in larger countries. In Quebec, 34% of mothers referred to a fetal cardiology service travel more than 100 km (Cloutier and Finley, 2004).

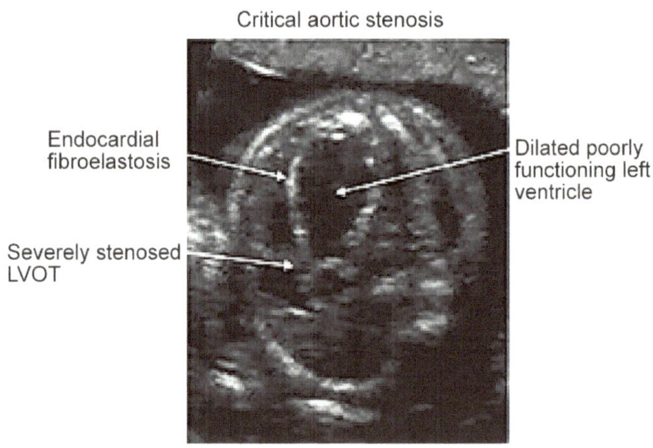

Fig. 42.18: *Example of severe congenital heart disease accurately diagnosed via tele-link in this study*

Table 42.1: *How congenital heart disease presents and the potential for telemedicine to support district general hospitals within a clinical network*

	Presentation	*Urgency*	*Potential for telemedicine*
Antenatal	Suspected CHD on routine anomally scan Risk factor for CHD	Nonurgent	Support sonographers Streamline antenatal screening
Neonate	Cyanosis Murmur Clinical shock Abnormal femoral pulses Risk factor for CHD	Usually an emergency	Immediate diagnosis or exclusion of CHD Institute potentially life-saving therapy Decide upon need for transfer
Infant and child	Hepatomegaly Abnormal femoral pulses Failure to thrive	Usually less urgent	Virtual clinics could help to recognize workload for peadiatric cardiologist

3. The summary of fetal cardiology literature demonstrates that timely, antennal diagnosis of CHD is important for improving outcomes for fetus and family by facilitating: parental counselling, elective delivery at an appropriate centre, parental choice in terms of termination and permitting fetal intervention in terms of pharmacotherapy for dysrhythmias and catheter intervention for severe complex lesions (Bonnet et al. 1999; Allan, 2000; Tworetzky et al. 2001; Gardiner, 2008).
4. The vast majority of fetuses with CHD are born from pregnancies without a recognisable antenatal risk factor. Obviously, formal evaluation by a fetal cardiologist cannot be offered to every single pregnancy. Therefore, in order to maximize antenatal detection of CHD, greater proficiency, from the non-specialist, is required at confirming normality and identifying pathology.

In the UK, the most practicable method of promoting antenatal detection of CHD is by improving cardiac evaluation during the routine anomaly scan. Previous studies have demonstrated the benefit and relative ease with which more detailed imaging of the heart may be incorporated into routine anomaly scanning (Stumpflen et al. 1996). However, such reports often reflect working practices immediately after the introduction of a training program. As the teaching study from Hunter et al demonstrated, there is a danger that if support from paediatric cardiology is not ongoing then the initial efficacy of training may diminish (Hunter et al. 2000). Telemedicine has the potential to facilitate earlier diagnosis of CHD by offering increased and quicker access to specialist opinion. Telemedicine may also support sonographers' education and training.

Fetal cardiology is predominantly a speciality of medical imaging as physical examination of the fetal cardiovascular system is obviously not possible and fetal catheter and surgical interventions are limited to a handful of centres worldwide. As is well documented, telemedicine lends itself to areas where medical imaging is crucial to diagnosis (Casey, 1999).

It may be suggested that performing fetal tele-echocardiography is much the same as tele-echocardiography in neonates but fetal echocardiography is significantly different from neonatal echocardiography:

1. The fetal heart is smaller and beats faster which may exacerbate motion artefact.
2. The fetus is surrounded by the mother so that ultrasound has to travel through more tissue impacting on image quality.
3. The fetus may move.
4. The fetus may be in a disadvantageous position e.g. back up. Experience of telemedicine in fetal cardiology is still in its infancy. The fetal cardiology telemedicine programs that are currently y active appear to have developed from centres with a major interest in telemedicine and fetal medicine. Whilst an acceptable bandwidth (384 kbps) has been established for neonatal tele-echocardiography. This is not the case with fetal tele-echocardiography. Therefore, research is required in this area.

Evidence for Fetal Telecardiology

a. Despite a potential role for telemedicine in fetal cardiology, there are very few studies investigating its potential. Only one study is reported to date that investigates the feasibility and acceptability of performing remote, real-time 2D fetal echocardiography. Sharma et al performed a study in two phases. Phase one was a laboratory study, investigating the effect of bandwidth on image quality and overall adequacy of scan. Sixty-four fetal echocardiograms were performed and randomly assigned to transmission across 128, 384 and 768 kbps and recorded on super VHS videotape for subsequent review. Six studies were excluded due to the presence of CHD. Of the 58 real-time studies interpreted, 15/58 were transmitted across 128 kbps, 21 across 384 kbps and 22 across 768 kbps. The image quality was felt to be significantly poorer at 128 kbps. At 128 kbps, the mean Likert score was 1.1/5 compared with 3.1/5 at 384 kbps ($p < 0.01$) and 3.4/5 at 768 kbps ($p < 0.01$). There was no significant difference in perceived image quality in transmission across 384 kbps compared with 768 kbps (p = 0.08). Similarly, there was no significant difference in the adequacy of studies transmitted across 384 kbps compared with 768 kbps. In this first phase, Sharma et al conclude that 384 kbps is an adequate bandwidth for the identification of normal heart structures.

In the second phase of the study, 34 fetal echocardiograms were successfully transmitted and interpreted in real-time. In four cases (11%), technical problems prevented transmission.

The fetal echocardiogram was performed by a fetal cardiac sonographer or a paediatric cardiology fellow with experience in fetal echocardiography. This was compared with a video recording of the study made at the transmitting site. Mothers were followed up with a face-to-face fetal echocardiogram if a concern was identified on the transmitted fetal echocardiogram. In order to evaluate patient satisfaction, a questionnaire was completed by all 34 expectant mothers and a control group of 195 patients referred from peripheral hospitals to the regional fetal cardiology clinic. There was no significant difference in the completeness of each study between the telefetal echocardiogram and the recorded fetal echocardiogram. CHD was identified correctly in two transmitted fetal echocardiograms with a third case of CHD being suspected but only confirmed on direct fetal echocardiography.

The satisfaction survey results were very positive. In all nine questions, the mean patient satisfaction score indicated high levels of satisfaction with the telemedicine consultation. In eight questions, there was no significant difference in patient satisfaction between the telemedicine and control groups. In addition, only 6% of patients stated that they felt uncomfortable talking to the doctor across the tele-link and only 3% felt it was difficult to ask questions. In this important study, the authors conclude that transmission of fetal echocardiograms across 384 kbps is feasible and adequate for the interpretation of screening fetal echocardiograms. Community acceptance of telemedicine screening and counselling is not adversely affected by a lack of direct personal contact with the specialist. Whilst this study is valuable there are some limitations. The majority of transmitted fetal echocardiograms were not followed up with a face-to-face fetal echocardiogram which is the gold standard. The proportion of fetuses with CHD was small in this cohort. Therefore, the diagnostic accuracy of the telemedicine process was not adequately assessed. The fetal echocardiograms were performed by an operator already skilled in fetal echocardiography. This may falsely enhance the adequacy and quality of the fetal echocardiogram being transmitted. It is suggested that most difficulties in interpreting echocardiograms transmitted via a tele-link are related to image acquisition rather than transmission (Cloutier, 2000). Eleven percent of studies were terminated due to technical difficulties.

A routine clinical service would be significantly limited if 11% of consultations were aborted due to technical difficulties. There are also reports of telemedicine facilitating 3D fetal echocardiography by spatiotemporal image correlation (STIC) and datasets transmitted across an ADSL link. STIC is a relatively new approach for clinical assessment of the fetal heart. It is an easy technique for acquiring data from the fetal heart (a single, automatic volume sweep) and produces a 4D cine sequence (Michailidis et al. 2001). A group from Chile conducted a similar study STIC transmitted across an ADSL connection with bandwidths of 300 and 600 kbps. In total, 50 scans were transmitted from two peripheral hospitals to the regional centre. On average complete fetal echocardiograms could be interpreted in 92% (Vinals et al. 2005). However, these isolated studies have not been followed up in the literature.

In a study conducted in our own department we evaluated fetal echocardiography, performed by sonographers with little training in fetal cardiology, but guided by a fetalcardiologist and transmitted in real-time across ISDN 6. The remote consultation concluded with a videoconference in which the fetal cardiologist explained the diagnosis and answered any questions from the prospective parents. This fetal-telecardiology consultation was compared with the subsequent "face-to-face" fetal cardiology consultation at the regional centre. Sixty-eight fetal tele-echocardiograms were performed and followed up. The diagnostic accuracy was very high (ê – statistic = 0.89, sensitivity = 0.92, specificity = 0.98, ppv = 0.92, npv = 0.98). Sonographers were very positive regarding their involvement in the study and reported significantly improved levels of confidence in performing fetal echocardiography. A significant positive feature of real-time fetal tele-echocardioghraphy is the continued support provided to radiographers performing fetal anomaly scans in DGHs. Patients were very positive about the telemedicine process and were equally satisfied with the remote consultation as the face-to-face consultation. Patients were equally satisfied with each consultation but consistently replied that they would prefer to have the fetal cardiology consultation performed at the local hospital facilitated by a telelink rather by a face-to-face consultation at the regional centre.

Counselling parents during the study it was noted that the received fetal echocardiographic images were of poorer quality following an upgrade in the ultrasound scanner. This did not appear to affect diagnostic accuracy. With the superior imaging, this deterioration in received picture quality was probably due to excess data being transmitted down the 384 kbps connection with resulting package loss and pixellation. This problem would likely be reduced if a larger bandwidth was employed. Extensions to inter-hospital networks make this a realistic option. Alternatively SDSL links (2MBps) can be installed at much cheaper rates than corresponding ISDN bandwidths. The introduction of a remote fetal cardiology service would have attendant costs which are not offset by savings in interhospital transfers. However, the possible establishment of a "one-stop-shop" for "high-risk" pregnancies in which the routine fetal anomaly scan is followed by a remote fetal echocardiogram confidently identifying all relevant cardiac-structures (55% in this cohort) could potentially be cost neutral, relieve pressure on the regional unit and present time and cost savings to the patient. Ultimately, the aim of future work should be aimed towards the establishment of a regional fetal tele-echocardiography service.

Tele-Applications in Cardiology and Radiology in India

A country like India , owing to it's vast geographical spread and the enormous population, requires tremendous resources and well-trained medical personnel so as to be able to deliver emergency medical care within a life-saving time frame in every nook and corner of the country. This may not always be possible given the fact that majority of the specialists are concentrated in urban areas with a significant paucity of trained specialists amongst the rural population. In a patient with a cardiac illness, the timing of medical intervention is crucial and dictates the outcome of treatment often proving to be the difference between life and death.

A typical example being the initiation of treatment early in a patient suffering a heart attack (golden hour), which can save life and have an important bearing on the quality of life post event (1) considering the fact that a significant proportion of the *Infant Mortality Rate* of 63.19 per 1,000 births (2) in our country could be attributed to the mortality associated with congenital heart defects, the burden posed by heart disease in the paediatric age group assumes enormous significance.

An estimated 48,000 to 1,28,000 babies are born every year with heart defects in India. This is based on the statistics that there are 16 million live births in India in a year and the incidence of heart disease in newborns is 8–12 per 1,000 live births. Only a bare 5% of these obtain medical attention and surgical care. Nearly 65% will die below 1 year of age and only 15% will survive beyond the age of 5 years. With at least 50,000 new cases of *Rheumatic fever* every year, it is estimated that there are currently more than 1 million patients with rheumatic heart disease in the country, which only adds to the disease burden. To compound these problems, there are less than 15 trained pediatric cardiologists in the country and less than 10 institutions in the country with the requisite infrastructure and manpower to offer surgical correction for neonates and infants with heart defects. There are, also, not more than 10 dedicated pediatric cardiothoracic surgeons.

The mismatch between the medical need and the availability of specialist care in our country is thus clearly evident. As mentioned earlier, this is because there is an estimated 620 million population living in the villages and the availability of specialist doctors there is inadequate. For

Table 42.2: *Potential measurements for heart failure monitoring*

Patient-report data

Signs and symptoms of congestion

Signs: Jugular venous distension, peripheral edema, pulmonary congestion/rales, pleural effusions, S3 gallop

Symptoms: Dyspnea on exertion, orthopnea, paroxysmal nocturnal dyspnea, fatigue, abdominal fullness, anorexia, nausea, vomiting

Daily weight

Sodium intake

Medication adherence/persistence

Laboratory data

- INR
- Natriuretic peptides (BNP and NT-proBNP)
- Other biomarkers

Directly recorded data

- Heart rate
- Blood pressure
- Atrial/ventricular arrhythmias
- Percentage pacing
- Pressure sensor data
- RV outflow
- Left atrial
- Pulmonary artery
- Device parameters
- Battery
- Alerts
- Leads
- Calculated/derived data
- Heart rate variability

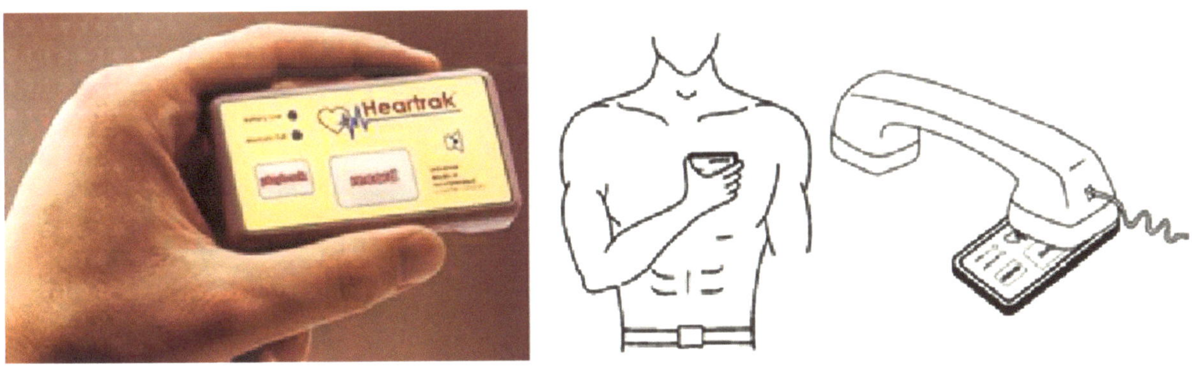

Fig. 42.19: *Left showing heartrak monitor, middle, shows patient placing the same over the heart area for record of ECG and right, shows a telephone through which the recorded information is transmitted*

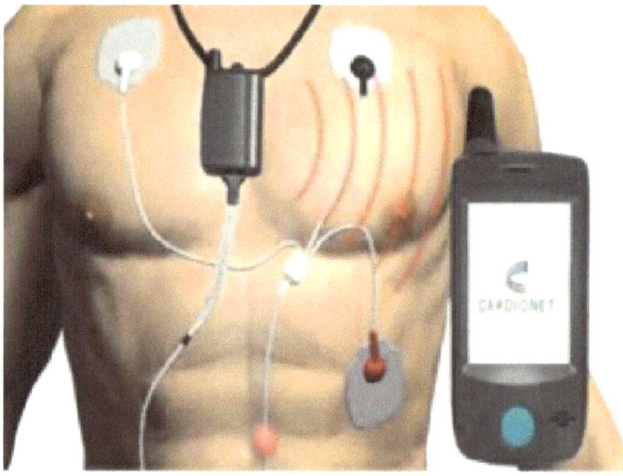

Fig. 42.20: *The sensor sends ECG information about every heart beat to a small portable monitor*

this reason, the rural population is known to be at twice the risk of death when compared to the urban population, for the same illness. Telemedicine can play a tremendous role in bridging the great divide between the patient and the medical specialist, especially in a country like India. By bringing together the patient and the specialist face to face and by its ability to allow the specialist to conduct an examination and view investigations both in report format and in real-time, telemedicine allows a comprehensive medical consultation in the initial stages of the disease presentation without requiring the patient to travel long distances.

Telecardiology in India

The basic requirement for telecardiac consultation is for a computer with a web camera, a modem and a standard telephone connection at the remote site with ISDN (Integrated Services Digital Network) or broadband capacity.

All aspects of a comprehensive cardiac consultation, such as

- A detailed history of the illness from the patient or the patient's attenders
- Visual general assessment of the patient's clinical status
- Auscultation of the patient's heart and lungs
- Reading the patient's ECG, chest X-ray and echocardiography
- Advising appropriate management including initiation of emergency life-saving treatment can be done to the

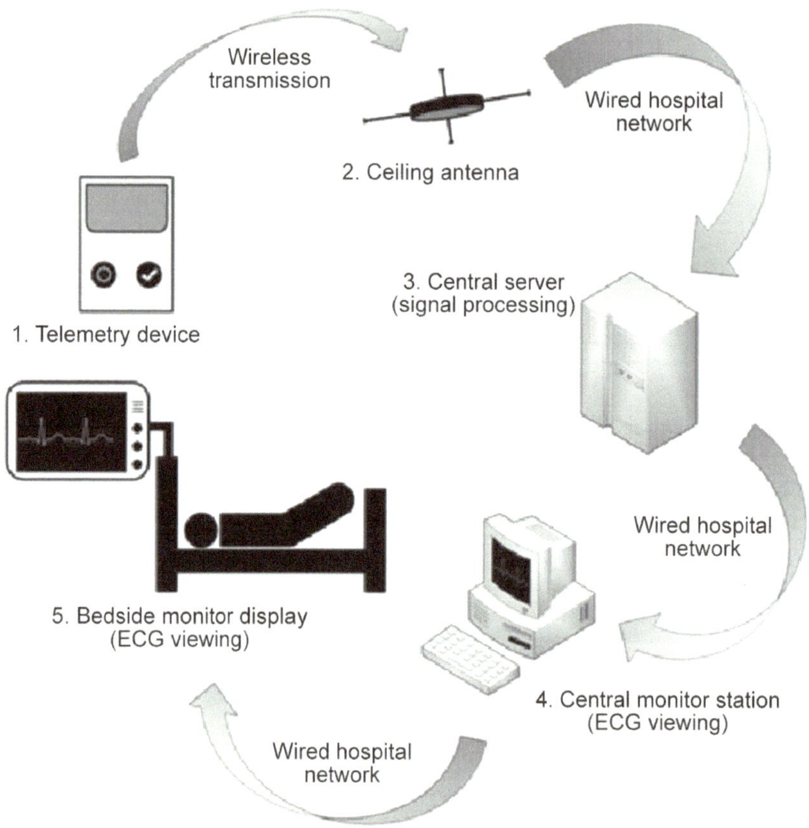

Fig. 42.21: *Illustration of configuration of a typical networked wireless telemetry system. This schematic is for illustrative purposes and does not represent the system of any single manufacturer. The patient's ECG signal is acquired with electrodes and lead wires connected to the telemetry device (1) and transmitted to ceiling antennae (2) via radio frequencies federally allocated to wireless medical telemetry services. The ECG is then transmitted directly over computer cables that link the ceiling antennae, central server (3), and central monitor station (4). The bedside monitor display typically receives the data from the central server or monitor station via a wired hospital network. There may be significant delays of up to several seconds from the time that a heart rhythm is experienced by the patient (step 1) to the time that the rhythm is displayed on the bedside monitor (step 5)*

satisfaction of the clinician and the patient through teleconferencing.

Auscultatory findings play a crucial part in diagnosing cardiac ailments, especially in those with congenital heart disease. Recent technological aids such as electronic stethoscope makes it possible for the clinician to hear the patients' heart sounds for himself across many miles and come to an accurate clinical diagnosis. This eliminates the risk of error associated with having to rely on the attending persons clinical auscultation. Even a narrow bandwidth (analog) telephonic stethoscope has been proven to be effective in distinguishing accurately between an innocent and a pathological murmur. The clinical diagnosis, thus arrived at, can then be confirmed by reviewing investigations such as electrocardiogram (ECG), chest X-ray, echocardiogram, treadmill test, angiocardiography, cardiac CT scan, cardiac MRI scan, ambulatory ECG monitoring, pacemaker evaluation, and relevant blood tests. Most of these test results are reviewed using a ***store and forward*** technique from the remote site, where the tests are initially performed, captured and stored in the computer which is then forwarded as still frames to the specialist for review. Transtelephonic ECG provides the means of transmitting an electrocardiogram recorded in a patient with rhythm disorders or a myocardial infarction, enabling immediate initiation of treatment. Having connectivity between an ultrasound (echocardiography) equipment and the computer, enables the transmission of streaming video pictures of the heart scan in real time to the specialist. This is particularly useful in situations where a child is brought in with a complex cardiac lesion. The primary doctor or technician may not be skilled to perform a detailed scan of the heart of the child and interpret them accurately, and in such cases the specialist is required to view the test ***live*** to be able to make an accurate diagnosis. Telemedicine can be effectively used to transmit fetal echocardiography images as identifying fetal cardiac anomalies early on in gestation prepares the parents and the attending doctor towards care immediate post-partum thus greatly enhancing the outcome of management for that baby. As not many are trained to identify cardiac anomalies in early pregnancy, a technician could be directed by the clinical specialist at the referral center to show the required views to enable a diagnosis of fetal cardiac problem.

Chest X-ray and Echocardiography as Transmitted by Internet

The practice of diagnosing complex congenital heart defects by transmission over an ISDN line is well established. However, in our experience, it was found that broadband or VSAT connectivity was superior to ISDN connectivity in that it enhanced the quality of the transmitted images as well as ensured an uninterrupted transmission, especially when transmitting streaming images such as online echocardiography. This is crucial for ensuring accuracy of the diagnosis, particularly in the case of a complex congenital cardiac anomaly. There are previous studies

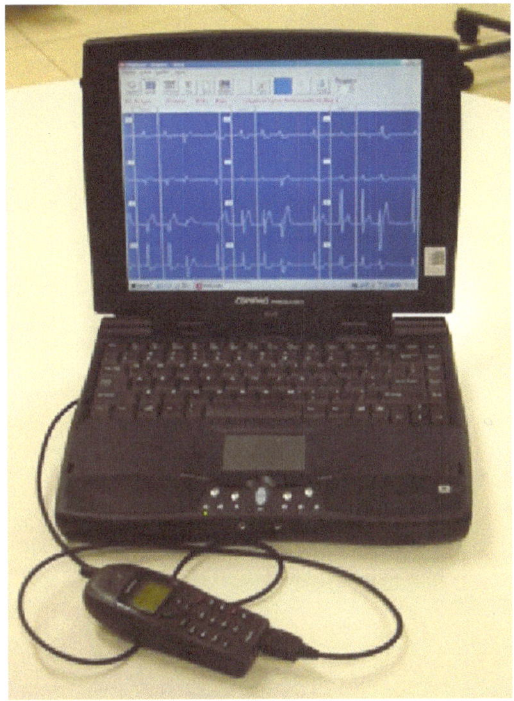

Fig. 42.22: Remote computer connected to a mobile phone of the digital tele-ECG system. The PC anywhere 32 is the telecommunication software, which is installed in the host and the remote computers, a system that allows data transmission via phone for remote analysis

corroborating the accuracy of a diagnosis by telemedicine as compared to one by personal clinical examination.

Specialist Viewing Transmitted Live Echocardiography from a Remote Centre

In acute cardiac events, telecardiology provides the means by which the specialist is able to guide the primary doctor or the paramedical personnel at the scene to undertake measures which would help save the life of the cardiac patient based on the history provided, and the investigation findings. An extremely important aspect of telecardiology is that it achieves shared care of the patient by the primary physician and the specialist and also in the process entrains the primary physician in the ways of specialist management for the specific condition. Telemedicine can also be effectively utilized to propagate the knowledge of the specialist to primary care physicians and the public through teleconferencing continuing medical education (CME) programs.

Applications in Radiology

Images in radiology are predominantly plain X-ray pictures, ultrasound scan images and images of CT scans, MRI scans, cine angiography, etc. These images can be digitally scanned and stored in an archival server in DICOM (digital imaging and communications in medicine) format even if they are previously in non-DICOM format. Subsequently, the images can be stored in the web server in either compressed or noncompressed form and be available for

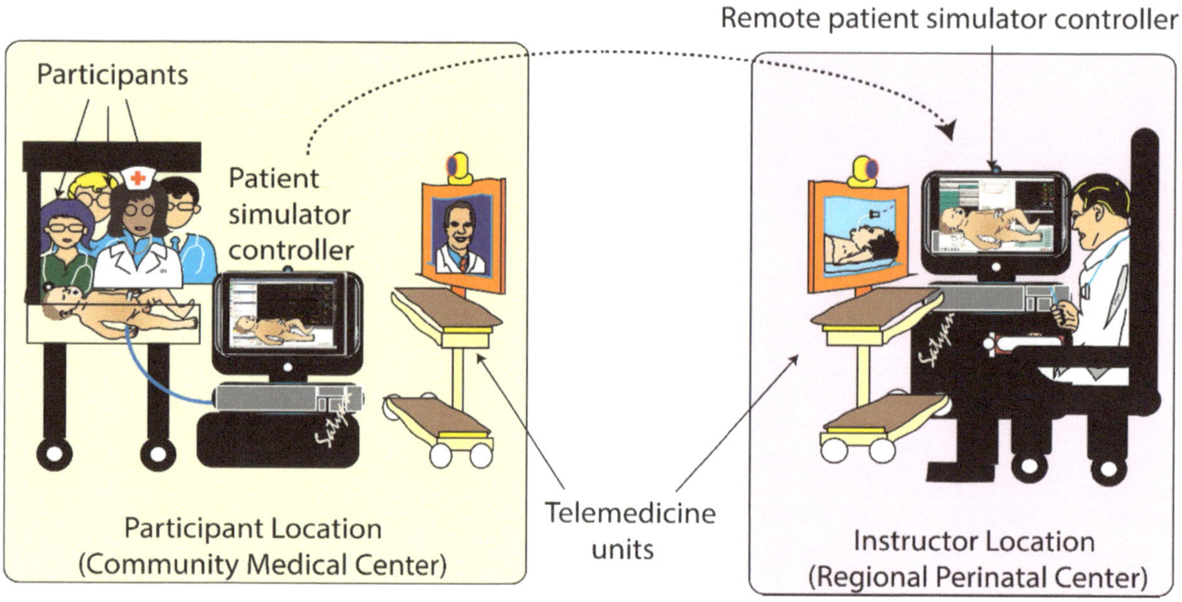

Fig 42.23 **Primary care pediatrician is taking consultation from remotely placed specialised pediatric cardiac center**

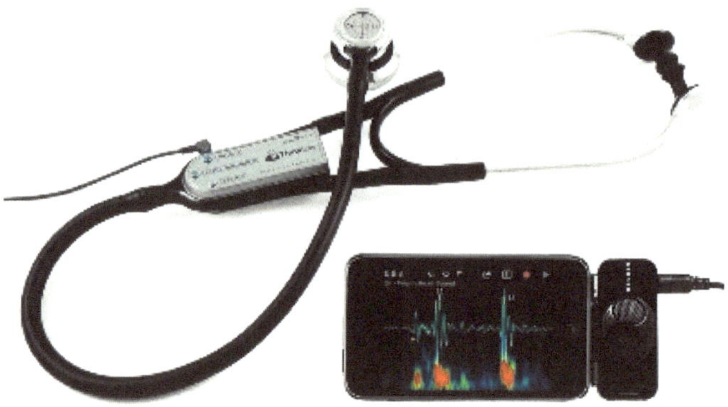

Fig.42.24 Digital Stethoscope Complete Touch System from Thinklabs

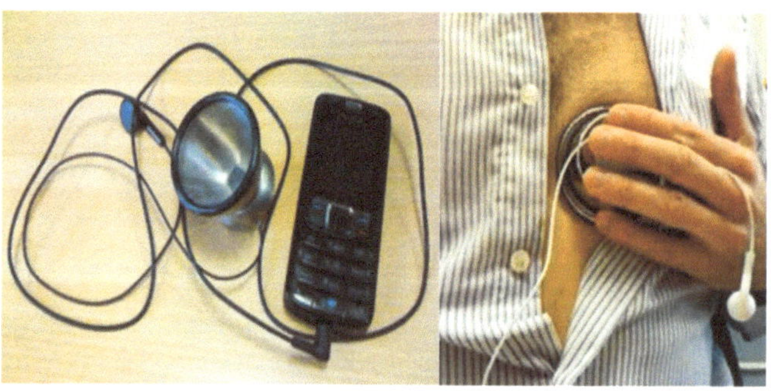

Fig 42.25 Showing Mobile Phone appratus (left) and its applicability over the chest of the patient (right).

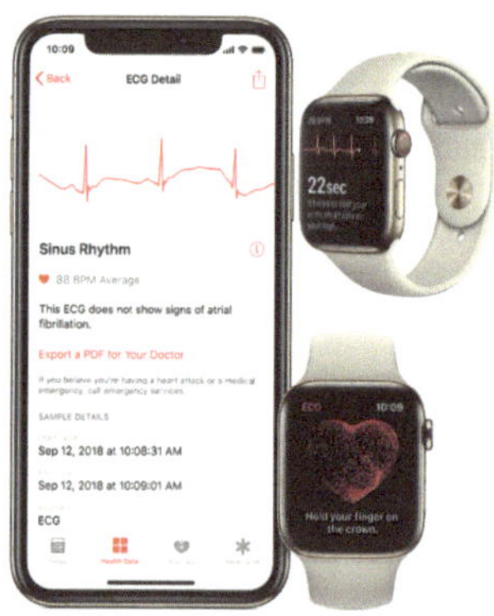

Fig.42.26 Apple Watch Series 4 used to obtain single-lead electrocardiograms (ECGs) that represent lead 1 on a standard 12-lead ECG.

A Fetal ECG Monitoring System Based on the Android Smartphone

Cognitive and exercise impairment caused by fetal hypoxia during the perinatal period remains a serious health problem worldwide . Physicians track fetal growth and development during the perinatal period by monitoring changes in of heart sounds, heart rate, and fetal electrocardiogram (ECG). The fetal ECG reflects the electrophysiological activity of the fetal heart. Using fetal ECG waveform analysis, fetal abnormalities during fetal development, such as fetal distress and intrauterine hypoxia, may be detected

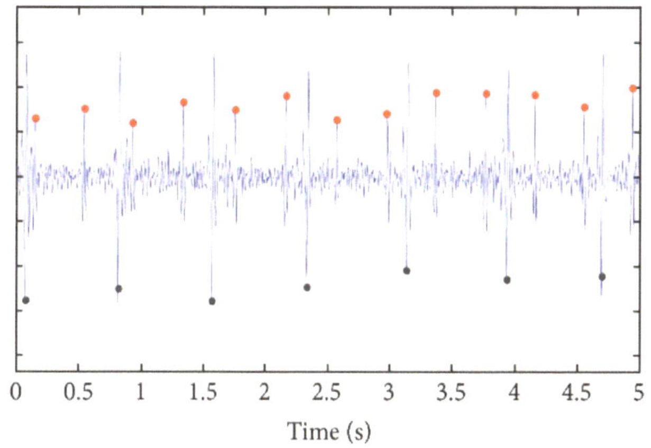

Fig 42.27 Example of ECG recording taken from the Tele fetal care system. The identification of maternal (gray dots, down) and fetal (red dots, up) heart beats is computed off-line by a novel algorithm implemented in Matlab..

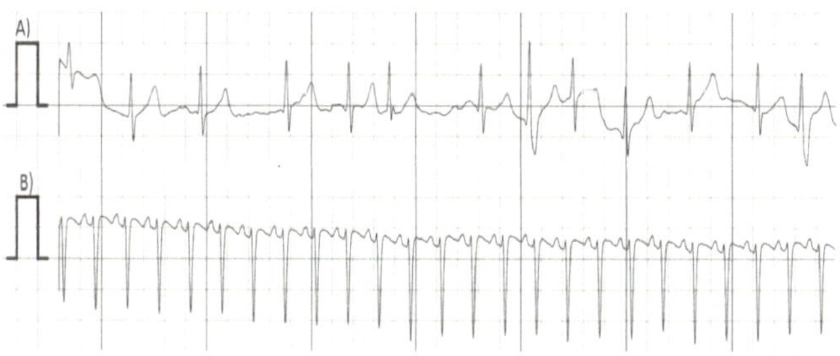

Fig 42.28 Samples of transmitted ECG tracings. A) Atrial fibrillation. B) Supraventricular tachycardia.

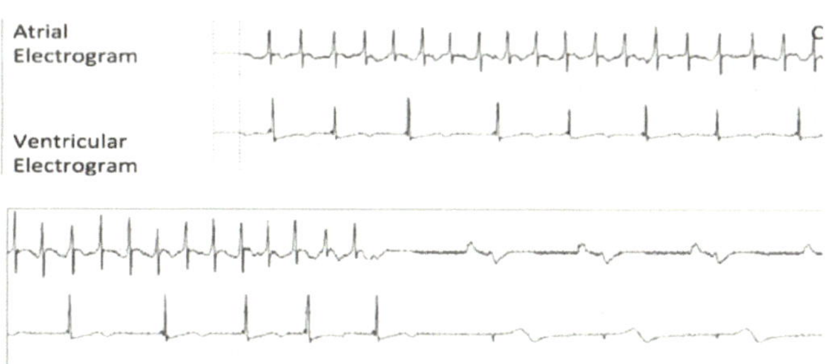

Fig 42.29 Example of atrial tachycardia from interrogation of an implantable device in a patient who was recurrent episodes of asymptomatic (silent) AF.

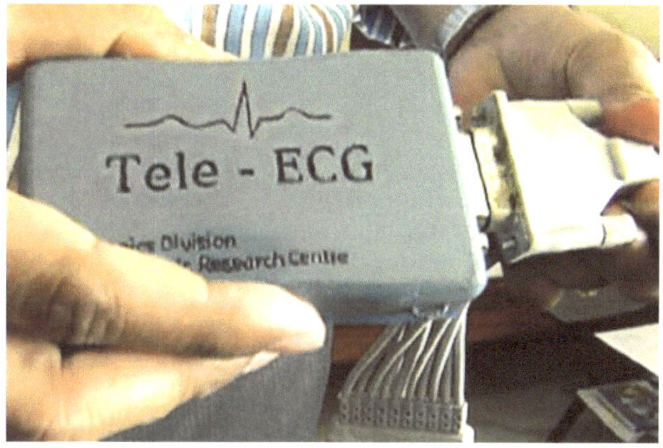

Fig.42.30 Currently, Indian scientists at Bhaba Research Center have developed a credit card sized low priced Tele ECG Machine.

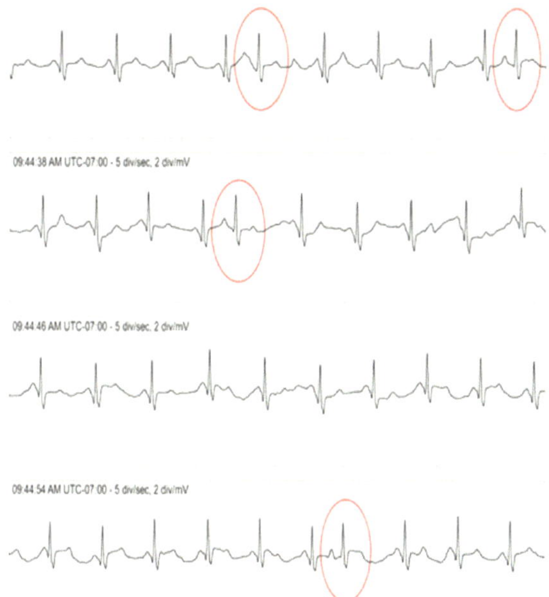

Fig.42.31 AliveCor #ECG from earlier, recorded after symptoms. Turns out those were #supraventricular #ectopic beats

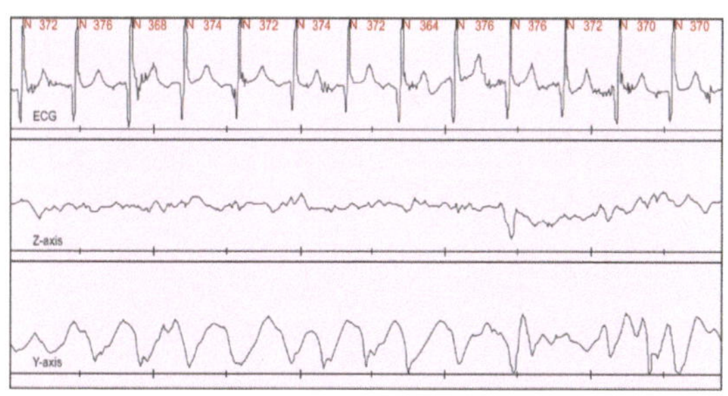

Fig. 42.32 Recordings obtained with the wireless ECG sensor system during outdoor football game training, where the upper curve shows the ECG signal, while the two lower curves show a signal from an accelerometer in Z-axis (sideways) and Y-axis (upwards) directions indicating the level of physical activity. The actual heart rate is approx. 160 b/min.

acquisition either within the institution through internet or worldwide through internet. It is important to adhere to the DICOM-ACR-NEMA-3 standard for storing images and also important not to alter or edit the image during acquisition. Telemedicine plays a crucial role of networking whereby technicians in rural settings can acquire radiological images and transmit to a central hub where it can be reported on by a qualified radiologist and the report sent back to the primary physician in the rural center within a matter of minutes. Complicated imaging procedures or ultrasound-guided procedures can be undertaken confidently in remote settings while being guided by a specialist from elsewhere be it within the country or from abroad.

Specifications for Setting Up a Telemedicine Unit

The World Health Organization defines telemedicine as "The delivery of health care services, where distance is a critical factor, by all healthcare professionals using information and communication technologies for the exchange of valid information for diagnosis, treatment and prevention of disease and injuries, research and evaluation, and for the continuing education of healthcare providers, all in the interests of advancing the health of individuals and their communities".

Required Infrastructure

An **air-conditioned, sound-proof room** with electrical outlets for connecting various equipments and a very good earthing pit.

Recommendation

Five 15 amps Sockets for UPS, five 5 amps socket for other diagnostic equipments, UPS of atleast 3 KVA capacity.

Curtains/walls preferably light blue or gray in colour to give good contrast for video conferencing.

Video Conferencing Hardware (Fig. 53.1, 53.2 and 53.7)

A **television** preferably with 29″ screen. Alternatively, if Tele CMEs (Continuing Medical Education) are planned a LCD projection on to a big screen.

A video conferencing system—these can be:

1. Stand-alone code based system **(recommended)**
2. PC based using PC add-on card codec
3. PC based with in-camera codec
4. PC based web camera and software only codec.

IT Hardware

A computer with printer and a scanner (capable of scanning X-ray films also or alternatively a X-ray digitizer).

Data such as images and video pictures that are NOT in digital format require to be converted to digital format for transmission. This is done using **"codec"** units. (short for coder/decoder).

Compression softwares help transmit large files in shorter time. Digital Imaging and Communications in Medicine (DICOM) compression is the recommended standard for transmitting medical images.

Connectivity Hardware

It can be either terrestrial or satellite based.

- Terrestrial communication can be through analog modems, DSL modems, ISDN and broadband.
- Satellite communication is usually through Very Small Aperture Terminals (VSATs). It provides much better image transfer quality than terrestrial mode of communication as well as instantaneous global coverage.

Medical Hardware

Various instrumentation that can be connected to the video-conferencing unit to directly relay data from the patient are: Digital 12 lead ECG, electronic stethescope, digital microscope, digital blood pressure monitor, skin camera, doppler ultrasound and echocardiography equipment, etc. Stored images such as X-rays, ultrasound images, CT/MRI images or pathology slide images can be scanned into a computer and transmitted. Moving video images of echocardiography can be transmitted by connecting the video player/DVD player to the video-conferencing system (Figs 53.1–53.5, 53.7–53.12, 53.16–53.17).

Recommendations in Telemedicine

Accessibility to telemedicine centers can be enhanced if such models as the one in this study are developed on a larger scale networking the entire length and breadth of the country. This could be done with government and private sector partnership nurturing the way to establishment of a platform for dispensing uniform healthcare to one and all in the country despite the geographical restrictions.

Risk v Benefit in Telecardiology

The earlier diagnosis and initiation of appropriate treatment that can be achieved using telemedicine links should reduce morbidity and mortality but as yet there are no published controlled trials measuring this benefit. A further significant benefit is that unnecessary transfers are avoided. In our series of 63 cases, the need for transfer to obtain a diagnosis was avoided in 47. There are therefore potentially significant financial savings for the referring hospital.

For the paediatric cardiologist the concern about participating in diagnosis by telemedicine is that a serious lesion may be missed and false reassurance given. The medicolegal aspects of patient responsibility after remote consultation in this way are still unclear. In our series of 61 transmitted studies using ISDN2, there were four errors in diagnosis: three small ventricular septal defects and one moderate pulmonary valvar stenosis were not detected. Twenty eight major lesions were accurately diagnosed. In the series reported by Finlay et al, patients in whom a diagnosis was made by using their telemedicine link had follow-up echocardiography by "paediatric cardiology echocardiography staff".

No significant diagnostic discrepancies were found. Sobczyk et al reported their experience of remote diagnosis in 47 patients from prerecorded images transmitted transtelephonically studies were normal. Lesions accurately diagnosed included persistent ductus arteriosus (PDA) (n = 8), ventricular septal defect (n = 6), and ventricular septal defect with interrupted aortic arch (n = 1). They reported an inappropriate clinical decision causing delay in transfer of a patient with a PDA requiring ligation due to an inconclusive transmitted study.

The available evidence thus suggests that remote echocardiography can be used to diagnose or exclude major lesions with accuracy. The diagnosis made on the transmitted scan should not, however, be considered the definitive cardiac consultation. This is not an issue for patients transferred to the regional centre on the basis of the remote consultation as they will all have a "hands on" consultation and echocardiography. I would advocate that babies considered to be normal or to have minor lesions on the transmitted scan should also electively have a follow-up direct consultation by a paediatric cardiologist.

Conclusion

It is likely that with further improvements in, and increasing availability of the equipment necessary to transmit good quality echocardiographic images, an increasing number of telemedicine links will be established from neonatal units to paediatric cardiology centres. It is not appropriate or necessary to apply this technology to the assessment of the child where an urgent clinical decision does not need to be made such as the evaluation of a murmur. Telemedicine links should be used to diagnose or exclude significant neonatal CHD and that over the next few years paediatric cardiologists will find that providing remote diagnosis in this way could become an increasingly important part of their workload.

BIBLIOGRAPHY

1. Boersma E, Maas AC, Deckers JW, Simoons ML. Early thrombolytic treatment in acute myocardial infarction: reappraisal of the golden hour. Lancet 1996 Nov 9;348(9037): 1312–3.
2. The world fact book 2001, CIA publication, Office of public affairs.
3. Belmont JM, Mattioli LF. Accuracy of analog telephonic stethoscopy for paediatric telecardiology. Pediatrics. 2003 Oct;112(4):780–6.
4. Fisher JB, Alboliras ET, Berdusis K, Webb CL: Rapid identification of serious congenital heart disease using real-time transtelephonic transmission of echocardiograms. Am Heart J 1996;131(6):1225–27.
5. Randolph GR, Hagler DJ, Khandheria BK, Lunn ER, Cook WJ, Seward JB, O'Leary PW: Remote telemedical interpretation of neonatal echocardiograms: Impact on clinical management in a primary care setting. J Amer Coll Cardiol 1999;34(1):241–245.
6. Stevenson JG. Evolution of echocardiography in neonatal diagnosis. Acta Paediatr Suppl. 1995;410:8–14.
7. Du ZD, Roguin N, Barak M. Clinical and echocardiographic evaluation of neonates with heart murmurs. Acta Paediatr. 1997;86:752–756.
8. Hurwitz RA, Caldwell RL. Should pediatric echocardiograms be performed in adult laboratories? Pediatrics. 1998;102(2).
9. Afset JE, Lunde P, Rasmussen K. Accuracy of routine echocardiographic measurements made by an inexperienced examiner through teleinstruction. J Telemed Telecare. 1996;2:148–154.
10. Casey F, Brown D, Corrigan N, et al. Value of a low-cost telemedicine link in the remote echocardiographic diagnosis of congenital heart defects. J Telemed Telecare. 1998;4(suppl 1):46–48.
11. Casey F, Brown D, Craig BG, Rogers J, Mulholland HC. Diagnosis of neonatal congenital heart defects by remote consultation using a lowcost telemedicine link. J Telemed Telecare. 1996;2:165–169.
12. Finley JP, Sharratt GP, Nanton MA, et al. Pediatric echocardiography by telemedicine—nine years' experience. J Telemed Telecare. 1997;3:200–204.
13. Fisher JB, Alboliras ET, Berdusis K, Webb CL. Rapid identification of congenital heart disease by transmission of echocardiograms. Am Heart J. 1996;131:1225–1227.
14. Hassol A, Irvin C, Gaumer G, Puskin D, Mintzer C, Grigsby J. Rural applications of telemedicine. Telemed J. 1997;3:215–225.
10. Randolph GR, Hagler DJ, Khandheria BK, et al. Remote telemedical interpretation of neonatal echocardiograms: impact on clinical management in a primary care setting. J Am Coll Cardiol. 1999;34:241–245.
11. Sable C, Roca T, Gold J, Gutierrez A, Gulotta E, Culpepper W. Live transmission of neonatal echocardiograms from underserved areas: accuracy, patient care, and cost. Telemed J. 1999;5:339–347.
12. Sobczyk WS, Solinger RE, Rees AH, Elbl F. Transtelephonic echocardiography: successful use in a tertiary pediatric referral center. J Pediatr. 1993;122:S84–S88.
13. Colton T. Statistics in Medicine. Boston, MA: Little, Brown and Company; 1974:237–250.
14. Finley JP, Human DG, Nanton MA, et al. Echocardiography by telephone—evaluation of pediatric disease at a distance. Am J Cardiol. 1989;63:1475–1477.
15. Trippi JA, Kopp G, Lee KS, et al. The feasibility of dobutamine stress echocardiography in the emergency department with telemedicine interpretation. J Am Soc Echocardiogr. 1996;9:113–118.
16. Trippi JA, Lee KS, Kopp G, Nelson D, Kovacs R. Emergency echocardiography telemedicine: an efficient method to provide 24-hour consultative echocardiography. J Am Coll Cardiol. 1996;27:1748–1752.
17. Trippi JA, Lee KS, Kopp G, Nelson DR, Yee KG, Cordell WH. Dobutamine stress tele-echocardiography for evaluation of emergency department patients with chest pain. J Am Coll Cardiol. 1997;30:627–632.
18. Houston A, McLeod K, Richens T, et al. Assessment of the quality of neonatal echocardiographic images transmitted by ISDN telephone lines. Heart. 1999;82:222–225.
19. Rendina MC, Downs SM, Carasco N, Loonsk J, Bose CL. Effect of telemedicine on health outcomes in 87 infants requiring neonatal intensive care. Telemed J. 1998;4:345–351.
20. Rendina MC, Long WA, deBliek R. Effect size and experimental power analysis in a pediatric cardiology telemedicine system. J Telemed Telecare. 1997;3(suppl 1):56–57.
21. Sable C. Telecardiology: potential impact on acute care. Crit Care Med. 2001;29:N159–N165.

22. Scholz TD, Kienzle MG. Optimizing utilization of pediatric echocardiography and implications for telemedicine. Am J Cardiol. 1999;83: 1645–1648.
23. Thomas JD, Main ML. Digital echocardiographic laboratory: where do we stand? J Am Soc Echocardiogr. 1998;11:978–983.
24. Egan EA, Eitzman DV. Umbilical vessel catheterization. Am J Dis Child. 1971;121:213–218.
25. Ades A, Sable C, Cummings, Martin G. Echocardiographic assessmentof umbilical venous catheter placement. Pediatr Res. 2000;47:383A.
26. Dunn PM. Localization of the umbilical catheter by post-mortem measurement. Arch Dis Child. 1966;41:69–7527.

Burdussis K. Tele-echocardiography and telecardiology. Telemed Today. 1999;7:25–26, 35–36.
28. Jenkins KJ, Newburger JW, Lock JE, Davis RB, Coffman GA, Iezzoni LI. In-hospital mortality for surgical repair of congenital heart defects: preliminary observations of variation by hospital caseload. Pediatrics. 1995;95:323–330.
29. Millman DS, Kiesel AB. Telecardiology: legal issues and new developments. Telemed Today. 1999;7:27–29.
30. States where Medicaid reimbursement of services utilizing telemedicine is available, June 27, 2000, Health Care Financing Administration.

43

Cardiovascular Drug Therapy

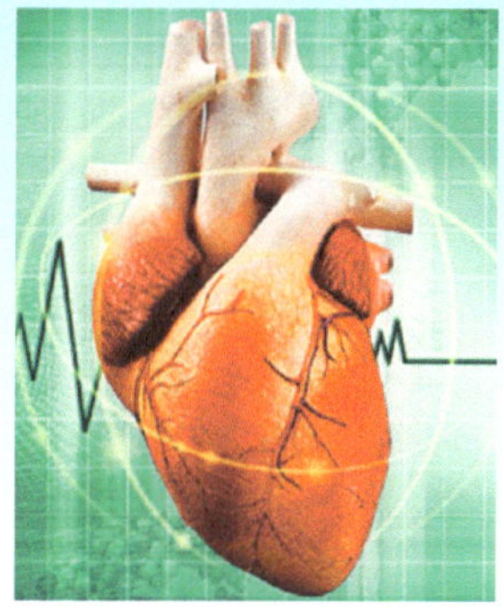

Advances in cardiology, surgical techniques, postoperative care, and medications have improved the chances of long-term survival of the neonatal and pediatric patient with complex congenital cardiac anomalies. Rather than undergoing palliative repair, these children are now frequently taken to the operating room for complete repair. As complete repair becomes the norm, collaborative management and a thorough understanding of the pre- and postoperative medications used become essential to the care of these patients. The nurse's ability to understand preop, postop, and management medications is enhanced by an understanding of the principles of cardiac anatomy and physiology, as well as developmental changes in cardiac function. All of these are reviewed. In addition, since the safe and effective administration of these drugs depends on the pediatric intensive care unit (PICU) and neonatal intensive care unit (NICU) nurse's thorough knowledge of these medications and their effects on the cardiovascular system, a brief review of these medications is presented. While new technology and techniques are improving survival rates for children with congenital heart anomalies, it is the postoperative care that these children receive that enhances the patient's survival even more.

Antihypertensive Drugs

Drug category: **Diuretics**

Cause diuresis, which decreases plasma volume and edema, thereby decreasing cardiac output and blood pressure.

Drug: Hydrochlorothiazide (esidrix, hydroDIURIL, microzide).

Description: Inhibits reabsorption of sodium in distal tubules, causing increased excretion of sodium, water, potassium and hydrogen ions.

Adult dose: 25–100 mg PO qd; not to exceed 200 mg/kg/d.

Pediatric dose: < 6 months: 2–3 mg/kg/d PO divided bid, > 6 months: 2 mg/kg/d PO divided bid.

Contraindications: Documented hypersensitivity; anuria; renal decompensation.

Interactions: May decrease effects of anticoagulants, antigout agents, and sulfonylureas; may increase toxicity of allopurinol, anesthetics, antineoplastics, calcium salts, loop diuretics, lithium, diazoxide, digitalis, amphotericin B, and nondepolarizing muscle relaxants.

Table 43.1: *Presents normal hemodynamics and oxygen consumption in children*

Age (weight/BSA)	*Cardiac output (mL/min)*	*Heart rate*	*Stroke volume (mL)*	*Oxygen consumption (mL/min*	*mL/min/m*
Newborn (3.2 kg/0.2 m)	700–800	145	5	36–54	180–270
6 months (8 kg/0/42 m)	1000–1600	120	10	70–100	167–238
1 year (10 kg/0/5 m)	1300–1500	115	13	85–110	170–220
2 years (13 kg/0.59 m)	1500–2000	115	18	91–123	154–211
4 years (17 kg/0.71 m)	2300–2375	105	27	110–150	155–211
5 years (19 kg/0.77 m)	2500–3000	95	31	115–170	149–221
8 years (28 kg/0.96 m)	3400–3600	83	42	150–208	156–200
10 years (35 kg/1.1 m)	3800–4000	75	50	190–250	122–227
15 years (50 kg/1.4 m)	5000–6000	70	85	300–400	120–200

Table 43. 2: *Drug therapy in children*

Medication	*Indication for use*	*Dosing*	*Onset*	*Side-effects*	*Half-life*	*Metabolism*	*Contraindications*
Dopamine	Pre- and postoperatively to increase cardiac output, blood pressure, and urine output. Volume depletion should be corrected prior to starting dopamine	Renal and mesentetric vasodilation: 2–5 mcg/kg/min (beta) effect: 5–10 mcg/kg/min Vasoconstriction and pressor (alpha) effect. >10 mcg/kg/min IV infusion	Within 5 mins	Tachydysthythmias, vasocontriction, gangrene of the extremities, anginal pain and palpitations	2 mins	Metabolized in the plasma kidney and liver	Hypersensitivity to sulfiters, phechromocytoma or ventricular fibrilation. Care must be given to ensure that extravasation does not occur. Extravasation causes severe tissue necrosis. In the event of extravasation, phentolamine should be instilled locally
Dobutamine	Pre-and postoperatively to increase cardiac output and to manage short-term cardiac decompensation. Volume depletion should be corrected prior to starting dobutamine	2–20 mcg/kg/min IV infusion. Transient hypotension may occur when starting this medication	1–10 mins	Ectopic heart beats, increased heart rate chest pain, headche, nausea and vomiting dyspnea, and in higher doses, ventricular dysrhythmias	2 mins	Metabolized in the tissues and liver	Hypersensitivity to sulfiltes and idiopathic hypertophic subaortic stenosis
Epinephrine	Pre- and postoperatively to increase cardiac output and blood pressure. Care must be taken when using this drug. The benefits of increased cardiac output and blood pressure must be weighed against the effects of increased consumption of myocardial oxygen, tachycardia, and decreased renal blood flow	0.1 to 1 mcg/kg/min IV infusion	5 mins	Pallor, tachycardia hypertension, increased myocardial oxygen consumption, anxiety, headache, dilated pupils, nausea, acute urinary retention, weakness, tremor, and decreased renal blood flow	3 mins	Metabolized in the liver and tissues	Hypersensitivity to epinephrine, cardiac dysrhythmias, and angle-closure glaucoma
Mllrinone amrinone	Postoperatively to treat low cardiac output syndrome and congestive heart failure. Both drugs increase cardiac output and stroke volume, decrease intracardiac filling pressure, and decrease systemic vascular resistance without changing heart rate or myocardial oxygen consumption. Milrinone has fewer side effects.	Loading dose: 50 mcg/kg IV over at least 10 mins Maintenance infusion: 0.2 to 1 mcg/kg	5–15 mins	Headache, ventricular dysthythmias, hypotension, and chest pain	1–5 hours	Excretion by the kidneys	Severe pulmonary or aortic obstructive disease and hypersensitivity to milrinone
Digoxin	Most frequently used in chronic heart failure, its primary use is to increase the force of contraction in the myocardium thus increasing cardiac output. May be given IV or PO	Digitalizing: 30–50 mcg/kg IV (Q 8 hrs: 1/2, 1/4. 1/4) Maintenance: 2–12 mcg/kg/day must be individualized according to age	5–30 mins	Sinus bradycardia, A-V and S-A block, ventricular dyrhythmias lethargy, confusion, nausea, vomiting, feeding intolerance, blurred vision	18–36 hours	Excretion by kidneys, removed by dialysis, dose must be adjusted for renal failure patients (follow levels closely)	Hypersensitivity to digoxin, ventricular fibrilation, A-V block, idiopathic hypertrophic subaortic stenosis, or constrictive pericarditis

(Contd...)

Table43.2: *Drug therapy in children (Contd...)*

Medication	*Indication for use*	*Dosing*	*Onset*	*Side-effects*	*Half-life*	*Metabolism*	*Contraindications*
Nitroglycerin	Postoperatively to dilate the coronary arteries, improving oxygenation of the myocardial tissues. As a venous dilator, nitroglycerine reduces left ventricular diastolic pressure and systemic vascular resistance, reducing myocardial oxygen demand	Initial dose: 0.25–0.5 micrograms/kg/min via infusion. May titrate by 0.5 to 1 microgram/kg/min every 3–5 min to a maximum dose of 5–10 mcg/min Caution: when mixing nitroglycarin, the maximum concentration is 400 micrograms/mL, it must be diluted in glass, and special non-polyviryl chloride tubing must be used	1–2 min	Severe hypotension, headache, dizziness, reflex tachycardia, nausea, and vomiting	1–4 min	Extensively during first-pass and excreted in the urine	Hypersensitivity to nitroglycerin, organic nitrates, glucoma, severe anemia, increased ICP, pericardial tamponae, constrictive pericarditis and hypotension
Nitroprusside	Indicated preoperatively and postoperatively for hypertensive crisis. Nitroprusside, a peripheral vasodilator, increases cardiac output by decressing afterload and systemic vascular resistance	Starting dose: 0.3 to 0.5 micrograms/kg/min IV infusion, titrating to effect to a maximum of 8 of 10 micrograms/kg/min. Nitroprusside must be protected from light (light greatly increases decomposition) D_5W should be used for dilution	Within 2 min	Profound hypotension, metabolic acidosis, increased ICP, thyroid suspression, and CNS toxicity. Cyanide and thiocyanate toxicity may occur if nitroprusside is used for greater than 4 days, if the infusion is > 4 micrograms/kg/min or in the presence of renal dysfunction. Monitor thiocyanate and cyanide levels keeping	Less than 10 min	Metabolized in the liver and excreted in the urine	Hypersensitivity to nitropresside and decreased cerebral perfusion
Lidocaine	A class IB antiarrhythmic indicated pre- and post operatively for ventricular dysrthythmias. Lidocaine suppresses automaticity of conduction tissues by increasing the electrical threshold of the ventricles	Loading: 1 mg/kg IV, may be repeated in 10–15 min times 2 doses, followed by a continuous infusion of 10–50 mcg/kg/min Lower loading doses: 0.5 mg/kg IV and lower infusion rates may be required in patients with CHF or hepatic disease.	45–50 sec after single IV bolus dose	Bradycardia, hypoten sion, heart block, lethargy, coma, agitation slurred speech, seizures, hallucinations, nausea, vomiting, muscle twiching, blurred vision, respiratory depression or arrest	Biphasic ranging from 7 min to 3.2 hours	Metabolized in the liver and excreted in the urine	Hypersensitivity to lidocaine Adams-strokes syndrome, or severe degree of S-A or A-V or ventricular heart block without a pacemaker

(Contd...)

Table 43 2: *Drug therapy in children (Contd...)*

Medication	*Indication for use*	*Dosing*	*Onset*	*Side-effects*	*Half-life*	*Metabolism*	*Contraindications*
Amiodarone	A class III antiarrhythmic indicated postoperatively for life-threatening ventricular dysthythmias and junctional ectopic tachycardia (JET). Amiodarone decreases A-V and S-A node conduction and prolongs the refractory period.	Loading: 5 milligram/kg IV over 1 hour followed by a maintance infusion of 0.3 to 1 milligram/kg/hr Aminodarone must be mixed with D_5W and in a glass bottle	Within hours of the loading dose	Worsening A-V block, bradycardia, hypotension. With long-term use hypothyroidism, liver toxicity	Extremely long 5 days	Metabolized in the liver and is excreted in the biliary tract and urine	Hypersensitivity to amiodarone, sinus bradycaria, second and third degree A-V block and cardiogenic shock. Many drug inter-actions; amiodarone is a very potent inhibitor of P450 liver enzymes
Precainamide	A class 1A antiarrhythmic indicated postoperatively for SVT, ventricular tachycardias, and atrial tachycardia. Procainamide inhibits the sodium pump decreases myocardial excitability and conduction velocity and depresses myocardial contractility.	*Loading:* 5–15 milligram/kg IV over 5 min to a maximum dose of 100 milligrams followed by a maintenance infusion of 20–80 microgram/kg/min to a maximum dose of 2 gm/24 hrs	10–30 min	Prolongation of the QT interval (stop infusion if QT increases by 50% of premedication length), hypotension, A-V block, confusion, tachycardia, nausea, and vomiting. Long-term side effects systemic lupus	1.7 hours	Metabolized in the liver and excreted in the urine	Complete heart block, A-V block, long QT interval, hypersensitivity to procainamide, and torsades de pointe
Furosemide	A loop diuretic indicated postoperatively to reduce preload, and in patients with postperfusion syndrome. Postperfusion syndrome is a systemic inflammatory response to cardiopulmonary bypass. This syndrome manifests itselft, in part, as renal insufficiency. Renal insuffciency (oliguria and fluid retention) affects 5% to 30% of all children after pediatric cardiac surgeries with the aid of cardiopulmonary bypass. Furosemide as either a continuous drip or intermittent boluses can be given. The study indicates that a constant infusion yields comparable urine output at a lower dose of furosemide while decreasing the fluctuations in urinary output and the need for volume replacement.	IV infusions: 0.05 mg/kg/hrs thrated to clinical effect. intermittent IV: 1–2 mg/kg/dose every 6–12 hrs	IV 5 min PO: 30–60 min	Hypotension, dizziness, utcaria, electrolyte imbalances, potential ototoxicity with high doses, and jaundice	Normal renal function 30 min, with renal failure 9 hrs	Metabolized by the liver and 80% excreted in the urine	Indomethacin decreases effect

(Contd...)

Table 43.2: *Drug therapy in children (Contd...)*

Medication	*Indication for use*	*Dosing*	*Onset*	*Side-effects*	*Half-life*	*Metabolism*	*Contraindications*
Bumetanide	A loop diuretic is indicated postoperatively to reduce preload	0.015–0.1 mg/kg/ dose given every 6–24 hrs IV	Within a few min when given IV	Hypotension, chest pain dizziness, rash, hyperglycemia, electrolyte imbalance, elevated liver enzymes, ototoxicity and elevated serum creatinine	Ranges from 1 hr to 2-1/2 hrs	Partially metabolized in the liver and excreted in the urine	Hypersensitivity to bumetanide and anuria or increasing azotemia
Ethacrynic acid	A loop diuretic is indicated postoperatively to reduce preload	1 mg/kg/dose given once. If necessary may be repeated every 8–12 hrs	5 min when given IV	Hypotension, chest pain, dizziness, rash, hyperglycemia, electrolyte imbalance, elevated liver enzymes, ototoxicity, and elevated serum creatinine	Range from 1 hr to 2½ hrs	Partially metabolized in the liver and excreted in the urine	Hypersensitivity to bumetanide and anuria or increasing azotemia
Ethacrynic acid	A loophdiuretic is indicated postoperatively to reduce preload	1 mg/kg/dose given once. If necessary may be repeated every 8–12 hrs	5 min when given IV	Hypotension, electrolyte imbalance, rash, hyperglycemia, abdominal pain, and renal injury	2 hrs if given IV	Metabolized in the liver and excreted in the bile and urine	Hypersensitivity to etacrynic acid, hypotension, hyponatremic dehydration, metabolic alkalosis with hypokalemia and anuria
Spironolactone	A potassium-sparing diuretic acting on the distal collecting duct of the nephron This drug is indicated for treatment of CHF. May be used in conjunction with lasix and digoxin	1–3 mg/kg/day, given once a day or divided into two doses given every 12 hours	1–3 hrs	Dysrhythmias, lethargy confusion, ataxia, rash electrolyte imbalance, dehydration, and decreased renal function		Metabolized in the liver and excreted in the urine and biliary tracts	If given with potassium supplements may increase potassium serum levels. Spironolactone, when given with potassium supplements, may potentiate inotropic affect of digoxin while decreasing digoxin clearance.
Calcium Chloride Calcium Gluconate	Often indicated in the postoperative cardiovascular patient to increase contractility of the myocardium. when choosing which calcium supplement to use, attention must be paid to the strength of the supplement and the purpose for using it. For example, calcium chloride has three times more elemental calcium than calcium gluconate. Since the body will be able to utilize the calcium from calcium chloride much more	Calcium chloride: 10 to 20 mg/kg/IV dose Calcium gluconate: 50–100 mg/min IV infusion		Vasodilation hypotension bradycardia, dysrhythmias ventricular fibrilation, syncope, headache, confusion, lethargy, coma constipation, nausea, vomiting and elevated serum amylase. Ionized calcium (amount of calcium) available for use) levels should be used instead of serum calcium (total amount of calcium in body) levels when monitoring calcium supplementation			Hypercalcemia, renal calculi ventricular fibrilation

(Contd...)

Table 43.2: *Drug therapy in children*

Medication	*Indication for use*	*Dosing*	*Onset*	*Side-effects*	*Half-life*	*Metabolism*	*Contraindications*
	Quickly, calcium chloride is used during emergent situations. Calcium gluconate releases the calcium more slowly and is utilized, via infusion, for long-term correction.						
Esmolol	A beta-blocker indicated postoperatively for the treatment of systemic hypertension, right or left-sided outflow tract obstruction, and is a class II antiarrhythmic	200–500 mcg/kg/ IV over 1–2 min followed by a maintenance infusion of 50–250 mcg/kg/min	1–2 min after loading dose	Heart failure, bradycardia, hypotension, nausea, and vomiting	3–5 min	Metabolized in the blood and excreted in the urine	Bradycardia, heart block, uncompensated heart failure, cardiogenic shock, and hypersensitivity to esmolol or any other beta-blocker
Indomethacin	A nonsteroidal antiinflammatory drug (NSAID) that inhibits the production of prostaglandin. It is indicated for pharmacological closure of a patent ductus arteriosus.	0.2 mg/kg intravenously if the ductus does not dose with the initial dose, two additional doses may be given. The amount and timing of those closes are determined by postnatal age, urine output, clinical assessment, and/or echocardiography. A second series of indomethacin may be necessary in some neonates to assure ductal closure		Transient renal dysfunction (decreased urine output, decreased urine sodium and chloride excretion, free water clearance, hyponatremia, transient hypoglycemia, decreased platelet aggregation and increased risk of hemorrhage, necrotizing enterocolitis, and gastric perforation. These side effects will usually dissipate 72 hrs after the last dose of indomethacin	Ranges from 15–50 hrs and is partially dependent on postnatal age	Metabolized in the liver and excreted in the urine and feces	Bleeding, necrotizing enterocolitis, platelet count < 50,000 and impaired renal function Use with caution in patients with diabetes mellitus and/or insipidis as symptoms may become exaggerated. Contraindicated with recent MI, uncorrected adrenal insufficiency, thyrotoxicosis and hypersensitivity to liothyronine
Liothyronine (continued)	On the heart, increased systemic vascular resistance, and an association with increased morbidity in the postoperative period						
Prostaglandin E_1	An endogenous fatty acid indicated preoperatively to the ductus arteriosus. This is vitally important with ductal dependent lesions such as severe coarctation of the aorta, critical pulmonary stenosis, and transposition of the great arteries	0.05 mcg/kg/min may be doubled every 15–30 minutes up to a maximum dose of 0.2 mcg/kg min until desired effect is obtained. The infusion may be decreased to the lowest effective close once ductal pattency is achieved	Relatively short with immediate effects	Apnea, hypotension seizures, flushing and elevated temperature		Metabolized rapidly in the pulmonary circulation and excreted by the kidneys	

Pregnancy: C-fetal risk revealed in studies in animals but not established or not studied in humans; may use if benefits outweigh risk to fetus.

Precautions: Caution in renal and hepatic disease, gout, diabetes mellitus, and lupus erythematosus.

Drug: Spironolactone (Aldactone).

Description: Used for management of hypertension. May block effects of aldosterone on arteriolar smooth muscles.

Adult dose: 25–200 mg/d PO qd or divided bid.

Pediatric dose: 1.5–3.5 mg/kg/d PO in divided doses q6–24h.

Contraindications: Documented hypersensitivity; anuria; renal failure; hyperkalemia.

Interactions: May decrease effect of anticoagulants; potassium and potassium-sparing diuretics may increase toxicity of spironolactone.

Pregnancy: D-fetal risk shown in humans; use only if benefits outweigh risk to fetus.

Precautions: Caution in renal and hepatic impairment.

Drug: Amiloride (Midamor)

Description: l-carbonyl-guanidine unrelated chemically to other known antikaliuretic or diuretic agents. Potassium-conserving (antikaliuretic) drug that, compared with thiazide diuretics, possesses weak natriuretic, diuretic, and antihypertensive activity.

Adult dose: 5–20 mg PO qd.

Pediatric dose: Not established.

Contraindications: Documented hypersensitivity; elevated serum potassium levels > 5.5 mEq/L; impaired renal function, acute or chronic renal insufficiency, and evidence of diabetic nephropathy.

Interactions: Concomitant therapy with potassium supplementation may increase serum potassium levels (if concomitant use indicated because of demonstrated hypokalemia, use caution and monitor serum potassium frequently); lithium generally should not be administered with diuretics because may reduce renal clearance and increase risk of lithium toxicity; administration of nonsteroidal antiinflammatory agents can reduce diuretic, natriuretic, and antihypertensive effects of loop, potassium-sparing, and thiazide diuretics (when used concomitantly, observe patient closely to determine if desired effect of diuretic achieved); indomethacin and potassium-sparing diuretics including amiloride, may be associated with increased serum potassium levels, so consider potential effects on potassium kinetics and renal function.

Pregnancy: B-fetal risk not confirmed in studies in humans but has been shown in some studies in animals.

Precautions: Potassium retention associated with use of an antikaliuretic agent accentuated in presence of renal impairment and may result in rapid development of hyperkalemia; monitor serum potassium level; mild hyperkalemia usually not associated with abnormal ECG findings; monitor electrolytes closely if evidence of renal functional impairment present, BUN > 30 mg/100 mL, or serum creatinine levels >1.5 mg/100 mL.

Drug: Furosemide (lasix)

Description: Increases excretion of water by interfering with chloride-binding cotransport system, which, in turn, inhibits sodium and chloride reabsorption in ascending loop of Henle and distal renal tubule. Dose must be individualized to patient. Depending on response, administer at increments of 20–40 mg no sooner than 6–8 h after previous dose until desired diuresis occurs. When treating infants, titrate with 1-mg/kg per dose increments until satisfactory effect achieved.

Adult dose: 20–80 mg/d PO/IV/IM; titrate up to 600 mg/d for severe edematous states.

Pediatric dose: 1–2 mg/kg/dose PO; not to exceed 6 mg/kg/dose; not to administer more often than q6h Alternatively, 1 mg/kg IV/IM slowly under close supervision; not to exceed 6 mg/kg.

Contraindications: Documented hypersensitivity; hepatic coma; anuria; state of severe electrolyte depletion.

Interactions: Metformin decreases furosemide concentrations; furosemide interferes with hypoglycemic effect of antidiabetic agents and antagonizes muscle-relaxing effect of tubocurarine; auditory toxicity appears to be increased with coadministration of aminoglycosides and furosemide; hearing loss of varying degrees may occur; anticoagulant activity of warfarin may be enhanced when taken concurrently with this medication; increased plasma lithium levels and toxicity possible when taken concurrently.

Pregnancy: C-fetal risk revealed in studies in animals but not established or not studied in humans; may use if benefits outweigh risk to fetus.

Precautions: Perform frequent serum electrolyte, CO_2, glucose, creatinine, uric acid, calcium, and BUN determinations during first few mo of therapy and periodically thereafter.

Drug: Alpha1-adrenergic blockers

Selectively block postsynaptic alpha1-adrenergic receptors. Dilate arterioles and veins, thus lowering blood pressure.

Drug: Prazosin (Minipress), Terazosin (Hytrin)

Description: Prazosin treats prostatic hypertrophy. Improves urine flow rates by relaxing smooth muscle, which is caused by blocking alpha1-adrenoceptors in bladder neck and prostate. When increasing dose, administer first dose of each increment at bedtime to reduce syncopal episodes. Although doses > 20 mg/d usually do not increase efficacy, some patients may benefit from as much as 40 mg/d. Terazosin decreases arterial tone by allowing peripheral postsynaptic blockade. Has minimal alpha2 effect.

Adult dose: Prazosin: 1 mg PO bid/tid initial; 6–15 mg/d PO bid/tid maintenance. Terazosin: 1 mg PO hs; increase slowly to effect; not to exceed 20 mg/d.

Pediatric dose: Prazosin: not established; suggested dose is 0.5-7 mg PO tidTerazosin: not established.

Contraindications: Documented hypersensitivity.

Interactions: Acute postural hypotensive reaction from beta-blockers may worsen; indomethacin may decrease antihypertensive activity; verapamil may increase serum levels and may increase patient's sensitivity to drug-induced postural hypotension; may decrease anti-hypertensive effects of clonidine.

Pregnancy: C-fetal risk revealed in studies in animals but not established or not studied in humans; may use if benefits outweigh risk to fetus.

Precautions: Caution in renal impairment; may cause marked hypotension following first dose and coadministration with beta-blockers.

Drug: Beta-adrenergic blocking agents
Used to treat hypertension as initial agents or in combination with other drugs (e.g., thiazides).

Drug: Atenolol (tenormin), metoprolol (lopressor, toprol XL), propranolol (inderal), nebivolol (bystolic).

Description: Atenolol and metoprolol selectively block beta1-receptors with little or no effect on beta2 types. Propranolol is a class II antiarrhythmic, nonselective, beta-adrenergic receptor blocker with membrane-stabilizing activity that decreases automaticity of contractions. Nebivolol actions depend on metabolic factors and dose. In extensive metabolizers (majority of the population) and doses ≤10 mg, preferentially elicits beta1 selective inhibition whereas in poor metabolizers and at higher doses, inhibits both beta1- and beta2-receptors.

Adult dose: Atenolol: 50 mg PO qd; increase to 100 mg/d, if necessary. Metoprolol: 100 mg/d PO qd or divided bid/tid initial; increase at 1-wk intervals prn to a total of 450 mg/d if necessary. Propranolol: 40–80 mg PO bid initial; increase to 160–320 mg/d (may require up to 640 mg/d). Nebivolol: 5 PO qd initially if further blood pressure. reduction required after 2 wk, may increase dose at 2 wk intervals, not to exceed 40 mg/d; decrease initial dose to 2.5 mg/d for CrCl <30 mL/min and moderate hepatic impairment.

Pediatric dose: Atenolol: 1–2 mg/kg/dose PO qd Metoprolol: 1–5 mg/kg/d PO divided bid. Propranolol: 0.5 mg/kg/d PO divided bid/qid; increase gradually q3–7d; range is 2–4 mg/kg/d divided bid; not to exceed 2 mg/kg/d. Nebivolol: not established.

Contraindications: Documented hypersensitivity; congestive heart failure; pulmonary edema; cardiogenic shock; AV conduction abnormalities; heart block (without a pacemaker).

Interactions: Coadministration with aluminum salts, barbiturates, calcium salts, cholestyramine, NSAIDs, penicillins, and rifampin may decrease effects; haloperidol, hydralazine, loop diuretics, and MAOIs may increase toxicity; coadministration with myocardial depressants, AV conduction inhibitors (e.g. verapamil, diltiazem), or antiarrhythmic agents (e.g. disopyramide) may increase risk for bradycardia; if coadministered with clonidine, discontinue nebivolol several days before gradually tapering clonidine

Pregnancy: C-fetal risk revealed in studies in animals but not established or not studied in humans; may use if benefits outweigh risk to fetus.

Precautions: Beta-adrenergic blockade may reduce signs and symptoms of acute hypoglycemia and may decrease clinical signs of hyperthyroidism; abrupt withdrawal may exacerbate symptoms of hyperthyroidism including thyroid storm; monitor patient closely and withdraw drug slowly during IV administration, carefully monitor blood pressure, heart rate and ECG.

Drug: Alpha/beta-adrenergic blocking agents

Block alpha-, beta1-, and beta2-adrenergic receptor sites, thus decreasing blood pressure.

Drug: Labetalol (normodyne, trandate), carvedilol (coreg).

Description: Nonselective beta- and alpha-adrenergic blockers. Do not appear to have intrinsic sympathomimetic activity. May reduce cardiac output and decrease peripheral vascular resistance. Use in aortic dissection not advisable when titratable drugs, such as esmolol and nitroprusside, available.

Adult dose: Labetalol: 20–30 mg IV over 2 min followed by 40–80 mg at 10-min intervals; not to exceed 300 mg/dose. Carvedilol: 6.25 mg PO bid; maintain for 1–2 wk if tolerated and increase to 12.5 mg bid to maximum 25 mg bid.

Pediatric dose: Labetalol: not established; suggested dose is 0.4-1 mg/kg/h; not to exceed 3 mg/kg/h. Carvedilol: not established.

Contraindications: Documented hypersensitivity; cardiogenic shock; pulmonary edema; bradycardia; AV block; uncompensated congestive heart failure; reactive airway disease; severe bradycardia.

Interactions: Labetalol decreases effect of diuretics and increases toxicity of methotrexate, lithium and salicylates; may diminish reflex tachycardia resulting from nitroglycerin use without interfering with hypotensive effects; cimetidine may increase labetalol and carvedilol blood levels; glutethimide may decrease labetalol effects by inducing microsomal enzymes; rifampin, barbiturates, cholestyramine, colestipol, NSAIDs, salicylates, and penicillins may decrease carvedilol effects; carvedilol may increase effects of antidiabetic agents, digoxin, and calcium channel blockers; concurrent administration with clonidine may increase blood pressure and decrease heart rate; carvedilol may decrease effect of sulfonylureas; fluoxetine, paroxetine, and propafenone may increase carvedilol levels

Pregnancy: C-fetal risk revealed in studies in animals but not established or not studied in humans; may use if benefits outweigh risk to fetus.

Precautions: Caution in impaired hepatic function; discontinue therapy if signs of liver dysfunction present; in elderly patients, a lower response rate and higher incidence of toxicity may be observed; caution in congestive heart failure being treated with digitalis, diuretics, or ACE inhibitors (AV conduction may be slowed); caution in peripheral vascular disease, hyperthyroidism, and diabetes mellitus.

Drug category: Peripheral vasodilators
Relax blood vessels to improve blood flow, thus decreasing blood pressure.

Drug: Hydralazine (apresoline), minoxidil (rogaine loniten)

Description: Hydralazine decreases systemic resistance through direct vasodilation of arterioles. Minoxidil relaxes arteriolar smooth muscle, causing vasodilation, which, in turn, may reduce blood pressure.

Adult dose: Hydralazine: 10–20 mg/dose IV/IM q 4–6h prn initial; increase to 40 mg/dose if necessary; change to PO as soon as possible. Minoxidil: 5 mg PO qd; increase gradually q3d; 10–40 mg/d PO qd or divided bid maintenance; not to exceed 100 mg/d.

Pediatric dose: Not established.

Contraindications: Documented hypersensitivity; mitral valve, rheumatic heart disease (hydralazine); pheochromocytoma (minoxidil).

Interactions: MAOIs and beta-blockers may increase hydralazine toxicity; pharmacologic effects of hydralazine may be decreased by indomethacin; concurrent use of minoxidil with guanethidine, diuretics, or hypotensive agents may result in additive hypotension.

Pregnancy: C-fetal risk revealed in studies in animals but not established or not studied in humans; may use if benefits outweigh risk to fetus.

Precautions: Hydralazine has been implicated in MI; minoxidil may exacerbate angina pectoris; caution in pulmonary hypertension, congestive heart failure, coronary artery disease, and significant renal failure.

Drug category: Calcium channel blockers
May be a more effective class of medication for black patients.

Drug: Diltiazem (cardizem, dilacor), verapamil (calan, covera-HS), nifedipine (adalat).

Description: During depolarization, inhibits calcium ion from entering slow channels or voltage-sensitive areas of vascular smooth muscle and myocardium.

Adult dose: Diltiazem: cardizem SR: 60–120 mg PO bid. Cardizem CD: 180–240 mg PO qd.

Hypertension: 180–240 mg PO qd. Angina: 120 mg/d PO; titrate slowly over 7–14 d up to 480 mg/d prn; not to exceed 540 mg/d. Verapamil: 240–480 mg/d PO divided tid/qid. Nifedipine: 10–30 mg IR cap PO tid; not to exceed 120–180 mg/d 30–60 mg SR tab PO qd; not to exceed 90–120 mg/d.

Pediatric dose: Diltiazem: not established. Verapamil: Not established. Nifedipine: 0.25–0.5 mg/kg/dose PO tid/qid prn.

Contraindications: Documented hypersensitivity; severe CHF; sick sinus syndrome; second- or third-degree AV block; hypotension (<90 mmHg systolic).

Interactions: May increase carbamazepine, digoxin, cyclosporine, and theophylline levels; when administered with amiodarone, may cause bradycardia and a decrease in cardiac output; when administered with beta-blockers, may increase cardiac depression; cimetidine may increase levels.

Pregnancy: C-fetal risk revealed in studies in animals but not established or not studied in humans; may use if benefits outweigh risk to fetus.

Precautions: Caution in impaired renal or hepatic function; may increase LFTs, and hepatic injury may occur; nifedipine may cause lower extremity edema.

Drug category: Angiotensin-converting enzyme (ACE) inhibitors
Competitive inhibitors of ACE. Reduces angiotensin II levels, thus decreasing aldosterone secretion.

Drug: Captopril (capoten), enalapril (vasotec), lisinopril (zestril), ramipril (altace).

Description: Prevents conversion of angiotensin I to angiotensin II, a potent vasoconstrictor, resulting in lower aldosterone secretion.

Adult dose: Captopril: 12.5–25 mg PO bid/tid; may increase by 12.5–25 mg/dose at 1- to 2-wk intervals up to 50 mg tid. Enalapril: 2.5–5 mg/d PO (increase as necessary); range is 10–40 mg/d PO in 1–2 divided doses 1.25 mg/dose IV over 5 min q6h. Lisinopril: 10 mg/d PO; increase 5–10 mg/d at 1- to 2-wk intervals; not to exceed 40 mg. Ramipril: 2.5–5 mg PO qd; not to exceed 20 mg/d.

Pediatric dose: Captopril: 6.25–12.5 mg/dose PO q 12–24 h; not to exceed 6 mg/kg/d. Enalapril: not established. Lisinopril: not established. Ramipril: not established.

Contraindications: Documented hypersensitivity; history of angioedema.

Interactions: NSAIDs may reduce hypotensive effects; ACE inhibitors may increase digoxin, lithium, and allopurinol levels; rifampin decreases levels; probenecid may increase levels; hypotensive effects of ACE inhibitors may be enhanced when administered concurrently with diuretics.

Pregnancy: C-fetal risk revealed in studies in animals but not established or not studied in humans; may use if benefits outweigh risk to fetus.

Precautions: Category D in second and third trimester of pregnancy; caution in renal impairment, valvular stenosis, or severe congestive heart failure.

Drug category: Angiotensin II receptor antagonists. For patients unable to tolerate ACE inhibitors.

Drug: Losartan (cozaar), valsartan (diovan).

Description: Nonpeptide angiotensin II receptor antagonists that block vasoconstrictor and aldosterone-secreting effects of angiotensin II. May induce more complete inhibition of renin-angiotensin system than ACE inhibitors, do not affect response to bradykinin, and are less likely to be associated with cough and angioedema.

Adult dose: Losartan: 25–100 mg PO qd/bid. Valsartan: 80 mg/d PO; may increase to 160 mg/d if needed.

Pediatric dose: Not established.

Contraindications: Documented hypersensitivity.

Interactions: Ketoconazole, troleandomycin, sulfaphenazole, and phenobarbital may decrease effects; cimetidine may increase effects.

Pregnancy: C-fetal risk revealed in studies in animals but not established or not studied in humans; may use if benefits outweigh risk to fetus.

Precautions: Category D in second and third trimester of pregnancy; caution in unilateral or bilateral renal artery stenosis, severe hepatic insufficiency, biliary cirrhosis or obstruction, primary hyperaldosteronism, and hyperkalemia.

Drug: Eprosartan (teveten), olmesartan (benicar).

Description: Angiotensin receptor antagonist that binds to AT1 angiotensin II receptor, blocking vasoconstrictor and aldosterone-secreting effects of angiotensin II. May induce a more complete inhibition of renin-angiotensin system than ACE inhibitors and do not affect response to bradykinin and, thus, is less likely to be associated with cough and angioedema. For patients unable to tolerate ACE inhibitors.

Adult dose: Eprosartan (teveten): 400–800 mg PO qd or divided bid. Olmesartan (benicar): 20 mg PO qd initially; may increase to 40 mg/d after 2 wk if further BP reduction required. Note: lower dose in volume- or salt-depleted patients.

Pediatric dose: Not established.

Contraindications: Documented hypersensitivity; bilateral renal artery stenosis and preexisting renal insufficiency; significant aortic/mitral stenosis.

Interactions: May increase toxicity of lithium; may decrease angiotensin II antagonist efficacy; may increase risk of hyperkalemia if taken concurrently with potassium supplements.

Pregnancy: C-fetal risk revealed in studies in animals but not established or not studied in humans; may use if benefits outweigh risk to fetus.

Precautions: Pregnancy category D in second and third trimester of pregnancy; avoid use or use lower dose in patients who are volume depleted (correct volume depletion first); renal deterioration can occur with initiation of therapy; caution in unilateral renal artery stenosis and preexisting renal insufficiency; caution in aortic/mitral stenosis.

Drug category: Aldosterone antagonists

Compete with aldosterone receptor sites, reducing blood pressure and sodium reabsorption.

Drug: Eplerenone (INSPRA).

Description: Selectively blocks aldosterone at the mineralocorticoid receptors in epithelial (e.g. kidney) and nonepithelial (e.g. heart, blood vessels, brain) tissues, thus decreasing blood pressure and sodium reabsorption.

Adult dose: 50 mg PO qd; may increase dose after 4 wk, not to exceed 100 mg/d.

Pediatric dose: Not established.

Contraindications: Documented hypersensitivity; hyperkalemia or coadministration with drugs causing increased potassium; type 2 diabetes with microalbuminuria; moderate-to-severe renal insufficiency [i.e. CrCl < 50 mL/min or serum creatinine >2 mg/dL (males) or > 1.8 mg/dL (females)].

Interactions: CYP450 3A4 substrate; potent CYP3A4 inhibitors (e.g. ketoconazole) increase serum levels about fivefold, less potent CYP3A4 inhibitors (e.g. erythromycin, saquinavir, verapamil, fluconazole) increase serum levels about twofold; grapefruit juice increases serum levels about 25%; coadministration with potassium supplements, salt substitutes, or drugs known to increase serum potassium (e.g. amiloride, spironolactone, triamterene, ACE inhibitors, angiotensin II inhibitors) increases risk of hyperkalemia.

Pregnancy: B-fetal risk not confirmed in studies in humans but has been shown in some studies in animals.

Precautions: May cause hyperkalemia, headache, or dizziness; caution with hepatic insufficiency.

Drug category: Alpha-adrenergic agonists.

Stimulate presynaptic alpha2-adrenergic receptors in the brain stem which reduces sympathetic nervous activity.

Drug: Methyldopa (aldomet).

Description: Stimulates central alpha-adrenergic receptors by a false transmitter, resulting in decreased sympathetic outflow. This results in inhibition of vasoconstriction.

Adult dose: 250 mg PO bid/tid; increase q2d prn; not to exceed 3 g/d.

Pediatric dose: 10 mg/kg/d PO divided bid/qid; increase q2d prn to maximum 65 mg/kg/d; not to exceed 3 g/d.

Contraindications: Documented hypersensitivity; acute liver disease.

Interactions: Effects may decrease with concurrent administration of barbiturates and tricyclic antidepressants; increase in blood pressure may occur with coadministration of iron supplements, MAOIs, sympathomimetics, phenothiazines and beta-blockers.

Pregnancy: C-fetal risk revealed in studies in animals but not established or not studied in humans; may use if benefits outweigh risk to fetus.

Precautions: Caution in previous history of liver disease; hemolytic anemia and liver disease may occur; reduce dose in renal disease.

Table 43.3: *Medications for pediatric resuscitation and arrhythmias*

Medication	*Dose*	*Remarks*
Adenosine	0.1 mg/kg (maximum 6 mg) Repeat: 0.2 mg/kg (maximum 12 mg)	Monitor ECG Rapid IV/IO bolus
Amiodarone	5 mg/kg IV/IO; repeat up to 15 mg/kg Maximum: 300 mg	Monitor ECG and blood pressure Adjust administration rate to urgency (give more slowly when perfusing rhythm present) Use caution when administering with other drugs that prolong QT (consider expert consultation)
Atropine	0.02 mg/kg IV/IO 0.03 mg/kg ET* Repeat once if needed Minimum dose: 0.1 mg Maximum single dose Child 0.5 mg Adolescent 1 mg	Higher doses may be used with organophosphate poisoning
Calcium chloride (10%)	20 mg/kg IV/IO (0.2 mL/kg)	Slowly
Epinephrine	0.01 mg/kg (0.1 mL/kg 1:10,000) IV/IO 0.1 mg/kg (0.1/kg 1:1,000) ET* Maximum dose: 1 mg IV/IO; 10 mg ET	Adult dose: 5–10 mL
Glucose	0.5–1 g/kg IV/IO	D10W: 5–10 mL/kg D25W: 2–4 mL/kg D50W: 1–2 mL/kg
Lidocaine	Bolus: 1 mg/kg IV/IO Maximum dose: 100 mg Infusion: 20–50 1/4 g/kg per minute ET*: 2–3 mg	
Magnesium sulfate	25–50 mg/kg IV/IO over 10–20 min faster in torsades Maximum dose: 2 g	
Naloxone	< 5 y or 20 kg: 0.1 mg/kg IV/IO/ET* 5 y or > 20 kg: 2 mg IV/IO/ET*	Use lower doses to reverse respiratory depression associated with therapeutic opioid use (1–15 1/4 g/kg)
Procainamide	15 mg/kg IV/IO over 30–60 min Adult dose: 20 mg/min IV infusion upto total maximum dose 17 mg/kg	Monitor ECG and blood pressure Use caution when administering with other drugs that prolong QT (consider expert consultation)
Sodium bicarbonate	1 mEq/kg per dose IV/IO slowly	After adequate ventilation

IV indicates intravenous; IO intraosseous; and ET, via endotracheal tube.
*Flush with 5 mL of normal saline and follow with 5 ventilations.

Drug: Clonidine (catapres)

Description: Stimulates alpha2-adrenoreceptors in brain stem, activating an inhibitory neuron, which, in turn, results in reduced sympathetic outflow. These effects result in a decrease in vasomotor tone and heart rate.

Adult dose: 0.1 mg PO bid initial; 0.2–1.2 mg/d divided bid/qid maintenance; not to exceed 1.2 mg/d.

Pediatric dose: Not established.

Contraindications: Documented hypersensitivity.

Interactions: Tricyclic antidepressants inhibit hypotensive effects of clonidine; coadministration of clonidine with beta-blockers may potentiate bradycardia; tricyclic anti-depressants may enhance hypertensive response associated with abrupt clonidine withdrawal; hypotensive effects of clonidine are enhanced by narcotic analgesics.

Pregnancy: C-fetal risk revealed in studies in animals but not established or not studied in humans; may use if benefits outweigh risk to fetus.

Precautions: Caution in cerebrovascular disease, coronary insufficiency, sinus node dysfunction and renal impairment.

Drug category: Renin inhibitor

Newest class of antihypertensive drugs. Acts by disrupting the renin-angiotensin-aldosterone system feedback loop.

Drug: Aliskiren (tekturna)

Description: Direct renin inhibitor. Decreases plasma renin activity and inhibits conversion of angiotensinogen to angiotensin I (as a result, also decreasing angiotensin II) and, thereby, disrupts the renin-angiotensin-aldosterone system (RAAS) feedback loop. Indicated for hypertension as monotherapy or in combination with other antihypertensive drugs.

Adult dose: 150 mg PO qd initially; if needed, may increase to 300 mg/d.

Pediatric dose: <18 years: not established.

Contraindications: Documented hypersensitivity.

Interactions: Coadministration with irbesartan decreases C_{max} by 50%; coadministration with atorvastatin increases C_{max} and AUC by 50%; ketoconazole increases plasma levels by about 80%; does not inhibit CYP450 isoenzymes or induce CYP3A4; coadministration with furosemide decreases furosemide C_{max} and AUC by 30% and 50%, respectively; high-fat meals substantially decrease absorption; use with maximal dose of ACE inhibitors has not been studied.

Pregnancy: D-fetal risk shown in humans; use only if benefits outweigh risk to fetus.

Precautions: Discontinue use in pregnancy as soon as possible because use of drugs affecting the renin-angiotensin system during second and third trimesters has been associated with fetal and neonatal injury including hypotension, neonatal skull hypoplasia, anuria, renal failure, and fetal death; may cause angioedema; dose-related GI adverse effects may occur.

Drug category: Anticoagulants

Unfractionated IV heparin and fractionated low molecular weight SC heparins are the two choices for initial anticoagulation therapy. Warfarin therapy may be initiated after 1–3 days of effective heparinization.

Drug: Heparin.

Description: Usually administered as CIV infusion for the treatment of acute thrombosis. For prevention of thrombosis, unfractionated heparin is administered SC.

Adult dose: Initial dose: 80 U/kg IV bolus. Maintenance: 18 U/kg/h CIV infusion (See discussion under introduction to medications section regarding target aPTT and dose monitoring).

Pediatric dose: Administer as in adults.

Contraindications: Documented hypersensitivity; subacute bacterial endocarditis; active bleeding; history of heparin-induced thrombocytopenia; relative contraindications include recent surgery (especially ocular and neurosurgical procedures) and hereditary bleeding disorders.

Interactions: Digoxin, nicotine, tetracycline, and antihistamines may decrease effects; NSAIDs, aspirin, dextran, dipyridamole, and hydroxychloroquine may increase heparin toxicity.

Pregnancy: B-fetal risk not confirmed in studies in humans but has been shown in some studies in animals.

Precautions: Bleeding is most frequent complication; occurrence of thrombocytopenia during heparin therapy may indicate onset of heparin immune reaction, termed heparin-induced thrombocytopenia (HIT); syndrome can be life-threatening and can be associated with new-onset paradoxical arterial or venous thrombosis; elevations of liver enzymes have been observed during heparin therapy; heparin is not indicated for IM injection; IM medications should be administered by alternate route; in neonates, preservative-free heparin is recommended to avoid possible toxicity (gasping syndrome) by benzyl alcohol, which is used as preservative; caution in severe hypotension and shock.

Drug: Enoxaparin (lovenox).

Description: Enhances inhibition of factor Xa and thrombin by increasing antithrombin III activity. In addition, preferentially increases inhibition of factor Xa. Average duration of treatment is 7–14 d.

Adult dose: Treatment of established DVT with or without PE: 1 mg/kg SC q12h can be administered in the hospital or in an outpatient setting under supervision. Alternatively, 1.5 mg/kg SC once qd, administered at same time qd is approved for in-hospital treatment of DVT without symptomatic PE. Prevention of DVT: 30 mg SC q12h or 40 mg qd. These two regimens differ by indication, i.e. hip replacement versus knee surgery, and in use as extended prophylaxis; in acutely ill patients at high risk for DVT/PE, a dose of 40 mg SC once qd has reported efficacy.

Pediatric dose: Not established. Suggested dose: 0.75 mg/kg/dose SC bid for <2 mo; 0.5 mg/kg/dose SC bid if > 2 mo.

Contraindications: Documented hypersensitivity; major bleeding; thrombocytopenia.

Interactions: Platelet inhibitors or oral anticoagulants (e.g. dipyridamole, salicylates, aspirin, NSAIDs, sulfinpyrazone, ticlopidine) may increase risk of bleeding.

Pregnancy: B-fetal risk not confirmed in studies in humans but has been shown in some studies in animals.

Precautions: LMWH is cleared by renal mechanisms; LMWHs should be used with caution, if at all, in patients with renal impairment (i.e. CrCl <30 mL/min); if thromboembolic event occurs despite LMWH prophylaxis, discontinue drug and initiate alternate therapy; elevation of hepatic transaminases may occur but is reversible; heparin-associated thrombocytopenia may occur with fractionated LMWHs; 1 mg of protamine sulfate reverses effect of approximately 1 mg of enoxaparin if significant bleeding complications develop; however, protamine sulfate provides incomplete reversal of the anti-Xa effect of LMWHs including Lovenox. LMWHs are safe and effective in preventing or treating thrombosis during pregnancy; prophylactic regimens are preferred in patients with no history of thrombosis; guidelines for the use of LMWHs in pregnancy are still formative; some authors recommend monitoring LMWH blood levels to maintain trough anti-Xa activity of 0.15–0.2 U/mL and 2 h postinjection peak levels of 0.4–0.6 U/mL; levels are checked monthly during pregnancy; most women may require dosage increase at 20.5 wk gestation (SD 8.2 wk); in women with prosthetic valves, heparin use during pregnancy presents additional challenges and extreme caution with close monitoring is needed; reports exist of thrombosis of cardiac valves while on usual doses of LMWH; this is an evolving field and clinical trials are required to determine optimal dosage and safety in this setting; recommended to continue treatment with LMWH for 4–6 wk postpartum. Cases of epidural hematoma have been described following epidural/spinal anesthesia and concomitant LMWH heparin administration; these events occurred with prophylactic doses of LMWH; risk of hematoma is increased by indwelling catheters, concomitant NSAID use, and traumatic or repeated epidural or spinal puncture; current guidelines suggest LMWH therapy be started 24 h after epidural anesthesia; epidural catheter removal should be: (1) > 2 h before first dose of LMWH or (2) no less than 12 h after the last dose of LMWH.

Drug: Dalteparin (fragmin)

Description: Enhances inhibition of factor Xa and thrombin by increasing antithrombin III activity. In addition, preferentially increases inhibition of factor Xa. Average duration of treatment is 7–14 d.

Adult dose: 2,500–5,000 U SC qd for prevention of DVT; current recommended dose in patients undergoing abdominal surgery is 2,500 U SC qd.

Pediatric dose: Not established.

Contraindications: Documented hypersensitivity; major bleeding; thrombocytopenia.

Interactions: Platelet inhibitors or oral anticoagulants, such as dipyridamole, salicylates, aspirin, NSAIDs, sulfinpyrazone and ticlopidine, may increase risk of bleeding.

Pregnancy: C-fetal risk revealed in studies in animals but not established or not studied in humans; may use if benefits outweigh risk to fetus.

Precautions: LMWH is cleared by renal mechanisms; LMWHs should be used with caution, if at all, in patients with renal impairment (i.e. CrCl <30 mL/min); if thromboembolic event occurs despite LMWH prophylaxis, discontinue drug and initiate alternate therapy; elevation of hepatic transaminases may occur but is reversible; heparin-associated thrombocytopenia may occur with fractionated LMWHs; 1 mg of protamine sulfate reverses effect of approximately 1 mg of enoxaparin if significant bleeding complications develop; however, protamine sulfate provides incomplete reversal of the anti-Xa effect of LMWHs including Fragmin. Cases of epidural hematoma have been described following epidural/spinal anesthesia and concomitant LMWH administration; these events occurred with prophylactic doses of LMWH; the risk of hematoma is increased by indwelling catheters, concomitant NSAID use, and traumatic or repeated epidural or spinal puncture; current guidelines suggest LMWH therapy be started 24 h after epidural anesthesia; epidural catheter removal should be (1) >2 h before the first dose of LMWH or (2) no less than 12 h after the last dose LMWH.

Drug: Fondaparinux sodium (arixtra).

Description: Only synthetic compound in this class of LMW heparins. This compound is a novel pentasaccharide capable of inhibiting factor Xa via the action of antithrombin (AT) but devoid of anti-factor IIa (thrombin) activity. Interestingly, this compound does not appear to cross-react with HIT antibodies. Approved for use in hip fracture surgery, knee replacement surgery, and hip replacement surgery. Only FDA-approved anticoagulant drug for hip fracture surgery. Also used and approved for extended prophylactic dosing for 21 d following hip fracture surgery.

Adult dose: Symptomatic DVT and acute symptomatic PE:<50 kg BW: 5 mg SC qd for 5 d50–100 kg BW: 7.5 mg SC qd for 5 d>100 kg BW: 10 mg SC qd for 5d. Treatment should be continued until therapeutic oral anticoagulant effect is established (INR 2-3) with at least two determinations. For prophylaxis of VTE: 2.5 mg SC qd; initial dose recommended to be given 6–8 h following surgery, after hemostasis established; administration <6 h after surgery associated with increased risk of major bleeding.

Pediatric dose: Not established.

Contraindications: Documented hypersensitivity; seriously impaired kidney function or patients who weigh <110 lb; patients given spinal anesthesia or spinal puncture; major bleeding; thrombocytopenia.

Interactions: None reported; increased risk of bleeding possible with concurrent administration of platelet inhibitors, oral anticoagulants, or thrombolytic agents.

Pregnancy: C-Fetal risk revealed in studies in animals but not established or not studied in humans; may use if benefits outweigh risk to fetus.

Precautions: When spinal anesthesia or spinal puncture used, blood clot in spine may develop, which can result in long-term or permanent paralysis (holding 2 doses prior to LP or surgery is recommended); major bleeding risk increased when initiated before 6 h following surgery; elimination decreased in elderly persons and in those with renal impairment. Use caution in patients with severe renal impairment (i.e. CrCl <30 mL/min); if thromboembolic event occurs despite LMWH prophylaxis, discontinue drug and initiate alternate therapy; elevation of hepatic transaminases may occur but is reversible; no known antidote exists for this drug. Protamine sulfate does not appear to reverse effect of this compound; if significant bleeding complications develop; some authors have recommended the use of recombinant factor VIIa as a means of hemostasis. Cases of epidural hematoma have been described following epidural/spinal anesthesia and concomitant LMWH administration; these events occurred with prophylactic doses of LMWH; risk of hematoma is increased by indwelling catheters, concomitant NSAID use, and traumatic or repeated epidural or spinal puncture; current guidelines suggest LMWH therapy be started 24 h after epidural anesthesia; epidural catheter removal should be (1) >2 h before first dose of LMWH or (2) no less than 12 h after last dose of LMWH.

Drug: Tinzaparin (innohep).

Description: Enhances inhibition of factor Xa and thrombin by increasing antithrombin III activity. In addition, preferentially increases inhibition of factor Xa. Average duration of treatment is 7–14 d.

Adult dose: 175 U/kg SC qd, at same time qd, for treatment of DVT/PE.

Pediatric dose: Not established; adult dose suggested.

Contraindications: Documented hypersensitivity; major bleeding; thrombocytopenia.

Interactions: Platelet inhibitors or oral anticoagulants, such as dipyridamole, salicylates, aspirin, NSAIDs, sulfinpyrazone, and ticlopidine, may increase risk of bleeding.

Pregnancy: B-fetal risk not confirmed in studies in humans but has been shown in some studies in animals.

Precautions: LMWH is cleared by renal mechanisms; LMWHs should be used with caution, if at all, in patients with renal impairment (i.e. CrCl <30 mL/min); if thromboembolic event occurs despite LMWH prophylaxis, discontinue drug and initiate alternate therapy; elevation of hepatic transaminases may occur but is reversible; heparin-associated thrombocytopenia may occur with fractionated LMWHs; 1 mg of protamine sulfate reverses effect of approximately 1 mg of enoxaparin if significant bleeding complications develop; however, protamine sulfate provides incomplete reversal of anti-Xa effect of LMWHs including Lovenox. Cases of epidural hematoma have been described following epidural/spinal anesthesia and concomitant LMWH administration; these events occurred with prophylactic doses of LMWH; the risk of hematoma is increased by indwelling catheters, concomitant NSAID use, and traumatic or repeated epidural or spinal puncture; current guidelines suggest LMWH therapy be started 24 h after epidural anesthesia; epidural catheter removal should be (1) >2 h before the first dose of LMWH or (2) no less than 12 h after the last dose of LMWH.

Drug: Warfarin (coumadin).

Description: Oral anticoagulant that antagonizes action of vitamin K in normal synthesis of clotting factors II, VII, IX, and X. Safe and effective for long-term oral management of thrombotic disorders. See articles on deep venous thrombosis or pulmonary embolism (discussed in Treatment section) for additional details on dosing and monitoring of warfarin. Therapy is initiated without a loading dose at a dose range of 5–10 mg qd for 70 kg adult. Monitor PT/INR daily during initiation of therapy to measure anticoagulation effect. After initial 5–10 d and stabilization of warfarin dose, measure PT/INR 2–3 times qwk for 2–4 wk, then monthly thereafter.

Adult dose: 5–10 mg PO qd; adjust dose according to desired INR.

Pediatric dose: 0.05–0.34 mg/kg/d PO qd; adjust dose according to desired INR.

Contraindications: Documented hypersensitivity; severe liver or kidney disease; open wounds or GI ulcers.

Interactions: Drugs that may decrease anticoagulant effects include griseofulvin, carbamazepine, glutethimide, estrogens, nafcillin, phenytoin, rifampin, barbiturates, cholestyramine, colestipol, vitamin K, spironolactone, oral contraceptives, and sucralfate; medications that may increase anticoagulant effects include oral antibiotics, phenylbutazone, salicylates, sulfonamides, chloral hydrate, clofibrate, diazoxide, anabolic steroids, ketoconazole, ethacrynic acid, miconazole, nalidixic acid, sulfonylureas, allopurinol, chloramphenicol, cimetidine, disulfiram, metronidazole, phenylbutazone, phenytoin, propoxyphene, sulfonamides, gemfibrozil, acetaminophen, and sulindac.

Pregnancy: D-fetal risk shown in humans; use only if benefits outweigh risk to fetus.

Precautions: Contraindicated in first trimester; warfarin skin necrosis (see Medical/Legal Pitfalls); do not switch brands after achieving therapeutic response; caution in active tuberculosis or diabetes; patients with protein C or S deficiency are at risk of developing skin necrosis.

Drug category: Antiplatelet agents—these agents prevent formation of thrombi associated with MI and inhibit platelet function by blocking aggregation. Antiplatelet therapy has been shown to reduce mortality by reducing the risk of fatal MIs, fatal strokes and vascular death. Pooled data from over 2,000 patients revealed reduction of death or MI from 11.8% to 6% with aspirin in cases of unstable angina. A recent randomized clinical trial involving 12,562 patients showed a reduction of cardiovascular death, MI, or stroke from 11.4% to 9.3% by adding clopidogrel to aspirin therapy.

Drug: Aspirin (anacin, bayer buffered aspirin, ecotrin)—administer as soon as possible. Inhibits cyclo-oxygenase, which produces thromboxane A2, a potent platelet activator. Early administration has been shown to reduce mortality.

Adult dose: 160–324 mg PO qd.

Pediatric dose: Not established.

Contraindications: Documented hypersensitivity; liver damage; hypoprothrombinemia; vitamin K deficiency; bleeding disorders; asthma; patients <16 y with influenza (because of association of aspirin with Reye syndrome).

Interactions: Effects may decrease with antacids and urinary alkalinizers; corticosteroids decrease salicylate serum levels; additive hypoprothrombinemic effects and increased bleeding time may occur with coadministration of anticoagulants; may antagonize uricosuric effects of probenecid and increase toxicity of phenytoin and valproic acid; doses > 2 g/d may potentiate glucose-lowering effect of sulfonylurea drugs.

Pregnancy: D-unsafe in pregnancy.

Precautions: May cause transient decrease in renal function and aggravate chronic renal disease; avoid use in patients with severe anemia, those with history of blood coagulation defects, or those taking anticoagulants.

Drug name: Clopidogrel (plavix)—selectively inhibits adenosine diphosphate (ADP) binding to platelet receptor and subsequent ADP-mediated activation of glycoprotein llb/llla complex, thereby inhibiting platelet aggregation.

This agent is used as an alternative to aspirin or in addition to aspirin after coronary stenting (CAPRIE Steering Committee, 1996 #158). The recently concluded randomized clinical trial clopidogrel in unstable angina to prevent recurrent events (CURE) showed an absolute risk reduction in cardiac death, MI, or stroke of 2.1% (11.4% down to 9.3% at 1-y) at the cost of increased major bleeding by 1.0% (3.7% versus 2.7%).

Adult dose: CURE protocol for unstable angina patients within 24 h of symptom onset: 300 mg loading dose PO followed by 75 mg PO qd for 3–12 mo (mean = 9 mo) in conjunction with aspirin 75–325 mg/d PO.

Pediatric dose: Not established.

Contraindications: Documented hypersensitivity; active pathological bleeding, such as peptic ulcer, or intracranial hemorrhage.

Interactions: Coadministration with naproxen is associated with increased occult GI blood loss; clopidogrel prolongs bleeding time; safety of coadministration with warfarin not established.

Pregnancy: C-safety for use during pregnancy has not been established.

Precautions: Caution in patients at increased risk of bleeding from trauma, surgery, or other pathological conditions; caution in patients with lesions with propensity to bleed (e.g. ulcers).

Drug category: HMG-CoA reductase inhibitors used to treat hypercholesterolemia. Highly efficacious and very well tolerated.

Drug: Atorvastatin (lipitor) can provide up to 60% reduction in LDL-C. Inhibits 3-hydroxy-3-methylglutaryl coenzyme A (HMG-CoA reductase), which in turn inhibits cholesterol synthesis and increases cholesterol metabolism. The half-life of atorvastatin and active metabolites is longer than that of all the other statins (i.e. approximately 48 h compared to 3–4 h). The myocardial ischemia reduction with aggressive cholesterol lowering (MIRACL) randomized clinical trial randomized 3,086 patients with unstable angina to high-dose atorvastatin versus placebo. Therapy resulted in a reduction in the primary end-point (i.e., death, MI, resuscitated cardiac arrest, severe recurrent symptomatic ischemia) from 17.4% to 14.8% (P = .048) within a relatively short period of 4 mo. The benefit was mostly for recurrent symptomatic ischemia with objective evidence and requiring emergency rehospitalization (8.4% down to 6.2%, P = .02).

Adult dose: 10 mg PO qd in the evening; titrate to a maximum 80 mg/d prn. MIRACL protocol: 80 mg PO qd commenced within 1–4 d after admission for unstable angina, continue for at least 16 wk.

Pediatric dose: Not established.

Contraindications: Documented hypersensitivity; significant hepatic impairment; pregnancy; breastfeeding.

Interactions: Toxicity increases when coadministered with triazole antifungals, CNS depressants, macrolide antibiotics, and mibefradil; atorvastatin increases the action of anticoagulants and levothyroxine.

Pregnancy: Contraindicated in pregnancy.

Precautions: Thirty-one cases of rhabdomyolysis (out of 1.33 million total prescriptions) were reported in Canada, resulting in 1 death associated with concomitant use of gemfibrozil, a fibric acid derivative; concomitant use with nicotinic acid (niacin) also advised. Stop drug use or decrease doses for elevations of transaminases more than 3 times the upper limit of the reference range; elevations generally resolve upon withdrawal of drug; if symptoms of myopathy and rhabdomyolysis occur, stop the drug and obtain a CKDo not exceed daily dose; caution in patients receiving drugs that prolong QRS or Q-T interval; monitor transaminase levels before treatment, at 6 wk and 12 wk, then q6mo.

Drug category: Glycoprotein IIb/IIIa receptor antagonists Up to 80,000 copies of these integrins on the platelet cell surface serve as ligands for fibrinogen cross-linkage, the final common pathway for platelet aggregation and thrombus formation, even under arterial shear stress conditions. To date, more than 40,000 patients have been enrolled in randomized clinical trials evaluating glycoprotein IIb/IIIa antagonists in ACS. These trials have shown 30 day relative risk reductions of 22–56% in composite end-points, with beneficial trends in each of the component outcomes, largely in association with percutaneous coronary intervention.

Drug: Tirofiban (aggrastat)—nonpeptide antagonist of platelet GP IIb/IIIa receptor that reversibly prevents von Willebrand factor, fibrinogen, and other adhesion ligands from binding to the GP IIb/IIIa receptor, thereby inhibiting platelet aggregation. Effects persist over the duration of maintenance infusion and are reversed after stopping the infusion. Approved by the FDA for use in combination with heparin for patients with ACS who are being managed medically and for those undergoing PCI. Dose should be halved in patients with severe renal insufficiency (CrCl <30 mL/min).

Adult dose: 0.4 mcg/kg/min IV for 30 min, followed by 0.1 mcg/kg/min for up to 72 h. If CrCl <30 mL/min, then reduce dose by 50%.

Pediatric dose: Not established.

Contraindications: Documented hypersensitivity; severe hypertension (systolic BP >200 mmHg); active internal bleeding; history of intracranial hemorrhage, intracranial neoplasm, arteriovenous malformation, or aneurysm; acute pericarditis; bleeding diathesis; trauma or stroke within previous 30 d; platelet count <100,000/mm^3; history of thrombocytopenia following exposure to this product; serum creatinine >2 mg/dL (for 180 mcg/kg bolus and 2 mcg/kg/min infusion) or > 4 mg/dL (for 135 mcg/kg bolus and 0.5 mcg/kg/min infusion); history of bleeding diathesis within 30 d; intracranial hemorrhage; history of hemorrhagic stroke; severe hypertension (systolic BP >200 mmHg or diastolic BP >110 mmHg); major surgical procedure within past mo.

Interactions: Possible increased risk of bleeding with coadministration of heparin or aspirin; closely monitor when using concurrently with drugs that affect hemostasis (e.g., warfarin)

Pregnancy: B-usually safe but benefits must outweigh the risks.

Precautions: Bleeding events are the most common complications encountered during therapy with eptifibatide; caution with platelet count <150,000/mm³ and hemorrhagic retinopathy; prior to treatment, monitor platelet counts, serum creatinine, hemoglobin, hematocrit, and PT/aPTT within 6 h after loading infusion and at least daily thereafter (more frequently if evidence of significant decline); because these agents inhibit platelet aggregation, caution when using concurrently with drugs that affect hemostasis (e.g. thrombolytics, ticlopidine, NSAIDs, warfarin, dipyridamole, clopidogrel); measure ACT and maintain aPTT 50–70 seconds unless a PCI needs to be performed; maintain ACT 300–350 seconds during PCI; if platelet count decreases to <100,000/mm³, perform additional platelet counts to exclude pseudothrombocytopenia; if thrombocytopenia is confirmed, discontinue GP IIb/IIIa inhibitors and heparin and appropriately monitor and treat the condition; to monitor unfractionated heparin, monitor aPTT 6 h after beginning heparin infusion; adjust to maintain aPTT higher than 2 times baseline.

Drug: Eptifibatide (integrilin)—cyclic heptapeptide antagonist of the platelet GP IIb/IIIa receptor that reversibly prevents von Willebrand factor, fibrinogen, and other adhesion ligands from binding to the GP IIb/IIIa receptor, thereby inhibiting platelet aggregation. Effects persist over duration of maintenance infusion and are reversed when infusion ends. Approved by the FDA for use in combination with heparin for patients with ACS, patients who are being managed medically, and for those undergoing PCI.

Adult dose: Unstable angina: 180 mcg/kg IV bolus, followed by continuous infusion of 2 mcg/kg/min for up to 72 h. Undergoing PCI: additional 180 mcg/kg IV bolus 10 min after the first bolus. For patients with serum Cr >2 mg/dL: Lower dose to 135 mcg/kg bolus and 0.5 mcg/kg/min infusion.

Pediatric dose: Not established.

Contraindications: Documented hypersensitivity; severe hypertension (systolic BP >200 mmHg); active internal bleeding; history of intracranial hemorrhage, intracranial neoplasm, arteriovenous malformation or aneurysm, acute pericarditis, or bleeding diathesis; trauma or stroke within previous 30 d; platelet count <100,000/mm³; history of thrombocytopenia following prior exposure to this product; serum Cr >4 mg/dL.

Interactions: Possible increased risk of bleeding with coadministration of heparin, warfarin, or aspirin; closely monitor when using other drugs that affect hemostasis.

Pregnancy: B-usually safe but benefits must outweigh the risks.

Precautions: Bleeding events are the most common complications encountered during therapy with eptifibatide; caution in platelet count <150,000/mm³ and hemorrhagic retinopathy; because agent inhibits platelet aggregation, caution when using concurrently with drugs that affect hemostasis (e.g. thrombolytics, ticlopidine, NSAIDs, warfarin, dipyridamole, clopidogrel); measure ACT and maintain aPTT 50-70 seconds unless a PCI needs to be performed; maintain ACT 250-350 seconds during a PCI; if platelets decrease to <100,000/mm³, perform additional platelet counts to exclude possibility of pseudothrombocytopenia; if thrombocytopenia is confirmed, discontinue GP IIb/IIIa inhibitors and heparin and appropriately monitor and treat the condition; monitor aPTT 6 h after start of heparin infusion and at least daily thereafter.

Drug category: Platelet aggregation inhibitors inhibit platelet aggregation.

Drug: Abciximab (ReoPro)—chimeric human-murine monoclonal antibody approved for use in elective/urgent/emergent PCI. Binds to receptor with high affinity and reduces platelet aggregation by 80% for up to 48 h following infusion. The recently concluded GUSTO-4 randomized clinical trial did not show any benefit for abciximab in medically treated patients who do not undergo PCI. In fact, longer duration of abciximab use was associated with a negative trend in event rates. On the other hand, in the context of PCI, it has been shown to be superior to tirofiban.

Adult dose: 0.25 mg/kg IV bolus, followed by 10 mcg/min IV for 12 h after PCI.

Pediatric dose: Not established.

Contraindications: Documented hypersensitivity; severe hypertension (systolic BP >200 mmHg); active internal bleeding; history of intracranial hemorrhage, intracranial neoplasm, arteriovenous malformation or aneurysm, acute pericarditis, or bleeding diathesis; trauma or stroke within previous 30 d; platelet count <100,000/mm³; history of thrombocytopenia following prior exposure to this product.

Interactions: Possible increased risk of bleeding with coadministration with heparin, warfarin, or aspirin; closely monitor when using other drugs that affect hemostasis.

Pregnancy: B-usually safe but benefits must outweigh the risks. Bleeding events are the most common complications encountered during therapy with abciximab; caution in platelet count <150,000/mm³ and hemorrhagic retinopathy; because agent inhibits platelet aggregation, caution when using concurrently with drugs that affect hemostasis (e.g. thrombolytics, ticlopidine, NSAIDs, warfarin, dipyridamole, clopidogrel); measure ACT and maintain aPTT 50–70 seconds unless a PCI needs to be performed; maintain ACT 250–350 seconds during a PCI; if platelets decrease to <100,000/mm³, perform additional platelet counts to exclude possibility of pseudothrombocytopenia; if thrombocytopenia is confirmed, discontinue GP IIb/IIIa inhibitors and heparin and appropriately monitor and treat condition; monitor aPTT 6 h after start of heparin infusion and at least daily thereafter; abciximab is associated with an incidence of thrombocytopenia in approximately 2% of patients.

Drug category: Beta-adrenergic blocking agents—limit heart rate and reduce blood pressure to decrease myocardial oxygen demand, oppose effects of elevated catecholamines, and produce antiarrhythmic properties. Clinical trials of beta-adrenoreceptor blockers in cases of unstable angina have shown decreases in ischemic symptoms and in occurrence of MIs. In vitro studies have shown inhibition of platelet aggregation with this drug class. Infrequent situations in which beta-blocker therapy should be avoided in patients with unstable angina include nonischemic exacerbation of heart failure, cocaine-induced coronary vasoconstriction, and vasospastic angina.

Drug: Metoprolol (lopressor, toprol XL)—selective beta1-adrenergic receptor blocker that decreases automaticity of contractions. During IV administration, carefully monitor blood pressure, heart rate and ECG.

Adult dose: 5 mg IV slow infusion q5min up to 3 times until resolution of angina or titrate to reduce heart rate to 50–70 bpm.

Pediatric dose: Not established.

Contraindications: Documented hypersensitivity; uncompensated congestive heart failure; bradycardia; asthma; cardiogenic shock; AV conduction abnormalities.

Interactions: Aluminum salts, barbiturates, NSAIDs, penicillins, calcium salts, cholestyramine, and rifampin may decrease bioavailability and plasma levels of metoprolol, possibly resulting in decreased pharmacologic effects; toxicity of metoprolol may increase with coadministration of sparfloxacin, phenothiazines, astemizole, calcium channel blockers, quinidine, flecainide and contraceptives; may increase toxicity of digoxin, flecainide, clonidine, epinephrine, nifedipine, prazosin, verapamil, and lidocaine.

Pregnancy: B-usually safe but benefits must outweigh the risks.

Precautions: Beta-adrenergic blockade may reduce signs and symptoms of acute hypoglycemia and may decrease clinical signs of hyperthyroidism; abrupt withdrawal may exacerbate symptoms of hyperthyroidism including thyroid storm; closely monitor patient and slowly withdraw the drug; caution in patients taking other negative chronotropes or inotropes (e.g. verapamil).

Drug: Esmolol (brevibloc)—shown to reduce episodes of chest pain and clinical cardiac events compared to placebo. The very short half-life (8 min) allows a large degree of dosing flexibility, such that cardiovascular benefits are comparable to PO propranolol, yet adverse effects can be managed promptly. It is particularly useful for patients at risk for complications with beta-blockade (e.g. reactive airway disease or COPD, severe bradycardia, or poor left ventricular function).

Adult dose: 0.05 mg/kg/min IV over 1 min initially; 0.1 mg/kg/min IV maintenance; titrate in increments of 0.05 mg/kg/min q10–15 min until resolution of angina, until heart rate of 50–70 bpm is attained, or until maximum dose of 0.2 mg/kg/min is reached.

Pediatric dose: Not established.

Contraindications: Documented hypersensitivity; uncompensated congestive heart failure; bradycardia; asthma; cardiogenic shock; AV conduction abnormalities.

Interactions: Aluminum salts, barbiturates, NSAIDs, penicillins, calcium salts, cholestyramine, and rifampin may decrease bioavailability and plasma levels of metoprolol, possibly resulting in decreased pharmacologic effects; toxicity of metoprolol may increase with coadministration of sparfloxacin, phenothiazines, astemizole, calcium channel blockers, quinidine, flecainide and contraceptives; metoprolol may increase toxicity of digoxin, flecainide, clonidine, epinephrine, nifedipine, prazosin, verapamil and lidocaine.

Pregnancy: C-safety for use during pregnancy has not been established.

Precautions: Beta-adrenergic blockade may mask signs and symptoms of acute hypoglycemia and may decrease clinical signs of hyperthyroidism; abrupt withdrawal may exacerbate symptoms of hyperthyroidism including thyroid storm; closely monitor patient and slowly withdraw the drug; during IV administration, carefully monitor blood pressure, heart rate and ECG.

Drug: Propranolol (inderal)—nonselective beta-blocker that is lipophilic (penetrates CNS). Although generally short-acting agent, long-acting preparations are also available.

Adult dose: IR: 40–160 mg PO bid; SR: 60–320 mg PO qd.

Pediatric dose: Not established.

Contraindications: Documented hypersensitivity; history of bronchospasm; uncompensated congestive heart failure; bradycardia; cardiogenic shock; AV conduction abnormalities.

Interactions: Coadministration with aluminum salts, barbiturates, NSAIDs, penicillins, calcium salts, cholestyramine, and rifampin may decrease propranolol effects; calcium channel blockers, cimetidine, loop diuretics, and MAOIs may increase toxicity of propranolol; toxicity of hydralazine, haloperidol, benzodiazepines, and phenothiazines may increase with propranolol.

Pregnancy: C-safety for use during pregnancy has not been established.

Precautions: Beta-adrenergic blockade may hide signs of acute hypoglycemia and hyperthyroidism; abrupt withdrawal may exacerbate symptoms of hyperthyroidism, including thyroid storm; slowly withdraw drug and closely monitor patient; adverse effects include bronchial constriction, Raynaud phenomenon, hypotension, decreased libido, impotence, lethargy, depression, and decreased HDL; caution in Wolff-Parkinson-White syndrome and renal or hepatic dysfunction.

Drug: Nadolol (corgard)—competitively blocks beta-1 and beta-2 receptors. Does not exhibit membrane stabilizing activity or intrinsic sympathomimetic activity.

Adult dose: 40 mg/d PO initially; gradually increase dose by 40–80 mg increments at 3–7 d intervals up to 160–240 mg/d.

Pediatric dose: Not established.

Contraindications: Documented hypersensitivity; congestive heart failure; pulmonary edema; cardiogenic shock; AV conduction abnormalities; heart block (without a pacemaker).

Interactions: Coadministration with aluminum salts, barbiturates, calcium salts, cholestyramine, NSAIDs, penicillins, and rifampin may decrease effects; haloperidol, hydralazine, loop diuretics, and MAOIs may increase toxicity of nadolol.

Pregnancy: C-safety for use during pregnancy has not been established.

Precautions: Beta-adrenergic blockade may reduce symptoms of acute hypoglycemia and mask signs of hyperthyroidism; abrupt withdrawal may exacerbate symptoms of hyperthyroidism and cause thyroid storm; closely monitor patients and slowly withdraw drug; during an IV, carefully monitor BP, heart rate and ECG.

Drug category: Antithrombotic agents—thrombin, the end product of the coagulation mechanism, initiates transformation of fibrinogen to a fibrin clot and activates platelets. Its antagonist, antithrombin III, is the major endogenous inhibitor of the coagulation cascade and is the essential cofactor for heparin.

Drug: Heparin (hep-lock)—catalyzes the effect of antithrombin III on coagulative proteinases (e.g. factors II, XII, XI, IX, and X; tissue factor VIIa). Prevents reaccumulation of clot after endogenous fibrinolysis. Meta-analysis shows modest benefit (when compared to aspirin alone) and slight increase in bleeding. Reactivation of unstable angina after discontinuation of heparin has been documented among subjects not receiving concomitant aspirin therapy. When unfractionated heparin is used, the aPTT should not be checked until 6 h after initial heparin bolus.

Table 43.4: *Treatment of hypercyanotic spells in tetralogy of fallot*

Knee to chest position
Supplemental oxygen
Morphine sulfate (0.1 mg/kg 1 m or SC)
If not responding to above:
Obtain IV access
Repeat morphine sulfate if agitated
IV fluid bolus 00 mL/kg
Phenylephrine infusion 0.5–5.0 (~kg/min fitrate to effect)
$NaHCO_3$ (1 mEq/kg IV)
Propraolol (0.5–0.10 mg/kg IV maximum dose 1 mg)
If remains criticat:
Consider general anethesia and paralytic agent.
Urgent consultation with cardiothoracic surgery is needed for

Adult dose: 80 U/kg IV bolus, followed by infusion of 18 U/kg/h; titrate to maintain aPTT 1.5-2.5 times control; decrease initial bolus dose to 50 U/kg IV when used in conjunction with GP IIb/IIIa antagonist.

Pediatric dose: Not established.

Contraindications: Documented hypersensitivity; subacute bacterial endocarditis; active bleeding; history of heparin-induced thrombocytopenia.

Interactions: Digoxin, nicotine, tetracycline, and antihistamines may decrease effects; NSAIDs, aspirin, dextran, dipyridamole, and hydroxychloroquine may increase heparin toxicity.

Pregnancy: B-usually safe but benefits must outweigh the risks.

Precautions: Most important risk with unfractionated heparin is ineffectiveness because of insufficient dose; may cause hemorrhagic complications; if significant bleeding complications develop, 15 mg protamine sulphate (infused over 3 min) usually reverses anticoagulant effect; can trigger immune thrombotic thrombocytopenia 1–2 wk after beginning of treatment; heparin-associated thrombocytopenia is serious, causes widespread thrombosis refractory to treatment, and can be fatal if not recognized quickly and managed appropriately; some preparations contain benzyl alcohol as a preservative, which can be associated with fetal toxicity (gasping syndrome) when used in large amounts; use of preservative-free heparin is recommended in neonates; caution in shock or severe hypotension.

Drug: Enoxaparin (lovenox) or dalteparin (fragmin)—enoxaparin: only LMWH now approved by the FDA both for treatment and for prophylaxis of deep venous thrombosis and pulmonary embolism. LMWH has been widely used in pregnancy, although clinical trials are not yet available to demonstrate that it is as safe as unfractionated heparin. Except in overdoses, checking PT or aPTT is not useful because aPTT does not correlate with the anticoagulant effect of fractionated LMWH. Dalteparin: LMWH with many similarities to enoxaparin but with a different dosing schedule. Except in overdoses, checking PT or aPTT is not useful because aPTT does not correlate with the anticoagulant effect of fractionated LMWH. Approved for deep venous thrombosis and pulmonary embolism prophylaxis for patients undergoing orthopedic and abdominal surgery.

Adult dose: Enoxaparin: 1 mg/kg SC q12h or 1.5 mg/kg SC qd. Prophylaxis against DVT: 30 mg SC q12h. Dalteparin: 120 IU/kg SC q12h; not to exceed 10,000 IU for at least 5 d or until revascularization is performed (FRISC-2 regimen).

Pediatric dose: Not established.

Contraindications: Documented hypersensitivity; major bleeding; thrombocytopenia.

Interactions: Platelet inhibitors or PO anticoagulants (e.g. dipyridamole, salicylates, aspirin, NSAIDs, sulfinpyrazone, ticlopidine) may increase risk of bleeding.

Pregnancy: B-usually safe but benefits must outweigh the risks.

Precautions: If thromboembolic event occurs despite LMWH prophylaxis, discontinue drug and initiate alternate therapy; elevation of hepatic transaminases may occur but is reversible; heparin-associated thrombocytopenia may occur with fractionated LMWHs; 1 mg of protamine sulfate reverses effect of approximately 1 mg of enoxaparin if significant bleeding complications develop; if necessary, 1 mg of protamine can neutralize 100 U dalteparin.

Drug category: Thrombin inhibitors—lepirudin and bivalirudin are direct thrombin inhibitors. Advantages over heparin are efficacy against clot-bound thrombin, resistance to inactivation by platelet factor 4 and thrombospondin, and nondependence on antithrombin III pathways. Data to date suggest only a modest reduction in adverse events at the cost of increased nonmajor bleeding complications. GUSTO IIB investigators compared recombinant hirudin and heparin in 12,142 patients, a third of whom had ST elevation MI. The hirudin group had a 9% relative risk reduction in 30-d death or MI rates (8.9% vs 9.8%), but more moderate bleeding events occurred (8.8% vs 7.7%).

OASIS-2 was an international randomized clinical trial that involved 10,141 patients. Patients were randomized between heparin (aPTT maintained between 60 and 100 seconds) or lepirudin, which is recombinant hirudin (0.4 mg/kg bolus followed by 0.15 mg/kg/h 72-h IV infusion). Unlike for GP IIb/IIIa antagonists, no evidence indicates attenuation of myocardial necrosis (based on CK or troponin measurements). Approved by the FDA in patients with heparin-induced thrombocytopenia and associated thrombotic disease. Goal is 1.5-2.5 times the control aPTT values. Dose needs to be adjusted for patients with renal impairment. Bivalirudin (angiomax) is a thrombin inhibitor used for anticoagulation in patients with unstable angina undergoing PTCA.

Drug: Bivalirudin (angiomax) used for anticoagulation in patients with unstable angina undergoing PTCA. Synthetic analogue of recombinant hirudin. Inhibits thrombin. Potential advantages over conventional heparin therapy include more predictable and precise levels of anticoagulation, activity against clot-bound thrombin, absence of natural inhibitors (e.g. platelet factor 4, heparinase), and continued efficacy following clearance from plasma (due to binding to thrombin).

Adult dose: 1 mg/kg IV bolus initially; followed by 2.5 mg/kg/h IV for 4 h; may administer additional IV infusion at 0.2 mg/kg/h (not to exceed 20 h); administer with 300–325 mg/d aspirin.

Pediatric dose: Not established.

Contraindications: Documented hypersensitivity; cerebral aneurysm; intracranial hemorrhage; general uncontrollable hemorrhage; active major bleeding.

Interactions: Coadministration with antiplatelets (other than aspirin) or other anticoagulants not fully evaluated (use caution)

Pregnancy: B-usually safe but benefits must outweigh the risks.

Precautions: Adjust dose in renal impairment; caution in recent surgery, trauma, or GI ulceration; bleeding may occur; may cause back pain, nausea, headache and hypotension.

Drug: Lepirudin (refludan)—recombinant hirudin derived from yeast cells. Highly specific direct inhibitor of thrombin. Natural hirudin is produced in trace amounts as a family of highly homologous isopolypeptides by the leech *Hirudo medicinalis.* Biosynthetic lepirudin is identical to natural hirudin except for substitution of leucine for isoleucine at the *N*-terminal end of the molecule and the absence of a sulfate group on the tyrosine at position 63. Activity of lepirudin is measured in a chromogenic assay. One antithrombin unit (ATU) is the amount of lepirudin that neutralizes one unit of World Health Organization preparation 89/588 of thrombin. Specific activity of lepirudin is >16,000 ATU/mg. Mode of action is independent of antithrombin III. Platelet factor 4 does not inhibit lepirudin. One molecule of lepirudin binds to one molecule of thrombin and thereby blocks the thrombogenic activity of thrombin. As a result, all thrombin-dependent coagulation assays are affected (e.g. aPTT values increase in a dose-dependent fashion).Goal is 1.5-2.5 times the control aPTT values. Dose needs to be adjusted for patients with renal impairment.

Adult dose: 0.4 mg/kg IV bolus over 15–20 seconds, followed by continuous infusion of 0.15 mg/kg/h.

Pediatric dose: Not established.

Contraindications: Documented hypersensitivity; major bleeding; thrombocytopenia.

Interactions: Intracranial bleeding may be life-threatening following concomitant fibrinolytic therapy.

Pregnancy: B-usually safe but benefits must outweigh the risks.

Precautions: Associated with increased need for transfusion (vs unfractionated heparin) and slightly increased risk of intracranial hemorrhage; no specific antidote.

Drug category: Vasodilators—relieve chest discomfort by improving myocardial oxygen supply, which in turn dilates epicardial and collateral vessels, improving blood supply to the ischemic myocardium. Opposes coronary artery spasm, which augments coronary blood flow and reduces cardiac work by decreasing preload and afterload. Effective in the management of symptoms in acute MI but may reduce mortality only slightly. Nitroglycerin can be administered sublingually by tablet or spray, topically, or IV. In acute MI, topical administration is a less desirable route because of unpredictable absorption and onset of clinical effects.

Drug: Nitroglycerin (minitran, nitrogard, nitrol, nitrolingual, nitrostat, nitro-dur)—causes relaxation of vascular smooth muscle by stimulating intracellular cyclic guanosine monophosphate production. Whether administered topically, SL, PO, or IV, nitrates ameliorate several pathways of unstable angina and reduce the incidence of symptomatic ischemia. Nitrates lower systemic arterial pressure and decrease venous return to the heart, both of which reduce myocardial wall stress. Similarly, nitrates are excellent coronary vasodilators. Other possible beneficial effects include transient inhibition of platelet aggregation, increase in coronary collateral blood flow, and a favorable redistribution of regional flow. Of note, induction of heparin resistance has been reported.

Adult dose: 400 mcg SL tab or spray q5min, repeated up to 3 times; if symptoms persist, infuse IV at a rate of 5–10 mcg/min; titrate dose to a 10% reduction in mean arterial pressure.

Pediatric dose: Not established.

Contraindications: Documented hypersensitivity; severe anemia; shock; postural hypotension; head trauma; closed-angle glaucoma; cerebral hemorrhage; known right ventricular infarct.

Interactions: Aspirin may increase nitrate serum concentrations; marked symptomatic orthostatic hypotension may occur with coadministration of calcium channel blockers (dose adjustment of either agent may be necessary).

Pregnancy: C-safety for use during pregnancy has not been established.

Precautions: Caution in CAD and low systolic blood; limiting adverse effects include hypotension (>30% reduction in mean arterial pressure or systolic BP < 90).

Treatment and Prevention of GAS

Treatment and prevention of GAS pharyngitis outlined here are based on the current recommendations of the Committee on Infectious Disease (American Academy of Pediatrics). Medical therapy is directed toward elimination of GAS pharyngitis (if still present), suppression of inflammation from the autoimmune response, and supportive treatment of CHF. Attempts are being made to produce vaccines against GAS infection, but the vaccines will not be available for years.

Antibiotics for endocarditis prophylaxis are administered to patients with certain cardiac conditions, such as carditis caused by rheumatic fever before procedures that may cause bacteremia are performed. For more information:

Drug category: Antibiotics—the roles for antibiotics are to (1) initially treat GAS pharyngitis, (2) prevent recurrent streptococcal pharyngitis, RF, and RHD, and (3) provide prophylaxis against bacterial endocarditis.

Drug: Penicillin VK (Beepen-VK, Pen.Vee K, V-Cillin K, Veetids)—DOC for treatment of GAS pharyngitis. Although ampicillin or amoxicillin may be used instead, they have no microbiologic advantage. Do not use tetracyclines and sulfonamides to treat GAS pharyngitis. For recurrent GAS pharyngitis, a second 10-d course of same antibiotic may be repeated. Alternate drugs include narrow-spectrum cephalosporins, amoxicillin-clavulanate, dicloxacillin, erythromycin, or other macrolides.

Adult dose: 500 mg PO bid/tid for 10 d.

Pediatric dose: Children: 250 mg (400,000 U) PO bid/tid for 10 d. Adolescents: administer as in adults.

Contraindications: Documented hypersensitivity.

Interactions: Probenecid may increase effectiveness by decreasing clearance; tetracyclines are bacteriostatic, causing decrease in effectiveness of penicillins when administered concurrently.

Pregnancy: B-usually safe but benefits must outweigh the risks.

Precautions: Renal impairment, anaphylaxis, thrombocytopenia.

Drug: Benzathine (Bicillin L-A)/procaine penicillin (Crysticillin A.S., Wycillin) used when PO administration of penicillin is not feasible or dependable. IM therapy with penicillin is painful, but discomfort may be minimized if penicillin G is brought to room temperature before injection or combination of benzathine penicillin G and procaine penicillin G is used. Initial course of antibiotics administered to eradicate streptococcal infection also serves as first course of prophylaxis. An injection of benzathine penicillin G IM q4wk is recommended regimen for secondary prevention for most United States patients. Administer same dosage q3wk in areas where RF is endemic, in patients with residual carditis, and in high-risk patients.

Adult dose: Eradication: 1.2 million U of benzathine penicillin G or a combination of 900,000 U of benzathine penicillin G with 300,000 U of procaine penicillin G IM as a single dose. Secondary prevention: administer eradication dose q3wk (in high-risk areas, high-risk patients) or q4wk (for most areas in United States).

Pediatric dose: Eradication <60 lb: 600,000 U of benzathine penicillin G IM as a single dose. Secondary prevention: Administer eradication dose q3wk (in high-risk areas, high-risk patients) or q4wk (for most areas in United States)

Contraindications: Documented hypersensitivity.

Interactions: Increases risk of bleeding when administered concurrently with warfarin; ethacrynic acid, aspirin, indomethacin, and furosemide may compete with penicillin G for renal tubular secretion, increasing penicillin serum concentrations.

Pregnancy: B-usually safe but benefits must outweigh the risks.

Precautions: Never use IV route to administer penicillin G procaine; impaired renal function; anaphylaxis; thrombocytopenia.

Drug: Erythromycin (EES, E-Mycin, Eryc, Ery-Tab, Erythrocin)—used for patients who are allergic to penicillin. Other options include clarithromycin, azithromycin, or a narrow-spectrum cephalosporin (i.e., cephalexin). As many as 15% of penicillin-allergic patients also are allergic to cephalosporins.

Adult dose: 250 mg erythromycin stearate/base (or 400 mg ethylsuccinate) q6h PO 1 h ac for 10 d.

Pediatric dose: 20-40 mg (as base, estolate, or stearate)/ kg/d PO divided bid/qid for 10 d; not to exceed 1 g/ dAlternatively, 40 mg (as ethylsuccinate)/kg/d PO divided bid/qid for 10 d.

Contraindications: Documented hypersensitivity; with terfenadine (off US market) or astemizole (use in combination with erythromycin may cause prolongation of QT interval, with increased risk of ventricular arrhythmias and sudden death).

Interactions: Coadministration may increase toxicity of theophylline, digoxin, carbamazepine and cyclosporine; may potentiate anticoagulant effects of warfarin; coadministration with lovastatin and simvastatin increases risk of rhabdomyolysis.

Pregnancy: B-Usually safe but benefits must outweigh the risks.

Precautions: Caution in liver disease; estolate formulation may cause cholestatic jaundice; GI adverse effects are common (administer doses pc); discontinue use if nausea, vomiting, malaise, abdominal colic, or fever occurs.

Drug: Clarithromycin (biaxin)—alternate antibiotic for treating GAS pharyngitis in patients allergic to penicillin.

Adult dose: 250–500 mg PO bid for 10 d.

Pediatric dose: 7.5 mg/kg PO bid for 10 d.

Contraindications: Documented hypersensitivity; coadministration of pimozide; patients taking terfenadine (off US market); patients with long QT syndrome.

Interactions: CYP450 1A2 and 3A4 inhibitor; toxicity increases with coadministration of fluconazole and pimozide; clarithromycin effects decrease and GI adverse effects may increase with coadministration of rifabutin or rifampin; may increase toxicity of anticoagulants, cyclosporine, tacrolimus, digoxin, omeprazole, carbamazepine, ergot alkaloids, triazolam, and HMG CoA-reductase inhibitors; plasma levels of certain benzodiazepines may increase, prolonging CNS depression; arrhythmias and increase in QTc intervals occur with disopyramide; coadministration with omeprazole may increase plasma levels of both agents.

Pregnancy: C-safety for use during pregnancy has not been established.

Precautions: Coadministration with ranitidine or bismuth citrate is not recommended with CrCl <25 mL/min; administer one half dose or increase dosing interval if CrCl <30 mL/min; diarrhea may be sign of pseudomembranous colitis; superinfections may occur with prolonged or repeated antibiotic therapies.

Drug: Azithromycin (zithromax)—alternate antibiotic for treating GAS pharyngitis in patients allergic to penicillin.

Adult dose: 12 mg/kg (not to exceed 500 mg) PO qd for 5 d.

Pediatric dose: Administer as in adults.

Contraindications: Documented hypersensitivity; hepatic impairment; do not administer with pimozide.

Interactions: May increase toxicity of theophylline, warfarin, and digoxin; effects are reduced with coadministration of aluminum and/or magnesium antacids; nephrotoxicity and neurotoxicity may occur when coadministered with cyclosporine.

Pregnancy: B-usually safe but benefits must outweigh the risks.

Precautions: May increase hepatic enzymes and cholestatic jaundice; caution in patients with impaired hepatic function, prolonged QT intervals, or pneumonia; caution in patients who are hospitalized, geriatric, or debilitated.

Drug: Cephalexin (keflex, biocef, keftab)—alternate antibiotic for treating GAS pharyngitis in patients allergic to penicillin.

Adult dose: 250–500 mg PO qid for 10 d.

Pediatric dose: 25–50 mg/kg/d PO divided qid for 10 d.

Contraindications: Documented hypersensitivity.

Interactions: Coadministration with aminoglycosides increases nephrotoxic potential.

Pregnancy: B-Usually safe but benefits must outweigh the risks.

*Precautions:*Adjust dose in renal impairment.

Drug: Amoxicillin (amoxil, biomox, trimox)—DOC used for bacterial endocarditis prophylaxis. Administered as single PO dose 1 h before dental work or surgery.

Adult dose: 2 g PO once as a single dose.

Pediatric dose: 50 mg/kg PO once as a single dose.

Contraindications: Documented hypersensitivity.

Interactions: None significant for prophylaxis.

Pregnancy: B-usually safe but benefits must outweigh the risks.

Precautions: Adjust dose in renal impairment.

Drug category: Antiinflammatory agents—manifestations of acute RF (including carditis) typically respond rapidly to therapy with anti-inflammatory agents. Aspirin, in anti-inflammatory doses, is DOC. Prednisone is added when evidence of worsening carditis and heart failure exists.

Drug: Aspirin (anacin, ascriptin, bayer aspirin)—begin administration immediately after diagnosis of RF. Initiation of therapy may mask manifestations of disease.

Adult dose: 4–8 g/d PO divided q4-6h; maintain aspirin levels in 20-25 mg/dL range until all symptoms have resolved and APRs have returned to normal.

Pediatric dose: 80–100 mg/kg/d PO divided q4–6h; maintain aspirin levels in 20–25 mg/dL range until all symptoms have resolved and APRs have returned to normal.

Contraindications: Documented hypersensitivity; liver damage; hypoprothrombinemia, vitamin K deficiency; bleeding disorders; asthma.

Interactions: Effects may decrease with antacids and urinary alkalinizers; corticosteroids decrease salicylate serum levels; additive hypoprothrombinemic effects and increased bleeding time may occur with coadministration of anticoagulants; may antagonize uricosuric effects of probenecid and increase toxicity of phenytoin and valproic acid; doses > 2 g/d may potentiate glucose-lowering effect of sulfonylurea drugs.

Pregnancy: D-unsafe in pregnancy.

Precautions: Risk of salicylate intoxication and poisoning; watch for hyperventilation with prolonged expiratory phase with respiratory alkalosis and metabolic acidosis; risk of tinnitus, GI discomfort, and ulceration; when taken during pregnancy, increased risk of pulmonary hypertension exists in fetus in neonatal period.

Drug: Prednisone (deltasone, orasone) if moderate-to-severe carditis is present as indicated by cardiomegaly, CHF, or third-degree heart block, use 2 mg/kg/d PO prednisone in addition to or in lieu of salicylate therapy. Continue prednisone for 2–4 wk depending on severity of carditis and taper during last week of therapy. Discontinuing prednisone therapy after 2 wk while adding or maintaining salicylates for additional 2–4 wk may minimize adverse effects.

Adult dose: 2 mg/kg/d PO for 2–4 wk.

Pediatric dose: Administer as in adults.

Contraindications: Documented hypersensitivity; viral infection; peptic ulcer disease; hepatic dysfunction; connective tissue infections; fungal or tubercular skin infections; GI disease.

Interactions: Coadministration with estrogens may decrease prednisone clearance; concurrent use with digoxin may cause digitalis toxicity secondary to hypokalemia; phenobarbital, phenytoin, and rifampin may increase metabolism of glucocorticoids (consider increasing maintenance dose); monitor for hypokalemia with coadministration of diuretics.

Pregnancy: C-safety for use during pregnancy has not been established.

Precautions: Abrupt discontinuation of glucocorticoids may cause adrenal crisis; hyperglycemia, edema, osteonecrosis, myopathy, peptic ulcer disease, hypokalemia, osteoporosis, euphoria, psychosis, myasthenia gravis, growth suppression, and infections may occur with glucocorticoid use.

***Drug category:* Therapy for congestive heart failure**—heart failure in RHD probably is related in part to severe insufficiency of the mitral and aortic valves and in part to pancarditis. Therapy traditionally has consisted of an inotropic agent (digitalis) in combination with diuretics (furosemide, spironolactone) and afterload reduction (captopril).

Drug: Digoxin (lanoxin, lanoxicaps)—inotropic agent widely used in past. Its efficacy in CHF is under review. Potential for toxicity is present. Therapeutic levels and clinical effects are observed more quickly if loading doses of digitalis are administered before routine maintenance doses. Acts directly on cardiac muscle, increasing myocardial systolic contractions. Indirect actions result in increased carotid sinus nerve activity and enhanced sympathetic withdrawal for any given increase in mean arterial pressure. Therapeutic digoxin levels are present at trough levels of 1.5–2 ng/mL.

Adult dose: Total digitalizing dose (TDD) to be administered over 24 h; first dose is one half the TDD; second dose is one-fourth the TDD, given 8 h later; third dose is one-fourth the TDD, given 8 h after the second. TDD: 0.75–1.5 mg PO. Maintenance dose: 0.125–0.5 mg PO qd.

Pediatric dose: TDD to be administered over 24 h; first dose is one half the TDD; second dose is one-fourth the TDD, given 8 h later; third dose is one-fourth the TDD, given 8 h after the second TDD: preterm infant: 20–30 mcg/kg PO, Term infant: 25–35 mcg/kg PO. 1 month to 2 years:

Table 43.5: *Medications to maintain cardiac output and for postresuscitation stabilization*

Medication	*Dose range*	*Comment*
Inamrinone	0.75–1 mg/kg IV/IO over 5 minutes; may repeat × 2 then: 2–20 μg/kg per minute	Inodilator
Dobutamine	2–20 mg/kg per minute IV/IO	Inotrope; vasodilator
Dopamine	2–20 mg/kg per minute IV/IO	Inotrope; chronotrope; renal and splanchnic vasodilator in low doses; pressor in high doses
Epinephrine	0.1–1 mg/kg per minute IV/IO	Inotrope; chronotrope; vasodilator in low doses; pressor in higher doses
Milrinone	50–75 μg/kg IV/IO over 10–60 min then 0.5–0.75 μg/kg per minute	Indilator
Norepinephrine	0.1–2 μg/kg per minute	Inotrope; vasopressor
Sodium nitroprusside	1–8 μg/kg per minute	Vasodilator; prepare only in D5W

IV, intravenous; IO, intraosseous

Alternative formula for calculating an infusion:

Infusion rate (mL/h) - [weight (kg) × dose (μg/kg/min) × 60 (min/h)]/concentration μg/mL.

Table 43.6 *Meanings of terms used in pediatric cardiology*

Adrenergic: Activating the sympathetic nervous system
Afterload: The resistance against which the myocardium must eject
Agonist: Acting positively toward an action
Alpha: Vasoconstriction
Antagonist: Opposite in action
Beta1: Increasing contractility, heart rate
Beta2: Vasodilation and bronchodilation
Cardiac output: (Heart rate) × (Stroke volume)
Cholinergic: Activating the parasympathetic nervous system
Chronotropic: Affecting heart rate
Contractility: The intrinsic ability of the myocardial fibers to contract
Dopaminergic: Renal perfusion
Half-life: The time required for 50% of a dose to be excreted, used to determine intervals for dosing
Heart rate: The rate of ventricular contraction
Inotropic: Affecting contractility
Preload: The amount of blood distending the ventricles prior to contraction
Stroke volume: Determined by preload, afterload, and contracility

35–60 mcg/kg. PO_2-5 years: 30–40 mcg/kg PO. 5–10 years: 20–35 mcg/kg PO>10 years: Administer as in adults. Maintenance dose: preterm infant: 5–7.5 mcg/kg/d PO divided bid. Term infant: 6–10 mcg/kg/d PO divided bid 1 month to 2 years: 10–15 mcg/kg/d PO divided bid 2–5 years: 7.5–10 mcg/kg/d PO divided bid 5–10 years: 5–10 mcg/kg/d PO divided bid > 10 years: Administer as in adults.

Contraindications: Documented hypersensitivity; beri beri heart disease; idiopathic hypertrophic subaortic stenosis; constrictive pericarditis; carotid sinus syndrome.

Interactions: Medications that may increase digoxin levels include alprazolam, benzodiazepines, bepridil, captopril, cyclosporine, propafenone, propantheline, quinidine, diltiazem, aminoglycosides, PO amiodarone, anticholinergics, diphenoxylate, erythromycin, felodipine, flecainide, hydroxychloroquine, itraconazole, nifedipine, omeprazole, quinine, ibuprofen, indomethacin, esmolol, tetracycline, tolbutamide, and verapamil. Medications that may decrease serum digoxin levels include aminoglutethimide, antihistamines, cholestyramine, neomycin, penicillamine, aminoglycosides, PO colestipol, hydantoins, hypoglycemic agents, antineoplastic treatment combinations (e.g. carmustine, bleomycin, methotrexate, cytarabine, doxorubicin, cyclophosphamide, vincristine, procarbazine), aluminum or magnesium antacids, rifampin, sucralfate, sulfasalazine, barbiturates, kaolin/pectin, and aminosalicylic acid.

Pregnancy: C-safety for use during pregnancy has not been established.

Precautions: Hypokalemia may reduce positive inotropic effect of digitalis; IV calcium may produce arrhythmias in patients receiving digitalis; hypercalcemia predisposes patient to digitalis toxicity, and hypocalcemia can make digoxin ineffective until serum calcium levels are normal; magnesium replacement therapy must be instituted in patients with hypomagnesemia to prevent digitalis toxicity; patients diagnosed with incomplete AV block may progress to complete block when treated with digoxin; caution in hypothyroidism, hypoxia, and acute myocarditis; initiate digoxin only after checking electrolytes and correcting abnormalities in serum potassium.

Drug: Captopril (capoten)—systemic afterload reduction may be helpful in improving cardiac output, particularly in setting of mitral and aortic valve insufficiency. Some patients have unusually large hypotensive response. Use small starting dose, particularly with hypovolemia.

Adult dose: Starting dose: 6.25–12.5 mg PO tid. Typical dose: 50–100 mg PO tid.

Pediatric dose: Starting dose: 0.1–0.5 mg/kg/d PO divided tid; typically 1–2 mg/kg/d PO divided tid.

Contraindications: Documented hypersensitivity; renal impairment.

Interactions: NSAIDs may reduce hypotensive effects of captopril; ACE inhibitors may increase digoxin, lithium, and allopurinol levels; rifampin decreases captopril levels; probenecid may increase captopril levels; hypotensive effects of ACE inhibitors may be enhanced when administered concurrently with diuretics.

Pregnancy: C-safety for use during pregnancy has not been established.

Precautions: Pregnancy category D in second and third trimesters; caution in renal impairment, valvular stenosis, or severe CHF.

Drug: Furosemide (lasix)—diuretics frequently are used in conjunction with inotropic agents for patients with CHF. When used aggressively, may result in hypokalemia and hypovolemia. Risk of hearing loss in premature infants. Increases excretion of water by interfering with chloride-binding cotransport system, which, in turn, inhibits sodium and chloride reabsorption in ascending loop of Henle and distal renal tubule.

Adult dose: 20–40 mg PO/IV/IM bid/tid.

Pediatric dose: 1–2 mg/kg/dose PO/IV/IM qd/tid.

Contraindications: Documented hypersensitivity; hepatic coma; anuria; state of severe electrolyte depletion.

Interactions Metformin decreases furosemide concentrations; furosemide interferes with hypoglycemic effect of antidiabetic agents and antagonizes muscle-relaxing effect of tubocurarine; auditory toxicity appears to be increased with coadministration of aminoglycosides and furosemide; hearing loss of varying degrees may occur; anticoagulant activity of warfarin may be enhanced with concurrent administration; increased plasma lithium levels and toxicity are possible with concurrent administration.

Pregnancy: C-safety for use during pregnancy has not been established.

Precautions: Obtain frequent serum electrolyte, carbon dioxide, glucose, creatinine, uric acid, calcium, and BUN determinations during first few months of therapy and periodically thereafter.

Drug: Spironolactone (aldactone) used in conjunction with furosemide as potassium-sparing diuretic. Competes with aldosterone for receptor sites in distal renal tubules, increasing water excretion while retaining potassium and hydrogen ions.

Adult dose: 100 mg PO divided qd/bid.

Pediatric dose: 2–4 mg/kg/d PO divided bid.

Contraindications: Documented hypersensitivity; anuria; renal failure; hyperkalemia.

Interactions: May decrease effect of anticoagulants; potassium and potassium-sparing diuretics may increase toxicity of spironolactone.

Pregnancy: D-unsafe in pregnancy.

Precautions: Caution in renal and hepatic impairment mmHg or severe headache.

BIBLIOGRAPHY

1. Bailey JM, Miller BE, Lu, W, Tosone, SR, Kanter, KR, & Tam, VK (1999). The pharmacokinetics of milrinone in pediatric patients after cardiac surgery. Anesthesiology, 90, 1012–1018.
2. Bell SG. (1998). Neonatal cardiovascular pharmacology. Neonatal Network, 17, 7–15.
3. Berg RA, & Padbury JF. (1997). Sulphoconjugation and renal excretion contribute to the interpatient variation of exogenous catecholamine clearance in critically ill children. Critical Care Medicine, 25, 1247–1251.
4. Bindler RM, & Howry, LB (1997). Pediatric drugs and nursing implications (2nd ed.). Upper Saddle River, NJ: Pearson Education.
5. Chowdhury C, Parnell VA, Ojamaa K, Boxer R., Cooper, R., & Klein, I. (1999). Usefulness of triodothyronine (T3) treatment after surgery for complex congenital heart disease in infants and children. The American Journal of Cardiology, 84, 1107–1109.
6. Fineman JR, & Soifer SJ (1998). The fetal and neonatal circulations. In AC Chang, FL Hanley, G Wernovsky, & C.L. Wessel (Eds.), Pediatric cardiac intensive care (pp. 17–20). Baltimore: Williams & Wilkins.
7. Hazinski MF (1999). Cardiovascular disorders. The manual of pediatric critical care (pp. 112, 284–288). St. Louis: Mosby.
8. Kohr LM, & Sims SL (1998). Alterations of cardiovascular function in children. Pathophysiology: The biologic basis for disease in adults and children (3rd ed.) (pp. 1093–1101). St. Louis: Mosby.
9. McCance KL (1998). Structure and function of the cardiovascular and lymphatic systems. Pathophysiology: The biologic basis for disease in adults and children (3rd ed.) (pp. 968–988). St. Louis: Mosby.
10. Noerr, B. (1999). Pointers in practical pharmacology: Spironolactone. Neonatal Network, 18, 43–46.
11. Rosen DA (1996). Effects of T3 to treat postoperative cardiac failure in congenital cardiac surgery patients. Critical Care Medicine, 24 (1), A121.
12. Taketomo CK, Hodding, JH, & Kraus, CK (2000). Pediatric dosage handbook (7th ed.). Hudson, OH: Lexi-Comp, Inc.

APPENDIX

The Neonatal Intensive Care Unit (NICU)

Technological Developments including Artificial intelligence

The Neonatal Intensive Care Unit (NICU)

Technological Developments including Artificial intelligence

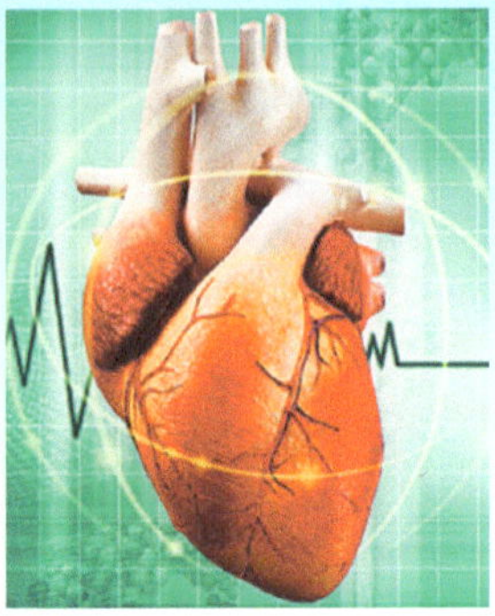

The birth of a baby is a wonderful and very complex process. Many physical and emotional changes occur for both mother and baby. A baby must make many physical adjustments to life outside the mother's body. Leaving the uterus means that a baby can no longer depend on the mother's blood supply and placenta for important body functions.

bodyf unctions

Your baby's body systems must work together in a new way. In some cases, a baby has trouble making the transition outside the womb. Preterm birth, a difficult birth, or birth defects can make these changes more challenging. But a lot of special care is available to help newborn babies.

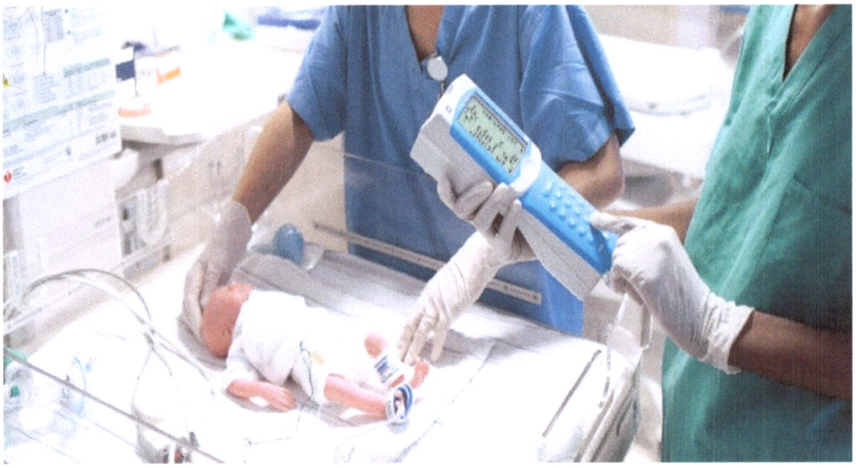

Fig. A1 **Evaluation of i-STAT portable clinical analyzer in a neonatal and pediatric intensive care unit**

Before birth, the baby depends on functions from the mother. These include breathing, eating, elimination of waste, and immune protection. When a baby leaves the womb, its body systems must change. For example:

- The lungs must breathe air.
- The cardiac and pulmonary circulation changes.
- The digestive system must begin to process food and excrete waste.
- The kidneys must begin working to balance fluids and chemicals in the body and excrete waste.
- The liver and immune systems must begin working on their own.

What is the neonatal intensive care unit (NICU)?

Newborn babies who need intensive medical care are often put in a special area of the hospital called the neonatal intensive care unit (NICU). The NICU has advanced technology and trained healthcare professionals to give special care for the tiniest patients. NICUs may also care areas for babies who are not as sick but do need specialized nursing care. Some hospitals don't have the staff for a NICU and babies must be moved to another hospital. Babies who need intensive care do better if they are born in a hospital with a NICU than if they are moved after birth.

Some newborn babies will require care in a NICU. Giving birth to a sick or premature baby can be unexpected for any parent. The NICU can be overwhelming. This information is to help you understand why a baby may need to be in the NICU. You will also find out about some of the procedures that may be needed for the care of your baby

Which babies need special care?

Most babies admitted to the NICU are preterm (born before 37 weeks of pregnancy), have low birth weight (less than 5.5 pounds), or have a health condition that needs special care. In the U.S., nearly half a million babies are born preterm. Many of these babies also have low birth weights. Twins, triplets, and other multiples often are admitted to the NICU. This is because they tend to be born earlier and smaller than single birth babies. Babies with health conditions such as breathing trouble, heart problems, infections, or birth defects are also cared for in the NICU

Below are some factors that can place a baby at high risk and increase the chances of being admitted to the NICU. But each baby must be assessed to see if he or she needs the NICU. High-risk factors include the below.

Maternal factors include:

- Being younger than age 16 or older than age 40
- Drug or alcohol use
- Diabetes
- High blood pressure (hypertension)
- Bleeding
- Sexually transmitted diseases
- Multiple pregnancy (twins, triplets, or more)
- Too little or too much amniotic fluid
- Premature rupture of membranes (also called the amniotic sac or bag of waters)

Delivery factors include:

- Changes in a baby's organ systems due to lack of oxygen (fetal distress or birth asphyxia)
- Buttocks delivered first (breech birth) or other abnormal position
- The baby's first stool (meconium) passed during pregnancy into the amniotic fluid
- Umbilical cord wrapped around the baby's neck (nuchal cord)
- Forceps or cesarean delivery

Baby factors include:

- Baby born at gestational age of less than 37 weeks or more than 42 weeks
- Birth weight less than 5 pounds, 8 ounces (2,500 grams) or over 8 pounds, 13 ounces (4,000 grams)
- Small for gestational age
- Medicine or resuscitation in the delivery room
- Birth defects
- Respiratory distress including rapid breathing, grunting, or stopping breathing (apnea)Infection such as herpes, group B streptococcus, chlamydia
- Seizures
- Low blood sugar (hypoglycemia)
- Need for extra oxygen or monitoring, IV (intravenous) therapy, or medicine
- Need for special treatment or procedures such as a blood transfusion

Who will care for your baby in the NICU

Some of the specially-trained healthcare providers who may care for your baby include

Neonatologist. This is a pediatrician with extra training in the care of sick and premature babies. The neonatologist (often called the attending physician) supervises pediatric fellows and residents, nurse practitioners, and nurses who care for babies in the NICU.

Neonatal fellow. This is a pediatrician getting extra training in the care of sick and premature babies. He or she may do procedures and direct your child's care

Pediatric resident. This is a doctor who is getting extra training in the care of children. He or she may do or assist in procedures and help direct your child's care

Neonatal nurse practitioner. This is a registered nurse with extra training in the care of newborn babies. He or she can do procedures and help direct your child's care.

Respiratory therapist. This is a person with special training in giving respiratory support. This includes managing breathing machines and oxygen

Physical,occupational, and speech therapists. These types of therapists make sure a baby is developing well. They also help with care including positioning and soothing methods. Speech therapists help babies learn to eat by mouth

Dietitians. Dietitians ensure the babies are growing well and getting good nutrition. They watch your baby's intake of calories, protein, vitamins, and minerals

Lactation consultants. These are healthcare providers with extra training and certification in helping women and babies breastfeed. They can help with pumping, maintaining milk supply, and starting and continuing breastfeeding

Pharmacists. Pharmacists help in the NICU by assisting the care providers choose the best medicines. They check medicine doses and levels. They keep the team aware of possible side effects and monitoring that may be needed

Social workers. Social workers help families cope with many things when a child is ill. They give emotional support. They help families get information from healthcare providers. They support the family with other more basic care needs, too. These can include money problems, transportation, or arranging home healthcare.

Hospital chaplain. The hospital chaplain may be a priest, minister, lay pastor, or other religious advisor. The chaplain can give spiritual support and counseling to help families cope with the stress of the NICU.
NICU team members work together with parents to create a plan of care for high-risk newborns. Ask about the NICU's parent support groups and other programs designed to help parents.

What types of equipment are used in the NICU?

Neonatal Intensive Care Units (NICUs) have complex machines and devices for the unique needs of tiny babies. The NICU can be overwhelming to a new parent. Learning about what to expect in the NICU can help ease your concerns.
Some of the equipment often used in the NICU includes:

Heart or cardiorespiratory monitor. This monitor displays a baby's heart and breathing rates and patterns on a screen. Wires from the monitor are attached to adhesive patches on the skin of the baby's chest, and abdomen

Blood pressure monitor. Blood pressure is measured using a small cuff placed around the baby's upper arm or leg. Periodically, a blood pressure monitor pumps up the cuff and measures the level of blood pressure. Some babies need continuous blood pressure monitoring. This can be done using a catheter (small tube) in 1 of the baby's arteries. **Temperature.** A temperature probe is placed on the baby's skin with an adhesive patch. A wire connects the temperature probe to the overhead warmer (or incubator) to help regulate the heat needed to keep the baby warm.

Pulse oximeter. This machine measures the amount of oxygen in the baby's blood through the skin. A tiny light is taped to the baby's foot or hand. A wire connects the light to the monitor where it displays the oxygen saturation or "sat." This refers to the amount of hemoglobin in the baby's red blood cells that is saturated with oxygen

X-ray. Portable X-ray machines may be brought to the baby's bedside in the NICU. X-rays use invisible electromagnetic energy beams to produce images of internal tissues, bones, and organs on film X-rays are taken for many reasons including checking the placement of catheters and other tubes, looking for signs of lung problems, such as respiratory distress syndrome or pneumothorax, and checking for signs ofbowelproblems

CT scan. A CT scan is a diagnostic imaging procedure that uses a combination of X-rays and computer technology to produce horizontal, or axial, images (often called slices) of the body. A CT scan shows detailed images of any part of the body, including the bones, muscles, fat, and organs. CT scans are more detailed than general X-rays. CT scans are sometimes done to assess bleeding inside a baby's head. A CT scan is done in a special room and the baby may need a sedative medication so that he or she will be motionless for the exam. MRI. MRI is a procedure that uses a large magnet, radio waves, and a computer to make detailed images of organs and other tissues in the body. Like a CT scan, MRI is done in a special area of the hospital. It is often done to examine a baby's brain stem, spinal cord, and soft tissues. The baby will need a sedative medicine so that he or she will lie still for the exam

Endotracheal tube (ET). This tube is placed through the baby's mouth or nose into the trachea (windpipe). The ET tube is held in place with special tape and connects to a mechanical ventilator (breathing machine) with flexible tubing. An X-ray is used to check the tube's placement. When a baby has an ET tube, he or she is unable to make sounds or cry. **Respiratoror mechanical ventilator.** This machine helps babies who can't breathe on their own or who need help taking bigger breaths. High frequency ventilators give hundreds of very fast puffs of air to help keep a baby's airways open. Ventilators can also give extra oxygen to the baby.

Continuous positive airway pressure (CPAP). Through small tubes that fit into the baby's nostrils, called nasal CPAP, this machine pushes a continuous flow of air to the airways to help keep tiny air passages in the lungs open. CPAP can give extra oxygen as well. It may also be given through an ET tube

Extracorporeal membrane oxygenation (ECMO). This is a special treatment for babies with respiratory disease that does not respond to maximum medical care. With ECMO, blood from the baby's vein is pumped through an artificial lung where oxygen is added and carbon dioxide is removed. The blood is then returned back to the baby. ECMO is only used in specialized NICUs

Developmental Care for Babies in the NICU

Advances in the care of sick and premature babies include new technology and medicine. There are treatments that focus on the special emotional and developmental needs of these babies. Babies in the neonatal intensive care unit (NICU) face many tests, procedures, noises, and lights. This is very different from the warm, dark, comfort of the mother's womb. Some babies are too sick to be held. Or they may have trouble comforting themselves when not being held. Premature babies need special support to help them continue to mature and develop as they would in their mother's womb.

What is developmental care?

This type of care is used in many NICUs to meet babies' special needs. Developmental care includes many aspects such as:

- o Meeting babies' comfort needs
- o Helping babies feel secure
- o Helping babies develop normal sleep patterns
- o Decreasing stimulation from noise, lights, or procedures

Research into this kind of care is showing many benefits for babies, especially for premature babies. These include:

- o Shorter hospital stays
- o Fewer complications
- o Improved weight gain
- o Better feeding
- o Enhanced parent and infant bonding

Developmental care includes:

- o Changing the baby's surroundings to provide normal day/night cycles and decrease noise and stress
- o Using cushions to support the baby and keep the baby's arms and legs in good position to help with development and comfort
- o Using cues from the baby to plan care at times when he or she is awake and least stressed rather than disturbing sleep or doing procedures when the baby is at a high stress level

What is kangaroo care?

Kangaroo care is a practice that started in Colombia in the late 1970s. It has been used worldwide. This is because it is very helpful for premature babies. Kangaroo care means holding a NICU baby skin-to-skin, against the parent's chest. Premature and sick babies who have this contact appear to relax and become content. Several studies show that kangaroo care has many health benefits. These include

- o Higher blood oxygen levels
- o Better sleep
- o Better breastfeeding
- o More weight gain

Kangaroo care also helps parents feel close to their baby. This gives the parents confidence in their ability to meet their baby's needs. Mothers who use kangaroo care also tend to make more breast milk. Many of these effects in parents and babies are because skin-to-skin contact increases levels of oxytocin. Oxytocin is a hormone that naturally causes milk release. It also causes feelings of relaxation and connection

Intravenous (IV) Line and Tubes

Because most babies in the NICU are too small or sick to take full milk feedings, medicines, and fluids are often given through their veins or arteries. Babies may also need frequent lab tests and measurements of blood oxygen levels. There are several ways a baby may get fluids and medicines and have blood drawn. These include the following:

Intravenous (IV) line. Babies may have an IV placed in a hand, foot, or scalp, where veins are easily accessed. Tubing connects the IV to a bag of fluids that are carefully given to the baby with a pump. **Umbilical catheter (UVC or UAC).** After the umbilical cord is cut at birth, a newborn baby has the short stump of the cord still in place. Because the umbilical cord stump is still connected to their blood and circulatory system, a catheter (small flexible tube) can be inserted into 1 of the 2 arteries or the vein of the umbilical cord. Medicines, fluids, and blood can be given through this catheter. Sometimes blood may be drawn from it as well. After placement of the umbilical catheter, X-rays are taken to check that it's in the right place.

Percutaneous line. A catheter is placed in a deep vein or artery in the baby's arm or leg. It is used instead of an IV in the hand or scalp if a baby has longer-term needs.

A baby may need IV lines or catheters for just a short time or for many days. Once a baby is well enough to take milk feedings and is gaining weight, IV lines may be removed. In some cases, an IV may be needed for giving a baby antibiotics or other medicine even when the baby can be fed normally.

The Evolution of Neonatal Care Equipment

Neonatal care has come a long way in the past few decades, with significant advancements in technology and equipment that have greatly improved the care and outcomes for premature and critically ill newborns. In this blog, we will explore the evolution of neonatal care equipment, including the latest innovations and trends in NICU (Neonatal Intensive Care Unit) technology.

Neonatal care equipment manufacturers have been at the forefront of developing cutting-edge devices and tools to support the delicate needs of newborns. From infant care devices and neonatal monitors to incubators and pediatric equipment, the range of specialized medical devices for neonatal care is extensive. These manufacturers have been continuously innovating to improve the safety, comfort, and outcomes for premature and sick infants.

One of the most significant trends in NICU technology is the development of advanced respiratory support systems for neonates. Neonatal respiratory support is crucial for premature babies with underdeveloped lungs, and manufacturers have been introducing state-of-the-art devices to provide optimal respiratory care for these vulnerable patients. This includes advanced ventilators, high-frequency oscillatory ventilators, and non-invasive respiratory support systems.

Another important innovation in neonatal care equipment is the use of LED phototherapy units for newborns with jaundice. These devices provide effective and safe treatment for neonatal jaundice, helping to reduce the risk of complications associated with high levels of bilirubin in the blood.

In addition to specialized medical devices, manufacturers have also been focusing on developing equipment for infection control and hygiene in the NICU. Surface disinfection systems and medical-grade measuring tapes are essential tools for maintaining a clean and safe environment for neonates, helping to prevent the spread of infections and ensure the highest standards of care.

The cost of NICU equipment has been a significant consideration for healthcare facilities, and manufacturers have been working to develop cost-effective solutions without compromising on quality and safety. This has led to the introduction of more affordable yet reliable neonatal care equipment, making it more accessible for healthcare providers around the world.

Some of the common NICU equipment includes infant incubators, radiant warmers, eye pads, gonad protectors, and infantometers. These devices play a crucial role in providing a controlled and supportive environment for premature and sick newborns, helping to regulate their body temperature, protect their delicate eyes, and ensure their overall well-being.

As technology continues to advance, we can expect to see further innovations in neonatal care equipment, with a focus on enhancing the precision, efficiency, and safety of devices used in the NICU. Manufacturers will continue to collaborate with healthcare professionals to develop solutions that meet the evolving needs of neonatal care, ultimately improving the outcomes for the tiniest and most vulnerable patients.

In conclusion, the evolution of neonatal care equipment has been driven by a commitment to innovation, safety, and quality in the NICU. Manufacturers have been instrumental in developing advanced devices and tools that have revolutionized the care of premature and critically ill newborns, and the future holds even more promising advancements in neonatal care technology

5 Advances in NICU Equipment and Medical Technology for Neonatal Nurses

Neonatal nurse practitioners (NNPs) deliver services and treatment to millions of women in the United States each year.

[1] Unfortunately, many expectant mothers miss out on the vital services provided by NNPs. To mitigate potentially harmful complications, neonatal nurse practitioners conduct treatment and interventions that aim to bring services to expectant mothers in their communities.

Births that occur before the appropriate gestation period typically result in newborns with low birth weights and other health complications.

[2] While not all premature births result in complications, this event can cause short- and long-term health problems. Conditions may present at birth or later in the child's lifespan and may include some of the following ailments. Breathing complications may arise due to underdeveloped respiratory organs. Heart problems are another common condition that presents among premature children. Early births can also lead to interventricular hemorrhaging, which is bleeding in the tissue of the brain. Finally, premature births might result in a condition where newborns' bodies cannot compensate for normal heat loss.

The following five innovations aid neonatal nurse practitioners in diagnosing and treating conditions that commonly present among premature children.

1.Phototherapy

Phototherapy is the most common treatment that neonatal nurse practitioners use to treat jaundice in newborns, which occurs due to an excess of a chemical called bilirubin..A typical phototherapy session

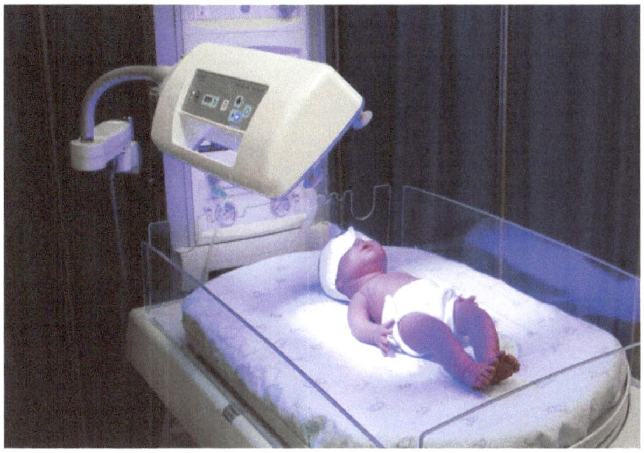

Fig A2 Photography machine in INCU

encompasses placing an infant in a bassinet or incubator and bathing them with florescent light. The procedure causes a change in the infant's bilirubin, which they then excrete in their stool or urine. During this safe procedure, NPPs expose as much of the infant's skin as possible, protect the baby's eyes, ensure that the child maintains a proper diet, and measure the patient's bilirubin level daily.

Another phototherapy treatment is the fiber-optic blanket or band, which caregivers wrap around the baby – typically in the home setting. Although the practice has proven successful, this method takes longer than the fluorescent light treatment.

2.Artificial Womb

The average gestation period for a human being is forty weeks. However, nearly 30,000 infants enter the world after only twenty-six weeks. The artificial womb is an important, relatively recent, development in treating infants who were born too early. Researchers report conducting a study where they successfully nurtured eight lambs through their gestation periods, mimicking the function a mother's womb in an artificial environment. The scientists revealed that the lambs developed properly and some went on to live through adulthood. Researcher Alan Flake of the Children's Hospital of Philadelphia reports that the lambs are normal in every way. The researchers' next objective is to repeat this success with premature babies to help them develop in full health.

3.The Heart Rate Observation System (HeRO)

Infection is the leading cause of mortality events among premature infants. [6] A Neonatal Intensive Care Unit (NICU) innovation allows NNPs to predict host infections twenty-four hours in advance. The Heart Rate Observation System (HeRO) uses an

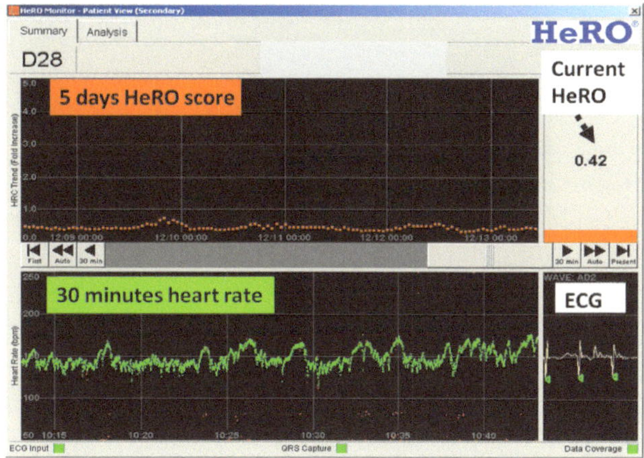

Fig A3 HeRO monitor showing normal heart rate characteristics

algorithm to detect heart beat irregularities that might indicate a major oncoming infection, a serious health threat for infants that weigh less than three pounds. It's difficult to identify the subtle symptoms that might indicate the beginning stages of a condition. However, HeRO allows practitioners to intervene before an infection occurs.

4.Artificial Surfactant

Researcher John Clements discovered a concept about lung function in 1953 that would later save the lives of millions of infants. Three years earlier, Clements – a United States Army Sargent – wanted to enter the biochemistry field. However, his commanding officer steered him toward physiology. His work led to a finding by Dr. Mary Ellen Avery of Harvard Medical School that the lungs of premature infants do not produce surfactant, a chemical compound the reduces surface tension.

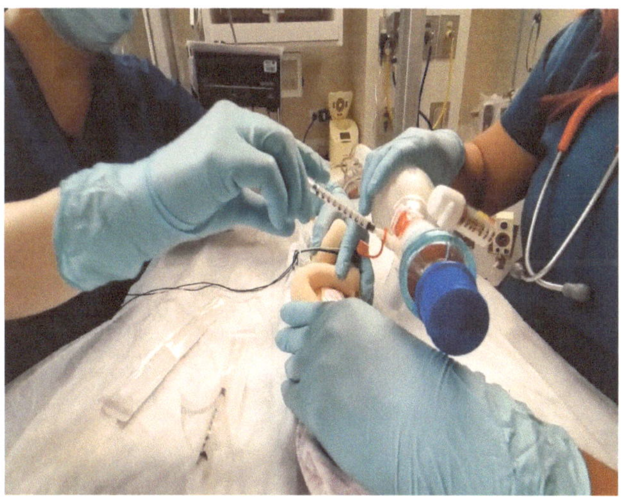

Fig. A4 The Federal Food and Drug Administration (FDA) has approved synthetic surfactant to prevent RDS among the infant population.

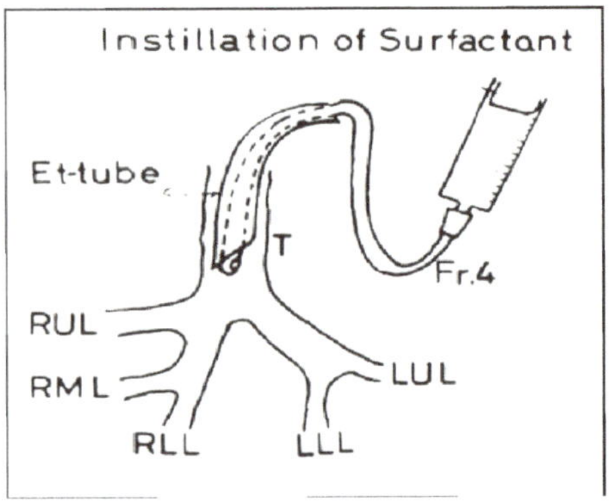

Fig.A 5 Diagrammatic represtation of technique of surfactant instalation in to the lungs with the help of endotracheal tube .

At the time, respiratory distress syndrome (RDS) was a leading cause of infant mortalities. Since then, the Federal Food and Drug Administration (FDA) has approved synthetic surfactant to prevent RDS among the infant population.

5.Pea Pod

A product overview published by medical equipment manufacturer COSMED explains that their Pea Pod density measurement apparatus uses air displacement to identify the body mass of infants who weigh roughly 2.5 to 17.5 pounds. The manufacturer proclaims that Pea Pod sets the global benchmark for body mass assessments.The entire process only takes about seven minutes. The device, which guides practitioners through the assessment process with prompts, is relatively simple to use and performs favorably when compared to techniques outlined in medical research publications.

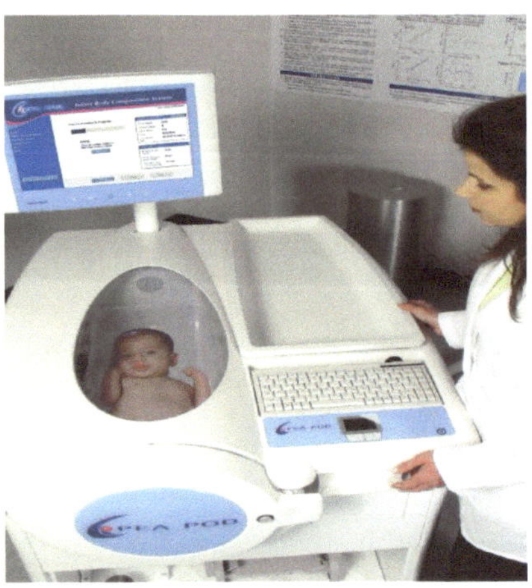

Fig. A6 Pea Pod uses air displacement to identify the body mass of infants who weigh roughly 2.5 to 17.5 pounds. The manufacturer proclaims that Pea Pod sets the global benchmark for body mass assessments

Modern neonatal nurse practitioners promote preventative education to encourage expectant mothers to live healthy lives. NNPs also identify genetic traits that could lead to birth complications. America's future mothers need a continuing supply of qualified neonatal nurse practitioners to promote wellness among newborns and lead the population in living healthy, satisfying lives.

Incubators and innovators: Tech transforming Neonatal baby care

Premature babies usually require an extended hospital stay after they're born, where they need to be closely monitored to make sure they receive the best possible start in life. Caring for this uniquely vulnerable population has always been a challenge, but new technologies mean neonates are receiving better medical treatment than ever before. Chloe Kent rounds up the smart tech helping to keep premature babies alive and healthy.

Neonates are a population that has been historically underserved by the medtech industry. Very few devices are authorised for patients younger than two years old each year, despite their unique medical needs.

Premature babies, or preemies, are a particularly vulnerable part of the neonatal population. These babies, born before 37 weeks gestation, typically require special care after they are born as they haven't had the chance to fully develop, and aren't always ready for life outside the womb.

Fortunately, advances in neonatal care have come a long way and premature babies now have access to better medical care than they ever have before. Medical Technology takes a closer look at some of the most exciting developments in the field of preemie care.

A smart mattress could soon be helping keep premature babies warm

Premature babies are at an increased risk of complications if their body temperature isn't maintained, but they can lose heat rapidly. Researchers at Nottingham Trent University have developed a smart warming system that can provide enough heat to ensure premature babies are kept warm. Active warming like this can avoid the need for more intensive intervention down the line and improve a baby's early development.

The mattress, which is made from polyurethane elastomers and foam, applies uniform and precisely controlled heating characteristics. In its current prototype form, it has to be precisely controlled to ensure that it delivers the correct amount of heat.

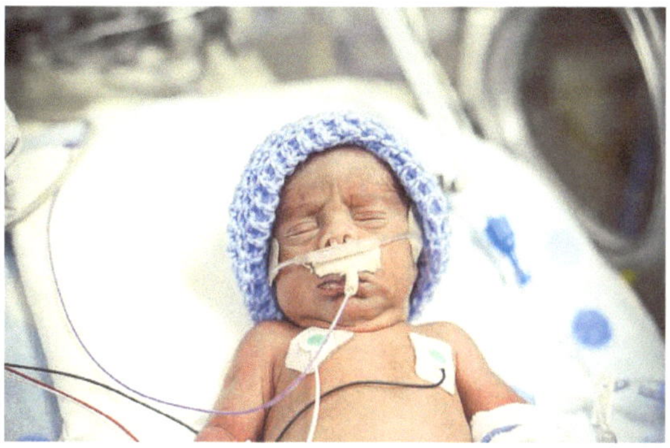

Fig.A7 Smart mattress for premature babies for temperature regulation

The prototype is now expected to undergo testing before any open market release. The project has been completed in collaboration with Rober, a company that manufactures 'zero pressure' mattresses to help bedbound people avoid pressure ulcers.

Incubation innovations are improving care for babies and families

Premature babies in special incubators are something most of us are familiar with, even if this is via film and TV rather than personal experience, and the technology inside of them is becoming more advanced every year.
Keeping a premature or very ill baby in an incubator allows them to put all their energy into growing rather than keeping warm. If the baby needs to have surgery, being kept in an incubator will improve their potential outcomes as the device allows doctors to prepare them in the best possible environment.
The Dräger BabyLeo represents the very latest in neonatal care technology, designed around the needs of both the baby and their family to ensure the child receives the best possible treatment.

The device is designed to keep a baby warm as an incubator, a radiant warmer and during the transition between close and open care. Its connected heater, dual radiant warmer and heated mattress are all synchronised to maintain a stable temperature at all times, regardless of which setting needs to be used.
What sets the BabyLeo apart are its family-focused features. The large variable height adjustment range helps breastfeeding parents nurse their newborn even if they're in a wheelchair, making the device more accessible for both disabled parents and those temporarily in a wheelchair while they recover from giving birth.Newborns in a BabyLeo can also nurse with the lid of the incubator open or closed depending on what procedures are being performed, meaning there's no risk of any treatment they're undergoing being disrupted while they feed.
The device also comes with a personalised Family View display which displays information about the baby's therapy status and progress into an easy-to-understand format, helping to integrate parents into their child's care.

Video messaging is keeping families connected during the pandemic

During the Covid-19 pandemic, many neonatal intensive care units in the UK are limiting who can physically visit their baby. Some units are only allowing one parent to see their child at a time or implementing visiting time limits.
For parents who cannot be with their baby, vCreate allows them to stay connected to their child. The secure video messaging service allows hospital staff to send regular video and photo messages to parents, so they don't miss crucial moments of their child's first weeksThe messages can be accessed on any device, whenever the parents want, and can be downloaded and kept forever. vCreate's security protocols mean that parents and staff

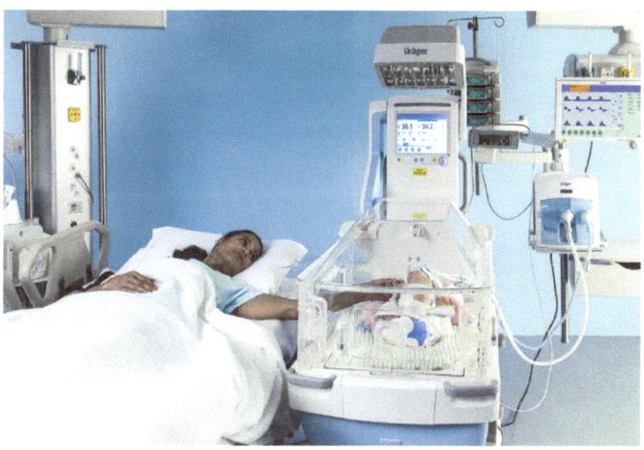

Fig.A 8 Showing the Dräger BabyLeo incubator for neonatal care

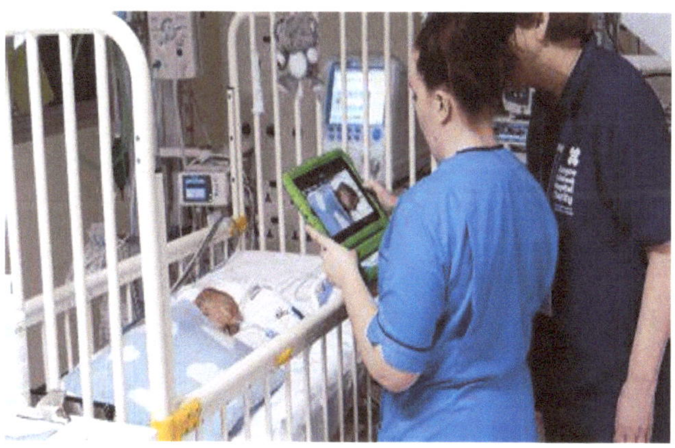

Fig. A 9 Showing the vCreate system which allows parents/care takers to stay connected to their child. with videos

have full control of the videos, and only they can access them.

Even before Covid-19, it was understood that preemie parents couldn't be with their children 24/7, and technologies like vCreate can help them feel more connected with their baby's care process.

The software is available globally to all neonatal units and is NHS Trusted in the UK. vCreate's sponsor-led funding model means the service is free to all parents and comes at no cost to the units.

Medtronic is paving the way for neonatal kidney therapy

Critically ill neonates are particularly vulnerable to fluid overload, a condition where there is too much fluid in the blood, and acute kidney injury. It's one of the most critical things to avoid during those first few weeks, as the mortality rate for neonates with acute kidney injuries has been estimated to be as high as 60%.The US Food and Drug Administration has now approved Medtronic's Carpediem Cardio-Renal Paediatric Dialysis Emergency Machine for clinical use. The Carpediem system is designed to provide continuous renal replacement therapy (CRRT) for neonatal patients from 2.5kg to 10kg, enabling more precise treatment and reducing risks.

CRRT is one of the most common blood purification therapies used for patients with kidney injuries. The patient's blood is pumped through a haemofilter to remove waste and excess fluid, maintaining cardiac stability and minimising the risk of low blood pressure.

However, CRRT for neonatal patients hasn't always been delivered in optimal circumstances, as traditional dialysis machines aren't designed for their small bodies. As younger children have less blood, the effect of errors is amplified when they use a machine designed for an adult, putting their safety at risk.

Medtronic is now rolling out the device across the US, with its first successful deployment occurring at the Cincinnati Children's Hospital Medical Center in December last year.

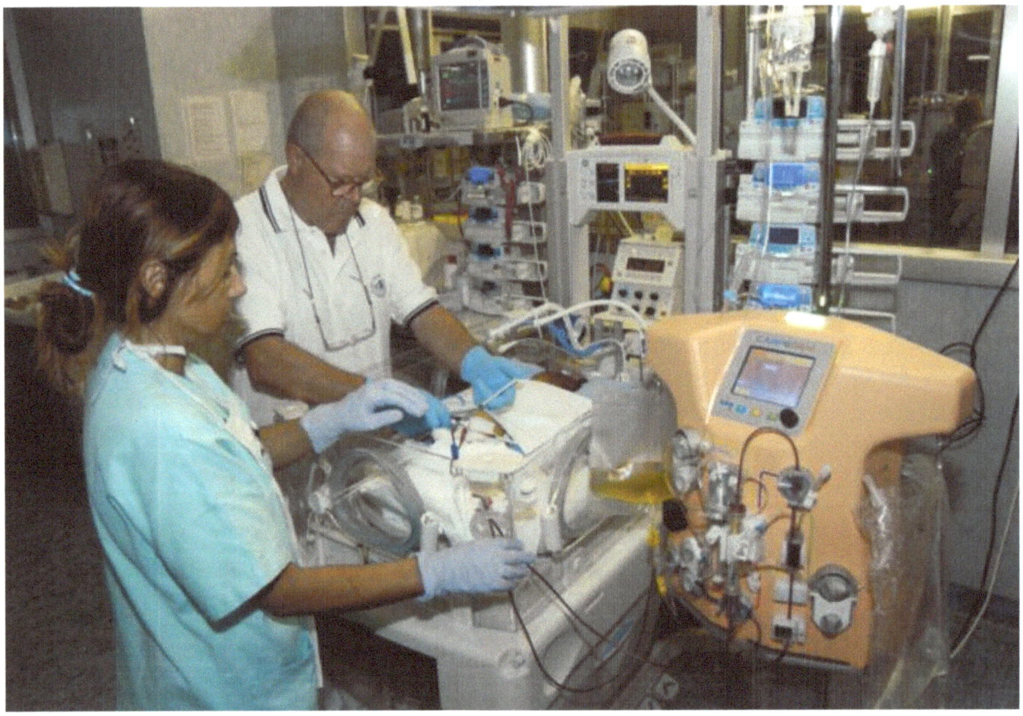

Fig. A 10 Pictured is the CARPEDIEM machine in action. The device successfully treated a 2.9-kg newborn with multiple organ failure.

Neonatal intensive care units with artificial intelligence: a systematic review

Machine learning and deep learning are two subsets of artificial intelligence that involve teaching computers to learn and make decisions from any sort of data. Most recent developments in artificial intelligence are coming from deep learning, which has proven revolutionary in almost all fields, from computer vision to health sciences. The effects of deep learning in medicine have changed the conventional ways of clinical application significantly. Although some sub-fields of medicine, such as pediatrics, have been relatively slow in receiving the critical benefits of deep learning, related research in pediatrics has started to accumulate to a significant level, tooHence, in this chapter the review of recently developed machine learning and deep learning-based solutions for neonatology applications is discussed . One can systematically evaluate the roles of both classical machine learning and deep learning in neonatology applications, define the methodologies, including algorithmic developments, and describe the remaining challenges in the assessment of neonatal diseases by using PRISMA 2020 guidelines. To date, the primary areas of focus in neonatology regarding AI applications have included survival analysis, neuroimaging, analysis of vital parameters and biosignals, and retinopathy of prematurity diagnosis.

What are the needs in clinics? Clinicians are concerned about the healthcare system's integration with AI: there is an exponential need for diagnostic testing, early detection, and alarm tools to provide diagnosis and novel treatments without invasive tests and procedures50. Clinicians have higher expectations of AI in their daily practices than before. AI is expected to decrease the need for multiple diagnostic invasive tests and increase diagnostic accuracy with less invasive (or non-invasive) tests. Such AI systems can easily recognize imaging patterns on test images (i.e., unseen or not utilized efficiently in daily routines), allowing them to detect and diagnose various diseases. These methods could improve detection and diagnosis in different fields of medicine.

The overall goal of this systematic review is to explain AI's potential use and benefits in the field of neonatology

We intend to enlighten the potential role of AI in the future in neonatal care. We postulate that AI would be best used as a hybrid intelligence (i.e., human-in-the-loop or mixed intelligence) to make neonatal care more feasible, increase the accuracy of diagnosis, and predict the outcome and diseases in advance. The rest of the paper is organized as follows: In results, we explain the published AI applications in neonatology along with AI evaluation metrics to fully understand their efficacy in neonatology and provide a comprehensive overview of DL applications in neonatology. In discussion, we examine the difficulties of AI utilization in neonatology and future research discussions. In the methods section, we outline the systematic review procedures, including the examination of existing literature and the development of our search strategy.

We review the past, current, and future of AI-based diagnostic and monitoring tools that might aid neonatologists' patient management and follow-up. We discuss several AI designs for electronic health records, image, and signal processing, analyze the merits and limits of newly created decision support systems, and illuminate future views clinicians and neonatologists might use in their normal diagnostic activities. AI has made significant breakthroughs to solve issues with conventional imaging approaches by identifying clinical variables and imaging aspects not easily visible to human eyes. Improved diagnostic skills could prevent missed diagnoses and aid in diagnostic decision-making. Briefly, our objectives in this systematic review are:

- to explain the various AI models and evaluation metrics thoroughly explained and describe the principal features of the AI models,
- to categorize neonatology-related AI applications into macro-domains, to explain their sub-domains and the important elements of the applicable AI models,
- to examine the state-of-the-art in studies, particularly from the past several years, with an emphasis on the use of ML in encompassing all neonatology,
- to present a comprehensive overview and classification of DL applications utilized and in neonatology,
- to analyze and debate the current and open difficulties associated with AI in neonatology, as well as future research directions, to offer the clinician a comprehensive perspective of the actual situation.

AI covers a broad concept for the application of computing algorithms that can categorize, predict, or generate valuable conclusions from enormous datasets. Algorithms such as Naive Bayes, Genetic Algorithms, Fuzzy Logic, Clustering, Neural Networks (NN), Support Vector Machines (SVM), Decision Trees, and Random Forests (RF) have been used for more than three decades for detection, diagnosis, classification, and risk assessment in medicine as ML methods.. Conventional ML approaches for image classification involve using hand-engineered features, which are visual descriptions and annotations learned from radiologists, that are encoded into algorithms Images, signals, genetic expressions, EHR, and vital signs are examples of the various unstructured data sources that comprise medical data. Due to the complexity of their structures, DL frameworks may take advantage of this heterogeneity by attaining high abstraction levels in data analysis.Unstructured data such as medical images, vital signals, genetic

Unfortunately, many end-users do not have an easy time comprehending these measurements. In addition, it might be difficult to objectively compare models from different research models, and there is currently no method or tool available that can compare models based on the same performance measures. In this part, the common ML and DL evaluation metrics are explained so neonatologists
could adapt them into their research and understand of upcoming articles and research design.

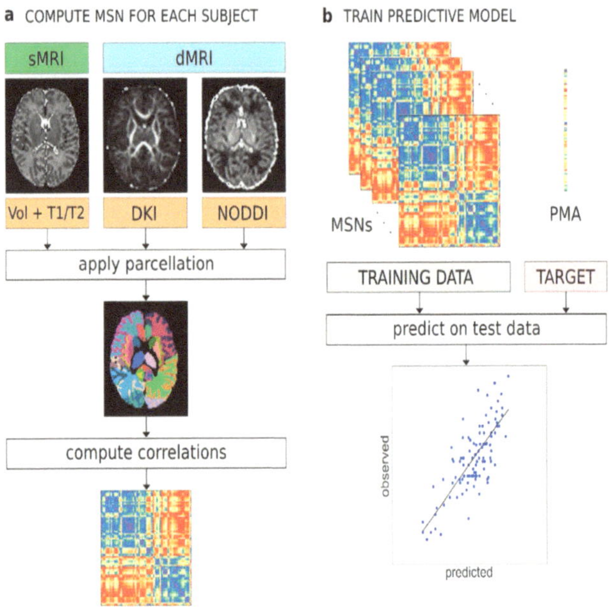

Fig.A11 a) Individual morphometric similarity networks (MSN) construction: Different metrics are extracted from structural and diffusion MRI data (sMRI, dMRI (such as diffusion kurtosis imaging (DKI) and Neurite Orientation Dispersion and Density Imaging (NODDI) models)). The same labelled atlas is applied to all image types and the average metric values are computed for 81 regions of interest. An MSN (represented here as a connectivity matrix) is built by computing the Pearson correlation between the vectors of metrics of each pair of ROIs. b) Training of a predictive model from individual MSNs: the inter-regional correlations are used as predictor variables in a machine learning model for chronological brain age. The performance of the model is evaluated on an independent test set. From Galdi P et al. Neuroimage Clin [20].

expressions, EHRs, and signal data contribute to the wide variety of medical information. Analyzing and interpreting different data streams in neonatology requires a comprehensive strategy because each has unique characteristics and complications.

While ML requires manual/hand-crafted selection of information from incoming data and related transformation procedures, DL performs these tasks more efficiently and with higher efficacy DL is able to discover these components by analyzing a large number of samples with a high degree of automation7. The literature on these ML approaches is extensive before the development of DL

It is essential for clinicians to understand how the suggested ML model should enhance patient care. Since it is impossible for a single metric to capture all the desirable attributes of a model, it is customarily necessary to describe the performance of a model using several different metrics.

AI is commonly utilized everywhere, from daily life to high-risk applications in medicine. Although slower compared to other fields, numerous studies began to appear in the literature investigating the use of AI in neonatology. These studies have used various imaging modalities, electronic health records, and ML algorithms, some of which have barely gone through the clinical workflow. Though there is no systematic review and future discussions in particular in this field.Many studies were dedicated to introducing these systems into neonatology. However, the success of these studies has been limited. Lately, research in this field has been moving in a more favorable direction due to exciting new advances in DL. Metrics for evaluations in those studies were the standard metrics such as sensitivity (true-positive rate), specificity (true-negative rate), false-positive rate, false-negative rate, receiver operating characteristics (ROC), area under the ROC curves (AUC), and accuracy

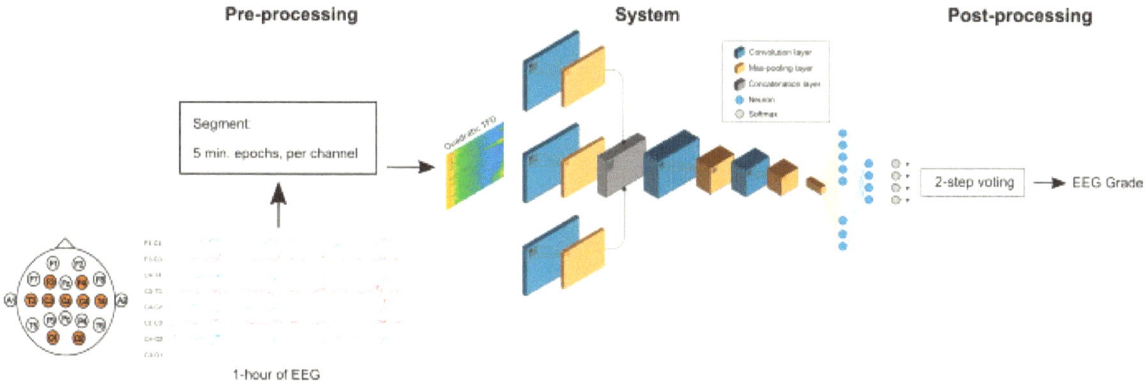

Fig. A 12: Overview of an AI system to grade the neonatal EEG. The system assigns a grade (1–4) based on 1 h of multi-channel EEG. Pre-processing: the EEG is filtered and downsampled to 64 Hz, then divided into 5-min segments. System model: each 5-min segment, per channel, is converted to a quadratic time-frequency distribution (TFD). This 2-dimensional image is passed through a pre-trained convolutional neural network (CNN). The CNN has parallel layers to extract information across time, frequency, and in the joint time-frequency direction of the TFD. The CNN produces a separate probability for each of the 4 grades. Post-processing: the probabilities from the CNN are combined over all 5-min segments and across channels to give a final grade prediction. Adapted from Raurale et al. J Neural Eng.

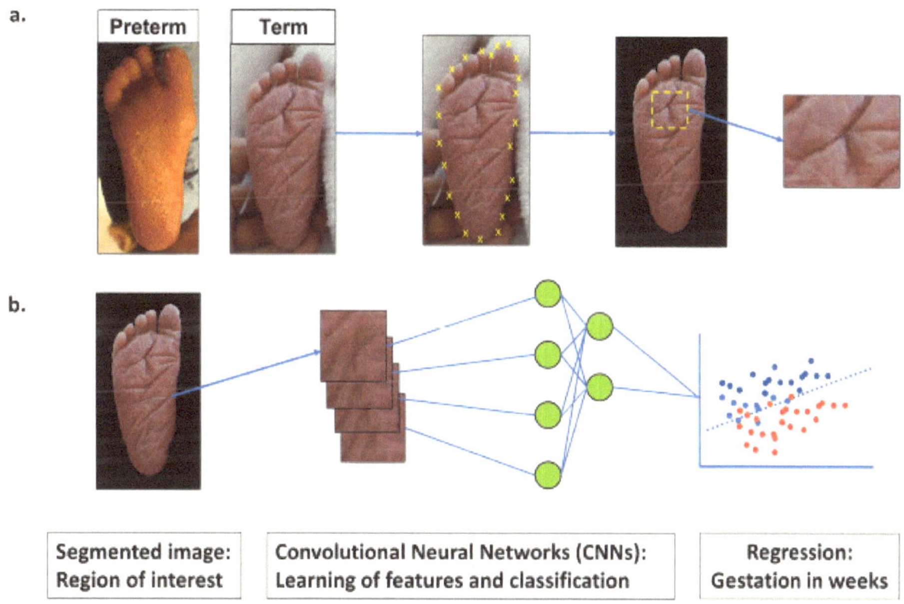

Fig.A 13: a) Plantar surface photograph of preterm and post-term infant. Manually labelled region of interest (ROI) used to train system to identify foot and remove background with subsequent plantar crease pattern recognition. This uses fully Convolutional Neural Networks (CNNs) to segment images and provide per-pixel classification. b) Images undergo deep machine learning, with CNNs passing through different layers, to be classified into one of five classes (extremely preterm, very preterm, moderate preterm, term and post-term). This probability vector is then combined with the weight of the infant to improve the decision-making process during regression and the output is an estimate of gestational age in weeks. Adapted from Torres et al. Image and Vision Computing.

ML applications in neonatal mortality

Neonatal mortality is a major factor in child mortality. Neonatal fatalities account for 47 percent of all mortality in children under the age of five, according to the World Health Organization It is, therefore, a priority to minimize worldwide infant mortality by 2030

ML investigated infant mortality, its reasons, and its mortality prediction. In a recent review, 1.26 million infants born from 22 weeks to 40 weeks of gestational age were enrolled67. Predictions were made as early as 5 min of life and as late as 7 days. An average of four models per investigation were neural networks, random forests, and logistic regression (58.3%) Two studies (18.2%) completed external validation, although five (45.5%) published calibration plots. Eight studies reported AUC, and five supplied sensitivity and specificity. The AUC was 58.3–97.0%. Sensitivities averaged 63 to 80%, and specificities 78 to 98%Linear regression analysis was the best overall model despite having 17 features. This analysis highlighted the most prevalent AI neonatal mortality measures and predictions. Despite the advancement in neonatal care, it is crucial that preterm infants remain highly susceptible to mortality due to immaturity of organ systems and increased susceptibility to early and late sepsis69. Addressing these permanent risks necessitates the utilization of ML to predict mortality. Early studies employed ANN and fuzzy linguistic models and achieved an AUC of 85–95% and accuracy of 90%New studies in a large preterm populations and extremely low birthweight infants found an AUC of 68.9–93.3%There are some shortcomings in these studies; for example, none of them used vital parameters to represent dynamic changes, and hence, there was no improvement in clinical practice in neonatology. Unsurprisingly, gestational age, birthweight, and APGAR scores were shown as the most important variables in the models Future research is suggested to focus on external evaluation, calibration, and implementation of healthcare applications.

Neonatal sepsis, which includes both early onset sepsis and late onset sepsis, is a significant factor contributing to neonatal mortality and morbidity73. Neonatal sepsis diagnosis and antibiotic initiation present considerable obstacles in the field of neonatal care, underscoring the importance of implementing comprehensive interventions to alleviate their profound negative consequences. The studies have predicted early sepsis from heart rate variability with an accuracy of 64–94%. Another secondary analysis of multicenter data revealed that clinical biomarkers weighed the ML decision by integrating all clinical and lab variables and achieved an AUC of 73–83%

ML applications in neurodevelopmental outcome

Recent advancements in neonatal healthcare have resulted in a decrease in the incidence of severe prenatal brain injury and an increase in the survival rates of preterm babies. However, even though routine radiological imaging does not reveal any signs of brain damage, this population is nonetheless at significant risk of having a negative outcome in terms of neurodevelopment It is essential to discover early indicators of abnormalities in brain development that might serve as a guide for the treatment of preterm children at a greater risk of having negative neurodevelopmental consequences.

The most common reason for neurodevelopmental impairment is intraventricular hemorrhage (IVH) in preterm infants.. Two studies predicted IVH in preterm infants. Both studies have not deployed the ultrasound images in their analysis, they only predicted IVH according to the clinical variables. Morphological studies have demonstrated that preterm birth is linked to smaller brain volume, cortical folding, axonal integrity, and microstructural connectivity.Studies concentrating on functional markers of brain maturation, such as those derived from resting-state functional connectivity (rsFC) analyses of blood-oxygen-level dependent (BOLD) fluctuations, have revealed further impacts of prematurity on the developing connectome, ranging from decreased network-specific connectivity.Many studies investigated brain connectivity in preterm infants. and brain structural analysis in neonates93 and neonatal brain segmentation94 with the help of ML methods. Similarly, one of the most important outcomes of neurodevelopment at 2-year-old-age is neurocognitive evaluations.The studies evaluated the morphological changes in the brain in relation to neurocognitive outcome and brain age prediction.It has been found that near-term regional white matter (WM) microstructure on diffusion tensor imaging (DTI) predicted neurodevelopment in preterm infants using exhaustive feature selection with cross-validation96 and multivariate models of near-term structural MRI and WM microstructure on DTI might help identify preterm infants at risk for language impairment and guide early intervention.One of the studies that evaluated the effects of PPAR gene activity on brain development with ML methods100 revealed a strong association between abnormal brain connectivity and implicating PPAR gene signaling in abnormal white matter development.

Inhibited brain growth in individuals exposed to early extrauterine stress is controlled by genetic variables, and PPARG signaling has a formerly unknown role in cerebral development. Alternative to morphological studies, neuromonitorization is shown to be an important tool for which ML methods have been frequently employed, for example, in automatic seizure detection from video .and EEG biosignals in infants and neonates with . The detection of artifacts.sleep states,, rhythmic patterns, burst suppression in extremely preterm infant from EEG records were studied with ML methods. EEG records are often used for HIE gradingtoo. It has been shown in those studies that EEG recordings of different neonate datasets found an AUC of 89% to 96%, accuracy 78–87% regarding seizure detection with different ML methods .

MLapplications in predictions of prematurity complications (BPD, PDA, and ROP)

Another important cause of mortality and morbidity in the NICU is PDA (Patent Ductus Arteriosus). The ductus arteriosus is typically present during the fetal stage, when the circulation in the lungs and body is regularly supplied by the mother; in newborns, the ductus arteriosus closes functionally by 72 h of age.20–50% of infants with a gestational age (GA) 32 weeks have the ductus arteriosus on day 3 of life, while up to 60% of neonates with a GA 29 weeks have the ductus arteriosus. The presence of PDA in preterm neonates is associated with higher mortality and morbidity, and physicians should evaluate if PDA closure might enhance the likelihood of survival vs. the burden of adverse effects.

ML methods were utilized on PDA detection from EHR and auscultation records such that 47 perinatal factors were analyzed with 5 different ML methods in 10390 very low birth weight infants' predicted PDA with an accuracy of 76% and 250 auscultation records were analyzed with XGBoost and found to have an accuracy of 74%.

Bronchopulmonary dysplasia (BPD) is a leading cause of infant death and morbidity in preterm births. While various biomarkers have been linked to the development of respiratory distress syndrome (RDS), no clinically relevant prognostic tests are available for BPD at birth.. There are ML studies aiming to predict BPD from birth gastric aspirate content and genetic data and it has been shown that BPD could be predicted with an accuracy of up to 86% in the best-case scenario, analysis of responsible genes with ML could predict BPD development with an AUC of 90% and combination of gastric aspirate after birth and clinical information analysis with SVM predicted BPD development with a sensitivity of 88%.In relation to published studies in BPD with ML-based predictions, long-term invasive ventilation is considered one of the most important risk factors for BPD, nosocomial infections, and increased hospital stay. There are ML-based studies aiming to predict extubation failure and optimum weaning time using long-term invasive ventilation information. It has been shown in those studies that predicted extubation failure with an accuracy of 83.2% to 87%.

Retinopathy of prematurity (ROP) is another area of interest in the application of machine learning in neonatology.ROP is a serious complication of prematurity that affects the blood vessels in the retina and is a leading cause of childhood blindness in high and middle-income countries, including the United States, among very low-birthweight (1500 g), very preterm (28–32 weeks), and extremely preterm infants (less than 28 weeks). Due to a shortage of ophthalmologists available to treat ROP patients, there has been increased interest in the use of telemedicine and artificial intelligence as solutions for diagnosing ROP.. Some ML methods, such as Gaussian mixture models, were employed to diagnose and classify ROP from retinal fundus images in studiesand it has been reported that the i-ROP system classified pre-plus and plus disease with 95% accuracy. This was close to the performance of the three individual experts (96%, 94%, and 92%, respectively), and much higher than the mean performance of 31 nonexperts (81%).

Other ML applications in neonatal diseases

EHR and medical records were featured in ML algorithms for the diagnosis of congenital heart defects.HIE (Hypoxic Ischemic Encephalopathy), IVH (Intraventricular Hemorrhage), neonatal jaundice,prediction of NEC (Necrotizing Enterocolitis), prediction of neurodevelopmental outcome in ELBW (extremely low birth weight) infants,, prediction of neonatal surgical site infections, and prediction of rehospitalization.

Electronically captured physiologic data are evaluated as signal data, and they were analyzed with ML to detect artifact patterns,late onset sepsis,, and predict infant morbidity.Electronically captured vital parameters (respiratory rate, heart rate) of 138 infants (≤34 weeks' gestation, birth weight ≤2000 gram) in the first 3 h of life predicted an accuracy of overall morbidity and an AUC of 91%.In addition to physiologic data, clinical data up to 12 h after cardiac surgery in HLHS (hypoplastic left heart syndrome) and TGA (transposition of great arteries) infants were analyzed to predict PVL (periventricular leukomalacia) occurrence after surgery.The F-score results for infants with HLHS and those without HLHS were 88% and 100%, respectively.Voice records were used to diagnose respiratory phases in infant cry,to classify neonatal diseases in infant cry,and to evaluate asphyxia from infant cry voice records.Voice records of 35 infants were analyzed with ANN, and accuracy was found 85%. Cry records of 14 infants in their 1st year of life were analyzed with SVM and GMM, and phases of respiration and crying rate were quantified with an accuracy of 86%.

SVM was the most commonly used method in the diagnosis of metabolic disorders of newborns, including MMA (methylmalonic acidemia), PKU (phenylketonuria),, MCADD (medium-chain acyl CoA dehydrogenase deficiency). During the Bavarian newborn screening program, dried blood samples were analyzed with ML and increased the positive predictive value for PKU (71.9% versus 16,2) and for MCADD (88.4% versus 54.6%).

Neonatology with deep learning

The main uses of DL in clinical image analysis are categorized into three categories: classification, detection, and segmentation. Classification involves identifying a specific feature in an image, detection involves locating multiple features within an image; and segmentation involves dividing an image into multiple parts.

Neuroradiological evaluation with AI in neonatology

Neonatal neuroimaging can establish early indicators of neurodevelopmental abnormality to provide early intervention during a time of maximal neuroplasticity and fast cognitive and motor development.. DL methods can assist in an earlier diagnosis than clinical signs would indicate.The imaging of an infant's brain using MRI can be challenging due to lower tissue contrast, substantial tissue inhomogeneities, regionally heterogeneous image appearance, immense age-related intensity variations, and severe partial volume impact due to the smaller brain size. Since most of the existing tools were created for adult brain MRI data, infant-specific computational neuroanatomy tools are recently being developed. A typical pipeline for early prediction of neurodevelopmental disorders from infant structural MRI (sMRI) is made up of three basic phases.

(1) Image preprocessing, tissue segmentation, regional labeling, and extraction of image-based characteristics
(2) Surface reconstruction, surface correspondence, surface parcellation, and extraction of surface-based features
(3) Feature preprocessing, feature extraction, AI model training, and prediction of unseen subjects.The segmentation of a newborn brain is difficult due to the decreased SNR (signal to noise ratio) resulting from the shorter scanning duration enforced by predicted motion restrictions and the diminutive size of the neonatal brain. In addition, the cerebrospinal fluid (CSF)-gray matter border has an intensity profile comparable to that of the mostly unmyelinated white matter (WM), resulting in significant partial volume effects. In addition, the high variability resulting from the fast growth of the brain and the continuing myelination of WM imposes additional constraints on the creation of effective segmentation techniques. Several non-DL-based approaches for properly segmenting newborn brains have been presented over the years. These methods may be broadly classified as parametric,, classification,multi-atlas fusion,and deformable models.The Dice Similarity Coefficient metric is used for image segmentation evaluation; the higher the dice, the higher the segmentation accuracy.

In the NeoBrainS12 2012 MICCAI Grand-Challenge (https://neobrains12.isi.uu.nl), T1W and T2W images were presented with manually segmented structures to assess strategies for segmenting neonatal tissue162. Most methods were found to be accurate, but classification-based approaches were particularly precise and sensitive. However, segmentation of myelinated vs. unmyelinated WM remains a difficulty since the majority of approaches, failed to consistently obtain reliable results.

Future research in neonatal brain segmentation will involve a more thorough neural segmentation network. Current studies are intended to highlight efficient networks capable of producing accurate and dependable segmentations while comparing them to existing conventional computer vision techniques. In the perspective of comparing previous efforts on newborn brain segmentation, the small sample size of high-quality labeled data must also be recognized as a significant restriction.The field of artificial intelligence in neonatology has progressed slowly due to a shortage of open-source algorithms and the availability of datasets

Future research should also focus on improving the accuracy of DL for diagnosing germinal matrix hemorrhage and figuring out how DL can help a radiologist's workflow by comparing how well sonographers identify studies that look suspicious. More studies could also look at how well DL works for accurately grading germinal matrix hemorrhages and maybe even small hemorrhages that a radiologist can see on an MRI but not on a head ultrasound. This could be useful in improving the diagnostic capabilities of head ultrasound in various clinical scenarios.

Evaluation of prematurity complications with DL in neonatology

In the above discussion, we have addressed the primary applications of DL in relation to disease prediction. These include DL for analyzing conditions such as PDA (patent ductus arteriosus), IVH (intraventricular ventricular hemorrhage),, BPD (bronchopulmonary dysplasia,, ROP (retinopathy of prematurity),, retinal hemorrhage,diagnosis. This also includes DL applications for analyzing MR images, and combined with EHR data, for predicting neurocognitive outcome and mortality. Additionally, DL has potential applications in treatment planning and discharge from the NICU,including customized medicine and follow-up.

Digital imaging and analysis with AI are promising and cost-effective tools for detecting infants with severe ROP who may need therapy.Despite limitations such as image quality, interpretation variability, equipment costs, and compatibility issues with EHR systems, AI has been shown to be effective in detecting ROP.. Studies comparing BIO (Binocular Indirect Ophthalmoscope) to telemedicine have shown that both methods have equivalent sensitivity for identifying zone disease, plus disease, and ROP. However, BIO was found to be slightly better at identifying zone III and stage 3 ROP.DL algorithms were applied to 5511 retinal images, achieving an AUC of 94% (diagnosis of normal) and 98% (diagnosis of plus disease), outperforming 6 out of 8 ROP experts.In another study, DL was used to quantify the clinical progression of ROP by assigning ROP vascular severity scores. A consecutive study with a large dataset showed in 4175 retinal images from 32 NICUs, resulting in an AUC of 98% for detecting therapy required ROP with DL. The use of AI in ROP screening programs may increase access to care for secondary prevention of ROP and enable the evaluation of disease epidemiology.

Signal detection for sleep protection in the NICU is another ongoing discussion. DL has been used to analyze infant EEGs and identify sleep states. Interruptions of sleep states have been linked to problems in neuronal development.Automated sleep state detection from EEG records and from ECG monitoring parameters1 were demonstrated with DL. The underperformance of the all-state classification (kappa score 0.33 to 0.44) was likely owing to the difficulties in differentiating small changes between states and a lack of enough training data for minority classes.

DL has been found to be effective in real-time evaluation of cardiac MRI for congenital heart disease. Studies have shown that DL can accurately calculate ventricular volumes from images rebuilt using residual UNet, which are not statistically different from the gold standard, cardiac MRI. This technology has the potential to be particularly beneficial for infants and critically ill individuals who are unable to hold their breath during the imaging process.

DL-based 3D CNN algorithms have been used to demonstrate the automated classification of brain dysmaturation from neonatal brain MRI.. In a study, brain MRIs of 90 term neonates with congenital heart diseases and 40 term healthy controls were analyzed using this method, which achieved an accuracy of 98%. This technique could be useful in detecting brain dysmaturation in neonates with congenital heart diseases.

DL algorithms have been used to classify neonatal diseases from thermal images.. These studies analyzed neonatal thermograms to determine the health status of infants and achieved good AUC scores.. However, these studies didn't include any clinical information . Two large scale studies showed breakthrough results regarding the effect of nutrition practices in NICU and wireless sensors in NICU.. A nutrition study revealed that nutrition practices were associated with discharge weight and BPD.This exemplifies how unbiased ML techniques may be used to effectively bring about clinical practice changes.Novel, wireless sensors can improve monitoring, prevent iatrogenic injuries, and encourage family-centered care. Early validation results show performance equal to standard-of-care monitoring systems in high-income nations. Furthermore, the use of reusable sensors and compatibility with low-cost mobile phones may reduce monitoring.

AI Ethics

While AI has great promise for enhancing healthcare, it also presents significant ethical concerns. Ethical concerns in health AI include informed consent, bias, safety, transparency, patient privacy, and allocation, and their solutions are complicated to negotiate.. In neonatology, crucial decision-making is frequently accompanied by a complicated and challenging ethical component. Interdisciplinary approaches are required for progress. The border of viability, life sustaining treatments and the different regulations worldwide made AI utilization in neonatology more complicated. How an ethics framework is implemented in an AI in neonatology has not been reported yet, and there is a need for transparency for trustworthy AI.

Bibliography and Acknowledgement

- A. Foran, D.K. Shah, et al. A machine-learning algorithm for neonatal seizure recognition: a multicentre, randomised, controlled trial Lancet Child Adolesc. Health, 4 (10) (2020), pp. 740-749
- A.A. Garvey, A.M. Pavel, D.M. Murray, G.B. Boylan, E.M. Dempsey Does early cerebral near-infrared spectroscopy monitoring predict outcome in neonates with hypoxic Ischaemic encephalopathy? A systematic review of diagnostic test accuracy Neonatology, 119 (1) (2022), pp. 1-9
- B. Moller, E. Bradley, S. Chakwera, L. Hussain-Alkhateeb, A. Lewin, et al. National, regional, and global estimates of preterm birth in 2020, with trends from 2010: a systematic analysisLancet, 402 (10409) (2023), pp. 1261-1271
- Bagci, U., Irmakci, I., Demir, U. & Keles, E. in AI in Clinical Medicine: A Practical Guide for Healthcare Professionals 56–65 (2023).
- Barekatain, A. Sadeghnia, M. Johari, M. Marofi, N. Tavakoli-Fard, M. Mehrkash Which site is better for skin sensor temperature probe in newborns under open care system for prevention of hypo – hyperthermia Int. J. Prev. Med., 13 (1) (2022), p. 132
- C.C. Roehr, G. Hansmann, T. Hoehn, C. Buhrer The 2010 Guidelines on Neonatal Resuscitation (AHA, ERC, ILCOR): similarities and differences—what progress has been made since 2005? Klin. Padiatr., 223 (5) (2011), pp. 299-307
- C.J. Morley, P.G. Davis, L.W. Doyle, L.P. Brion, J.M. Hascoet, J.B. Carlin Nasal CPAP or intubation at birth for very preterm infantsEngl. J. Med., 358 (7) (2008), pp. 700-708
- Cools, M. Offringa, L.M. Askie Elective high frequency oscillatory ventilation versus conventional ventilation for acute pulmonary dysfunction in preterm infants Cochrane Database Syst. Rev. (3) (2015), Article Cd000104
- D.V. Azzopardi, B. Strohm, A.D. Edwards, L. Dyet, H.L. Halliday, E. Juszczak, et al. Moderate hypothermia to treat perinatal asphyxial encephalopathy N. Engl. J. Med., 361 (14) (2009), pp. 1349-1358
- Dalley, K. Hodgson, J. Dawson, M. Tracy, P. Davis, M. Thio The NEOTRAIN study: introducing a novel respiratory function monitor for neonatal resuscitation training J. Paediatr. Child Health, 59 (Supplement 1) (2023), p. 70
- Desmond, S. Namachivayam Does near-infrared spectroscopy play a role in paediatric intensive care?BJA Edu., 16 (8) (2015), pp. 281-285
- Dimich, P.P. Singh, A. Adell, M. Hendler, N. Sonnenklar, M. Jhaveri Evaluation of oxygen saturation monitoring by pulse oximetry in neonates in the delivery system Can. J. Anaesth., 38 (8) (1991), pp. 985-988
- E.D. Johnston, B. Boyle, E. Juszczak, A. King, P. Brocklehurst, B.J. Stenson Oxygen targeting in preterm infants using the Masimo SET radical pulse oximeterArch. Dis. Child. Fetal Neonatal Ed., 96 (6) (2011), pp. F429-F433
- E.P. Fogtmann, A.M. Plomgaard, G. Greisen, C. Gluud Prognostic accuracy of electroencephalograms in preterm infants: a systematic reviewPediatrics, 139 (2) (2017)
- F.E. Wood, C.J. Morley, J.A. Dawson, P.G. Davis A respiratory function monitor improves mask ventilation Arch. Dis. Child. Fetal Neonatal Ed., 93 (5) (2008), pp. f380-f381
- Galderisi, A. Facchinetti, G.M. Steil, P. OrtizRubio, F. Cavallin
- W.V. Tamborlane, et al. Continuous glucose monitoring in very preterm infants: a randomized controlled trialPediatrics, 140 (4) (2017)

  Gerstmann, R. Berg, R. Haskell, C. Brower, K. Wood, B.
- Yoder, et al. Operational evaluation of pulse oximetry in NICU patients with arterial access J. Perinatol., 23 (5) (2003), pp. 378-383
- H.A. van Zanten, K. Kuypers, E.W. van Zwet, J.J. va Vonderen, C.O.F. Kamlin, L. Springer, et al. A multi-centre randomised controlled trial of respiratory function monitoring during stabilisation of very preterm infants at birth Resuscitation, 167 (2021), pp. 317-325
- Hsu, J. F. et al. Machine learning algorithms to predict mortality of neonates on mechanical intubation for respiratory failure. Biomedicines 9, 1377 (2021).
- J. Robertson, S. Mitra Role of optical neuromonitoring in neonatal encephalopathy-current state and recent advances Front. Pediatr., 9 (2021), Article 653676
- J. Singh, S.K. Sinha, P. Clarke, S. Byrne, S.M. Donn Mechanical ventilation of very low birth weight infants: is volume or pressure a better target variable?J. Pediatr., 149 (3) (2006), pp. 308-313
- Jeong, H. & Kamaleswaran, R. Pivotal challenges in artificial intelligence and machine learning applications for neonatal care. In Seminars in Fetal and Neonatal Medicine Vol. 27, 101393 (Elsevier, 2022)
- K. Faisst, W. Hannon, J.S. Jørgensen, V. König, H.U. Bucher, A. Huch, et al. Reflectance pulse oximetry in neonates Eur. J. Obstet. Gynecol. Reprod. Biol., 61 (2) (1995), pp. 117-122
- K. Lingappan, J.L. Arnold, C.J. Fernandes, M. Pammi Videolaryngoscopy versus direct laryngoscopy for tracheal intubation in neonates Cochrane Database Syst. Rev., 6 (6) (2018), Article Cd009975
- K.L. Zaleski, B.D. KussmanNear-infrared spectroscopy in pediatric congenital heart diseaseJ. Cardiothorac. Vasc. Anesth., 34 (2) (2020), pp. 489-500
- Khurshid, F. et al. Comparison of multivariable logistic regression and machine learning models for predicting bronchopulmonary dysplasia or death in very preterm infants. Front Pediatr. 9, 759776 (2021).
- Kwok, T. N. C. et al. Application and potential of artificial intelligence in neonatal medicine. Semin. Fetal Neonatal Med. 27, 101346 (2022).
- L. Pickup, A. Lang, L. Shipley, C. Henry, J. Carpenter, D. McCartney, et al.
- L. Shipley, C. Gale, D. Sharkey Trends in the incidence and management of hypoxic-ischaemic encephalopathy in the therapeutic hypothermia era: a national population studyArch. Dis. Child. Fetal Neonatal Ed., 106 (5) (2021), pp. 529-534
- L.M. Askie, D.J. Henderson-Smart, L. Irwig, J.M. Simpson Oxygen-saturation targets and outcomes in extremely preterm infants N. Engl. J. Med., 349 (10) (2003), pp. 959-967
- M. Durand, R. Ramanathan Pulse oximetry for continuous oxygen monitoring in sick newborn infants J. Pediatr., 109 (6) (1986), pp. 1052-1056
- M.D. Schreiber, K. Gin-Mestan, J.D. Marks, D. Huo, G. Lee, P. Srisuparp Inhaled nitric oxide in premature infants with the respiratory distress syndromeN. Engl. J. Med., 349 (22) (2003), pp. 2099-2107

- Mangold, C. et al. Machine learning models for predicting neonatal mortality: a systematic review. Neonatology 118, 394–405 (2021). McAdams, R. M. et al. Predicting clinical outcomes using artificial intelligence and machine learning in neonatal intensive care units: a systematic review. J. Perinatol. 42, 1561–1575 (2022).
- N.N. Finer, W.A. Carlo, M.C. Walsh, W. Rich, M.G. Gantz, A.R. Laptook, et al. Early CPAP versus surfactant in extremely preterm infants Engl. J. Med., 362 (21) (2010), pp. 1970-1979
- O'Currain, M. Thio, J.A. Dawson, S.M. Donath, P.G. Davis Respiratory monitors to teach newborn facemask ventilation: a randomised trialArch. Dis. Child. Fetal Neonatal Ed., 104 (6) (2019), pp. F582-F586
- P. Meier-Stauss, H.U. Bucher, R. Hurlimann, V. Konig, R. Huch Pulse oximetry used for documenting oxygen saturation and right-to-left shunting immediately after birth Eur. J. Pediatr., 149 (12) (1990), pp. 851-855
- P.A. Johnson, P.Y. Cheung, T.F. Lee, M. O'Reilly, G.M. Schmolzer Novel technologies for heart rate assessment during neonatal resuscitation at birth - a systematic reviewResuscitation, 143 (2019), pp. 196-207
- Perna, D. & Tagarelli, A. Deep auscultation: predicting respiratory anomalies and diseases via recurrent neural networks. in 2019 IEEE 32nd International Symposium on Computer-Based Medical Systems (CBMS) 50–55 (2019).
- Piccialli, F., Somma, V. D., Giampaolo, F., Cuomo, S. & Fortino, G. A survey on deep learning in medicine: Why, how and when? Inf. Fusion 66, 111–137 (2021).
- Q. Fei, Y. Lin, T.M. Yuan Lung ultrasound, a better choice for neonatal pneumothorax: a systematic review and meta-analysis Ultrasound Med. Biol., 47 (3) (2021), pp. 359-369
- R. Falsaperla, B. Scalia, F. Giaccone, A. Suppiej, A. Pulvirenti, J. Mailo, et al. aEEG vs cEEG's sensivity for seizure detection in the setting of neonatal intensive care units: a systematic review and meta-analysis Acta Paediatr., 111 (5) (2022), pp. 916-926
- R. Shah, J. Harding, J. Brown, C. McKinlay Neonatal glycaemia and neurodevelopmental outcomes: a systematic review and meta-analysis Neonatology, 115 (2) (2019), pp. 116-126
- R.E. Spitzmiller, T. Phillips, J. Meinzen-Derr, S.B. Hoath Amplitude-integrated EEG is useful in predicting neurodevelopmental outcome in full-term infants with hypoxic-ischemic encephalopathy: a meta-analysis Child Neurol., 22 (9) (2007), pp. 1069-1078
- Razak, M. Fade Neonatal lung ultrasonography to evaluate need for surfactant or mechanical ventilation: a systematic review and meta-analysis Arch. Dis. Child. Fetal Neonatal Ed., 105 (2) (2020), pp. 164-171
- S. Delin, K. Bošnjak Nađ, S. Martinec, D. Čokolić Petrović, A. Šimic Klarić, Bošnjak V. Mejaški Prognostic value of cranial ultrasonography in comparison with magnetic resonance imaging in children with cerebral palsy: a population-based study Acta Clin. Croat., 59 (2) (2020), pp. 260-269
- S. Hyttel-Sorensen, A. Pellicer, T. Alderliesten, T. Austin, F. van Bel, M. Benders, et al. Cerebral near infrared spectroscopy oximetry in extremely preterm infants: phase II randomised clinical trialBMJ, 350 (2015), Article g7635
- S. Shankaran, A.R. Laptook, R.A. Ehrenkranz, J.E. Tyson, S.A. McDonald, E.F. Donovan, et al. Whole-body hypothermia for neonates with hypoxic-ischemic encephalopathy N. Engl. J. Med., 353 (15) (2005), pp. 1574-1584
- S. Thangaratinam, K. Brown, J. Zamora, K.S. Khan, A.K. Ewer Pulse oximetry screening for critical congenital heart defects in asymptomatic newborn babies: a systematic review and meta-analysis Lancet, 379 (9835) (2012), pp. 2459-2464
- Sganga, R. Wallace, E. Kiehl, T. Irving, L. Witter A comparison of four methods of normal newborn temperature measurement MCN Am. J. Matern. Child Nurs., 25 (2) (2000), pp. 76-79 Shane, A. L., Sánchez, P. J. & Stoll, B. J. Neonatal sepsis. lancet 390, 1770–1780 (2017).
- Shi, M. Goodall, J. Dumville, J. Hill, G. Norman, O. Hamer, et al. The accuracy of pulse oximetry in measuring oxygen saturation by levels of skin pigmentation: a systematic review and meta-analysis BMC Med., 20 (1) (2022), p. 267
- Sandri, R. Plavka, G. Ancora, U. Simeoni, Z. Stranak, S. Martinelli, et al. Prophylactic or early selective surfactant combined with nCPAP in very preterm infants Pediatrics, 125 (6) (2010), pp. e1402-e1409
- Shipley, A. Mistry, D. Sharke Outcomes of neonatal hypoxic-ischaemic encephalopathy in centres with and without active therapeutic hypothermia: a nationwide propensity score-matched analysis Arch. Dis. Child. Fetal Neonatal Ed., 107 (1) (2022), pp.
- Sun, R. Cheng, W. Kang, H. Xiong, C. Zhou, Y. Zhang, et al.High-frequency oscillatory ventilation versus synchronized intermittent mandatory ventilation plus pressure support in preterm infants with severe respiratory distress syndromeRespir. Care, 59 (2) (2014), pp. 159-169

- Sganga, R. Wallace, E. Kiehl, T. Irving, L. Witter A comparison of four methods of normal newborn temperature measurement MCN Am. J. Matern. Child Nurs., 25 (2) (2000), pp. 76-79

- Schmidt, R.K. Whyte, E.V. Asztalos, D. Moddemann, C. Poets, Y. Rabi, et al. Effects of targeting higher vs lower arterial oxygen saturations on death or disability in extremely preterm infants: a randomized clinical trial JAMA, 309 (20) (2013), pp. 2111-2120
- T.C. Kwok, C. Henry, et al.Postmarketing trials and pediatric device approvals Pediatrics, 133 (5) (2014), pp. e1197-e1202
- T.J. Hwang, A.S. Kesselheim, F.T. Bourgeois Postmarketing trials and pediatric device approvals Pediatrics, 133 (5) (2014), pp. e1197-e1202
- V. Nair, P. Loganathan, M.K. Lal, T. BachmanAutomated oxygen delivery in neonatal intensive careFront. Pediatr., 10 (2022), Article 915312
- Van Reempts, C. Borstlap, S. Laroche, J.C. Van der Auwera Early use of high frequency ventilation in the premature neonate Eur. J. Pediatr., 162 (4) (2003), pp. 219-226
- W. Peng, H. Zhu, H. Shi, E. Liu Volume-targeted ventilation is more suitable than pressure-limited ventilation for preterm infants: a systematic review and meta-analysis Arch. Dis. Child. Fetal Neonatal Ed., 99 (2) (2014), pp. F158-F165
- W. TarnowMordi, B. Stenson, A. Kirby, E. Juszczak, M. Donoghoe, S. Deshpande, et al. Outcomes of two trials of oxygen-saturation targets in preterm infants N. Engl. J. Med., 374 (8) (2016), pp. 749-760
- Whole-body hypothermia for term and near-term newborns with hypoxic-ischemic encephalopathy: a randomized controlled trial Arch. Pediatr. Adolesc. Med., 165 (8) (2011), pp. 692-700
- Wilkinson, C. Andersen, C.P. O'Donnell, A.G. De Paoli, B.J. ManleyHigh flow nasal cannula for respiratory support in preterm infants Cochrane Database Syst. Rev., 2 (2) (2016),
- Zeballos Sarrato, M. Sanchez Luna, S. Zeballos Sarrato, A. Perez Perez, I. Pescador Chamorro, J.M. Bellon CanoNew strategies of pulmonary protection of preterm infants in the delivery room with the respiratory function monitoring Am. J. Perinatol., 36 (13) (2019), pp. 1368-1376
- Zernikow, B. et al. Artificial neural network for risk assessment in preterm neonates. Arch. Dis. Child.-Fetal Neonatal Ed. 79, F129–F134 (1998)

INDEX

A

B

C

D

E

F

G

H

M

N

O

P

Q

R

S

T

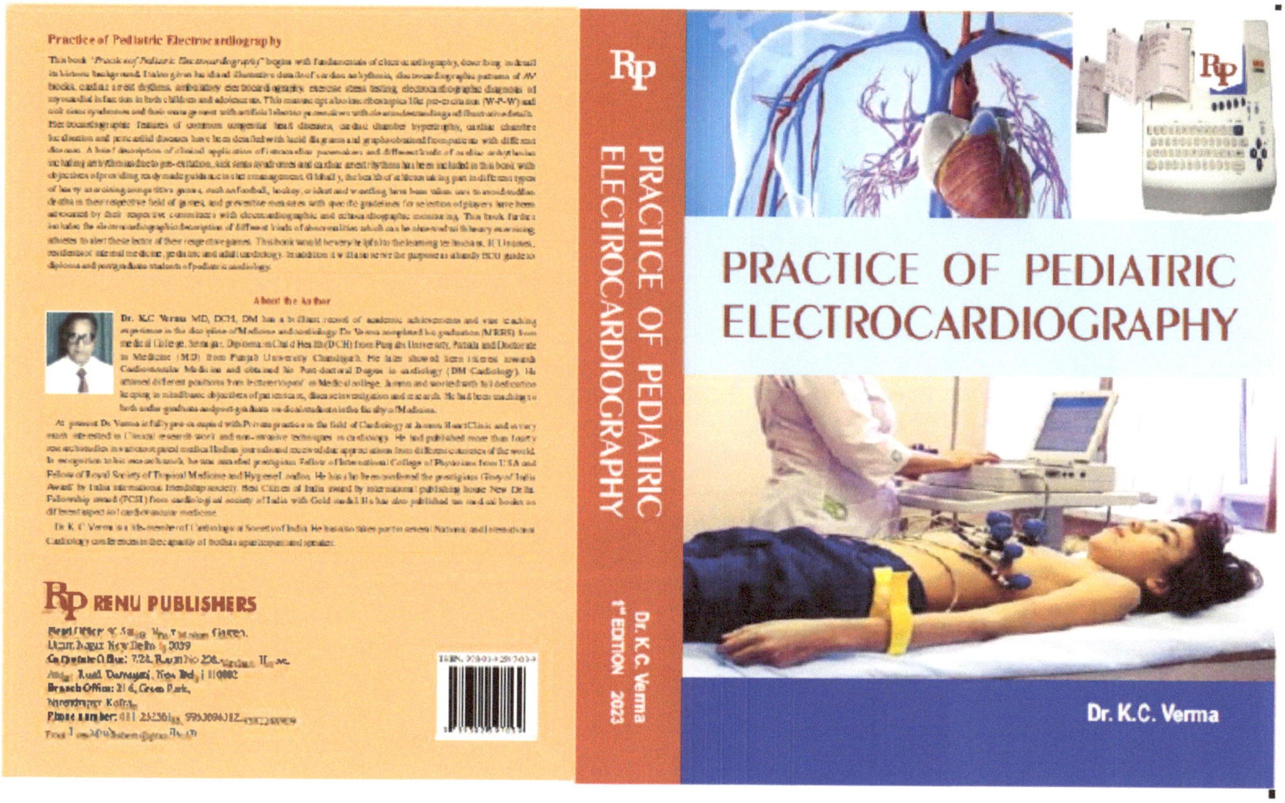
Practice of Pediatric Electrocardiography
About the Author
RENU PUBLISHERS
PRACTICE OF PEDIATRIC ELECTROCARDIOGRAPHY
Dr. K.C. Verma
1st EDITION 2023
PRACTICE OF PEDIATRIC
ELECTROCARDIOGRAPHY
Dr. K.C. Verma

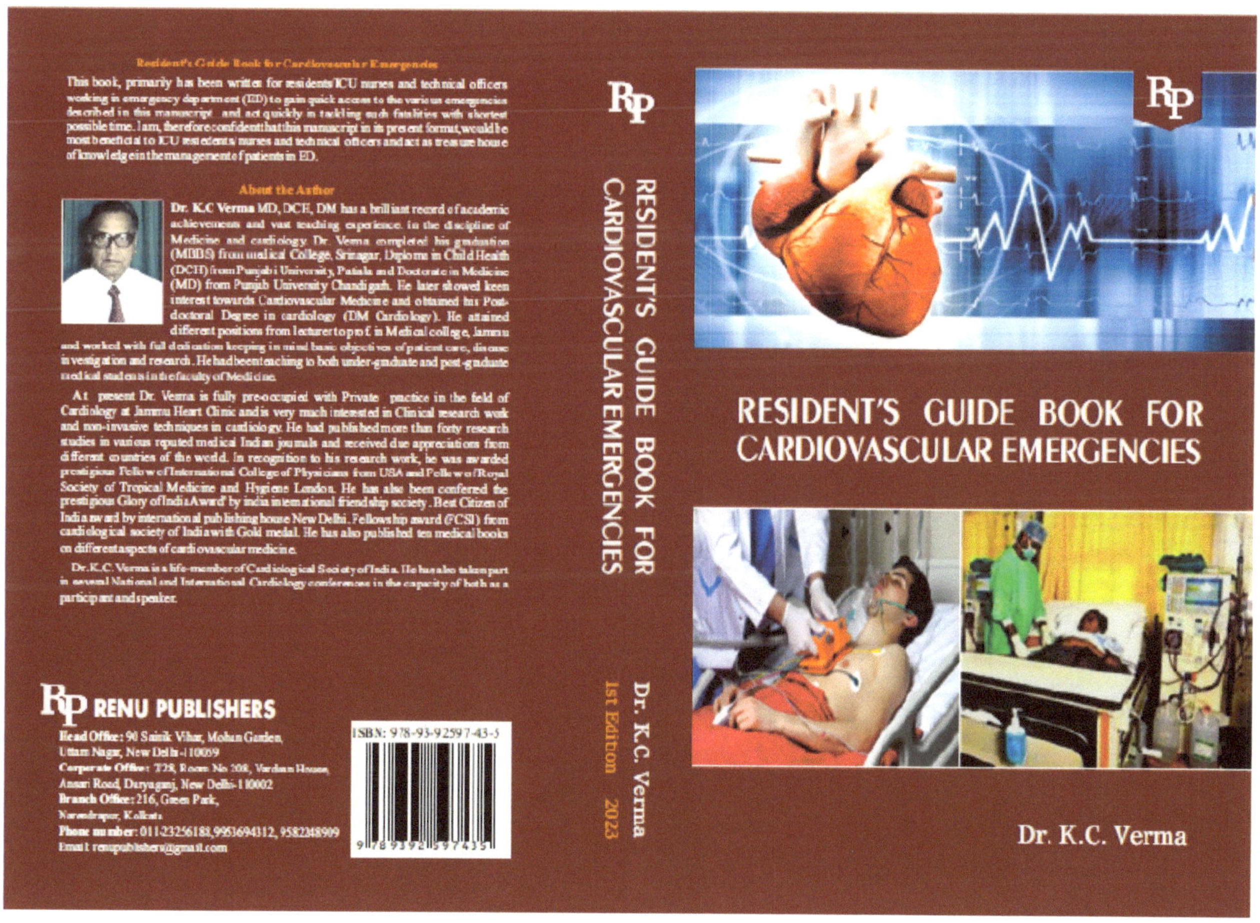
Resident's Guide Book for Cardiovascular Emergencies
This book, primarily has been written for residents/ICU nurses and technical officers working in emergency department (ED) to gain quick access to the various emergencies described in this manuscript and act quickly in tackling such fatalities with shortest possible time. I am, therefore confident that this manuscript in its present format, would be most beneficial to ICU residents/ nurses and technical officers and act as treasure house of knowledge in the management of patients in ED.
About the Author
Dr. K.C Verma MD, DCH, DM has a brilliant record of academic achievements and vast teaching experience in the discipline of Medicine and cardiology. Dr. Verma completed his graduation (MBBS) from medical College, Srinagar, Diploma in Child Health (DCH) from Punjabi University, Patiala and Doctorate in Medicine (MD) from Punjab University Chandigarh. He later showed keen interest towards Cardiovascular Medicine and obtained his Post-doctoral Degree in cardiology (DM Cardiology). He attained different positions from lecturer to prof. in Medical college, Jammu and worked with full dedication keeping in mind basic objectives of patient care, disease investigation and research. He had been teaching to both under-graduate and post-graduate medical students in the faculty of Medicine.
At present Dr. Verma is fully pre-occupied with Private practice in the field of Cardiology at Jammu Heart Clinic and is very much interested in Clinical research work and non-invasive techniques in cardiology. He had published more than forty research studies in various reputed medical Indian journals and received due appreciations from different countries of the world. In recognition to his research work, he was awarded prestigious Fellow of International College of Physicians from USA and Fellow of Royal Society of Tropical Medicine and Hygiene London. He has also been conferred the prestigious Glory of India Award' by india international friendship society. Best Citizen of India award by international publishing house New Delhi. Fellowship award (FCSI) from cardiological society of India with Gold medal. He has also published ten medical books on different aspects of cardiovascular medicine.
Dr. K.C. Verma is a life-member of Cardiological Society of India. He has also taken part in several National and International Cardiology conferences in the capacity of both as a participant and speaker.
RENU PUBLISHERS
Head Office: 90 Sainik Vihar, Mohan Garden,
Uttam Nagar, New Delhi-110059
Corporate Office: 7/28, Room No 208, Vardaan House,
Ansari Road, Daryaganj, New Delhi-110002
Branch Office: 216, Green Park,
Narendrapur, Kolkata
Phone number: 011-23256188, 9953694312, 9582248909
Email: renupublishers@gmail.com
ISBN: 978-93-92597-43-5
RESIDENT'S GUIDE BOOK FOR CARDIOVASCULAR EMERGENCIES
Dr. K.C. Verma
1st Edition 2023
RESIDENT'S GUIDE BOOK FOR
CARDIOVASCULAR EMERGENCIES
Dr. K.C. Verma

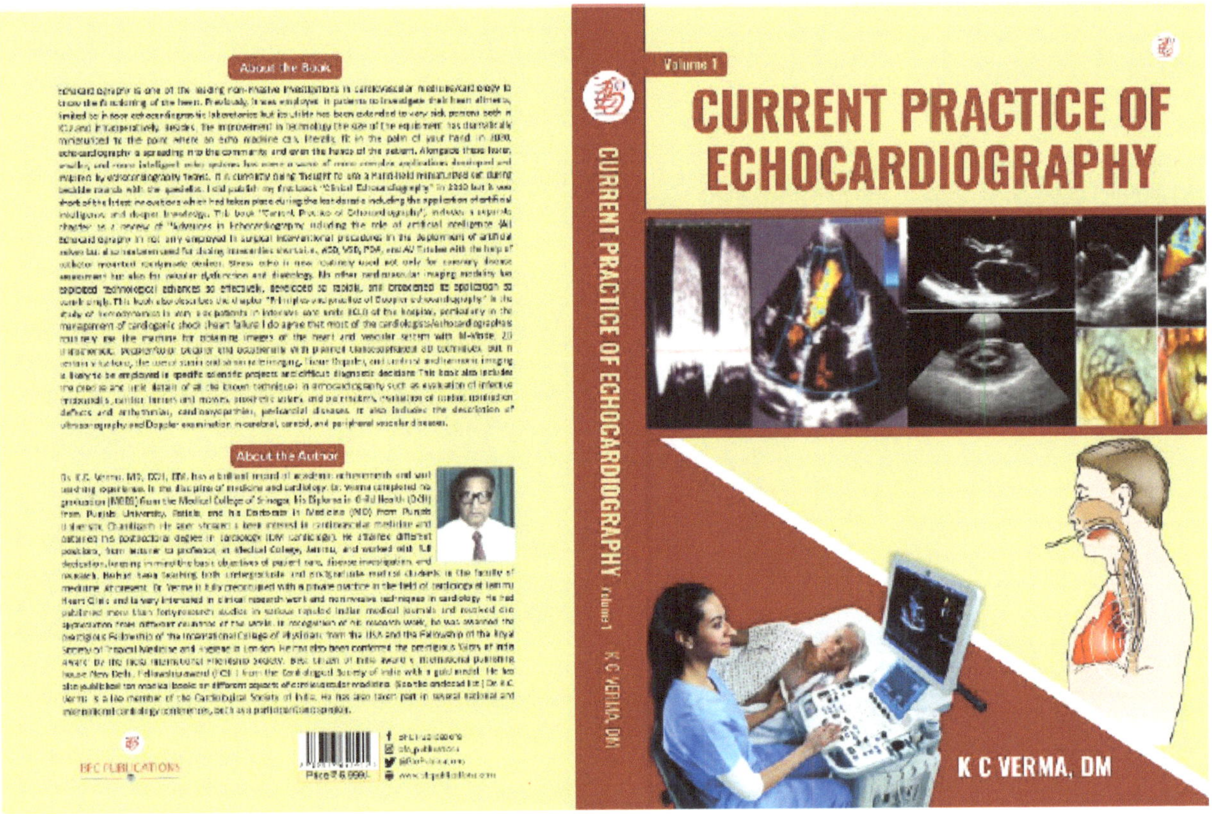
About the Book
About the Author
BFC PUBLICATIONS
Volume 1
CURRENT PRACTICE OF ECHOCARDIOGRAPHY
K C VERMA, DM

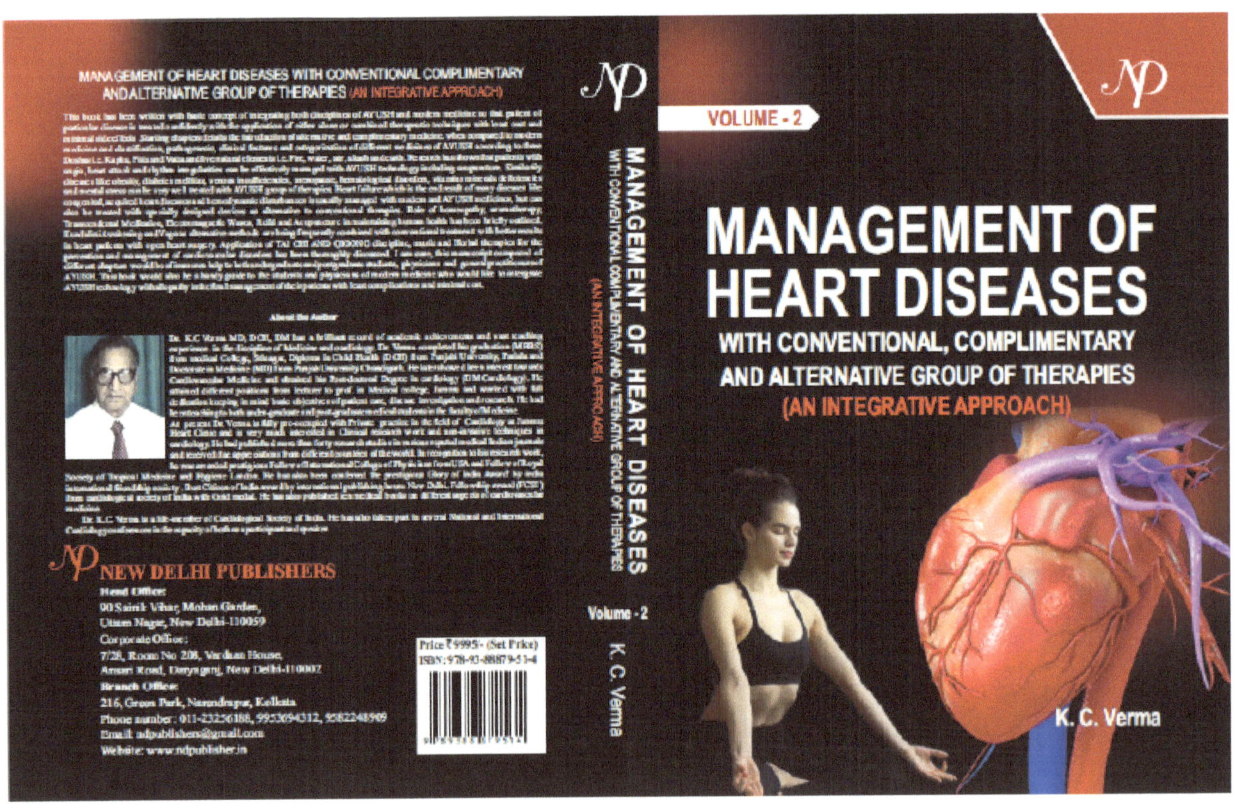
MANAGEMENT OF HEART DISEASES WITH CONVENTIONAL COMPLIMENTARY AND ALTERNATIVE GROUP OF THERAPIES (AN INTEGRATIVE APPROACH)
NEW DELHI PUBLISHERS
Head Office:
90 Sainik Vihar, Mohan Garden,
Uttam Nagar, New Delhi-110059
Corporate Office:
7/28, Room No 208, Vardhan House,
Ansari Road, Daryaganj, New Delhi-110002
Branch Office:
216, Green Park, Narendrapur, Kolkata
Website: www.ndpublisher.in
Price ₹ 9995/- (Set Price)
Volume - 2
K. C. Verma
VOLUME - 2
MANAGEMENT OF
HEART DISEASES
WITH CONVENTIONAL, COMPLIMENTARY
AND ALTERNATIVE GROUP OF THERAPIES
(AN INTEGRATIVE APPROACH)
K. C. Verma

www.ingramcontent.com/pod-product-compliance
Ingram Content Group UK Ltd.
Pitfield, Milton Keynes, MK11 3LW, UK
UKHW060039010826
14090UKWH00041B/254
* 9 7 9 8 8 9 5 1 9 8 1 1 7 *